Dietary Allowances (RDA), 1989[a]

		WEIGHT (kg)	WEIGHT (lb)	HEIGHT (cm)	HEIGHT (inches)	PROTEIN (g)	(RE) VITAMIN A	(µg) VITAMIN D	(mg) VITAMIN E	(µg) VITAMIN K	(mg) VITAMIN C	(mg) THIAMIN	(mg) RIBOFLAVIN	(mg equiv.) NIACIN	(mg) VITAMIN B_6	(µg) FOLATE	(µg) VITAMIN B_{12}	(mg) CALCIUM	(mg) PHOSPHORUS	(mg) MAGNESIUM	(mg) IRON	(mg) ZINC	(µg) IODINE	(µg) SELENIUM
Infants	0.0–0.5	6	13	60	24	13	375	7.5	3	5	30	0.3	0.4	5	0.3	25	0.3	400	300	40	6	5	40	10
	0.5–1.0	9	20	71	28	14	375	10	4	10	35	0.4	0.5	6	0.6	35	0.5	600	500	60	10	5	50	15
Children	1–3	13	29	90	35	16	400	10	6	15	40	0.7	0.8	9	1.0	50	0.7	800	800	80	10	10	70	20
	4–6	20	44	112	44	24	500	10	7	20	45	0.9	1.1	12	1.1	75	1.0	800	800	120	10	10	90	20
	7–10	28	62	132	52	28	700	10	7	30	45	1.0	1.2	13	1.4	100	1.4	800	800	170	10	10	120	30
Males	11–14	45	99	157	62	45	1000	10	10	45	50	1.3	1.5	17	1.7	150	2.0	1200	1200	270	12	15	150	40
	15–18	66	145	176	69	59	1000	10	10	65	60	1.5	1.8	20	2.0	200	2.0	1200	1200	400	12	15	150	50
	19–24	72	160	177	70	58	1000	10	10	70	60	1.5	1.7	19	2.0	200	2.0	1200	1200	350	10	15	150	70
	25–50	79	174	176	70	63	1000	5	10	80	60	1.5	1.7	19	2.0	200	2.0	800	800	350	10	15	150	70
	51+	77	170	173	68	63	1000	5	10	80	60	1.2	1.4	15	2.0	200	2.0	800	800	350	10	15	150	70
Females	11–14	46	101	157	62	46	800	10	8	45	50	1.1	1.3	15	1.4	150	2.0	1200	1200	280	15	12	150	45
	15–18	55	120	163	64	44	800	10	8	55	60	1.1	1.3	15	1.5	180	2.0	1200	1200	300	15	12	150	50
	19–24	58	128	164	65	46	800	10	8	60	60	1.1	1.3	15	1.6	180	2.0	1200	1200	280	15	12	150	55
	25–50	63	138	163	64	50	800	5	8	65	60	1.1	1.3	15	1.6	180	2.0	800	800	280	15	12	150	55
	51+	65	143	160	63	50	800	5	8	65	60	1.0	1.2	13	1.6	180	2.0	800	800	280	10	12	150	55
Pregnant						60	800	10	10	65	70	1.5	1.6	17	2.2	400	2.2	1200	1200	320	30	15	175	65
Lactating	1st 6 mo					65	1300	10	12	65	95	1.6	1.8	20	2.1	280	2.6	1200	1200	355	15	19	200	75
	2nd 6 mo					62	1200	10	11	65	90	1.6	1.7	20	2.1	260	2.6	1200	1200	340	15	16	200	75

[a]The allowances are intended to provide for individual variations among most normal, healthy people in the United States under usual environmental stresses. Diets should be based on a variety of common foods in order to provide other nutrients for which human requirements have been less well defined.

Source: Reprinted with permission from RECOMMENDED DIETARY ALLOWANCES: 10TH EDITION. Copyright 1989 by the National Academy of Sciences. Courtesy of the National Academy Press, Washington, D.C.

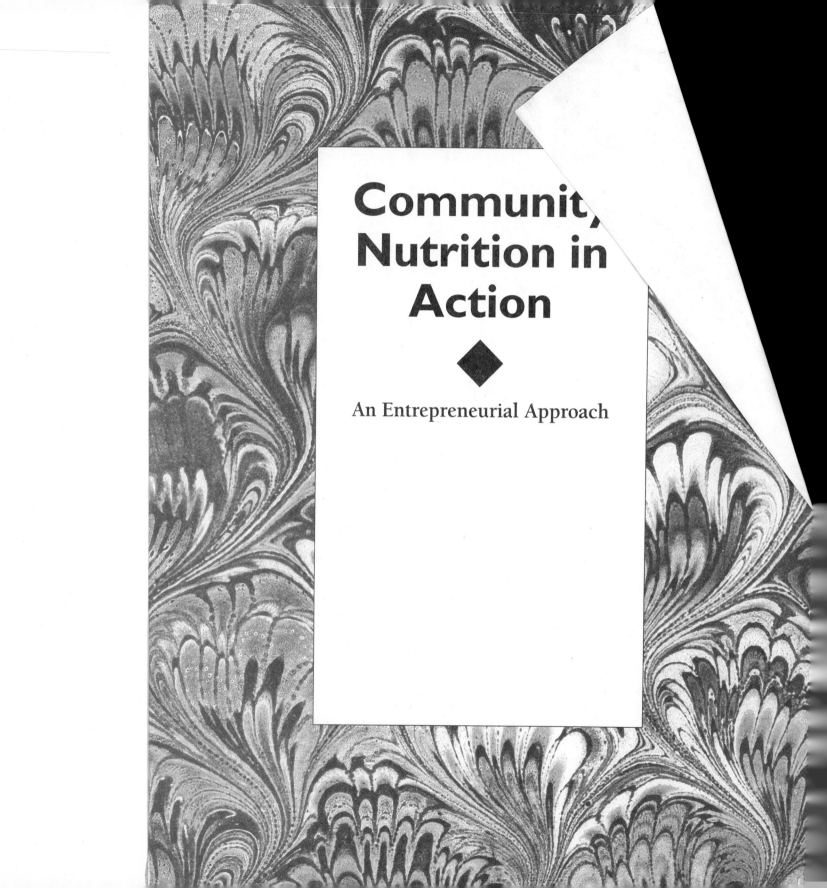

Community Nutrition in Action

◆

An Entrepreneurial Approach

Community Nutrition in Action

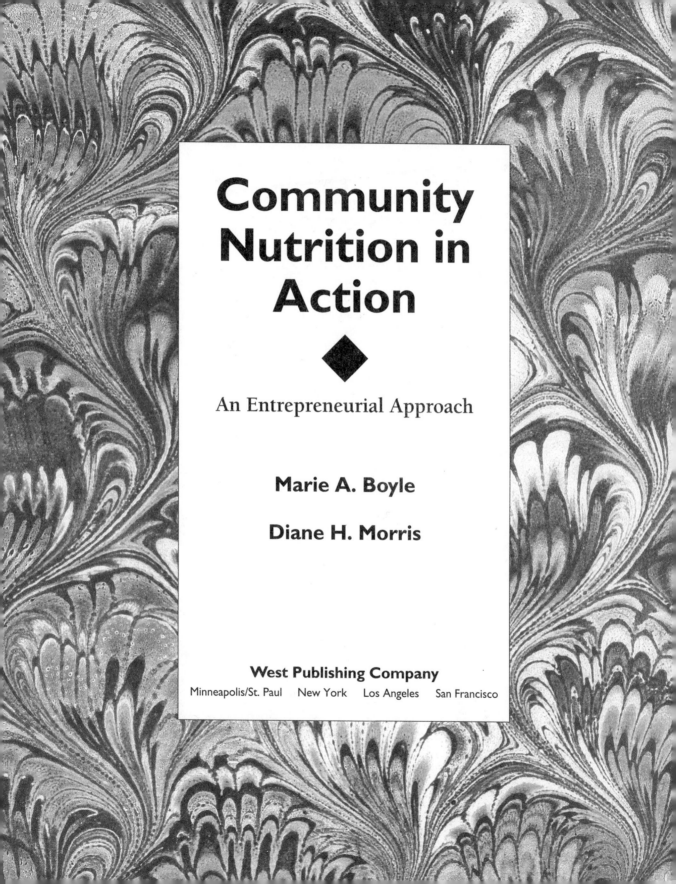

An Entrepreneurial Approach

Marie A. Boyle

Diane H. Morris

West Publishing Company

Minneapolis/St. Paul   New York   Los Angeles   San Francisco

◆ PRODUCTION CREDITS

Text Design: Roslyn Stendahl, Dapper Design

Copyediting: Patricia Lewis

Composition: Parkwood Composition Services, Inc.

Artwork: Randy Miyake

Cover Image: *Communion Celebration* by Montas Antoine. Photo © Van Hoorick/Superstock.

Cover Design: Roslyn Stendahl, Dapper Design

Index: Schroeder Indexing Services

WEST'S COMMITMENT TO THE ENVIRONMENT

In 1906, West Publishing Company began recycling materials left over from the production of books. This began a tradition of efficient and responsible use of resources. Today, up to 95 percent of our legal books and 70 percent of our college and school texts are printed on recycled, acid-free stock. West also recycles nearly 22 million pounds of scrap paper annually—the equivalent of 181,717 trees. Since the 1960s, West has devised ways to capture and recycle waste inks, solvents, oils, and vapors created in the printing process. We also recycle plastics of all kinds, wood, glass, corrugated cardboard, and batteries, and have eliminated the use of Styrofoam book packaging. We at West are proud of the longevity and the scope of our commitment to the environment.

Production, Prepress, Printing and Binding by West Publishing Company.

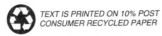 TEXT IS PRINTED ON 10% POST CONSUMER RECYCLED PAPER   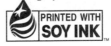 PRINTED WITH SOY INK™

Copyright ©1994   By WEST PUBLISHING COMPANY
610 Opperman Drive
P.O. Box 64526
St. Paul, MN 55164-0526

Printed in the United States of America

01 00 99 98 97 96 95 94   8 7 6 5 4 3 2 1 0

Library of Congress Cataloging-in-Publication Data

Boyle, Marie A. (Marie Ann)
     Community nutrition in action : an entrepreneurial approach /
  Marie A. Boyle, Diane H. Morris
        p. cm.
     Includes index.
     ISBN 0-314-02819-6
     1. Nutrition policy––United States.   2. Nutrition––United States.
  3. Community health services––United States.   I. Morris, Diane H.
  II. Title.
  TX360.U6B69   1994   94-8255

To my sister, Kathy,
for the love, confidence, and friendship
through all the times of our lives
—Marie Boyle

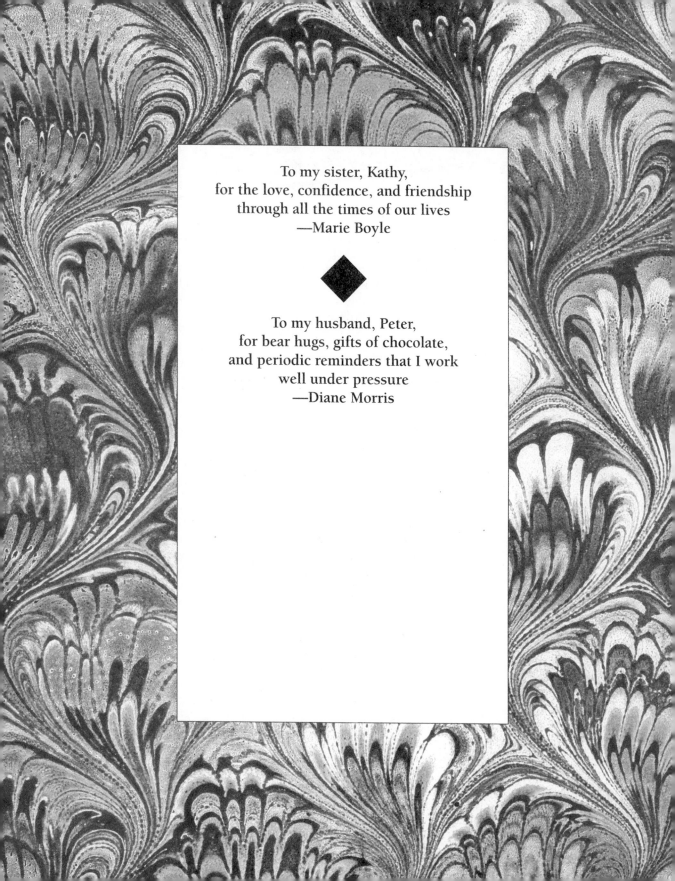

To my husband, Peter,
for bear hugs, gifts of chocolate,
and periodic reminders that I work
well under pressure
—Diane Morris

◆ About the Authors

Marie A. Boyle, Ph.D., R.D., received her B.A. in psychology from the University of Maine in 1975, her M.S. in nutrition from Florida State University in 1985, and her Ph.D. in nutrition from Florida State University in 1992. She has taught community nutrition and other undergraduate and graduate nutrition and health-related courses at the University of Florida in Gainesville and at Florida State University and Tallahassee Community College in Tallahassee. Her other professional activities include teaching a community-based "Culinary Hearts" cooking class for the American Heart Association, developing a community workshop on "Nutrition and Health Fraud," serving as chair of the local dietetic association's Hunger Committee, and acting as Administrator for the Florida Association of Professional Health Educators. She currently works as a consultant, writer, and nutrition educator and is preparing the third edition of her other textbook, *Personal Nutrition*.

Diane H. Morris, Ph.D., R.D., received her B.S. in nutrition science in 1972 and Ph.D. in nutrition in 1982 from the University of Tennessee at Knoxville. She has held faculty or staff positions with the American Medical Association, the Harvard School of Public Health, and the University of Massachusetts Medical School. She was a co-principal investigator on the Treatwell Program, a worksite-based nutrition education program to reduce cancer risk funded by the National Cancer Institute. She is currently a member of the Board of Directors of the Heart and Stroke Foundation of Manitoba and chairs two of its education committees. She is president of Mainstream Nutrition and works to educate other health professionals and the general public through her writing, public speaking, and volunteer service.

◆ Contents in Brief

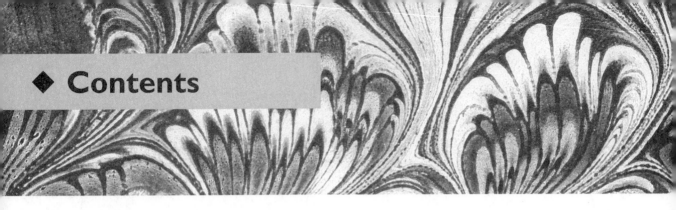

◆ Contents

SECTION II

Using the Tools: Designing and Implementing
Community Nutrition Programs   164

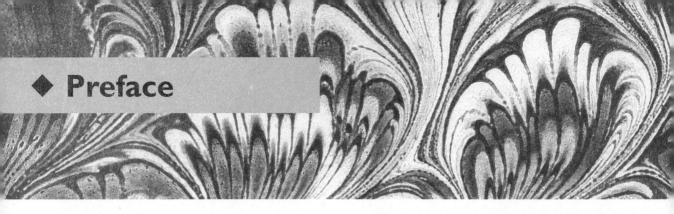

◆ Preface

We began this book with a vision. We wanted to share with students the challenges that go with helping consumers change their eating habits. We wanted to interest them in the creative aspects of program design. And we wanted to affirm our impression that the practice of community nutrition is changing—and changing rapidly. Whereas most students in community nutrition would have sought jobs in traditional public health settings such as state and city health departments a decade ago, today, students are looking for and creating jobs in other community settings: fitness centers, clinics, nonprofit health organizations, and schools.

More than ever before, community nutritionists are seeking new strategies for serving the public and improving community health. Their search has compelled them to draw on theories and methods from other disciplines such as marketing, management, and business. To succeed in today's changing economic and health care environment, community nutritionists must be skilled in many areas outside the science of foods and nutrition.

This textbook was written for students who seek public service, whether in government or the private sector. It was designed to develop leaders—nutrition entrepreneurs, if you will—who, through innovation and creativity, can guide individuals and communities to proper nutrition and good health. The book is organized into three sections. Section I lays the foundation for community work by describing the principles of public health, community nutrition, epidemiology, health care, legislation, and nutrition policy. It examines the principles of entrepreneurship and their application to the practice of community nutrition. Section II focuses on the tools of the community nutritionist: program planning, management, leadership, budgeting, social marketing, evaluation, principles of community needs assessment, and knowledge of consumer behavior. Section III describes current federal and nongovernment programs designed to meet the food and nutritional needs of pregnant and lactating women, infants, children, adolescents, and adults, including the elderly. It reviews some of the issues surrounding poverty and food insecurity in both the domestic and international arenas and considers how these contribute to nutritional risk and malnutrition.

The organization of this book is unique in some respects, for we have placed the discussions of policy and program planning *before* the description of nutrition and food assistance programs. We did this intentionally. We believe that students can better appreciate the complexities of a massive public program such as WIC after they have been exposed to the process by which "politics" and legislation shape program development and delivery, and after they have had a chance to experiment with the practical challenges of developing program goals, objectives, marketing strategies, dietary messages, and formats. Our intent is to expose students to policy and program planning on the front end of their studies so that they will be better positioned to critically evaluate the federal programs they study in this textbook and encounter in real life. The following outline summarizes the topics covered in each chapter:

◆ **Section I. Laying the Foundation: Understanding the Role of Nutrition in Public Health**

  ◆ Chapter 1 provides an overview of public health and the organization of public health services. It defines "community," describes the roles and responsibilities of the community nutritionist, and considers how the principles of entrepreneurship can be applied to community nutrition practice.

  ◆ Chapter 2 reviews the basic principles of epidemiology, the nature of dietary variation, and diet assessment methods.

  ◆ Chapter 3 describes the policy-making process and provides practical tips on how community nutritionists can influence legislation and public policy.

  ◆ Chapter 4 examines the U.S. health care system and the importance of securing reimbursement for nutrition services as part of health care reform.

  ◆ Chapter 5 describes the nation's nutrition agenda for improving the public's health, its nutrition monitoring system, and its dietary goals and guidelines.

◆ **Section II. Using the Tools: Designing and Implementing Community Nutrition Programs**

  ◆ Chapter 6 reviews the basic functions of management—planning, organizing, leading, and controlling.

  ◆ Chapter 7 explores the program planning process and how a community needs assessment is undertaken. It also discusses the challenges of setting priorities and designing programs.

  ◆ Chapter 8 focuses on the factors that influence consumer behavior and the theories and methods that community nutritionists can use to develop intervention strategies.

  ◆ Chapter 9 examines the fundamental principles of marketing—product, place, price, and promotion—and how a situational analysis can be used to market community-based programs.

  ◆ Chapter 10 reviews the various types of evaluation and how evaluation findings can be presented for maximum effect.

◆ **Section III. Raising the Roof: Programs for Promoting and Protecting the Public's Health**

◆ Chapter 11 discusses the causes and distribution of food insecurity in the United States and outlines the major domestic food assistance programs designed to help with food security.

◆ Chapter 12 reviews the nutrition assessment of pregnant and lactating women and infants and outlines the major domestic food and nutrition programs for this population.

◆ Chapter 13 reviews the nutrition assessment of children and adolescents and describes the food assistance and educational programs aimed at this group.

◆ Chapter 14 discusses the nutrition assessment of adults, including the elderly, and describes the major programs for this diverse and growing population group.

◆ Chapter 15 examines key global nutrition and health issues such as hunger, malnutrition, child survival activities, and sustainable development.

In addition to taking a new direction with the book's overall organization, we also included several unique features:

◆ **Focus on entrepreneurship.** Successful practitioners in community nutrition have a mind- and skill-set that opens them up to new ideas and ventures. They don't think, "This is how it has always been done." They think, "Let's try this. Let's do something different." We want the users of this textbook to begin thinking of themselves as "social entrepreneurs," as people who are willing to take risks, try new technologies, and use fresh approaches to improving the public's nutrition and health. Although the application of entrepreneurial principles to community nutrition practice is new, we anticipate a growing interest in social entrepreneurship as a tool for achieving change on the community level.

◆ **Focus on multiculturalism.** The growing ethnic diversity of our communities poses many challenges for community nutritionists. To increase students' awareness and appreciation of cultures beyond their own, we have woven examples and illustrations of various food-related beliefs and practices from different cultures throughout the text.

◆ **Professional Focus.** The ten Professional Focuses are designed to help students develop personal skills and attitudes that will boost their effectiveness and confidence in community settings. The topics range from goal setting and time management to writing, public speaking, negotiating, and mentoring. Where the material was complementary, we matched a particular Professional Focus with a particular chapter. This feature is meant to help students build their professional skills.

◆ **Entrepreneur in Action.** Five chapters include a short interview with an "entrepreneur" who offers a unique perspective on the practice of community nutrition. These five individuals—Kathy King Helm, Mary Kay

Hunt, Kathy Lauri, Rebecca Mullis, and Sally Temple—use their own words to describe the importance of entrepreneurship to the field of community nutrition, and each has a different message for students.

◆ **Program Spotlight.** Each chapter in Section III includes a Program Spotlight that describes one assistance program such as the Food Stamp Program, the National School Lunch Program, WIC, and the Congregate Meals Program. The Spotlights cover such topics as the policy issues underlying the program, current legislative issues affecting the program, and the program's effectiveness in reaching and meeting the needs of its intended audience.

◆ **Community Learning Activity.** At the end of every chapter is a Community Learning Activity designed to get students involved in learning about their community and its health and nutrition problems. While most activities can be completed independently, those in Section II are meant to be undertaken by teams. The purpose of the Section II activities is to give students some experience in designing a program, creating marketing strategies, choosing nutrition messages, and developing goals and objectives. Grouping students into teams will facilitate the planning process and allow them to benefit from other team members' experiences and ideas.

Finally, a word is needed about the use of the personal pronouns "he" and "she" in the text. On the advice of our reviewers and editors, we used gender-neutral terms whenever possible, recognizing that there are male community nutritionists and the involvement of men in community nutrition is likely to increase in the coming years. In some places, however, we used the pronouns "she" and "he" to make the text more personal and engaging for the reader and because we thought it was important to enhance the image of community nutritionists, particularly women, as leaders, managers, and entrepreneurs. We want the users of this text, whether they are men or women, to begin thinking of themselves as planners, managers, change agents, thinkers, and leaders—in short, nutrition entrepreneurs—who have the energy and creativity to open up new vistas for improving the public's health through good nutrition.

Marie Boyle
Diane Morris
April 1994

◆ ACKNOWLEDGMENTS

Many people contributed to the development of this book. Family and friends provided encouragement and inspiration. Colleagues shared their insights about the practice of community nutrition and the value of focusing on entrepreneurship. We thank all of these people for sharing in this adventure with us.

Special thanks go to our editorial team of Pete Marshall, Becky Tollerson, and Sandy Gangelhoff for ensuring the quality of this production, providing guidance, and making us laugh. Pat Lewis, the copy editor, deserves mention for her excellent editorial suggestions, as does Angela Musey, the permissions editor, whose good humor and persistence saved us on more than one occasion. We also owe much to the following professionals who provided expert reviews of the manuscript, not only for their ideas and suggestions, many of which made their way into the text, but also for supporting our view of entrepreneurship as a key component of community nutrition practice: Shawna Berenbaum, University of Saskatchewan; Patricia Brevard, James Madison University; Nancy Cohen, University of Massachusetts at Amherst; Norma Jean Downes, San Jose State University; Marie Dunford, California State University—Fresno; Sareen Gropper, Auburn University; Evette Hackman, Seattle Pacific University; Margaret Hedley, University of Guelph; Jana Kicklighter, Georgia State University; Barbara Kirks, California State University—Chico; Bernice Kopel, Oklahoma State University; Suzanne Little, San Jacinto College; Rosalie Mahoney, Youngstown State University; Deborah Marino, Kent State University; Kathleen McBurney, California Polytechnic State University—San Luis Obispo; Shortie McKinney, Drexel University; Nweze Nnakwe, Illinois State University; Martha Rew, Texas Woman's University.

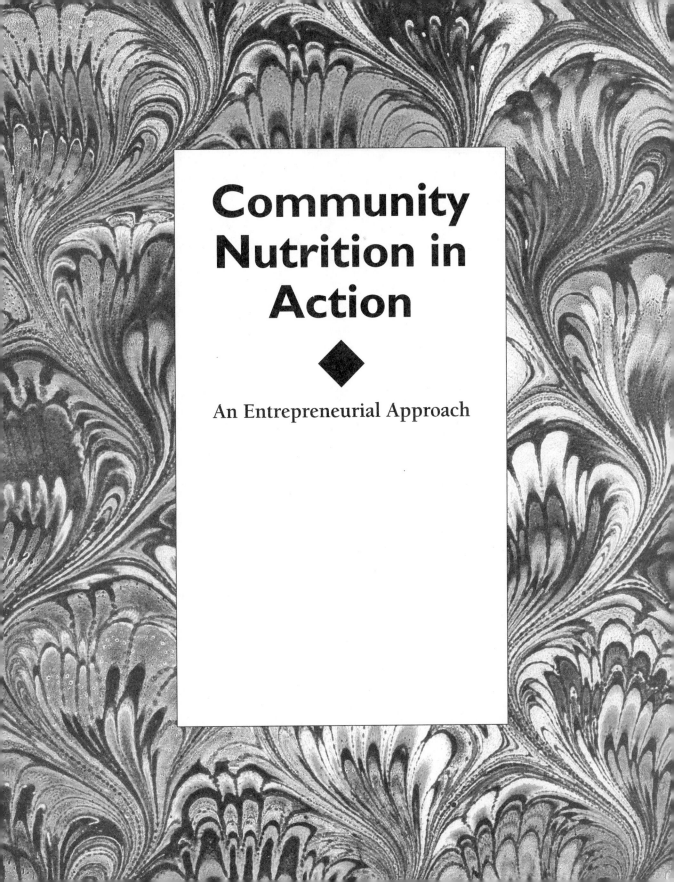

Community Nutrition in Action

◆

An Entrepreneurial Approach

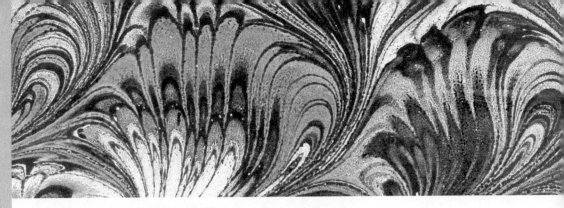

Laying the Foundation: Understanding the Role of Nutrition in Public Health

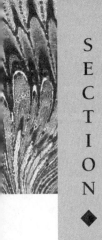

Any builder will tell you that you can't "raise high the roof beams"—to quote J. D. Salinger—or secure the brick-and-mortar walls before you lay the building's foundation. The foundation is the beginning, the bedrock upon which all of the other elements are built. Laying the foundation is no simple matter. The building site must be properly surveyed, the soil tested for composition and drainage capability, and the land excavated and graded according to the master plan. The grid for the foundation must be staked and situated appropriately in relation to other elements on the site. The masonry material must be carefully chosen, regardless of whether the foundation will ultimately support a modest house or a soaring skyscraper.

In much the same fashion, you are laying the groundwork for your sojourn into the field of community nutrition with the material in this section. Community nutritionists don't work in vacuums. They work with professionals in many diverse fields—social work, medicine, epidemiology, health education, regulatory affairs, marketing—to develop and deliver health messages and programs. When you become a community nutritionist, the success of your pro-

grams and services will depend on many things, including your knowledge of the following:

- ◆ The principles of entrepreneurship
- ◆ Public health
- ◆ Health promotion
- ◆ Health care
- ◆ Foods and food safety
- ◆ Nutrition
- ◆ Your clients—where they live; what they eat; their attitudes, values, and lifestyles
- ◆ Your community—its health needs and how it delivers public health services
- ◆ The policy-making process—how it affects your job and your ability to accomplish what you want to do

The material you master in this section will provide the legislative, policy, and health framework for the skills you acquire in the next section. Let's begin with a survey of the lay of the land.

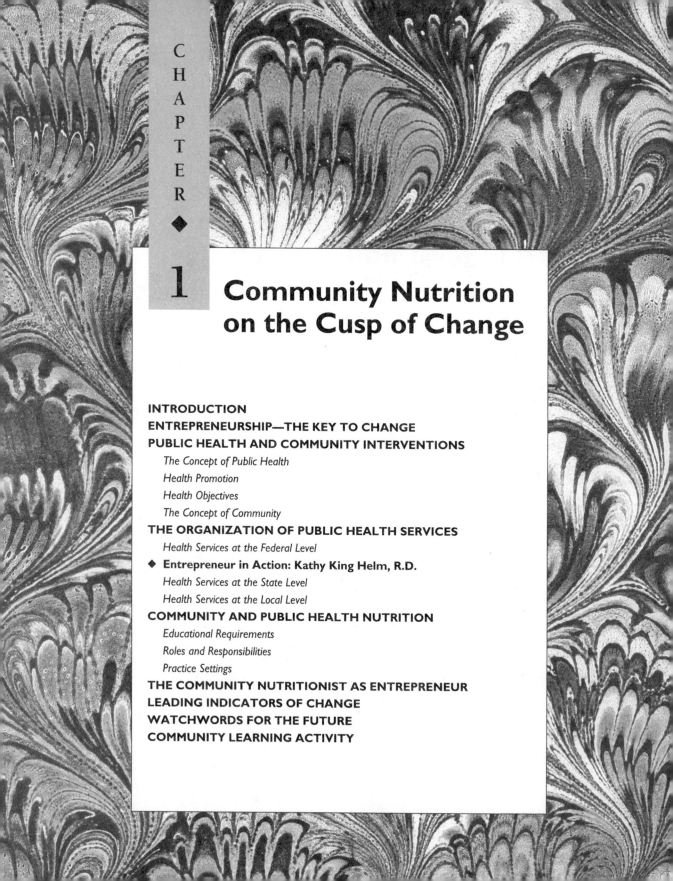

Community Nutrition on the Cusp of Change

Something to Think About . . .

Apart from hermits, people live and work in groups . . . so if you have it in mind to influence the way in which life goes on, you will not do it solely by trying to influence people-as-individuals, you will have also to think of people-in-groups.
—J. Yudkin and J. C. McKenzie, *Changing Food Habits*

Introduction

A worldwide sea change is taking place on a scale never before seen in the history of the human race. Through telephones, facsimile machines, electronic data systems, and 24-hour television news programming, we are instantly in touch with family members, friends, and coworkers and with historic events occurring around the world. A vast communications network spans continents and oceans, fueling the growth of the global marketplace. Transnational companies compete for global domination in a variety of product markets, from automobiles and computers to clothing and gourmet coffee.[1] National boundaries are no longer a barrier to marketing and sales, and the globalization of the workforce is altering the ethnic and cultural mix of many nations.[2]

The shifting currents of this final decade of the twentieth century stir us to think of the global community in new ways. In the business world, the 1990s have been called the entrepreneurial decade, a reference to the innovator's mandate to plan for consumers' changing values and practices in a global market.[3] Sociologists speak of the 1990s as the decade of global social innovation, a newly minted term that refers to new ways of organizing human and technological resources as tools for solving local and global problems.[4] In the health arena, the 1990s have been called the decade of death, a reference to the accelerating epidemic of the human immunodeficiency virus (HIV), which is believed to cause the acquired immunodeficiency syndrome (AIDS). This epidemic is expected to affect population growth worldwide.[5] On submitting the *Healthy People 2000* document to the secretary of health and human services, J. O. Mason, then the assistant secretary for health, indicated that the 1990s should be the decade of prevention in the United States. He cited the need to change the health focus from merely identifying and treating disease to preventing illness and disability.[6]

The challenge of improving the quality of life for humans is more complex than any previously experienced. And the mission is ambitious. As outlined by all the nations of the world in the 1978 conference on primary health care, convened by the World Health Organization and the United Nations Children's Fund (UNICEF), the goal of the world community is to "protect and promote the health of all people of the world."[7] Achieving this goal requires understanding the many physical, biologic, social, and behavioral factors that influence the health of individuals and communities. It requires innovative approaches to changing human behavior. Innovation, a key ingredient of the traditional scientific method, is being applied increasingly to the realm of human behavior and specifically to the challenge of helping people adopt healthful behaviors. Practitioners in the arena of health promotion and disease prevention, including community nutritionists, can use innovation as a tool for achieving the health of all peoples.

Entrepreneurship—The Key to Change

Peter Drucker, a business consultant and author of the book *Innovation and Entrepreneurship,* has said that change is the essence of entrepreneurship and the foundation of the entrepreneurial spirit.[8] Change is normal, healthy, and even desirable. It is a fundamental aspect of consumer behaviors, family structures, social norms, and community systems and organizations. Things change. Herb Kelleher, cofounder of Southwest Airlines, once remarked, "We tell our people all the time, 'You have to be ready for change.' In fact, sometimes only in change is there security."[9] A willingness to recognize and accept change is critical to entrepreneurship.

What is entrepreneurship? Who is an entrepreneur? How is entrepreneurship related to community nutrition? In the business world, entrepreneurship is sometimes defined as the act of starting a business or the process of creating new "values," be they goods, services, methods of production, technologies, or markets.[10] The essence of entrepreneurship is innovation, which doesn't have to be spectacular or heretofore unimagined. Consider the late Ray Kroc of McDonald's. He didn't invent the hamburger, but he did develop an entirely new way of marketing and delivering it to his customers. In the process, he revolutionized the foodservice industry. **Entrepreneurship**, then, is the creation of something of value, be it a product or service, through the creation of organization. In this context, organization refers to the orchestration of the materials, people, and capital required to deliver a product or service. This definition encompasses the myriad actions of individuals—the entrepreneurs—who "discover, invent, reveal, enact, and in other ways make manifest some new product, service, transaction, resource, technology, and/or market that has value to some community or marketplace."[11]

An **entrepreneur** is an enterpriser, innovator, initiator, promoter, and coordinator. Entrepreneurs are change agents who seek, recognize, and act on opportunities. They ask "What if?" and "Why not?" and translate their ideas into action. They tend to be creative, are able to see an old problem in a new light, and are willing to break new ground in delivering a product or service. When they spot an opportunity to fill a niche in the marketplace, they work to bring together the expertise, materials, labor, and capital necessary to meet the perceived want or need.

Some of the personality traits of individuals who practice entrepreneurship are listed in Table 1-1. These qualities are typically applied to the self-starting,

Entrepreneurship Creating something of value through the creation of organization.

Entrepreneur One who undertakes the risk of a business or enterprise.

◆ **Wants to achieve.** It is safe to say that all entrepreneurs have a desire to achieve. They all have the push to conquer problems and give birth to a successful venture.

◆ **Works hard.** Most entrepreneurs work hard; they have to work hard in order to achieve their goals.

◆ **Nurtures.** Entrepreneurs take charge of and watch over a venture until it can stand alone.

◆ **Accepts responsibility.** Entrepreneurs accept full responsibility for their ventures. They are morally, legally, and mentally accountable.

◆ **Is reward oriented.** Entrepreneurs want to achieve, work hard, and take responsibility; but they also want to be rewarded handsomely for their efforts. A reward can be other things besides money, such as recognition and respect.

◆ **Is optimistic.** Entrepreneurs live by the doctrine that this is the best of times and that anything is possible.

◆ **Seeks excellence.** Often entrepreneurs desire to achieve something that is outstanding and something that they can be proud of—something that is first-class.

◆ **Is a good organizer.** Most entrepreneurs are very good at bringing together all the components of a venture to make it achieve its goals. They are normally thought of as take-charge people.

◆ **Keeps financial rewards in perspective.** As surprising as it may seem, money takes a back seat to the nurturing quality and the desire to achieve. Entrepreneurs want to make a profit, but the profit serves more as a meter to gauge their degree of achievement and performance than as the end goal.

TABLE

1-1

A Personality Profile of the Entrepreneur
Source: J. G. Burch, *Entrepreneurship,* pp. 28–29. Copyright © 1986 by John Wiley & Sons, Inc. Reprinted by permission of John Wiley & Sons, Inc.

independent entrepreneur, but they also describe the **intrapreneur** or corporate employee who develops a business within a business. Intrapreneurs are seldom solely responsible for the financial risk associated with a new enterprise, but they share the same entrepreneurial spirit as their more independent counterparts. In this book, innovators in both the private (corporate) and public (government) sectors who embody the spirit and principles of entrepreneurship will be considered entrepreneurs.

Intrapreneur A risk taker whose job is located within a corporation, company, or other organization.

What do entrepreneurs do? One study of entrepreneurs identified at least 57 separate activities associated with launching a new venture, an indication of how complex entrepreneurial behavior can be. Entrepreneurs have a wide range of competencies in areas such as planning, marketing, networking, finance, and team building, as shown in Table 1-2. They turn their creative vision into intentional decision-making and problem-solving actions to accomplish specific goals. They are not just managers, although they typically "manage" themselves well. Their high self-esteem stems from a strong belief in their own personal worth, which strengthens their capacity for self-management. Successfully managing oneself means being in control (that is, having willpower), knowing one's personal strengths and weaknesses, and being willing to change one's own behavior and to receive feedback and criticism (another way of saying being self-directed).

What about failure? Do entrepreneurs experience failure, and if they do, how do they handle it? In one study, 80 percent of the 152 entrepreneurs interviewed admitted to making mistakes, especially during the start-up phase of their new ventures. Surprisingly, 20 percent reported making no mistakes![12] This result was unexpected, because entrepreneurial activities are fraught with opportunities to make mistakes. Given that key tactical or strategic mistakes can be made at any point in the entrepreneurial process—from product concept, design, and marketing to team building and capitalization—it is safe to say that entrepreneurs do make mistakes and suffer setbacks, just like everyone else. They differ from some of the rest of us, perhaps, in that they learn rapidly from their failures and are able to apply the insight gleaned from their mistakes to other problem areas and situations.

What relevance does entrepreneurship have to community nutrition? The answer to this question will become increasingly clear as you read the remaining chapters of this book. Suffice it to say at this point that entrepreneurship is the rubric under which many community-based nutrition activities and services can be organized and delivered. Consider the entrepreneurial activities listed in Table 1-2. Nearly all are relevant for the community nutritionist: recognizing an opportunity to deliver nutrition and health messages, developing an action plan for targeting a specific population group, building the team for delivering a nutrition program or service, developing a marketing plan, and evaluating the effectiveness of the nutrition program or service.

Nutrition educators who want to change people's eating habits must be able to see new ways to reach desired target groups. The strategy that works well with native young people living on a reservation will probably not work well with institutionalized elderly women or middle-aged men. Community nutritionists must be able to draw on theories and skills from the disciplines of sociology, educational psychology, medicine, communications, health education, and business to develop programs for improving people's eating patterns. The twin stanchions of entrepreneurship—creativity and innovation—will assist you as a community nutritionist in achieving the broad goal of improved health for all.

Public Health and Community Interventions

Most of us equate health with "feeling good," a concept we understand intuitively but cannot define exactly. Health can be viewed as the absence of disease and pain, a derivative of the old English word for "hale," which means whole, hearty, sound of mind and body.[13] Health can also be viewed as a continuum along which the total living experience can be placed, with freedom from disease or injury at one end of the spectrum and the presence of disease, impairment, or disability at the other. These views suggest, however, that existence in a state completely free from disease and stress is attainable. In *Mirage of Health,* R. J. Dubos remarked that "complete and lasting freedom from disease is but a dream remembered from imaginings of a Garden of Eden designed for the welfare of man."[14]

If complete freedom from disease and disability is not possible within the realm of human experience, then health is properly defined from an ecological viewpoint—that is, one that focuses on the interaction of humans among themselves and with their environment. In this sense, **health** is a state characterized by

Health The World Health Organization defines health as a state of complete physical, mental, and social well-being, not merely the absence of disease.

"anatomic integrity; ability to perform personally valued family, work, and community roles; ability to deal with physical, biological and social stress; a feeling of well-being; and freedom from the risk of disease and untimely death."[15] A healthy individual, then, has the physical, mental, and spiritual capacity to live, work, and interact joyfully with other human beings.

But how is good health achieved? Why does one child in a family become addicted to cocaine while another never touches illicit drugs? Why do people start smoking? Why do some women get breast cancer? Why is one 80-year-old healthy and vigorous, while a younger 70-year-old is infirm? The answers to these questions still elude epidemiologists and other scientists. We know that a myriad of biologic, environmental, and lifestyle factors influence health, including those listed in Table 1-3. The title of this table is somewhat misleading, for we know more about the factors that contribute to disease, injury, and disability than about the specific determinants of health. Understanding the causes of disease and ill health does not necessarily lead to an understanding of the causes of good health. We still have much to learn about how these factors interact to influence health. Nor is it clear precisely which of these factors are suitable for intervention on a public scale and which are more appropriately relegated to the realm of individual choice.

◆ THE CONCEPT OF PUBLIC HEALTH

In the nineteenth century, the scope of public health was generally restricted to matters of general sanitation and the control of infectious diseases. Building municipal sewer systems, purifying the water supply, and controlling food adulteration, particularly the handling and processing of perishable commodities such as milk, were major public health initiatives. Infectious diseases such as tuberculosis, smallpox, yellow fever, cholera, and typhoid were the leading causes of death and disability in North America a mere one hundred years ago. The morbidity and mortality linked with these disease outbreaks shaped public health practice for many years. Such runaway epidemics, which sometimes killed thousands of people in a single outbreak, are uncommon in North America today due to large-scale public efforts to improve water quality, control the spread of communicable diseases, and enhance personal hygiene and the sanitation of the environment. Currently, the leading causes of morbidity and mortality in North America tend to be chronic diseases such as heart disease and cancer, as shown in Table 1-4. Infectious diseases remain problematic, however. The AIDS epidemic continues to escalate. About 1 million people in the United States are infected with HIV, and nearly 250,000 people have received a diagnosis of AIDS. AIDS now ranks as one of the leading causes of premature death among American women and men.[16] Tuberculosis, whose incidence had been declining in the general U.S. population for several decades, has recently reemerged as a new health threat. Since 1985, the number of tuberculosis cases in the United States has increased 16 percent annually. The AIDS epidemic is partly responsible for the recent outbreaks of tuberculosis, although there are other causes, including increases in homelessness, drug abuse, immigration from other countries where tuberculosis is widespread, and crowded housing among the poor.[17]

TABLE

1-2

Entrepreneurial Activities

Identify an opportunity
Create the solution
Decide to go into business
Analyze individual strengths and weaknesses
Conduct market research
Assess potential share of the market
Establish business objectives
Set up organizational structure
Determine personnel requirements
Select the entrepreneurial team
Determine physical plant requirements
Prepare a financial plan
Locate financial resources
Prepare a production plan
Prepare a management plan
Prepare a marketing plan
Produce and test market the product
Build an organization
Respond to government and society

Source: From ENTREPRENEURIAL BEHAVIOR by Barbara J. Bird. Copyright © 1989 by Barbara J. Bird. Reprinted by permission of HarperCollins College Publishers.

TABLE 1-3	**Determinants of Health**

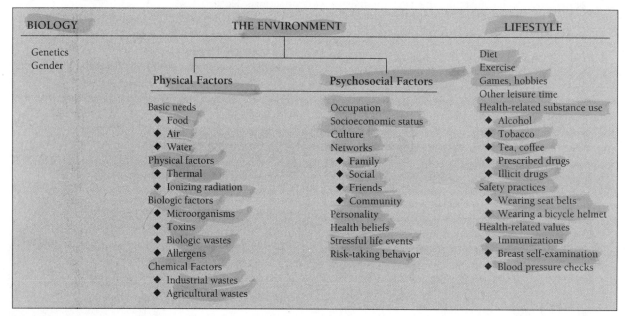

BIOLOGY	THE ENVIRONMENT		LIFESTYLE
Genetics			Diet
Gender			Exercise
	Physical Factors	**Psychosocial Factors**	Games, hobbies
			Other leisure time
	Basic needs	Occupation	Health-related substance use
	◆ Food	Socioeconomic status	◆ Alcohol
	◆ Air	Culture	◆ Tobacco
	◆ Water	Networks	◆ Tea, coffee
	Physical factors	◆ Family	◆ Prescribed drugs
	◆ Thermal	◆ Social	◆ Illicit drugs
	◆ Ionizing radiation	◆ Friends	Safety practices
	Biologic factors	◆ Community	◆ Wearing seat belts
	◆ Microorganisms	Personality	◆ Wearing a bicycle helmet
	◆ Toxins	Health beliefs	Health-related values
	◆ Biologic wastes	Stressful life events	◆ Immunizations
	◆ Allergens	Risk-taking behavior	◆ Breast self-examination
	Chemical Factors		◆ Blood pressure checks
	◆ Industrial wastes		
	◆ Agricultural wastes		

Source: Adapted, with permission, from G. Pickett and J. J. Hanlon, *Public Health: Administration and Practice* (St. Louis: Times Mirror/Mosby College Publishing, 1990), p. 50; and J. M. Last, *Public Health and Human Ecology* (East Norwalk, Conn.: Appleton & Lange, 1987), pp. 213, 224, and 229.

These changes in disease patterns over the past century have spawned changes in public health actions. Because the goals of public health reflect the values and beliefs of society and existing knowledge about disease and health, public health initiatives change as society's perception of health needs changes. **Public health** can be defined as an effort organized by society to protect, promote, and restore the people's health through the application of science, practical skills, and collective actions.

Public health is concerned with the health of the public.

◆ HEALTH PROMOTION

Some people do things that are not good for their health. They overeat, smoke, refuse to wear a helmet when riding a bicycle, never wear seat belts when driving, fail to take their blood pressure medication—the list is endless. These behaviors reflect personal choices, habits, and customs that are influenced and modified by social forces. We call these lifestyle behaviors, and they can be changed if the individual is so motivated. Educating people about healthy and unhealthy behaviors is one way to help them adopt positive health behaviors.

Health promotion is helping all people achieve their maximum potential for good health.

Health promotion focuses on getting people to behave healthfully: to eat healthful diets; adopt an active lifestyle; get regular rest; develop leisure-time hobbies for relaxation; achieve a balance among family, work, and play; and strengthen social networks with family and friends. It is a process of enabling people to improve their health by taking personal responsibility for their own

RANK	CAUSE OF DEATH	NUMBER OF DEATHS	PERCENTAGE OF TOTAL DEATHS
1[a]	Heart diseases	759,400	35.7
	(Coronary heart disease)	(511,700)	(24.1)
	(Other heart disease)	(247,700)	(11.6)
2[a]	Cancers	476,700	22.4
3[a]	Strokes	148,700	7.0
4[b]	Unintentional injuries	92,500	4.4
	(Motor vehicle)	(46,800)	(2.2)
	(All others)	(45,700)	(2.2)
5	Chronic obstructive lung diseases	78,000	3.7
6	Pneumonia and influenza	68,600	3.2
7[a]	Diabetes mellitus	37,800	1.8
8[b]	Suicide	29,600	1.4
9[b]	Chronic liver disease and cirrhosis	26,000	1.2
10[a]	Atherosclerosis	23,100	1.1
. . .	All causes	2,125,100	100.0

[a]Causes of death in which diet plays a part.
[b]Causes of death in which excessive alcohol consumption plays a part.

TABLE

1-4

The 10 Leading Causes of Death: United States, 1987

Source: U.S. Department of Health and Human Services, Public Health Service, *The Surgeon General's Report on Nutrition and Health* (Washington, D.C.: U.S. Government Printing Office, 1988), p. 22.

health.[18] The Canadian Ottawa Charter takes the definition one step further, stating that health promotion includes the creation of policies and environments that support healthful decisions and the tailoring of health services to promote preventive, and not just clinical, care.[19]

Although there are many unanswered questions about why people make the choices they make, the ways to promote good health are widely recognized. Born of decades, if not centuries, of scientific observation and testing, the strategies for promoting good health are outlined in Table 1-5. Although these strategies seem relatively straightforward, putting them into practice is a major challenge for most communities and nations.

◆ HEALTH OBJECTIVES

Nations differ in how they formulate health objectives for their peoples, although there are common themes. Working groups in the European Region of the World Health Organization (WHO), for example, outlined the following prerequisites for health:[20]

◆ Freedom from the fear of war—"the most serious of all threats to health"

◆ Equal opportunity for all peoples

◆ The satisfaction of basic needs for food, clean water and sanitation, decent housing, and education

◆ The right to find meaningful work and perform a useful role in society

TABLE

1-5

Ways to Promote Good Health

◆ Safe environment.	Control physical, chemical, and biologic hazards.
◆ Enhance immunity.	Immunize to protect individuals and communities.
◆ Sensible behavior.	Encourage healthy habits, and discourage harmful habits.
◆ Good nutrition.	Eat a well-balanced diet, containing neither too much nor too little.
◆ Well-born children.	Every child should be a wanted child, and every mother fit and healthy.
◆ Prudent health care.	Cautious skepticism is better than uncritical enthusiasm.

Source: Adapted, with permission, from J. M. Last, *Public Health and Human Ecology* (East Norwalk, Conn.: Appleton & Lange, 1987), p. 7.

Achieving these necessities requires both political will and public support, according to the working groups, which translated these prerequisites into specific targets for health. One such target, for example, aimed to reduce the gap in access to health care within and between countries. Another called for enhancing life expectancy by reducing disease, disability, and infant and maternal mortality. Other targets focused on enhancing social networks and promoting healthy behaviors, controlling water and air pollution, and improving the primary health care system.

In Canada, a new vision for promoting health and preventing disease among Canadians is taking shape through a document released by Health and Welfare Canada. Titled *Achieving Health for All: A Framework for Health Promotion*, this document hopes to promote a balance between individual and societal responsibilities for health. It cites three challenges to achieving health for all: reducing

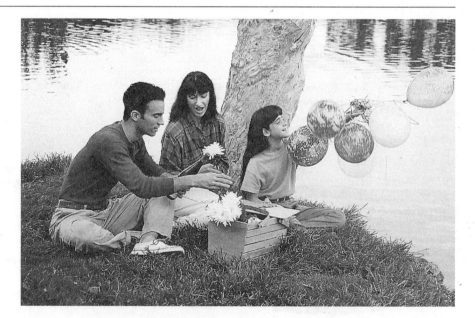

The goals of public health are set by our knowledge and the values of society, and they are directed toward the total ecologic relationship between people and their environment.

inequities in access to and use of the health care system; increasing prevention efforts to change unhealthy behaviors; and enhancing the individual's ability to cope with chronic illnesses, disabilities, and mental health problems. A key focus of the proposed implementation strategies is the strengthening of community-based health services, including worksite programs.[21] This new vision for health in Canada is a "window of opportunity" for community nutritionists to promote food and nutrition policies in all Canadian communities.[22]

The health objectives for the peoples of the United States differ slightly from those of the European and Canadian communities, reflecting the health needs of the U.S. population. A national strategy for improving the health of the nation was laid out in the publication, *Healthy People 2000: National Health Promotion and Disease Prevention Objectives.*[23] This document represents a national health agenda developed by a consortium of national health organizations, state health departments, the Institute of Medicine, and the U.S. Public Health Service. It grew out of a national health strategy that began in 1979 with the publication of *Healthy People: The Surgeon General's Report on Health Promotion and Disease Prevention*[24] and continued in 1980 with the release of the report *Promoting Health/Preventing Disease: Objectives for the Nation,* which established health objectives leading up to the year 1990.[25] The expert working groups of the *Healthy People 2000* consortium developed three broad goals designed to help Americans achieve their full potential:

- ◆ Increase the span of healthy life for Americans
- ◆ Reduce health disparities among Americans
- ◆ Achieve access to preventive services for all Americans

These goals represent the nation's hope for the improved health of its citizens, and they can serve as the foundation for all work toward health promotion and disease prevention. As stated, however, they are too broad to implement. Thus, the working groups also laid out specific, measurable targets or objectives to be achieved by the year 2000. These objectives are grouped into 22 broad categories, as shown in Table 1-6. Health promotion priorities include increasing daily physical activity, reducing cigarette smoking and alcohol consumption, and reducing child and spouse abuse, among others. Nutrition-related activities are considered essential, since 5 of the 10 leading causes of death in the United States are related to dietary imbalance and excess (coronary heart disease, some types of cancer, stroke, diabetes mellitus, and atherosclerosis), and another three are linked with the excessive consumption of alcohol (cirrhosis of the liver, accidents, and suicides). Diet also contributes to the development of other conditions, such as hypertension, osteoporosis, obesity, dental caries, and diseases of the gastrointestinal tract.[26] Some of the *Healthy People 2000* nutrition objectives focus on improving health status. For example, one health status objective calls for reducing coronary heart disease deaths to no more than 100 per 100,000 people. Nine objectives focus on risk reduction, including the following:[27]

- ◆ Reduce dietary fat intake to an average of 30 percent of calories or less and average saturated fat intake to less than 10 percent of calories among people aged 2 years and older.

TABLE
1-6

Priority Areas of the
Healthy People 2000
Initiative
Source: U.S. Department of Health
and Human Services, Public Health
Service, *Healthy People 2000:
National Health Promotion and Disease
Prevention Objectives* (Washington,
D.C.: U.S. Government Printing
Office, 1990), p. 7.

Health promotion
1. Physical activity and fitness
2. Nutrition
3. Tobacco
4. Alcohol and other drugs
5. Family planning
6. Mental health and mental disorders
7. Violent and abusive behavior
8. Educational and community-based programs

Health protection
9. Unintentional injuries
10. Occupational safety and health
11. Environmental health
12. Food and drug safety
13. Oral health

Preventive services
14. Maternal and infant health
15. Heart disease and stroke
16. Cancer
17. Diabetes and chronic disabling conditions
18. HIV infection
19. Sexually transmitted diseases
20. Immunization and infectious diseases
21. Clinical preventive services

Surveillance and data systems
22. Surveillance and data systems

Age-related objectives
    Children
    Adolescents and young adults
    Adults
    Older adults

◆ Increase complex carbohydrate and fiber-containing foods in the diets of adults to 5 or more daily servings for vegetables (including legumes) and fruits and to 6 or more daily servings for grain products.

◆ Increase to at least 50 percent the proportion of overweight people aged 12 years and older who have adopted sound dietary practices combined with regular physical activity to attain an appropriate body weight.

Health protection strategies encompass broad-based environmental measures, such as improving the workplace to reduce work-related injuries and reducing people's exposure to lead, air pollutants, and radon. Preventive services focus on areas of particular concern, such as maternal and infant health, and include screening, immunization, counseling, and other interventions for individuals in clinical settings. The primary objective for the surveillance and data systems is the systematic collection, analysis, interpretation, dissemination, and use of health data as a means of understanding a population's health status and planning prevention programs. Some of the health objectives outlined in the *Healthy People 2000* report address the special health needs of various age groups, such as children and adolescents, while others focus on special population groups, such as blacks, Hispanics, and Asians. The health objectives for these groups will be discussed in later chapters.

Many of the educational programs and services developed by public health practitioners to meet the objectives of *Healthy People 2000* focus on people in groups, whether they are in families, workplaces, or cities. Such strategies are directed toward people of all ages and segments within the community and occur over a sustained period of time. The ultimate objective of public health is to prevent increased risk and risky behaviors in the first place.[28]

◆ THE CONCEPT OF COMMUNITY

A prerequisite to delivering community-based public health and health promotion programs is understanding the community. In his analysis of 94 definitions of community, G. A. Hillery, Jr., concluded that "there is no complete agreement as to the nature of community."[29] Such diverse locales as isolated rural hamlets, mountain villages, prairie towns, state capitals, industrial cities, suburbs or ring ities, resort towns, and major metropolitan areas can all be lumped into a single category called "community."[30] In addition, the concept of community is not always circumscribed by a city limits sign or zoning laws. Sometimes it describes people who share certain interests, beliefs, or values, even though they live in diverse geographical locations. Thus, we refer to the academic community, the gay community, and the immigrant community. For our purposes, a **community** is a grouping of people who reside in a specific locality and who interact and connect through a definite social structure to fulfill a wide range of daily needs. By this definition, a community has four components: people, a location in geographical space, social interaction, and common ties.

It is possible to view the community on different scales: global, national, regional, and local. Each of these can be further segmented into specialized communities or groups, such as those individuals who speak Spanish, own VCRs, or observe Hanukkah. In the health arena, communities tend to be segmented around particular wellness, disease, or risk factors: for example, adults in the United States who exercise regularly; individuals worldwide who are infected with HIV; or black men in the Southeast who have high blood pressure.

Because communities consist of groups of people with particular characteristics, they can serve as the locus for specific interventions. The discipline of community medicine, for example, typically targets the health care needs of people living in their community environment—that is, outside the traditional hospital or clinic setting. In this context, the total community is the client or patient. Practitioners of community medicine, such as community physicians, do not merely respond to patients' health needs, as do their clinical counterparts; rather they are proactive, initiating interventions that work toward desired changes in the public's behavior.[31]

Community A group of people who live in the same geographical area, have common ties, and interact within a social system.

If we have no sense of community, the American dream will continue to wither.

—*President Bill Clinton*

An example of a community-based program is the Minnesota Heart Health Program, a research and demonstration project funded by the National Institutes of Health, an agency of the federal government. It was designed to reduce the risk of heart disease in three Minnesota communities. The educational initiatives undertaken by this 10-year program have included screening programs; education seminars for the lay public, physicians, and other health professionals; anti-smoking campaigns among school-aged children; and the use of environmental interventions (e.g., restaurant menu labeling, grocery shelf labeling) to reinforce positive health behavior changes.[32]

Another community-based program, implemented between 1980 and 1991, was the Pawtucket Heart Health Program, funded by the National Heart, Lung, and Blood Institute of the National Institutes of Health. This program used volunteers from the community of Pawtucket, Rhode Island, to deliver the program messages and services. Once again, the overall goal of this community-based health promotion effort was to lower the risk of cardiovascular disease (CVD), thus reducing the morbidity and mortality associated with CVD.[33]

The Organization of Public Health Services

In the United States, the delivery of services to meet public health needs is organized around three basic levels of government: federal, state, and local.[34] In the field of community nutrition, some of you will work within a government agency at one of these levels. Others of you will deliver nutrition programs and services through your own companies. Regardless of the setting in which you operate, you will be more effective if you understand how public health services are organized at these three levels of government.

◆ HEALTH SERVICES AT THE FEDERAL LEVEL

Public health services at the federal level are concerned with the policies and practices that affect the nation's health. To a lesser degree, some federal initiatives are also directed toward international health and related agencies, such as the WHO. In general, federal public health services include obtaining surveillance data on communicable diseases, providing health care for special population groups (e.g., the armed forces, native peoples, and government employees), conducting medical research, developing national policies for health promotion and occupational health, setting standards for health care, and obtaining health statistics on the population. In the United States, public health services are delivered through the three branches of government, as shown in Figure 1-1. The legislative branch enacts federal health laws, the judicial branch safeguards rights and settles disputes, and the executive branch approves the funding for services. The 13 executive departments are responsible for all major federal programs, and their chiefs, the departmental secretaries, report directly to the president.

At the federal level, two departments are important for our purposes: the Department of Health and Human Services (DHHS) and the Department of

FIGURE 1-1   The Organization of the U.S. Government

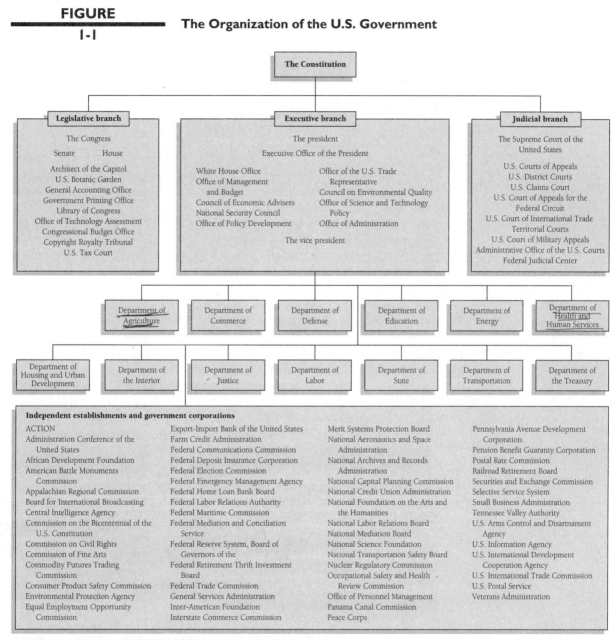

Source: Office of the Federal Register, National Archives and Records Administration, *The United States Government Manual 1988/89* (Washington, D.C.: U.S. Government Printing Office, 1988), p. 21.

Agriculture (USDA). The mission of the DHHS is to promote, protect, and advance the nation's physical and mental health. As shown on the organizational chart in Figure 1-2, the DHHS houses the Public Health Service, the premier agency for public health concerns at the national level. The Public Health Service

FIGURE 1-2

The Organization of the Department of Health and Human Services

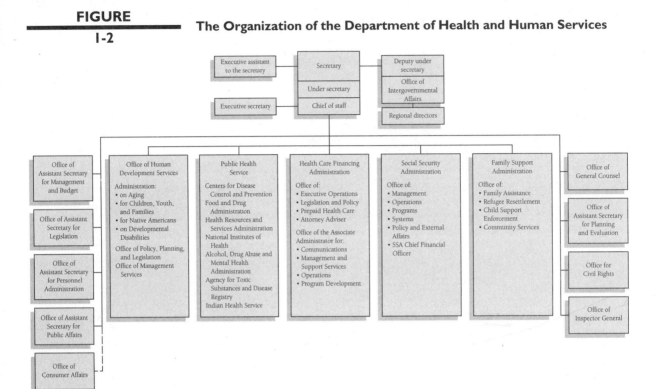

Source: Office of the Federal Register, National Archives and Records Administration, *The United States Government Manual 1988/89* (Washington, D.C.: U.S. Government Printing Office, 1988), p. 291.

is headed by the assistant secretary for health and is organized into seven units: (1) the Centers for Disease Control and Prevention; (2) the Food and Drug Administration; (3) the Health Resources and Services Administration; (4) the National Institutes of Health; (5) the Alcohol, Drug Abuse and Mental Health Administration; (6) the Agency for Toxic Substances and Disease Registry; and (7) the Indian Health Service. The Public Health Service coordinates national health policy, promotes intergovernmental relations, conducts medical and biomedical research, provides resources and expertise to the states in planning and delivering physical and mental health services, enforces laws to ensure the safety and efficacy of drugs, and protects the public against unsafe or impure foods, cosmetics, and medical devices.[35]

The USDA is also concerned with some important aspects of public health. Its organization is shown in Figure 1-3. The USDA's Food Safety and Inspection Service administers the federal meat inspection program, ensuring that meat and poultry products moved in interstate commerce are safe for consumption, wholesome, and properly labeled. The Food and Nutrition Service administers the following food assistance programs:

◆ The Food Stamp Program, which provides food coupons through local welfare agencies to needy people to increase their food-purchasing power.

**FIGURE
1-3**

The Organization of the Department of Agriculture

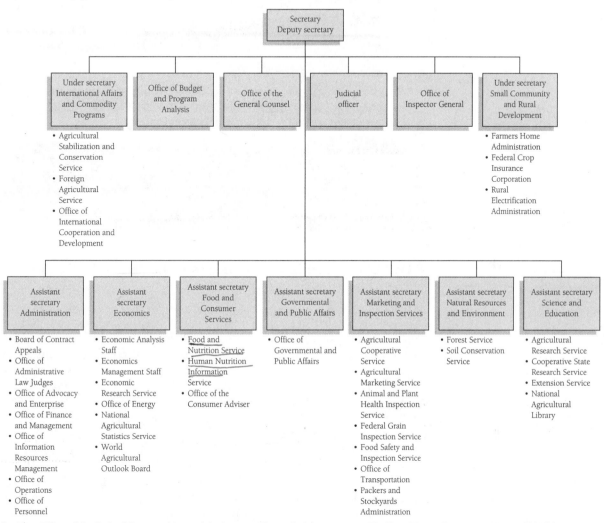

Source: Office of the Federal Register, National Archives and Records Administration, *The United States Government Manual 1988/89* (Washington, D.C.: U.S. Government Printing Office, 1988), p. 100.

◆ Programs designed to improve the nutrition of children such as the National School Lunch Program, the School Breakfast Program, the Summer Food Service Program for Children, the Child and Adult Care Food Program, and the Special Milk Program for Children.

◆ The Food Distribution Program, which makes foods available, in kind, to eligible persons. On native reservations, the program provides native peoples with access to a variety of donated foods, including meat, fruit, vegetables, and dairy and grain products.

◆ The Special Supplemental Food Program for Women, Infants, and Children (WIC), which provides nutritious supplemental foods to participants who are at nutritional risk.

◆ The Commodity Supplemental Food Program, which provides supplemental foods to infants and children and to pregnant, postpartum, and breastfeeding women with low incomes who are vulnerable to malnutrition and live in special districts.

◆ The Nutrition Education and Training program, which gives money to the states to assist them in providing nutrition education to children and in training foodservice and teaching personnel.

The USDA also houses the Human Nutrition Information Service, which conducts research in human nutrition, provides technical assistance to health professionals, and coordinates nutrition education activities. It carries out the national food consumption surveys and compiles data on the nutrient composition of foods through its Nutrient Data Bank; these food values are published in the Agriculture Handbook No. 8 series, *Composition of Foods.*

◆ HEALTH SERVICES AT THE STATE LEVEL

In the United States, the states are the basic unit for the delivery of public health services. They determine the form and function of local health agencies, select and appoint local health personnel, identify local health problems, and guarantee a minimum level of essential health services. State and federal public health services have a similar organization. A diagram of a generic state health agency appears in Appendix A.

State agencies provide many services, including services for maternal and child health, such as prenatal and postnatal programs, family planning, immunizations, and well-baby clinics; public and personal health education; control of communicable diseases, including immunizations, epidemiology, and laboratory services; preventive and general dental health; programs for handicapped children; population screening for chronic diseases; mental health, alcohol, and drug abuse programs; licensure of health professionals; and laboratory services to help identify and prevent disease. The state also governs the use of public hospital facilities for indigent patients, civil service programs, the control and management of toxic substances, social services, and the containment of health care costs. Altogether, as many as 30 different state agencies with some responsibility for public health have been identified. State health departments are credited with many public health initiatives in sanitation engineering, control of communicable diseases, and the development of strong networks of county health organizations. Many federal public health services actually originated in state health programs.

Each state has its own system for delivering public health services. Some states have a centralized organization, while others are decentralized to a greater or lesser extent. No two states have exactly the same organization, although common features do exist. Most states have an "umbrella" agency that allows for

◆ ENTREPRENEUR IN ACTION

Introducing Kathy King Helm, R.D.

◆ HER BACKGROUND . . .

Kathy King Helm began her business in 1972. She initially worked to build a counseling practice that focused on clinical and preventive nutrition. Later, she expanded her business to include giving talks on local and national television shows, counseling athletes with the Denver Bronco football team and the Denver Avalanche soccer team, and writing and teaching about wellness nutrition. In 1989 she hosted her own nationally syndicated radio talk show. She is the founder of Helm Seminars and the author of *The Entrepreneurial Nutritionist*, a book and home study course for the would-be entrepreneur.

◆ SHE HAS THIS TO SAY ABOUT ENTREPRENEURSHIP . . .

"Entrepreneurship is a way of thinking that becomes a style of living and a way to do business. Several words come to mind when I think of the word 'entrepreneurship': freedom, creativity, and energy. *Freedom* is necessary to explore the possibilities before evaluating all the limitations of an idea. *Creativity* is essential to making your product or service competitive in the marketplace. *Energy* makes it all happen or keeps it from happening. Entrepreneurship takes a lot of time and energy (in other words—hard work), and sometimes money. Community-based entrepreneurs take calculated risks financially and risk public scrutiny daily."

To Helm, entrepreneurship in nutrition has finally entered the mainstream. "Because the marketplaces where dietitians have worked traditionally have undergone dramatic changes in recent years, dietitians are looking for new career options and challenges. The window of opportunity for entrepreneurial community nutritionists is wide open, with plenty of opportunities in the field of nutrition."

Helm thinks that entrepreneurship is important to the practice of community nutrition, because it demands that practitioners keep abreast of the newest research findings, the current competition, and the latest gimmicks in the marketplace. She comments, "By understanding business and marketing, community nutritionists develop products, services, and social marketing campaigns that better address their consumers' needs. But they also need added flair and their own personal style to take on the competition and succeed!"

Helm believes that dietitians must work to become more visible and credible to the public and points out that while there are calculated risks to having one's own business, there are also many rewards. "I have learned," she says, "that when the tough decisions have to be made, no one can do it better than I. I find it still takes time and patience to break into new business arenas where I am unknown. Even so, I will continue in business, because I love the chance to be creative and to work with people. The difficulty of the challenge makes me appreciate the rewards even more."

greater coordination of public health programs and cost containment. Some have a board of health that formulates health policy; in others, the state health agency develops policy in cooperation with the governor's office.

◆ HEALTH SERVICES AT THE LOCAL LEVEL

The local health department is responsible for providing health protection directly to individuals within the community on a daily basis. It is usually, but not always, headed by a physician with special training in public health. (An example of an organizational chart for a local health department appears in Appendix A.) Other health professionals working in the local health department include nurses, dentists, nutritionists, health inspectors, social workers, health educators, hygienists, and epidemiologists.

The local health department has a wide range of duties. It conducts needs assessments to determine the community's existing health needs. It works to control communicable diseases by holding immunization clinics and identifying and recording cases of disease. It manages the community's environmental health by monitoring waste disposal and water and air pollution. The local health department also provides health education in schools and other settings, organizes special clinic services for families, delivers home care, coordinates disaster planning, and provides preventive screening to detect existing conditions such as hypertension, glaucoma, and tuberculosis. In the food arena, the local health department inspects restaurants and local food processing and production plants.

Community and Public Health Nutrition

Community nutrition A discipline that strives to prevent disease and enhance health by improving the public's eating habits.

Governments have ample reason to undertake public health initiatives to improve people's eating patterns, because adequate and proper nutrition is a key determinant of good health. **Community nutrition** is a discipline that strives to improve the nutrition—and, by extension, the health—of individuals and groups within communities. Nutrition programming can occur in many community settings, including worksites, hospitals, clinics, shopping malls, schools, churches, recreational and sports centers, and homes.

Community nutrition and public health nutrition are sometimes considered to be synonymous. In this book, *community nutrition* is the broader of the two terms and encompasses any nutrition program whose target is the community, whether the program is federally funded or sponsored by a private group (as in a worksite weight-management program). *Public health nutrition* refers to those community-based programs conducted by a government agency (federal, state, county, or city) whose official mandate is the delivery of health services to individuals living in a particular area.

The confusion over these terms stems partly from the traditional and somewhat distinct practice settings of community dietitians and public health nutritionists, as shown in Figure 1-4. Community dietitians, who are always registered dietitians (RDs), tend to be situated in hospitals, voluntary health organizations, worksites, and other nongovernment settings. Public health nutritionists, some of whom are RDs, provide nutrition services through government agencies. The public health nutritionist plans, coordinates, directs, manages, and evaluates the nutrition component of the agency's services.[36]

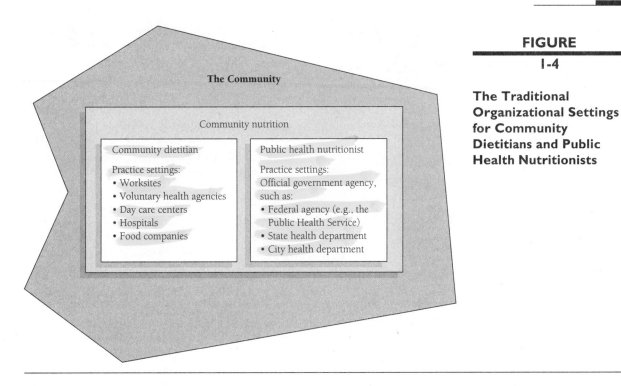

FIGURE

1-4

The Traditional Organizational Settings for Community Dietitians and Public Health Nutritionists

In today's practice environment, there is considerable overlap between these two designations, and practitioners in both areas share many goals, responsibilities, target groups, and practice settings. For our purposes, all nutritionists whose major orientation is community-based programming will be called community nutritionists, whether their official title is community dietitian, public health nutritionist, nutrition education specialist, or some other designation. The following section describes the educational requirements, roles and responsibilities, and practice settings of community nutritionists.

◆ EDUCATIONAL REQUIREMENTS

Community nutritionists have a solid background in the nutrition sciences. They have competencies in such areas as nutritional biochemistry, nutrition assessment, nutrition in health and disease, nutrition throughout the life cycle, food composition, and food habits and customs. They are knowledgeable about the theories and principles of health education, epidemiology, community organization, management, and social marketing. Marketing skills are especially important, as it is no longer sufficient merely to know *which* nutrition messages to deliver, it is also necessary to know *how* to deliver them effectively in a variety of media formats to a variety of audiences.

The minimum educational requirements for a community nutritionist include a bachelor's degree in community nutrition, foods and nutrition, or dietetics from an accredited college or university. Most community nutrition positions require registration as a dietitian by the American Dietetic Association (ADA). Some positions also require graduate-level training to obtain additional competencies in areas such as quality assurance, biostatistics, research methodology, survey design and analysis, and the behavioral sciences.

Although dietetic technicians registered (DTRs) are most often employed in the foodservice sector and in clinical settings, some do work in the community arena.[37] Community-based DTRs assist the community nutritionist in determining the community's nutritional needs and in delivering community nutrition programs and services. DTRs must have at least an associate's degree and pass the ADA registration examination.

TABLE

1-7

Activities of Dietitians Providing Nutrition Programs for Population Groups

Obtain screening data on groups

Obtain surveillance data on groups

Obtain data on community resources

Provide education programs to groups

Identify nutrition problems within groups

Prepare education materials for groups

Document program services

Disseminate information through the media

Lead support groups for clients

Teach community workers about nutrition

Assist community organizations with programs

Negotiate contracts for nutrition programs

Evaluate nutrition programs for groups

Provide health promotion programs

Source: © 1990 The American Dietetic Association. ROLE DELINEATION FOR REGISTERED DIETITIANS AND ENTRY-LEVEL DIETETIC TECHNICIANS. Used by permission.

◆ ROLES AND RESPONSIBILITIES

Community nutritionists have many roles: educator, counselor, coordinator, advocate, developer of standards, and supervisor. They are responsible for providing nutrition information to individuals, specialized groups, and the general population. They focus on normal nutrition, although they sometimes cover the principles of diet therapy and nutritional care in disease for certain groups (e.g., parents with HIV-positive children or people with diabetes).[38]

Community nutritionists are responsible for planning, evaluating, and managing nutrition services and programs. One survey of 350 community dietitians found that more than two-thirds had mid- to upper-level management responsibilities. Community dietitians in management positions reported spending more time planning, coordinating, and evaluating programs, and less time in actual interaction with clients, than did those in lower-level positions.[39] Managing people and resources is now viewed as an important role of the community nutritionist.

A role delineation study conducted by the ADA in 1989 found that RDs working in community settings also had advising, policy-setting, and supervising roles.[40] The community-wide activities of entry-level DTRs and RDs who participated in the role delineation study are listed in Table 1-7.* The time allocated to these activities varied somewhat by practice level. Community dietitians reported having major responsibility for teaching students, other dietitians, and health professionals; their roles overlapped significantly with those of RDs in clinical dietetics.

*The Dietetic Practice Inventory was a survey instrument developed by the ADA, the official organization of RDs responsible for determining "those major and specific responsibilities that a practitioner must assume and be held accountable for to provide quality care." In the early 1980s, the ADA recognized that the roles and functions of dietitians were becoming increasingly specialized.[41] Accordingly, it undertook three role delineation studies to define the practice of dietetics. Each of these studies focused on verifying the appropriate responsibilities and related knowledge required for competent entry-level practitioners in a specific area of practice: community dietetics, foodservice systems management, and clinical dietetics. Use of these study results was limited, however, because they were based on expert opinion about dietetic practice and not on the actual roles and responsibilities of practitioners in a variety of settings. Thus, in 1989, the ADA undertook a more comprehensive examination of dietetic practice. It developed the Dietetic Practice Survey to determine if there were common components of practice that cut across different levels of practice and different practice settings. A major objective was to describe the specific roles and activities of entry-level RDs, DTRs, and RDs beyond entry level.[42]

Community nutritionists who work for government agencies assist in developing policy, coordinating the collection of national data on food intake and dietary patterns, overseeing nutrition research projects, providing technical assistance to health professionals, and developing educational programs and materials for the public. In some state and territorial health agencies, they serve as the director or administrator of nutrition services.[43]

◆ PRACTICE SETTINGS

The practice settings of community nutritionists include worksites; universities, colleges, and medical schools; voluntary and nonprofit health organizations such as the American Heart Association; federal government agencies; public health departments; home health care agencies; day care centers; residential facilities; fitness centers; sports clinics; hospital outpatient facilities; and food companies. Some community nutritionists have their own business and work as consultants, providing nutrition expertise for government agencies, food companies, or other groups who are planning community-based interventions or education programs with a nutritional component.

Community nutritionists are also employed by world and regional health organizations. WHO's Division of Family Health, located in the headquarters office in Geneva, Switzerland, includes an office of nutrition. Likewise, the North American regional WHO office in Washington, D.C., which is known officially as the Pan American Sanitary Bureau and coexists with the Pan American Health Organization (PAHO), has a strong nutrition mandate. The PAHO directs its efforts toward solving nutritional problems in Latin America and the Caribbean.[44] Another prominent organization in global community nutrition is the Food and Agriculture Organization (FAO) of the United Nations. The programs of the Food Policy and Nutrition Division of the FAO are directed toward improving the nutrition status of at-risk populations and ensuring access to adequate supplies of safe, good-quality foods.[45]

The Community Nutritionist as Entrepreneur

We have just described the typical practice settings and activities of the traditional community nutritionist. Now, we would like to introduce a new activity—entrepreneurship. Entrepreneurship is as much an attitude as a cache of skills and insights. It is a way of thinking, a way of looking at the world. Although the entrepreneurial spark may be ignited by pure inspiration (the "Ah, ha" experience), successful new ventures more often than not are the result of planning, patience, and persistence.

Creativity and innovation—the essence of entrepreneurship—are as important to the discipline of community nutrition as to any other field. But, you may ask, in what way are they important? Both the skill set and the mind set required for entrepreneurship are relevant to the practice of community nutrition. As an

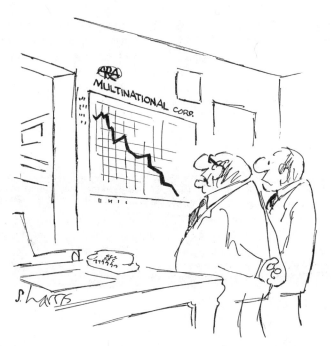

"It's not surprising. The production department is in Spain, the warehouse is in Korea, the accounting division is in Bolivia, the Board of Directors is in Canada . . ."

entrepreneurial community nutritionist, you seek new opportunities for nutrition education and explore new strategies for delivering nutrition messages. You tap into the ideas and trends of other disciplines to help develop, market, implement, and evaluate nutrition services and programs. You envision new ways of packaging and marketing traditional nutrition education materials, such as brochures, pamphlets, and fact sheets. Plus, you consider new technologies and alternative educational mediums—videos, computer software programs, compact disk technology, and the electronic highway, to name a few—as vehicles for disseminating nutrition information. You seek alliances with untraditional funding sources, perhaps forming partnerships with food or drug companies to sponsor new ventures. To create and innovate successfully in community nutrition, you must be alert for opportunities in a constantly changing environment. Indeed, the environment itself will shape the challenges you face in delivering nutrition information and the very nature of your practice in the community setting.

Leading Indicators of Change

The entrepreneurial community nutritionist monitors current trends affecting the marketplace. Ideas gleaned from television, radio, newspapers, magazines, scientific journals, advertising, grocery stores, shopping malls—from virtually everywhere—can be used to formulate strategies for reaching new and existing target markets. Some current trends have global implications for the health arena, and many have important consequences for community nutrition.

The trend toward globalization means, among other things, that the demographic profile of many communities is changing rapidly along with the client mix served by community nutritionists. Analysts predict that by the year 2000 the global workforce will likely experience massive relocations of people, including immigrants, refugees, retirees, temporary workers, and visitors, across national borders. Women are expected to enter the global workforce in unprecedented numbers in the coming decade, a trend that may lead to changes in traditional family norms, structures, and child rearing practices and thus affect the format and delivery of nutrition programs and services. A worldwide increase in the educational level of the workforce is also anticipated. Consequently, a variety of alternative educational strategies will be needed to reach consumers whose education, training, income, and economic potential will be highly diverse.[46]

In North America, the aging of the population, coupled with a more ethnically diverse society, will challenge community nutritionists to develop new products and services. In the United States, for example, the fastest-growing segment

By the Year 2000 . . .

◆ The U.S. population will have grown about 7 percent to nearly 270 million people.

◆ The average household size is expected to decline from 2.69 in 1985 to 2.48 in the year 2000, with husband-wife households decreasing from 58 to 53 percent of all households.

◆ The racial and ethnic composition of the American population will form a different pattern:

  ◆ Whites, not including Hispanic Americans, will decline from 76 to 72 percent of the population.

  ◆ Hispanics will rise from 8 to 11.3 percent, to more than 31 million Hispanic people.

  ◆ Blacks will increase their proportion from 12.4 to 13.1 percent.

  ◆ Other racial groups, including American Indians and Alaska Natives and Asians and Pacific Islanders, will increase from 3.5 to 4.3 percent of the total.

◆ The American population may increase by up to 6 million people through immigration. Certain states and cities, especially those on the East and West Coasts, can be expected to receive a disproportionately large number of these immigrants.

Source: U.S. Department of Health and Human Services, Public Health Service, *Healthy People 2000: National Health Promotion and Disease Prevention Objectives* (Washington, D.C.: U.S. Government Printing Office, 1990), pp. 2–3.

of the nation's population consists of people over 65 years of age. A large portion of this group has chronic health problems; nearly all will remain concerned about securing adequate food and shelter. The so-called baby boomers, those people born during or just after World War II, will reach their peak earning years in the next decade and are expected to be a leading market force. An interesting consequence of the influx of immigrants into Canada and the United States is an anticipated change in consumer marketing strategies due to the family-oriented shopping behaviors of Asian and Hispanic consumers. The cultural values and lifestyles of these ethnic groups tend to reinforce family decision-making and collective buying behavior. Marketers will have to change their strategies to appeal to the decision style of the extended family. They will need to market their products and services to groups rather than individuals.[47]

Watchwords for the Future

Several terms have surfaced repeatedly in this chapter: change, innovation, creativity, community, entrepreneurship. These watchwords herald the approach of a new century marked by unprecedented global social change. The world is growing smaller and its peoples seem to be moving toward the birth of a single, global nation. "Citizen of the world," a phrase popular during the mid-twentieth century, takes on added meaning with the approach of the twenty-first century. Where once a community was circumscribed by a distant ridge or the next valley, today the "informational city" links us via satellite and optic fibers to unseen faces on the other side of the earth. The growing connectedness of the human race promises to create new challenges for community nutritionists in their efforts to enhance the nutrition and health of all peoples.

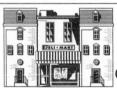

COMMUNITY LEARNING ACTIVITY

1. Interview an individual in your community who has been described as an entrepreneur or, in your view, captures the entrepreneurial spirit. You may locate this person in any number of ways—by reading your local newspaper, for example, or talking with other people in your community, such as your parents, a friend's parents, students you have met in other courses, or someone who lives in your building. This entrepreneur may be a nutritionist, but likely as not, she or he will be an inventor, artist, manufacturer, retailer, banker, farmer, chemist, carpenter, or other expert. A few of the questions you might ask this individual are listed here. You should be able to think of others.

   a. What factors contributed to your success?

b. What types of mistakes did you make and what did you learn from them?

c. Was there a point at which you thought about giving up? If so, what kept you going?

d. What advice would you give to a beginning entrepreneur?

2. Describe how you can use what you learned from this entrepreneur in your personal and professional life.

3. Search local community newspapers for articles describing health and nutrition issues.

a. For a designated period (e.g., one week), how many articles on health and nutrition did you find?

b. How many of these articles actually described *local* rather than national or international health and nutrition problems?

c. From your analysis of these articles, what appears to be the leading health problem in your community? How does nutrition status or intake contribute to this problem?

NOTES

1. D. W. Cravens and S. H. Shipp, Market-driven strategies for competitive advantage, *Business Horizons* 34 (1991): 53–61.
2. W. B. Johnston, Global work force 2000: The new world labor market, *Harvard Business Review* 69 (1991): 115–27.
3. L. Brokaw, Head of the class, *Inc.* 14 (1992): 63.
4. D. L. Cooperrider and W. A. Pasmore, Global social change: A new agenda for social science? *Human Relations* 44 (1991): 1037–55.
5. C. Gorman, Invincible AIDS, *Time* 140 (August 3, 1992): 18–22.
6. U. S. Department of Health and Human Services, Public Health Service, *Healthy People 2000: National Health Promotion and Disease Prevention Objectives* (Washington, D.C.: U.S. Government Printing Office, 1990), cover letter and pp. 1–8.
7. As cited in J. M. Last, *Public Health and Human Ecology* (East Norwalk, Conn.: Appleton & Lange, 1987), p. 16.
8. P. Drucker, *Innovation and Entrepreneurship* (New York: Harper & Row, 1985).
9. E. O. Welles, Captain Marvel, *Inc.* 14 (1992): 44–47.
10. The discussion of entrepreneurship was adapted from B. J. Bird, *Entrepreneurial Behavior* (Glenview, Ill.: Scott, Foresman, 1989), pp. 1-33, 57–76, and 349–75, and J. G. Burch, *Entrepreneurship* (New York: John Wiley & Sons, 1986), pp. 4–42.
11. Bird, *Entrepreneurial Behavior,* p. 3.
12. K. A. Egge and F. J. Simer, An analysis of the advice given by recent entrepreneurs to prospective entrepreneurs, in *Frontiers of Entrepreneurial Research* (Wellesley, Mass.: Babson College, 1988), pp. 119–33.
13. The discussion of the concepts of health and public health was adapted from Last, *Public Health and Human Ecology,* pp. 1–26, and G. Pickett and J. J. Hanlon, *Public Health: Administration and Practice* (St. Louis: Times Mirror/Mosby College Publishing, 1990), pp. 3–20.
14. R. J. Dubos, *Mirage of Health* (Garden City, N.Y.: Doubleday, 1959), pp. 13–14.
15. J. Stokes III and coauthors, Definition of terms and concepts applicable to clinical preventive medicine, *Journal of Community Health* 8 (1982): 33–41.
16. T. C. Quinn, Screening for HIV infection—benefits and costs (editorial), *New England Journal of Medicine* 327 (1992): 486–88.
17. D. E. Snider, Jr., and W. L. Roper, The new tuberculosis (editorial), *New England Journal of Medicine* 326 (1992): 703–5.
18. M. Minkler, Health education, health promotion, and the open society: An historical perspective, *Health Education Quarterly* 16 (1989): 17–30.
19. As cited in K. Glanz, F. M. Lewis, and B. K. Rimer, eds., *Health Behavior and Health Education* (San Francisco: Jossey-Bass, 1991), p. 9.

20. World Health Organization, *Targets for Health for All* (Copenhagen: World Health Organization Regional Office for Europe, 1985).

21. H. Nielsen, *Achieving Health for All:* A framework for nutrition in health promotion, *Journal of the Canadian Dietetic Association* 50 (1989): 77–80.

22. C. R. Connolly, A commentary on *Achieving Health for All: A Framework for Health Promotion, Journal of the Canadian Dietetic Association* 50 (1989): 89–92.

23. U.S. Department of Health and Human Services, Public Health Service, *Healthy People 2000.*

24. U.S. Department of Health and Human Services, Public Health Service, *Healthy People: The Surgeon General's Report on Health Promotion and Disease Prevention* (Washington, D.C.: U.S. Government Printing Office, PHS Pub. No. 79–55071, 1979).

25. U.S. Department of Health and Human Services, Public Health Service, *Promoting Health/Preventing Disease: Objectives for the Nation* (Washington, D.C.: U.S. Government Printing Office, 1980).

26. U.S. Department of Health and Human Services, Public Health Service, *The Surgeon General's Report on Nutrition and Health* (Washington, D.C.: U.S. Government Printing Office, DHHS Pub. No. 88–50210, 1988), pp. 1–20.

27. U.S. Department of Health and Human Services, Public Health Service, *Healthy People 2000,* pp. 117–19.

28. H. Blackburn, Research and demonstration projects in community cardiovascular disease prevention, *Journal of Public Health Policy* 4 (1983): 398–421.

29. G. A. Hillery, Jr., Definitions of community: Areas of agreement, *Rural Sociology* 20 (1955): 111–23.

30. The discussion of the concept of community was adapted from T. N. Clark, *Community Structure and Decision-Making: Comparative Analyses* (San Francisco: Chandler Publishing, 1968), pp. 83–89; A. D. Edwards and D. G. Jones, *Community and Community Development* (The Hague: Mouton & Co., 1976), pp. 11–39; R. M. MacIver, *On Community, Society and Power* (Chicago: University of Chicago Press, 1970), pp. 29–34; and D. E. Poplin, *Communities* (New York: Macmillan, 1979), pp. 3–25.

31. F. Eskin, The community physician as change agent, *Public Health in London* 94 (1980): 44–51.

32. U.S. Department of Health and Human Services, Public Health Service, National Institutes of Health, *With Every Beat of Your Heart: An Ideabook for Community Heart Health Programs* (Washington, D.C.: U.S. Government Printing Office, NIH Pub. No. 87–2641, 1987), p. 22.

33. R. C. Lefebvre and coauthors, Theory and delivery of health programming in the community: The Pawtucket Heart Health Program, *Preventive Medicine* 16 (1987): 80–95.

34. The discussion of the organization of public health services at the federal, state, and local levels was adapted from Last, *Public Health and Human Ecology,* pp. 281–300, and Pickett and Hanlon, *Public Health,* pp. 97–120.

35. Office of the Federal Register, National Archives and Records Administration, *The United States Government Manual 1988/89* (Washington, D.C.: U.S. Government Printing Office, Revised June 1, 1988), pp. 21, 97–126, and 282–309.

36. M. Kaufman, Preparing public health nutritionists to meet the future, *Journal of the American Dietetic Association* 86 (1986): 511–14.

37. American Dietetic Association, *Role Delineation for Registered Dietitians and Entry-Level Dietetic Technicians* (Chicago: American Dietetic Association, 1990).

38. L. M. Brown and M. F. Fruin, Management activities in community dietetics practice, *Journal of the American Dietetic Association* 89 (1989): 373–77.

39. Ibid.

40. American Dietetic Association, *Role Delineation for Registered Dietitians.*

41. The discussion of the role delineation study was taken in part from the *Journal of the American Dietetic Association* 90 (1990): 1117–21, 1122–23, and 1124–33.

42. American Dietetic Association, *Role Delineation for Registered Dietitians.*

43. M. Kaufman and coauthors, Survey of nutritionists in state and local public health agencies, *Journal of the American Dietetic Association* 86 (1986): 1566–70.

44. Pan American Health Organization, *Food and Nutrition Issues in Latin America and the Caribbean* (Washington, D.C.: Pan American Health Organization/Inter-American Development Bank, 1990).

45. Food and Agriculture Organization of the United Nations white paper on the Food Policy and Nutrition Division, pp. 24–29.

46. Johnston, Global work force 2000.

47. J. L. Zaichkowsky, Consumer behavior: Yesterday, today, and tomorrow, *Business Horizons* 34 (1991): 51–58.

Principles
of Epidemiology

Something to Think About . . .

The argument that we should wait for certainty [in making public health recommendations] is an argument for never taking action—we shall never be certain.

—M. G. Marmot

Introduction

In 1855, Dr. John Snow of London, England, wrote an account of his discovery of the link between contaminated water and a local outbreak of cholera, one of the greatest scourges of modern times. Snow observed that people who had drunk water from a pump on Broad Street in central London were attacked by the disease. He formulated a hypothesis about the mode of cholera transmission, suggesting that the intestinal discharges of people sick with cholera were seeping into the Thames River, the source of Broad Street drinking water, and were turning it into a cesspool. To test his hypothesis, he tracked down cholera cases and interviewed family members about their source of drinking water. He identified common events that linked cholera patients and established the ways in which they differed from healthy individuals in the same neighborhood. Snow observed that the rate of cholera was significantly lower in communities consuming water drawn from the Thames River upstream, which presumably was uncontaminated. His recommendation for stopping the cholera epidemic was simple: Remove the handle from the Broad Street pump so that it could not be used. Medical publishers were so skeptical of Snow's theory that he was forced to publish the particulars of his discovery at his own expense.[1]

Epidemiology From the Greek word meaning "upon the people"; the study of epidemics.

Snow described the mode of transmission of this dreaded infection nearly 30 years before the cholera bacterium, *Vibrio cholerae,* was discovered. Due, in part, to his careful observations, London took a major step toward controlling cholera epidemics and improving the public's health by installing new water supply systems. This story is an example of how the classic epidemiologic method was applied to determining the cause and course of a disease outbreak. In fact, the word **epidemiology** is derived from "epidemic," which translated from the Greek means "upon the people." As this derivation indicates, the epidemiologic method was initially used to investigate, control, and prevent epidemics of infectious diseases such as cholera, plague, smallpox, typhoid, tuberculosis, and poliomyelitis. Although investigating infectious disease outbreaks is still part of epidemiology, today it is also applied to the study of injuries, especially those occurring in the home and at work; chronic diseases such as cancer, coronary heart disease, and arthritis; and social problems such as teenage pregnancies, homicide, alcoholism, and cocaine abuse.

The Practice of Epidemiology

The discipline of epidemiology has expanded from its origin as the study of epidemics to include the control and prevention of all types of health problems. It is similar to clinical medicine and laboratory science in its concern with understanding the processes of health and disease in humans, but it differs from these disciplines in its focus on the health problems of populations rather than of individual patients. A panel of international experts recently arrived at the following definition of epidemiology:[2]

> Epidemiology is the study of the distribution and determinants of health-related states and events in specified populations and the application of this study to the control of health problems.

This definition requires some explanation. The term *distribution* refers to the relationship between the health problem or disease and the population in which it exists. The distribution includes the persons affected and the place and time of the occurrence. It also encompasses such population parameters as age, sex, race, occupational type, income and educational levels, exposure to certain agents, and other social and environmental features. Distribution is concerned with population trends or patterns of disease or exposure to a specific agent among groups of people.

The term *determinants* refers to the causes and factors that affect the risk of disease. Infectious diseases have a single, necessary cause. Shigellosis, for example, is an infection of the bowel caused by *Shigella* organisms. Rubella or German measles is a highly contagious disease caused by a virus spread by airborn droplets or close contact. Many conditions, however, have multiple determinants, as in the contribution of sex, race, dietary intake, and hormonal status to osteoporosis. Determinants of disease are typically divided into two groups: (1) host factors, such as age, sex, race, genetic makeup, nutrition status, and physiologic state, which determine an individual's susceptibility to disease; and (2) environmental factors, such as living conditions, occupation, geographical location, and lifestyle, which determine the host's exposure to a specific agent.

Whereas the clinician is concerned with an individual patient and the host and environmental factors that affect that patient's health status, the epidemiologist is concerned with groups of individuals or populations. The epidemiologist measures or counts those elements that are common to individuals, so that the magnitude and effects of individual variation within a population can be accounted for in studying a disease process. Differences in rates of disease in populations are then used to formulate hypotheses about the cause of a health problem or to assess exposure to a specific agent. Working closely with clinicians, laboratory scientists, biostatisticians, and other health professionals, the epidemiologist works to identify the causes of disease and to propose strategies for controlling or preventing health problems.[3]

In addition to enhancing our understanding of health and disease and searching for the causes of disease, epidemiology has several other uses. The epidemiologic method can be used to describe a community's particular health problems and to determine whether a community's overall health is improving or getting worse. "Diagnosing" a community's health problems is important to health agencies. The public health department, for example, may need to know whether the number of low birth weight infants born within the community decreased, increased, or remained the same compared with the previous year. The agency may want to compare the community's current rate of births of underweight infants with the rate from the previous decade or with the state or national average. This information can be used to evaluate the agency's current programs and services and determine whether they are meeting the health needs of pregnant women in the community. Potential health problems may also be spotted through this ongoing examination of a community's health status. For example, in the early 1980s, an unusual illness was observed mostly among gay men living in San Francisco, Los Angeles, and New York. The finding of an unusually high number of cases of Kaposi's sarcoma, a rare cancer affecting primarily middle-aged men of Jewish or Italian ancestry, led to the discovery of a new, fatal disease, the acquired immunodeficiency syndrome (AIDS).

Vital statistics Figures pertaining to life events, such as births, deaths, and marriages.

Based on the **vital statistics** (e.g., age at death, cause of death) recorded on death certificates, the epidemiologic method can also be used to calculate an individual's risk of dying before a certain age. This type of risk assessment is the foundation of the actuarial tables developed by life insurance companies. A related use occurs in clinical decision making when, for example, the effectiveness of a particular drug or surgical intervention in treating a certain condition is evaluated as well as whether its use is associated with side effects or other health risks. Sometimes the epidemiologic method is used to identify the characteristics of a disease and determine whether some syndromes are related to one another or

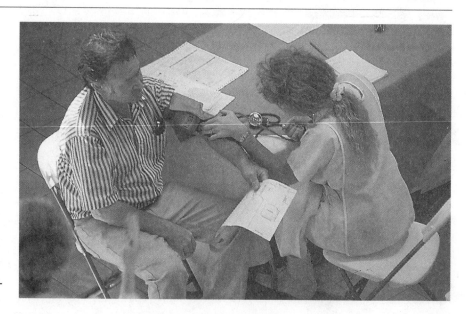

Health agencies screen people for high blood pressure and other conditions to help "diagnose" a community's health problems.

represent distinct conditions. A good example of this use was the development of a working case definition that outlined the clinical, behavioral, and physiological manifestations of the chronic fatigue syndrome.[4]

Basic Epidemiologic Concepts

Put simply, "the basic operation of the epidemiologist is to count cases and measure the population in which they arise" in order to calculate rates of occurrence of a health problem and compare the rates in different groups of people.[5] The primary reason for investigating and analyzing these health problems is to work toward controlling and preventing them, typically through the formulation of specific health policies. This section presents key epidemiologic concepts that illustrate how data about disease processes are obtained and analyzed.

◆ RATES AND RISKS

A middle-aged woman is admitted to the emergency room, complaining of chest pain, nausea, and dizziness. The attending physician orders a diagnostic workup, which confirms that the woman has had a heart attack. For the emergency room physician, this woman is a patient requiring immediate critical care. For the epidemiologist studying the factors that contribute to coronary heart disease, this woman is a **case**, a single individual with a confirmed diagnosis of myocardial infarction. The physician and the epidemiologist share a common concern about this woman—her risk status. Does she possess certain characteristics that placed her at high risk for heart attacks? If so, can the characteristics be modified to reduce her chance of having another one? If the woman does not appear to belong in a high-risk group, why did she have a heart attack at this particular time?

Case A particular instance of a disease or outcome of interest.

In epidemiology, **risk** refers to the likelihood that people who are without a disease, but exposed to certain **risk factors,** will acquire the disease at some point in their lives.[6] These risk factors may be inherited. Others are found in the physical environment in the form of infectious agents, toxins, or drugs. Some risk factors are derived from the social environment, that is, the family, community, or culture. Others are behavioral, such as not wearing seat belts or smoking.

Risk The probability or likelihood of an event occurring—in this case, the probability that people will acquire a disease.

Some of us are exposed to certain risk factors more than other individuals are. For example, workers in photographic laboratories, dry-cleaning establishments, and some industrial processing plants are exposed daily to chloroform, a highly volatile liquid that has been shown to cause tumors in mice and rats. Workers in office buildings and schools are typically not exposed to chloroform. These different exposure rates to a risk factor (in this case, chloroform) allow for basic comparisons of disease rates among individuals. One expression of how frequently a disease occurs in a population is **incidence**, the fraction or proportion of a group initially free of a disease or condition that develops the disease or condition over a period of time. Incidence is measured by a two-step process: (1) identify a group of susceptible people who are initially free of the disease or

Risk factor Clinically important signs associated with an increased likelihood of acquiring a disease.

Incidence *New* events in a given period.

Prevalence *All events in a given period.*

condition, and (2) examine them periodically over a period of time to discover and count the new cases of the disease that develop during that interval.

Another common measure of frequency of occurrence of an event is **prevalence,** or the fraction or proportion of a group possessing a disease or condition at a specific time. The prevalence rate is measured by a single examination or survey of a group. The characteristics of these two measures are summarized in Table 2-1. Incidence and prevalence rates describe the frequency with which particular events occur. By calculating and comparing rates, the strength of the association between risk factors and the health problem being studied can be determined.

◆ THE EPIDEMIOLOGIC METHOD

In its study of disease processes, epidemiology uses a variety of tools: clinical, microbiological, pathological, demographic, sociological, and statistical. None of these is exclusive to epidemiology, but the manner in which they are used uniquely defines the epidemiologic method. The following example uses the investigation of the "diet-heart" hypothesis to illustrate the rigorous, scientific approach of the epidemiologist:

1. **Observing.** Many years of investigation had shown that atherosclerosis could be induced in laboratory animals, particularly rabbits and monkeys, by feeding them a diet rich in fats and cholesterol. Physicians working in India, Africa, and Latin America also observed that coronary heart disease (CHD) was fairly rare in human populations whose diet tended to be high in vegetables and grains.[7]

2. **Counting cases or events.** Vital statistics obtained from the World Health Organization showed marked differences in deaths from CHD among countries, with Finland having one of the highest and Greece and Japan among the lowest CHD death rates, as shown graphically in Figure 2-1. The habitual diets of the peoples in these countries differed as well.

3. **Relating cases or events to the population at risk.** Public health officials in the United States became increasingly concerned about the number of

TABLE
2-1

Characteristics of Incidence Rates and Prevalence Rates

Source: R. H. Fletcher, S. W. Fletcher, and E. H. Wagner, *Clinical Epidemiology—The Essentials,* p. 78. © WILLIAMS & WILKINS 1982. Used with permission.

RATE	NUMERATOR	DENOMINATOR	TIME	HOW MEASURED
Incidence	New cases occurring during the follow-up period in a group initially free of the disease	All susceptible individuals present at the beginning of the follow-up period (often called the population at risk)	Duration of the follow-up period	Cohort study
Prevalence	All cases counted in a single survey or examination of a group	All individuals examined, including cases and noncases	Single point in time	Prevalence or cross-sectional study

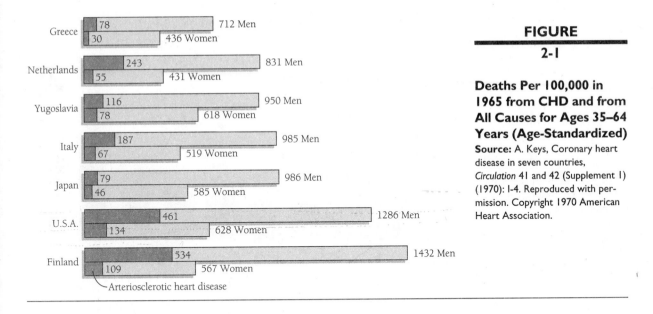

FIGURE

2-1

Deaths Per 100,000 in 1965 from CHD and from All Causes for Ages 35–64 Years (Age-Standardized)
Source: A. Keys, Coronary heart disease in seven countries, *Circulation* 41 and 42 (Supplement 1) (1970): I-4. Reproduced with permission. Copyright 1970 American Heart Association.

deaths attributable to CHD, which was (and remains) the leading cause of death in the U.S. population. Identifying the risk factors for CHD became a public health priority.

4. **Making comparisons.** One of the first large population studies to examine the relationship between blood cholesterol levels and risk of CHD was the Seven Countries Study.[8] This project was undertaken in the late 1950s to examine the effects of differences in lifestyle, culture, diet, and general health habits on risk factors such as serum cholesterol levels, morbidity, and mortality from CHD. Sixteen population groups, involving about 11,000 men aged 40 to 59 years, were studied in seven countries that had reliable census data and well-organized medical systems: Greece, the Netherlands, Yugoslavia, Italy, Japan, the United States, and Finland. The cohort of adult men was followed for 10 years. One of the main study findings, shown in Figure 2-2, was that the population risk of CHD death, after adjusting for age, rose in a stepwise manner with increasing total blood cholesterol levels.[9] In addition, an analysis of dietary intakes of the study population showed that the serum cholesterol level increased progressively as the level of saturated fat in the diet rose.

Figure 2-3 shows that Finland, with the highest reported intake of saturated fat (expressed as a percentage of total calories), had the highest mean population serum cholesterol level (about 260 mg/dL). (*Note:* The *"r"* value in the lower right-hand corner is the correlation coefficient. The correlation coefficient is a number between –1 and +1 that is used to quantify the strength of an association between two variables—in this case, dietary saturated fat and serum cholesterol level. The stronger the relationship of the two variables, the closer *r* is to 1; the weaker the relationship, the closer *r* is to 0. An *r* value of 0.89 means that while dietary saturated fat intake is

Cohort A group of people who have something in common.

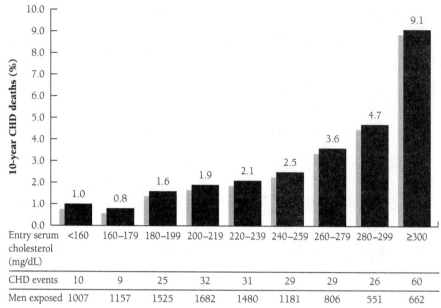

FIGURE
2-2

Total Blood Cholesterol and CHD Deaths in Men
(Note: A recent analysis of 30-year follow-up data revealed that longevity in men aged 50 years or more was not related to serum cholesterol in any of the cohorts.—Ancel Keys, personal communication)

Entry serum cholesterol (mg/dL)	<160	160–179	180–199	200–219	220–239	240–259	260–279	280–299	≥300
CHD events	10	9	25	32	31	29	29	26	60
Men exposed	1007	1157	1525	1682	1480	1181	806	551	662

Source: Reprinted by permission of the publishers from SEVEN COUNTRIES: A MULTIVARIATE ANALYSIS OF DEATH AND CORONARY HEART DISEASE by Ancel Keys, Cambridge, Mass.: Harvard University Press, Copyright © 1980 by the President and Fellows of Harvard College.

strongly correlated with serum cholesterol level, the relationship between the two variables isn't perfect due to measurement errors [e.g., in calculating the dietary intake of saturated fat or determining the serum cholesterol level] or other factors [e.g., genetic determinants].[10])

5. **Developing the hypothesis.** The results of animal studies and large-scale population studies such as the Seven Countries Study were used to formulate the hypothesis that a diet high in saturated fat increases blood cholesterol levels and contributes to the development of CHD.

6. **Testing the hypothesis.** Many different studies were undertaken to test this hypothesis. In one migration study, groups of Japanese living in Japan were compared with groups of Japanese who were originally from the same regions in Japan but who had emigrated to Hawaii or California.[11] The study design used standardized protocols for measuring blood cholesterol and the number of existing and new cases of CHD. It showed that the saturated fat intake as a percentage of total calories in the three populations varied widely, with Japanese living in Japan having a saturated fat intake of 7 percent of total calories and Japanese living in California having an intake of 26 percent. (The value for Japanese living in Hawaii was 23 percent.) Japanese living in Japan had the lowest blood cholesterol level, followed by those living in Hawaii; Japanese living in California had the highest blood cholesterol level. These differences in blood cholesterol paralleled the rates for CHD, suggesting that changes in diet after migra-

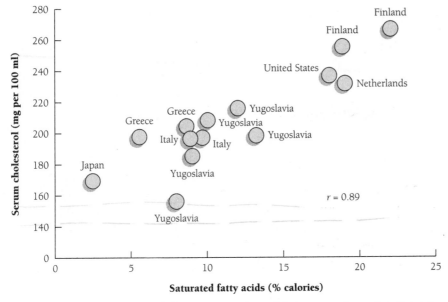

FIGURE

2-3

Median Serum Cholesterol Values of the Seven Countries Cohort Plotted Versus the Percentage of Total Calories from Saturated Fat

Source: Adapted from A. Keys, Coronary heart disease in seven countries, *Circulation* 41 and 42 (Supplement 1) (1970): I–170. Reproduced with permission. Copyright 1970 American Heart Association.

The Seven Countries cohort was drawn from the following regions and cities: Finland = east, west; Greece = Crete, Corfu; Italy = Crevalcore, Montegiorgio; Japan = Tanushimaru; Netherlands = Zutphen; U.S.A. = U.S. railroad; Yugoslavia = Belgrade, Dalmatia, Slavonia, Velika Krsna, Zrenjanin.

tion were partly responsible for the differences in blood cholesterol levels and the incidence of CHD.

Other population studies, such as the Western Electric Study[12] and the Puerto Rico Heart Health Program,[13] helped confirm the relationship of diet to blood cholesterol levels and CHD risk.

7. **Drawing scientific inferences.** The results of these and other large-scale population studies provided convincing evidence that the rates of CHD differ among populations and that these differences are due partly to environmental (diet) factors. However, the data have not been entirely consistent. The famous Ireland-Boston brothers study provided only weak support for the diet-heart hypothesis. This study did not find significant differences in CHD mortality between Irish brothers who were born and remained in Ireland and those who, although born in Ireland, had lived in Boston for at least 10 years. It did, however, underscore the increased risk of death from CHD among study subjects consuming a diet high in fat. Plus, it found that the consumption of a high-fiber, vegetable-rich diet decreased the risk of CHD death.[14]

It is unrealistic to expect total agreement among the results of epidemiologic or clinical studies. Many genetic, environmental, social, and experimental factors affect a study's outcome. On balance, however, many studies conducted over the last three decades have strengthened the diet–blood cholesterol–CHD link.

8. **Conducting experimental studies.** Studies with rabbits, pigs, and nonhuman primates showed that these species are susceptible to diet-induced

hypercholesterolemia. In addition, the blood cholesterol levels of some laboratory animals were affected by the type of fatty acids in the diet. In primates, for example, blood cholesterol levels rose when a diet rich in cholesterol and saturated fatty acids was consumed; a diet rich in polyunsaturated fatty acids lowered them.[15] Animal studies provided compelling support for a role of dietary fat and cholesterol in the atherogenic process.

9. **Intervening and evaluating.** One of the most ambitious interventions undertaken to modify CHD risk factors was the Multiple Risk Factor Intervention Trial (MRFIT), commonly called Mister Fit. This six-year clinical trial was directed toward the primary prevention of CHD among middle-aged men determined to be at high risk for CHD because they had hypertension or high blood cholesterol or smoked cigarettes. The 12,866 eligible men were randomly assigned to a special intervention group or a usual care group. Men in the special intervention group received extensive nutrition counseling to help them make dietary changes to reduce their fat and cholesterol intake. Participants in the special intervention group who smoked received counseling to help them stop smoking.[16] Although the mean reduction in blood cholesterol in the intervention group was less than the predicted response, MRFIT showed that serum cholesterol reductions and dietary changes could be sustained over a period of several years.[17]

The mounting experimental (animal) and epidemiologic evidence supporting the diet-heart hypothesis led to the formulation of dietary advice designed to reduce CHD risk in the general population. Voluntary and nonprofit health agencies, such as the American Heart Association[18] and the American Medical Association,[19] published statements for health professionals describing the known risk factors for CHD and strategies for reducing CHD risk. These were followed by the report of the National Cholesterol Education Program on the detection, evaluation, and treatment of high blood cholesterol in adults.[20] The science supporting the diet-heart link was eventually incorporated into the Dietary Guidelines for Americans, which advised the public to "choose a diet low in fat,

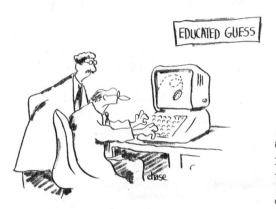

EDUCATED GUESS

Cartoon by John Chase.

saturated fat and cholesterol" as a means of reducing the risk of chronic disease and improving health.[21]

◆ HYPOTHESIS TESTING

Another precept of the epidemiologic method is hypothesis testing. Its importance to the experimental process cannot be understated. In planning an experimental trial, the investigator identifies a cause-effect comparison to be tested as the research hypothesis. A study might be designed to determine whether a vaccine for hepatitis A is effective among children or whether a protein in cow's milk is responsible for triggering insulin-dependent diabetes mellitus. In a community-based nutrition study, one hypothesis might be stated thus: There will be a significant decrease in the calories from fat and an increase in the grams of fiber consumed by employees in the eight intervention worksites receiving nutrition programming compared with employees in the eight control worksites.[22]

Once the specific research question (hypothesis) has been formulated, the investigators design a study to obtain information that will enable them to make inferences about the original hypothesis. In some epidemiologic studies, however, not all hypotheses are specified at the beginning. Rather, one or more hypotheses are generated retrospectively, after the research data have been collected and analyzed. The temptation to do this is compelling. A typical epidemiologic study produces reams of data about individuals (age, sex, race, educational level, occupation), specific agents (diet, vitamins, tobacco, alcohol, drugs, pesticides), and outcomes (death, heart attack, colon cancer, impairment of renal function). When the data are downloaded into a computer for statistical analysis, the investigator may consider rummaging among the data, searching for statistical associations among various groups that may suggest a cause-effect relationship. This activity, sometimes called "data dredging," is worth avoiding. The statement of a clear, precise hypothesis (or hypotheses) at the study outset ensures that the appropriate data are collected to answer the research question(s) and avoids the pitfall of drawing spurious conclusions from the data set.[23]

◆ EXPLAINING RESEARCH OBSERVATIONS

An important aspect of the epidemiologic method—and, indeed, of the scientific method in general—is determining whether the data are valid. That is, do the data represent the true state of affairs or are they distorted in some fashion? Research data can have three possible explanations, as shown in Table 2-2. Consider the following research project:

> A study was designed to determine whether a worksite-sponsored exercise program resulted in a lower percentage of body fat and lower blood lipids among overweight adults. Employees in two companies were invited to enroll in the three-month program. Those who agreed to participate underwent several clinical measurements at the beginning and end of the study: height, weight, skinfolds, and total blood cholesterol. The 156 employees who participated in the exercise program showed a reduction in percentage of body fat and total blood cholesterol compared with 210 adults who did not participate.

TABLE

2-2

Possible Explanations for Research Observations
Source: R. H. Fletcher, S. W. Fletcher, and E. H. Wagner, *Clinical Epidemiology—The Essentials*, p. 6. © WILLIAMS & WILKINS 1982. Used with permission.

Bias	The observation is incorrect because a systematic error was introduced by:
	◆ Selection bias—the method by which patients or study subjects were selected for observation
	◆ Measurement bias—the method by which the observation or measurement was made
	◆ Confounding bias—the presence of another variable that accounts for the observation
Chance	The observation is incorrect because of error arising from random variation.
Truth	The observation is correct. This explanation should be accepted only after the others have been excluded.

One explanation for these results is that the data are incorrect because they are biased; in other words, a systematic error was made in measuring one or more outcome variables, or there were systematic differences in the populations studied. Although there are probably dozens of possible biases, most fall into one of the three categories listed in Table 2-2. More than one bias may operate at one time. In the study just described, *selection bias* may have occurred because the study participants were self-selected, meaning that employees who were interested in improving their fitness level or losing weight were more inclined to join the program than those who were not. *Measurement bias* may have occurred if the technician responsible for obtaining skinfold measurements was an enthusiastic supporter of vigorous exercise and took more pains to make careful measurements in the exercising adults than in the sedentary adults. Finally, *confounding bias* may have existed in focusing on exercise as a sole determinant of changes in total blood cholesterol and body fat. It is possible that employees entering the exercise program made significant, but unconscious, alterations in their eating patterns that contributed to the changes in blood lipids and body composition. Thus, the presence of (unmeasured or unidentified) confounding factors may have influenced the study outcome.

Another explanation for the study results is that they are due simply to chance and do not represent the true state of affairs; that is, the observations made on these employees arose from random variation within the sample. Many factors could have contributed to the differences between the groups, including the manner in which the clinical or laboratory measurements were made or differences in the makeup of the workforce (e.g., a manufacturing plant versus a company that develops computer software programs). Random variation cannot be totally eliminated and usually occurs in tandem with some form of bias. The influence of these two sources of error can be reduced by careful study design and statistical analysis.

The final explanation for the study results is that they represent the truth: Participating in an exercise program resulted in reductions in body fat and total blood cholesterol among employees in these two companies. To say that the data are valid, then, means that they are neither biased nor incorrect due to chance and that they represent the true state of affairs regarding the physiologic effects of exercise.

Nutritional Epidemiology

The epidemiologic method lends itself to the study of the relationship of diet to health and disease. Historically, one of the first applications of epidemiology to nutrition science was James Lind's controlled trial investigating the curative effects of citrus fruits among sailors with scurvy.[24] Like Snow's proposed intervention to control cholera epidemics, Lind's suggestion that sea vessels carry a supply of limes, oranges, and other citrus fruits to prevent scurvy came 150 years before researchers proved in the laboratory that scurvy results from a dietary deficiency.[25] Similar investigations into the health effects of vitamin C and the other 40-odd essential nutrients are being conducted today.

Epidemiology has other applications in the nutrition arena. It can be used to describe the nutrition status of populations or specific subgroups of a population. The information obtained from large population surveys is then used to develop specific programs and services for groups whose nutrition status appears to be compromised. Furthermore, the epidemiologic method can be used to evaluate nutrition interventions. This usually involves monitoring the nutrition and health status of a high-risk group of individuals for a period of several months or even years.

Nutritional epidemiology is a fairly new area of study. Whereas its focus was once the deficiency diseases such as scurvy, beriberi, and rickets, today it is primarily concerned with the major, chronic diseases of the so-called Western world. Unlike nutritional deficiency states, chronic diseases tend to have many, sometimes interrelated, causes. One challenge to the study of the relationship of diet to disease is the complexity of our diets.

◆ THE NATURE OF DIETARY VARIATION

The foods we consume each day are complex mixtures of chemicals, some of which are known to be important to human health while others have not even been identified or measured. The chemicals found in or on foods include essential nutrients, structural compounds (e.g., cellulose), additives, microbes, pesticides, inorganic compounds such as heavy metals, natural toxins (e.g., nicotine), and other natural compounds such as DNA and RNA. The sheer diversity of the chemicals found in foodstuffs creates problems for investigators studying the relationship of diet to disease processes. When assessing the relationship of vitamin A intake to the development of lung cancer, for example, the population's intake of compounds with vitamin A activity—i.e., preformed vitamin A (retinol), retinal, retinoic acid, and the carotenoids—must be calculated. And not only must the intake of these compounds from foods be considered, but also the intake from vitamin supplements and other sources if they exist. In addition, for most epidemiologic investigations, it is the long-term dietary intake of foodstuffs that is important. In the case of a disease like lung cancer, which may take 10 to 20 years to develop, the lifelong intake of vitamin A must be estimated.

Another difficulty is that people don't eat the same foods every day. Work and school schedules, illnesses, holidays, the seasons of the year, weekends, personal preferences, availability of foods, social and cultural norms, and numerous other factors influence our daily food choices. As a result, our nutrient intake varies from day to day. The magnitude of the variation differs according to the nutrient.[26] Scientists with the Human Nutrition Information Service of the U.S. Department of Agriculture conducted a study to determine the number of days of food intake records needed to estimate the "true" average nutrient intake of a small number of adults.[27] The 29 men and women participating in the study completed detailed food records for 365 consecutive days. The ranges and average number of days of food records required to estimate the "true" average intake for individuals are shown in Table 2-3. Note the gender differences in the average values. For example, more food records were required to estimate the true average intake of calories by women than men. Note, too, that there were differences between nutrients. Compare the average values for calories with those for vitamins A and C, sodium, and fat. Finally, note the wide ranges in food records required to estimate true intakes. To estimate vitamin A intake, some men needed to complete 115 food records, while others required 1724 days or nearly five years! As these data demonstrate, a relatively large number of days of food intake records are required to achieve a certain level of statistical significance *for an individual.* If the individual data are combined into groups, however, fewer days of food intake records are required, as shown in Table 2-4.

The day-to-day variation in an individual's nutrient intake (called within-person variation) has important implications for nutritional epidemiologic studies. If only one day's intake is determined, then the true long-term nutrient intake may be misrepresented, and, for example, an individual whose vitamin C

TABLE 2-3	Ranges and Average Number of Days Required to Estimate the True Average Intake* for an Individual					
	RANGE AND AVERAGE NUMBER OF DAYS REQUIRED					
	Males (*n* = 13)			Females (*n* = 16)		
COMPONENT	*Minimum*	*Average*	*Maximum*	*Minimum*	*Average*	*Maximum*
Food energy	14	27	84	14	35	60
Protein	23	36	72	23	48	70
Fat	34	57	131	32	71	114
Carbohydrate	10	37	177	16	41	77
Iron	18	68	130	28	66	142
Calcium	30	74	140	35	88	168
Sodium	27	58	140	36	73	116
Vitamin A	115	390	1724	152	474	1372
Vitamin C	90	249	900	83	222	328
Niacin	27	53	89	48	78	126

*The "true" average intake was defined as the 365-day average for individuals.

Source: P. P. Basiotis and coauthors, Number of days of food intake records required to estimate individual and group nutrient intakes with defined confidence. © J. Nutr.: (Vol. 117, p. 1640), American Institute of Nutrition.

TABLE

2-4

Number of Days Required to Estimate the True Average Intake* for Groups of Individuals
Source: P. P. Basiotis and coauthors, Number of days of food intake records required to estimate individual and group nutrient intakes with defined confidence. © J. Nutr.: (Vol. 117, p. 1641), American Institute of Nutrition.

COMPONENT	ESTIMATED NUMBER OF DAYS REQUIRED FOR EACH GROUP	
	Males (n =13)	Females (n = 16)
Food energy	3	3
Protein	4	4
Fat	6	6
Carbohydrate	5	4
Iron	7	6
Calcium	10	7
Sodium	6	6
Vitamin A	39	44
Vitamin C	33	19
Niacin	5	6

*The "true" average intake was defined as the 365-day average for groups of individuals.

intake over a period of several days is in fact adequate may be classified as having a low vitamin C intake. The effects of within-person variation on dietary intake must be considered when designing and evaluating studies of the relationship of diet to disease.

◆ TYPES OF NUTRITIONAL EPIDEMIOLOGIC STUDIES

When a nutritional problem is suspected, an investigation is undertaken "to find out something." The hypothesis to be tested is defined, the population to be studied is selected, measurements are taken or cases are counted, and the data are analyzed to determine whether the established facts support the hypothesis. The type of investigation undertaken depends to a large extent on the research question being asked and the type of data needed to answer the question. The major types of nutritional epidemiological studies are described below.[28]

1. **Ecological or correlational studies.** Ecological or correlational studies compare the frequency of events (or disease rates) in different populations with the per capita consumption of certain dietary factors (e.g., saturated fat, total fat, beta-carotene). The dietary data collected in this type of study are usually _disappearance data_, that is, the national figures for food produced for human consumption minus the food that is exported, fed to animals, wasted, or otherwise not available for human consumption.

   An example of an ecological study is the investigation of the correlation between fish consumption and breast cancer incidence and mortality rates in humans.[29] In this study, incidence and mortality rates were derived from the cancer registries of various countries. Food consumption for each country was estimated from food availability data averaged over three years (1972–1974). Although there were some exceptions, as Figure 2-4 shows, the risk for breast cancer tended to be high in countries where the relative proportion of calories derived from fish was low and the con-

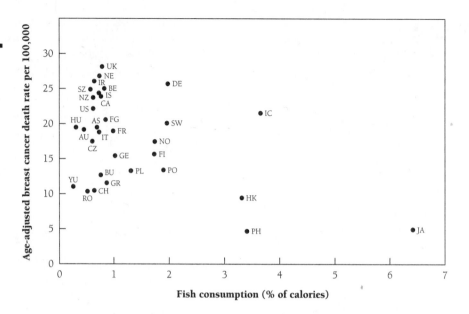

FIGURE 2-4

Breast Cancer Death Rate (Per 100,000) Plotted Versus Fish Consumption (Percentage of Caloric Intake)

Source: From "Fish Consumption and Breast Cancer Risk: An Ecological Study" by L. Kaizer, N. F. Boyd, V. Kriukov, and D. Tritchler, 1989, <u>Nutrition and Cancer, 12</u>, p. 63. Copyright 1989 by Lawrence Erlbaum Associates, Inc. Reprinted with permission.

Points include Australia (AS), Austria (AU), Belgium (BE), Bulgaria (BU), Canada (CA), Chile (CH), Czechoslovakia (CZ), Denmark (DE), Federal Republic of Germany (FG), Finland (FI), France (FR), German Democratic Republic (GE), Greece (GR), Hong Kong (HK), Hungary (HU), Iceland (IC), Ireland (IR), Israel (IS), Italy (IT), Japan (JA), Netherlands (NE), Norway (NO), New Zealand (NZ), Phillipines (PH), Poland (PL), Portugal (PO), Romania (RO), Sweden (SW), Switzerland (SZ), United Kingdom (UK), United States (US), Yugoslavia (YU).

sumption of animal fat was high, such as the United States, Canada, and Switzerland. In countries where fish was consumed frequently and the animal fat intake was low, such as Japan, the breast cancer death rate was low.

Do these results mean that diets high in animal fat *cause* breast cancer, while diets high in fish protect against cancer? No, the data from an ecological study cannot be used to draw conclusions about the role of foods or nutrients in the development of cancer (or other diseases). Why not? One reason is that the dietary data obtained in such a study are based on population food disappearance data and are therefore not particularly specific. Ecological studies can be used, however, to generate hypotheses about the relationship of dietary components to the disease process, which can then be tested with a more rigorous study design.

2. **Cross-sectional or prevalence studies.** Cross-sectional or prevalence studies examine the relationships among dietary intake, diseases, and other variables as they exist in a population at a particular time. This type of study is much like a camera snapshot. It gives a picture of what is happening within a particular population at a specific time.

An example of a cross-sectional study is the investigation of nutrient intakes and growth of predominantly breast-fed infants living in Capulhuac, Mexico, a farming community of about 5500 Otomi Indians. A representative sample of four- to six-month-old infants, together with their mothers, were enrolled in the study. The infants' weight, length, and intake of human breast milk were measured, and information about their health and morbidity (e.g., diarrhea or respiratory illness) was recorded. The study found that despite having milk intakes similar to or greater than those of infants from privileged populations (e.g., infants living in Houston, Texas), the nutrient intake from breast milk among the Otomi infants was not sufficient for normal growth. Growth faltering was evident by six months of age in this population.[30]

3. **Cohort or incidence studies.** Whereas cross-sectional studies are like a snapshot, cohort or incidence studies are like moving pictures of events occurring within populations. In these studies, a group of people free of the disease or condition of interest is identified and examined. This group is called the *cohort.* The members of the cohort are followed for months or even years, during which time they are examined periodically to determine which individuals develop the characteristics of interest and which do not. Cohort studies may look back in time to reconstruct exposures and health outcomes; such studies are called *retrospective cohort studies.* Those that follow a group into the future are called *prospective cohort studies.* Consult Table 2-5 for a list of the advantages and disadvantages of this type of study.

An example of a cohort study (in this case a prospective study) is the Framingham Heart Study, which was begun in 1949 in Framingham, Massachusetts. This study was undertaken to identify the factors associated with increased risk of coronary heart disease. A representative sample of 5209 men and women, 30 to 59 years of age, was selected from the

COHORT STUDIES	CASE-CONTROL STUDIES
Advantages	*Advantages*
Provides complete data on cases, stages	Excellent way to study rare diseases and diseases with long latency periods
Allows study of more than one effect of exposure	Relatively quick
Can calculate and compare rates in exposed and unexposed	Relatively inexpensive
Choice of factors available for study	Requires relatively few study subjects
Quality control of data	Can often use existing records
	Can study many possible causes of disease
Disadvantages	*Disadvantages*
Need to study large numbers	Relies on recall or existing records about past exposures
May take many years	Difficult or impossible to validate data
Circumstances may change during study	Control of extraneous factors incomplete
Expensive	Difficult to select suitable comparison group
Control of extraneous factors may be incomplete	Cannot calculate rates
Rarely possible to study mechanism of disease	Cannot study mechanism of disease

TABLE

2-5

Advantages and Disadvantages of Cohort and Case-Control Studies

Source: Adapted, with permission, from C. W. Tyler, Jr., and J. M. Last, Epidemiology, in *Maxcy-Rosenau-Last Public Health & Preventive Medicine,* 13th ed., ed. J. M. Last and R. B. Wallace (Norwalk, Conn.: Appleton & Lange, 1992), p. 25.

10,000 or so residents of that age group living in the Framingham community. Of these, 5127 were free of CHD when they were first examined. The cohort underwent complete physical examinations every two years for more than 30 years. The study has shown that the risk of developing CHD is associated with cigarette smoking, serum cholesterol, glucose intolerance, and blood pressure.[31] An analysis of the cohort's high-density lipoprotein cholesterol (HDL-C) levels taken over a period of 12 years revealed that HDL-C is a consistent predictor of CHD risk in both men and women. Individuals with a high HDL-C level (>60 mg/dL) had a low risk of CHD, regardless of their total cholesterol level, as shown in Figure 2-5.[32] Note that individuals with a low total blood cholesterol level (<200 mg/dL) had a high risk of CHD if their HDL-C levels were also low (<40 mg/dL). Thus, in the words of the investigators, "a low total cholesterol level per se does not necessarily indicate a low risk of developing CHD."

4. **Case-control studies.** In a case-control study, a group of persons or cases with the disease or condition of interest are compared with a group of persons without the disease or condition. Case-control studies are useful when a rare condition is being studied (see Table 2-5).

   One of the most thorough case-control studies of diet and cancer was a Canadian study published in 1978.[33] In this study, the diets of 400 Canadian women with breast cancer were compared with 400 women from similar neighborhoods who did not have breast cancer (the latter were called "neighborhood controls"). The investigators used three types of diet assessment techniques: the 24-hour recall, a four-day dietary record, and a diet history questionnaire. (These diet assessment methods are discussed in greater detail in the next section.) The investigators found that only the intake of total calories differed between cases and controls when the diet was analyzed by the 24-hour recall method. There were no differences in the intakes of total fat and saturated fat between cases and controls as a function of type of diet assessment method. This study did not support the hypothesis that fat composition of the diet is associated with the incidence of breast cancer. The investigators concluded that all three diet assessment methods may have been imperfect measures of dietary intake of fat.

5. **Controlled trials.** The randomized trial conducted as a double-blind experiment is the most rigorous evaluation of a dietary hypothesis. The primary drawback of the controlled trial is its expense. The MRFIT study cited earlier is an example of a controlled, clinical trial.

◆ DIET ASSESSMENT METHODS

A variety of methods are available for estimating dietary intake: food consumption survey, diet history, 24-hour recall, food record, and food frequency questionnaire. The method chosen for a particular research study or program evaluation depends on many factors, as shown in Table 2-6. None of the methods is perfect. All have strong and weak points, advantages and disadvantages. The trick

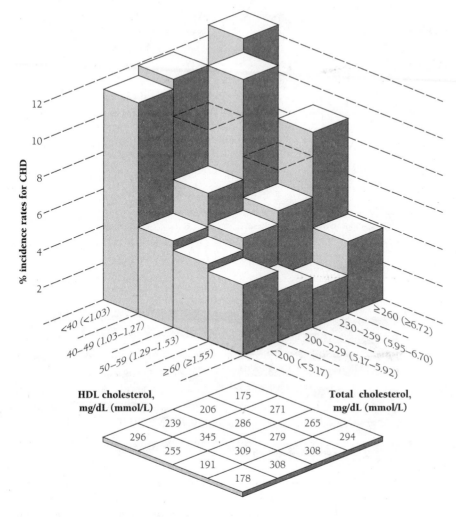

FIGURE

2-5

Incidence of CHD by High-Density Lipoprotein Cholesterol and Total Plasma Cholesterol Level for Men and Women Free of Cardiovascular Disease

Source: W. P. Castelli and coauthors, Incidence of coronary heart disease and lipoprotein cholesterol levels: The Framingham Study, *Journal of the American Medical Association* 256 (1986): 2835–38.

Dashed lines indicate two bars that are hidden from view: HDL–C less than 40 mg/dL (<1.03 mmol/L), total cholesterol 230 to 259 mg/dL (5.95 to 6.70 mmol/L), rate = 10.7%; HDL–C 40 to 49 mg/dL (1.03 to 1.27 mmol/L), total cholesterol greater than or equal to 260 mg/dL (6.72 mmol/L), rate = 6.6%. Diagram at bottom shows number of observations from combined sample that fell into each cell and were therefore at risk for CHD.

is to choose the most valid method, given the financial resources and personnel available to collect and analyze the dietary intake information.[34]

Two questions arise when evaluating diet assessment methods: one concerns the dietary instrument's validity, and the other its reliability or reproducibility. **Validity** refers to the ability of a diet assessment instrument to measure what it is intended to measure; that is, a valid instrument accurately measures an individual's usual or customary dietary intake over a period of time—one day, three days, seven days, one month, one year. An instrument's validity can be affected by many factors, as shown in the list that follows.[35]

Validity The accuracy of the diet assessment instrument.

TABLE

2-6

Criteria for Selecting a Dietary Intake Method

Source: J. M. Karkeck: Improving the use of dietary survey methodology. Copyright The American Dietetic Association. Reprinted by permission from JOURNAL OF THE AMERICAN DIETETIC ASSOCIATION, Vol. 87: 1987, p. 870.

Research or program objectives:

◆ Degree of accuracy needed

◆ Type of data needed—i.e., food intake, specific nutrient intake, dietary pattern, food pattern

Study population:

◆ Sample size

◆ Cooperation and ability of subjects

◆ Constraints on time

Expertise available:

◆ Skill of the interviewer

◆ Skill of the food coder

Resources available:

◆ Financial constraints

◆ Adequacy of the nutrient database

◆ Characteristics of the respondent—literacy level, education level, conscientiousness in completing the instrument, ability to follow instructions

◆ Questionnaire design—difficulty of instructions, ease of recording intake, number and type of foods listed, portion sizes given (if any)

◆ Adequacy of reference data—a sufficient number of days of intake data were obtained to estimate the "true" nutrient intake, completeness of the nutrient database used to calculate nutrient intake

◆ Accuracy of data input and management—quality control of keypunching or coding of food items

An individual's true usual diet cannot be known with certainty. It is not possible to follow respondents around all day and night and surreptitiously record every morsel they consume. And the very act of recording food intake can have a subtle influence, as the respondents may make choices they might not have made otherwise. (Although people's food and beverage intake can be monitored with precision on a metabolic ward, their dietary intake cannot be considered "usual" under these circumstances.) Attention to an instrument's validity ensures that respondents can be placed with a high degree of accuracy along a distribution of intake, from low to high consumption.

Reliability The repeatability or precision of the diet assessment instrument.

The second concern is the **reliability** or **reproducibility** of a diet assessment instrument, that is, its ability to produce the same estimate of dietary intake on two separate occasions, assuming the diet did not change in the interim. This issue is different from validity. It is possible for an instrument to give reproducible results that are also incorrect! An instrument's reliability can be affected by the respondents' ability to estimate their dietary intake reliably, by real dietary changes that occurred between the two assessment periods, and by inaccuracies in coding diet data.

Several methods are available for assessing dietary intake. Some of these are described on the following pages.

◆ **Food consumption at the national level.** The primary method of assessing the available food supply at the national level is based on **food balance sheets.** Food balance sheets do not measure the food actually ingested by a population. Rather they measure the food *available* for consumption from imports and domestic food production, less the food "lost" through exports, waste, or spoilage, on a per capita basis. The per capita figures are obtained from the population estimate for the country.

Food balance sheets National accounts of the annual production of food, changes in stocks, imports, and exports, and distribution of food over various uses within the country.

Food balance sheets tend to be affected by errors that arise in calculating production, waste, and consumption. Hence, they are not used to describe the nutritional inadequacies of countries. They can be used to formulate agricultural policies concerned with food production and consumption.[36]

◆ **Food consumption at the household level.** Methods of assessing **household food consumption** consider the per capita food consumption of the household, taking into account the age and sex of persons in the household (or institution), the number of meals eaten at home or away from home, income, shopping practices, and other factors. In most cases, no record is made of food obtained outside the household food supply or of food wasted, spoiled, or fed to pets. An exception is the U.S. Nationwide Food Consumption Survey (NFCS), where a trained interviewer asks the householder to use the *list-recall method* to recall all foods used from the home food supplies during the preceding seven days, including all food that has been eaten, discarded, and fed to pets.

Household food consumption The total amount of food available for consumption in the household, generally excluding food eaten away from home unless taken from home.

◆ **Food consumption by individuals.**

1. **Diet history method.** One of the earliest descriptions of diet analysis was reported by Bertha Burke with the Department of Child Hygiene of the Harvard School of Public Health. In studies of pregnant women and their infants and children, conducted during the 1930s, Burke and her colleagues developed a diet history questionnaire to assess usual dietary intake. Their studies showed statistically significant relationships between a mother's diet during pregnancy and the condition of her infant at birth. In addition, there was a correlation between the dietary ratings of the childrens' diets and objective measures of nutrition status, such as hemoglobin value.[37]

The diet history method has the advantage of being easy to administer, although it is time-consuming and requires a trained interviewer. For these reasons, it is not practical for large population studies. A true validation of the diet history method is probably not possible, although the method allows for reasonable confidence in classifying respondents according to some preset dietary criteria (e.g., the Recommended Dietary Allowances) or physiologic criteria (e.g., serum transferrin).[38] When undertaken repeatedly at different times, this method is fairly reliable. It is perhaps best used to provide qualitative, not quantitative, data.

2. **24-hour recall method.** The 24-hour recall method is one of the most widely used diet assessment methods. It is easy to administer, can be administered in person or by phone, and lends itself to large popula-

tion studies, mainly because it requires very little time from either the respondent or the interviewer. Its validity for assessing the intake of individuals has repeatedly been questioned, however.[39] There are indications that 24-hour recall data are subject to recall bias; that is, respondents cannot accurately recall the foods they ate during the previous 24-hour period and either over- or underestimate their dietary intakes. Gender differences in recalling dietary intakes have also been reported. Thus, a single 24-hour recall does not provide an accurate estimate of an individual's usual dietary intake.

The validity of 24-hour recall data can be improved by administering repeated recalls. Seven or eight 24-hour recalls of an individual's dietary intake over a period of two or three weeks are more likely to provide a reasonable estimate of that person's usual intake than a single recall. Even so, 24-hour recall data are best suited to describing the intakes of populations, not individuals.[40]

3. **Diet record method.** Diet records or food records have been considered the "gold standard" of diet assessment methods. Completed over a period of three, four, or seven days, or even as long as one year, they have the advantage of providing detailed information about food products, including brand names, and methods of food preparation, and they eliminate the uncertainty that goes with trying to recall the foods eaten. The amount of food consumed can be estimated or calculated by weighing. If the respondents are properly trained, diet records give a reasonably accurate picture of usual dietary intake. However, the diet record method replaces errors in recall with errors in recording, and the possibility always exists that the act of recording food intake changes the actual foods chosen for recording. Accurate food records can be obtained if the respondents are highly motivated, literate, and well trained.

4. **Food frequency method.** One of the first large-scale uses of the food frequency questionnaire was in the Nurses' Health Study, a study of a cohort of more than 95,000 female registered nurses being followed for the occurrence of CHD and cancer. A semiquantitative food frequency questionnaire was developed to categorize individuals by their intake of selected nutrients (e.g., vitamin A, vitamin C, animal fat). The validity and reproducibility of this instrument were evaluated using four sets of seven-day food records and a one-year diet record.[41]

The food frequency questionnaire offers several advantages: it is self-administered, requires only about 15 to 30 minutes to complete, and can be analyzed at a reasonable cost. Thus, it has been used in a variety of population studies where no other instrument could have been administered practically. It suffers, however, from the same limitations as any other recall method, in that the accurate reporting of intake depends on memory. In addition, the food list must necessarily be limited in scope and thus may overlook some foods commonly consumed by the population being surveyed. Controversy over the appropriate uses of the food frequency questionnaire continues.[42]

5. **Other diet assessment methods.** One recent innovation in the diet assessment arena is the use of photography to record and verify dietary intake. Food image processing reportedly has provided valid and reproducible results compared with food records. Telephone surveys of dietary intake have also been used to estimate dietary intake.[43]

Epidemiology and the Community Nutritionist

The science of epidemiology may seem far removed from the job responsibilities of the community nutritionist, but, in fact, it is absolutely essential to the delivery of effective nutrition programs and services. Recall from Chapter 1 that the key roles of the community nutritionist include *identifying* nutritional problems within the community and *interpreting* the scientific literature—especially experimental, clinical, and epidemiologic nutrition research findings—for the public and other health professionals. The community nutritionist must be able to critically evaluate the scientific literature before formulating new nutrition policies or altering eating pattern messages.

How is this accomplished, considering the magnitude of the research findings published and the complexity of the diet-disease relationship? As the criteria in Table 2-7 indicate, it helps to consider certain elements in judging the strength of epidemiologic associations. Interpreting epidemiologic data basically

Chronological Relationship	Exposure to the causative factor must occur before the onset of the disease.
Strength of Association	The association is strong if all those with a health problem have been exposed to the agent believed to be associated with this problem and only a few in the comparison group have been so exposed.
Intensity or Duration of Exposure	The association is likely to be causal if those with the most intense, or longest, exposure to the agent have the greatest frequency or severity of illness, while those with less exposure are not as ill. This is also referred to as a dose-response relationship.
Specificity of Association	The likelihood of a causal association is increased if an agent, or risk factor, can be isolated from others and shown to produce changes in the frequency of occurrence or severity of the disease.
Consistency of Findings	An association is consistent if it is confirmed by different investigators, in different populations, or using different methods of study.
Coherent and Plausible Findings	This criterion is met when a plausible relationship between the biological and behavioral factors related to the association support a causal hypothesis. Evidence from experimental animals and information from other experimental systems and forms of observation are among the kinds of evidence to be considered.

TABLE

2-7

Criteria for Evaluating the Strength of the Association between Variables or Outcomes
Source: Adapted, with permission, from C. W. Tyler, Jr., and J. M. Last, Epidemiology, in *Maxcy-Rosenau-Last Public Health & Preventive Medicine,* 13th ed., ed. J. M. Last and R. B. Wallace (Norwalk, Conn.: Appleton & Lange, 1992), p. 33.

involves two steps: (1) evaluate the criterion for a causal association carefully, and (2) assess the causal association critically for the presence of bias and the contribution of chance. Competence in this area is achieved to some degree by experience and dogged determination. The Professional Focus at the end of this chapter describes some of the journals and newsletters that will be important to you as a community nutritionist and explains how you can critically analyze a study's results.

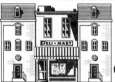 **COMMUNITY LEARNING ACTIVITY**

In Chapter 1's learning activity, you perused your local newspaper for articles on current health and nutrition issues, some of which may have dealt with local problems. As you probably realize, this is not the most precise way to obtain information about your community's health and nutritional problems. In this learning activity, you will become familiar with some of the surveillance data published by the Centers for Disease Control and Prevention and other groups that describe specific disease conditions in your county, state, and region.

To begin, locate the following publications in your school or local public library:

1. The *Morbidity and Mortality Weekly Report (MMWR)*. The MMWR reports case counts of diseases that are important nationally; aggregated case reports are compiled in tables for each state and a few other reporting areas.

2. If the MMWR itself is not available, check weekly issues of the *Journal of the American Medical Association,* which provide summaries of pertinent health data and disease conditions.

3. The *Monthly Vital Statistics Report,* published by the National Center for Health Statistics.

Examine the statistics published for your city or state over the last two years and then answer the following questions:

1. Which *five* conditions appear to be the leading health problems in your city (if available) or state?

2. Select *one* of these health conditions and describe its distribution in your community, including the population(s) most at risk. What are the primary host and environmental determinants of this problem? Do secondary determinants exist that could become important factors affecting the distribution of this problem at a later time?

3. What is the incidence rate of this condition? Is the incidence rate likely to change in the high-risk population? Why?

4. What is the prevalence rate of this condition? What does the prevalence rate tell you about the *future* cases of this health or nutritional problem?

◆ **PROFESSIONAL FOCUS**

The Well-Read Community Nutritionist

Here is a sobering statistic: More than 20,000 biomedical journals are published each month. If each journal published just 20 research articles, the conscientious community nutritionist would need to browse through 400,000 articles per month, or more than 13,000 articles per day, to stay abreast of current scientific findings! This figure doesn't even include editorials, review articles, and letters to the editor—all valuable reading. How can you, as a busy community nutritionist, handle this volume of information, keep informed, and maintain your sanity? While we don't have all the answers, we offer the following suggestions to help you cope with the onslaught of medical, health, and nutrition information. Let's begin with a few good reasons for reading the literature.

◆ TEN GOOD ARGUMENTS FOR READING JOURNALS

Consider the following 10 good reasons for reading journals regularly:[1]

1. To impress others
2. To keep abreast of professional news
3. To understand pathobiology
4. To find out how a seasoned health practitioner handles a particular problem
5. To find out whether to use a new or existing diagnostic test, survey instrument, or educational tool with your patients or clients
6. To learn the clinical features and course of a disorder
7. To determine etiology or causation
8. To distinguish useful from useless or even harmful therapy
9. To sort out claims concerning the need for and the use, quality, and cost-effectiveness of clinical and other health care
10. To be titillated by the letters to the editor

Regular reading of the literature, especially in your area of specialization, is a must. There is no other way to learn about the latest scientific findings, the merits of a particular intervention or assessment instrument, or current legislation and its potential impact upon your programs and clients. In short, to be an effective community nutritionist, you must constantly increase and update your knowledge base through regular perusal of journals, which brings us to our next question.

◆ WHICH JOURNALS SHOULD YOU READ?

There is no hard and fast rule about the "best" journals to read, since much depends on the type of work you are doing and the needs of your clients. Some journals will appear on your "must read regularly" list; others can be spot-checked every month or two. While nutrition journals will take priority, other speciality journals, particularly in the disciplines of epidemiology, health education, and medicine, are important. Check the boxed insert

Continued

◆ **PROFESSIONAL FOCUS**—*Continued*

Recommended Reading

Nutrition Journals

American Journal of Clinical Nutrition

British Journal of Nutrition

Human Nutrition: Applied Nutrition

Journal of the American College of Nutrition

Journal of the American Dietetic Association

Journal of the Canadian Dietetic Association

Journal of Nutrition

Journal of Nutrition Education

Nutrition Reviews

Nutrition Today

Nutrition Newsletters

Community Nutrition Institute's *Nutrition Week*

Dairy Council Digest

FDA Consumer

Harvard Health Letter

Nutrition Action

Nutrition and the M.D.

Ross Timesaver

Tufts University Diet & Nutrition Letter

University of California at Berkeley Wellness Letter

Speciality Journals

American Journal of Epidemiology

American Journal of Health Promotion

American Journal of Public Health

Family and Community Health

Health Education

Health Education Quarterly

Journal of the American Medical Association

Lancet

New England Journal of Medicine

Preventive Medicine

Continued

◆ PROFESSIONAL FOCUS—*Continued*

Recommended Reading
Public Health Reports
Science

Other Publications
American Council on Science and Health Reports
Science News

Anything You Can Get Your Hands On!

---

for a list of journals, newsletters, and other publications that will help you stay abreast of current developments that may be useful to you in delivering community programs.

◆ HOW TO GET THE MOST OUT OF A JOURNAL

There is no best way to "read" a journal. Although you will want to develop your own reading style, consider the following points. A glance at the table of contents will point you to pertinent research articles and briefs for in-depth reading. In journals that you subscribe to personally, highlight special-interest articles in the table of contents with a colored marking pen. (This simple act may make it easier for you to remember where you spotted that article on monounsaturated fat and non-insulin-dependent diabetes mellitus.)

After scanning the table of contents, check the professional updates and news features to keep informed about key players, committees, conferences, and events in your discipline. Consult review articles for extensive coverage of current issues. The journal's editorials will expose you to the controversies surrounding a study's findings or the implications of the findings for practitioners. Regular reading of the letters to the editor will help you appreciate the flaws in study designs and will expose you to the questions raised by scientists and practitioners in interpreting study results.

In choosing articles for in-depth reading, be selective and discriminating. You have only so much time. Select those articles that appear to be directly relevant to your needs, but allow time for other articles of interest. Refrain from beating yourself about the head because you don't have time to read as much as you think you should. Be organized and disciplined in your reading, but accept that no one can read everything.

◆ HOW TO TEASE APART AN ARTICLE

Most research articles have the same basic format with specific sections to help you assimilate the material:[2]

- ◆ **Abstract or summary.** Provides an overview of the study, highlights the results, and indicates the study's significance. It should contain a precise statement of the study's goal or purpose.

Continued

- ◆ **Introduction.** Presents background information such as the history of the problem or relevant clinical features. It reviews the work of other scientists in the area and describes the rationale for the study.

- ◆ **Methods.** Describes the study design, selection of subjects, methods of measurement (e.g., the diet assessment instrument used), specific hypotheses to be tested, and analytical techniques (e.g., the method used to measure blood cholesterol, method of statistical analysis).

- ◆ **Results.** Details the study's outcomes. The results are typically presented in tables, graphs, charts, and figures that help summarize the study's findings.

- ◆ **Discussion.** Provides an analysis of the meaning of the findings and compares the study's findings to those of other researchers. The discussion includes a critique of the work: What were the limitations of the study design? What problems occurred that may have affected the study outcome? What were the study's strengths?

- ◆ **Conclusions/implications.** Some, but not all, articles include a short section that summarizes the findings or considers how the study results can be applied in clinical practice; this section may also comment on directions for future research.

- ◆ **References/bibliography.** Cites the relevant work of other scientists that was considered in conducting the study or interpreting the results.

Reading an article involves more than simply scanning the abstract and flipping to the last paragraph of the discussion section for the authors' summary statements. If you have decided that the article is important to you, take time to read the methods section carefully, for the substance of the work is outlined here. Any new information presented in the article is only as good as the method by which it was obtained. Was the hypothesis clearly stated? Was the study design clearly described? Were the methods used appropriate for testing the hypothesis? How were the data collected and analyzed? Once you learn to critically review the methods section, you will find that in some cases you do not need to read further. The study was so poorly designed or seriously flawed that the results lack validity.

One other important precept remains. Learn to form your own opinions about the study findings presented in the articles you read. Do not automatically assume that the findings are valid merely because the study was published by a leading researcher or research team. Reading the letters to the editors and talking about the study results with your colleagues are good ways to help you assess the validity of a study.

◆ WHAT ELSE SHOULD YOU READ?

What else should you read to be an informed, effective community nutritionist? Everything! Well, everything you can get your hands on: newsletters, books, consumer magazines, food labels, newspapers, advertising, menus, junk mail.

Are we serious? Absolutely. We said at the outset (in Chapter 1) that one of your roles as a community nutritionist is to improve the nutrition and health of individuals living in communities. To do this well, you must be able to draw on many diverse elements within your community and culture to shape a program that meets a nutritional or health need. Let's say that you have been asked to design, implement, and evaluate a program to reduce the prevalence of obesity among schoolchildren in your community. To develop a

Continued

◆ PROFESSIONAL FOCUS—*Continued*

nutrition and fitness program that appeals to children, you must be able to speak their language and get inside *their* culture. Which reading material will help you find the right approach, the right colors, the right action figures, the right tone? Everything from the *Journal of the American Dietetic Association* to children's books, advertising inserts in your local newspaper, the newspaper comics, fast-food menus, T-shirt logos, a *Newsweek* article on latchkey children, a government publication on quick snack ideas—the list is endless. You never know when something you read in a totally unrelated area is the exact thing you need to help convey a nutrition message to your clients.

1. D. L. Sackett, How to read clinical journals. I. Why to read them and how to start reading them critically, *CMA Journal* 124 (1981): 555–58.
2. S. H. Gehlbach, *Interpreting the Medical Literature—A Clinician's Guide* (New York: Macmillan, 1982), pp. 1–15.

NOTES

1. V. Heiser, *An American Doctor's Odyssey* (New York: W. W. Norton, 1936), pp. 100–103.
2. The discussion of the uses and basic concepts of epidemiology were adapted from C.W. Tyler, Jr., and J. M. Last, Epidemiology, in *Public Health & Preventive Medicine,* 13th ed., ed. J. M. Last and R. B. Wallace (Norwalk, Conn.: Appleton & Lange, 1992), pp. 11–39.
3. R. I. Glass, New prospects for epidemiologic investigations, *Science* 234 (1986): 951–55.
4. G. P. Holmes and coauthors, Chronic fatigue syndrome: A working case definition, *Annals of Internal Medicine* 108 (1988): 387–89.
5. A. D. Langmuir, The territory of epidemiology: Pentimento, *Journal of Infectious Diseases* 155 (1987): 349–58.
6. The discussion of risk, risk factors, and the explanations for research results was adapted from R. H. Fletcher, S. W. Fletcher, and E. H. Wagner, *Clinical Epidemiology—The Essentials* (Baltimore: Williams & Wilkins, 1982).
7. U.S. Department of Health and Human Services, Public Health Service, *The Surgeon General's Report on Nutrition and Health* (Washington, D.C.: U.S. Government Printing Office, 1988), pp. 83–137.
8. A. Keys, Coronary heart disease in seven countries, *Circulation* 41 and 42 (Supplement 1) (1970): I-1–I-211.
9. National Cholesterol Education Program, *Report of the Expert Panel on Population Strategies for Blood Cholesterol Reduction* (Bethesda, Md.: National Institutes of Health, 1990), pp. 33–61.
10. S. A. Glantz, *Primer of Biostatistics,* 2d ed. (New York: McGraw-Hill, 1987), p. 221.
11. H. Kato and coauthors, Epidemiologic studies of coronary heart disease and stroke in Japanese men living in Japan, Hawaii, and California: Serum lipids and diet, *American Journal of Epidemiology* 97 (1973): 372–85.
12. R. B. Shekelle and coauthors, Diet, serum cholesterol, and death from coronary heart disease—the Western Electric study, *New England Journal of Medicine* 304 (1981): 65–70.
13. M. R. Garcia-Palmieri and coauthors, Relationship of dietary intake to subsequent coronary heart disease incidence: The Puerto Rico Heart Health Program, *American Journal of Clinical Nutrition* 33 (1980): 1818–27.
14. L. H. Kushi and coauthors, Diet and 20-year mortality from coronary heart disease—the Ireland-Boston Diet-Heart Study, *New England Journal of Medicine* 312 (1985): 811–18.
15. National Cholesterol Education Program, *Report of the Expert Panel.*
16. D. D. Gorder and coauthors, Dietary intake in the Multiple Risk Factor Intervention Trial (MRFIT): Nutrient and food group changes over 6 years, *Journal of the American Dietetic Association* 86 (1986): 744–51.
17. T. A. Dolecek and coauthors, A long-term nutrition intervention experience: Lipid responses and dietary adherence patterns in the Multiple Risk Factor Intervention Trial, *Journal of the American Dietetic Association* 86 (1986): 752–58.
18. S. M. Grundy and coauthors, Coronary risk factor statement for the American public: A statement of the nutrition committee of the American Heart Association, *Arteriosclerosis* 5 (1985): 678A–82A.
19. Council on Scientific Affairs, Dietary and pharmacologic therapy for the lipid risk factors, *Journal of the American Medical Association* 250 (1983): 1873–79.
20. The Expert Panel, Report of the National Cholesterol Education Program Expert Panel on detection, evaluation, and treatment of high blood cholesterol in adults, *Archives of Internal Medicine* 148 (1988): 36–69.
21. U.S. Department of Agriculture, U.S. Department of Health and Human Services, Food Marketing Institute, *Eating Right with the Dietary Guidelines* (Washington, D.C.: Food Marketing Institute, 1991).
22. G. Sorensen and coauthors, Work-site nutrition intervention and employees' dietary habits: The Treatwell Program, *American Journal of Public Health* 82 (1992): 877–80.
23. A. R. Feinstein, Scientific standards in epidemiologic studies of the menace of daily life, *Science* 242 (1988): 1257–63.
24. The discussion of the uses of epidemiology in the nutritional sciences was adapted from M. L. Burr, Epidemiology for nutritionists: 1. Some general principles, *Human Nutrition: Applied Nutrition* 37A (1983): 259–64.
25. H. E. Sauberlich, Ascorbic acid, in *Present Knowledge in Nutrition,* 6th ed., ed. M. L. Brown (Washington, D.C.: International Life Sciences Institute, 1990), p. 132.
26. W. Willett, *Nutritional Epidemiology* (New York: Oxford University Press, 1990), pp. 3–51.
27. P. P. Basiotis and coauthors, Number of days of food intake records required to estimate individual and group nutrient intakes with defined confidence, *Journal of Nutrition* 117 (1987): 1638–41.
28. The discussion of the types of epidemiologic studies was

adapted from G. D. Friedman, *Primer of Epidemiology,* 3d ed. (New York: McGraw-Hill, 1987), pp. 47–55, and Tyler and Last, *Public Health & Preventive Medicine.*

29. L. Kaizer and coauthors, Fish consumption and breast cancer risk: An ecological study, *Nutrition and Cancer* 12 (1989): 61–68.

30. N. F. Butte and coauthors, Human milk intake and growth faltering of rural Mesoamerindian infants, *American Journal of Clinical Nutrition* 55 (1992): 1109–16.

31. T. R. Dawber, *The Framingham Study: The Epidemiology of Atherosclerotic Disease* (Cambridge, Mass.: Harvard University Press, 1980).

32. W. P. Castelli and coauthors, Incidence of coronary heart disease and lipoprotein cholesterol levels: The Framingham Study, *Journal of the American Medical Association* 256 (1986): 2835–38.

33. A. B. Miller and coauthors, A study of diet and breast cancer, *American Journal of Epidemiology* 107 (1978): 499–509.

34. J. M. Karkeck, Improving the use of dietary survey methodology, *Journal of the American Dietetic Association* 87 (1987): 869–71.

35. G. Block and A. M. Hartman, Issues in reproducibility and validity of dietary studies, *American Journal of Clinical Nutrition* 50 (1989): 1133–38.

36. The discussion of food consumption was adapted from R. S. Gibson, *Principles of Nutritional Assessment* (New York: Oxford University Press, 1990), pp. 21–54.

37. B. S. Burke and coauthors, Nutrition studies during pregnancy, *American Journal of Obstetrics and Gynecology* 46 (1943): 38–52, and B. S. Burke and H. C. Stuart, A method of diet analysis, *Journal of Pediatrics* 12 (1938): 493–503.

38. The discussion of the validity and reliability of diet assessment methods was adapted from G. Block, A review of validations of dietary assessment methods, *American Journal of Epidemiology* 115 (1982): 492–505.

39. G. H. Beaton and coauthors, Sources of variance in 24-hour dietary recall data: Implications for nutrition study design and interpretation, *American Journal of Clinical Nutrition* 32 (1979): 2456–2559.

40. The discussion of the problems with the 24-hour dietary recall method was adapted from R-L. Karvetti and L-R. Knuts, Validity of the 24-hour dietary recall, *Journal of the American Dietetic Association* 85 (1985): 1437–42; S. M. Garn and coauthors, The problem with one-day dietary intakes, *Ecology of Food and Nutrition* 5 (1976): 245–47; and J. L. Forster and coauthors, Hypertension prevention trial: Do 24-h food records capture usual eating behavior in a dietary change study? *American Journal of Clinical Nutrition* 51 (1990): 253–57.

41. W. C. Willett and coauthors, Reproducibility and validity of a semiquantitative food frequency questionnaire, *American Journal of Epidemiology* 122 (1985): 51–65; and W. C. Willett and coauthors, Validation of a semiquantitative food frequency questionnaire: Comparison with a 1-year diet record, *Journal of the American Dietetic Association* 87 (1987): 43–47.

42. L. Sampson, Food frequency questionnaires as a research instrument, *Clinical Nutrition* 4 (1985): 171–78; S. N. Zulkifli and S. M. Yu, The food frequency method for dietary assessment, *Journal of the American Dietetic Association* 92 (1992): 681–85; R. R. Briefel and coauthors, Assessing the nation's diet: Limitations of the food frequency questionnaire, *Journal of the American Dietetic Association* 92 (1992): 959–62; and G. Block and A. F. Subar, Estimates of nutrient intake from a food frequency questionnaire: The 1987 National Health Interview Survey, *Journal of the American Dietetic Association* 92 (1992): 969–77.

43. G. P. Sevenhuysen and L. A. Wadsworth, Food image processing: A potential method for epidemiological surveys, *Nutrition Reports International* 39 (1989): 439–50, and T. A. Fox and coauthors, Telephone surveys as a method for obtaining dietary information: A review, *Journal of the American Dietetic Association* 92 (1992): 729–32.

The Art and Science of Policy Making

Something to Think About . . .

I make it a rule never to get involved with possessed people. Actually, it's more of a guideline than a rule.

—Bill Murray to Sigourney Weaver in *Ghostbusters*

The determination of what does and what does *not* become a matter of governmental action is, therefore, the supreme instrument of power.

—Dennis J. Palumbo, *Public Policy in America: Government in Action*

Introduction

During World War II, American and British military officers were stymied in their efforts to stop German submarine attacks on allied ships. In exasperation, they finally turned to an operations researcher for a solution. He thought for a moment and then responded, "That's easy, all you have to do is boil the ocean." The military officers queried, "But how do we do that?" To which the operations researcher replied, "I don't know. I only make policy. It's your job to implement it."[1] This story captures the essence of policy making: policies are developed to solve problems. At the same time, it illustrates the problem that arises when policy formulation is separated from policy implementation and evaluation: the policy may not be achievable.

Whether the issue is regulating the testing of new drugs, providing quality health care for all citizens, or controlling air pollution, policy making is an ongoing process that affects our lives daily. As a community nutritionist, both local and national policy issues will affect the way you work, how you deliver nutrition services, and the dietary messages you give to individuals in your community. Consider how you would respond to the following issues in the nutrition policy arena:

◆ Should all Americans reduce their dietary fat intake to 30 percent or less of total calories, considering that not everyone has a significant risk for heart disease?

◆ Are dietary guidelines developed for adults appropriate for children?

◆ Should U.S. manufacturers of baby formula be allowed to sell their products in developing countries where the use of such products may undercut breastfeeding practices?

◆ Should local health departments allow restaurants to donate their leftover food to local food banks?

◆ Based on evidence that an increased intake of folate during pregnancy reduces the risk of neural-tube birth defects, should the Food and Drug Administration authorize the addition of folate to flour and other foods, even though this action means that folate intake will increase for the entire population and not just pregnant women?

There are no simple answers to these difficult policy questions. This is not surprising, for public policy is much like a human shape-shifter: complex, elusive, and ever-changing. Although it is difficult to describe precisely, **policy** can be viewed as a process, a series of intentions, actions, and behaviors of governments, agencies, officials, and other participants over a period of time.[2] Policy is the guiding principle behind regulations and laws; the law itself is not policy. Rather, policy is what government *intends* to accomplish through its laws, regulations, and programs. The purpose of public policy is to fashion strategies for solving public problems. Consult Table 3-1 to help you distinguish among the various terms used in this discussion.

The Process of Policy Making

Policy making is a sequential process, beginning with the placement of a public need, problem, or issue on the policy agenda and proceeding through the stages of policy formulation, implementation, evaluation, and termination. The process can be viewed as a cycle, as shown in Figure 3-1. This diagram has the advantage of simplifying the policy-making process but also makes it a little too simple and neat. In reality, the various stages often overlap as a policy is fine-tuned and refined. Sometimes the stages occur out of sequence, as when agenda setting leads directly to evaluation. When the issue of hunger became a part of the national policy agenda in the 1960s, for example, existing nutrition and welfare

TABLE

3-1

Elements of Government and Public Policy

Source: Excerpts from PUBLIC POLICY IN AMERICA: GOVERNMENT IN ACTION by Dennis J. Palumbo, copyright © 1988 by Harcourt Brace & Company, reproduced by permission of the publisher.

◆ **Functions of government.** The general activities that are considered to be legitimate purposes of government, such as providing for the country's defense, regulating interstate commerce, and maintaining public safety.

◆ **Policies.** The intentions (contained in politicians' statements, party platforms, campaign promises, etc.) that guide action in pursuing these functions.

◆ **Agencies.** The governmental units (legislatures, courts, administrative agencies) responsible for formulating and implementing these policies.

◆ **Laws.** The specific acts passed by legislatures in pursuance of public policy.

◆ **Regulations.** The rules or orders issued by administrative agencies in pursuance of policy.

◆ **Decisions.** The particular choices made by government officials in formulating and implementing public policy.

◆ **Programs.** The specific activities engaged in by agencies in implementing public policy.

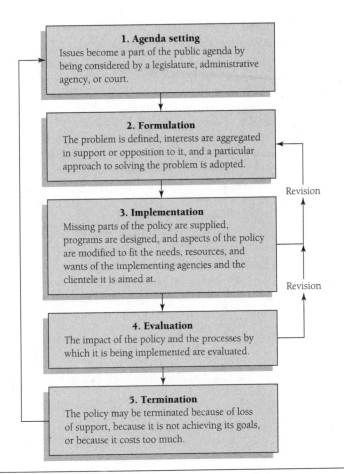

FIGURE

3-1

The Policy Cycle
Source: Excerpts from PUBLIC POLICY IN AMERICA: GOVERNMENT IN ACTION by Dennis J. Palumbo, copyright © 1988 by Harcourt Brace & Company, reproduced by permission of the publisher.

programs were evaluated to discover why they were not reaching hungry children. Nevertheless, viewing the policy-making process as a cycle allows us to see how policies evolve over time.

The discussion that follows focuses on policy making on the national level, because the laws that arise from federal policy making will affect some aspects of your job as a community nutritionist. As you study this section, think of ways in which the policy cycle can be applied to lower levels of government, such as your state or city government, and to other institutions, such as your college or university, place of employment, and even your home environment. As a student, for example, your life is affected by your school's policies on course requirements for graduation, parking on campus, residency, use of campus libraries, and many other activities. Consider how the policy cycle described here reflects the process by which your school formulated its policies:

1. **Agenda setting.** The first step in the policy cycle is to get an issue placed on the policy agenda. This **agenda** is not a written document or book, but a set of controversial issues that exist within society. There are two types

Agenda The set of problems to which policymakers give their attention.

Systemic agenda The issues that *can* become the subject of public policy.

Institutional agenda The issues that *are* the subject of public policy.

of agendas: systemic and institutional. The **systemic agenda** represents the broad set of issues that *can* become the subject of public policy. There are numerous systemic agendas in the United States, as each state, county, city, and community has its own systemic agenda. The **institutional agenda** represents those issues that actually *are* subjects for public policy. Institutional agendas are also numerous. Each legislative body in the United States (e.g., Congress, the state legislatures, city councils) has its own institutional agenda. Most issues move from the systemic to the institutional agenda by a process that is generally the same across government agencies.

The process of agenda setting is much like gatekeeping, with the gatekeepers deciding which items go onto the agenda and which do not. Actually getting policymakers to place a problem on the official agenda can be difficult. An issue may be so sensitive that policymakers or public attitudes work to keep it from reaching the agenda-setting stage. Consider, for example, the question of whether gay couples should be allowed to marry legally or adopt children. In the absence of widespread public support, some gay couples have taken this issue to the courts as a means of accessing the institutional agenda. In other situations, an issue may be perceived as a problem by only a small number of people who lack the political clout required to get the issue onto the institutional agenda. Sometimes a major catastrophe, such as an earthquake, assassination, riot, or an unusual human event, triggers a public outcry and pushes an issue onto the systemic agenda.

How can you access the policy agenda? The first step is to build widespread public interest for the issue you believe deserves government attention. One of the most effective ways to build public interest and support for an issue is to work through the media—radio, television, and newspapers. Because the media can both create and reflect public issues, they are one of the most useful tools for setting the public policy agenda. Photos of starving Somali children—"beyond hope, beyond life"—that were published in *Time* in the fall of 1992 helped to mobilize public support for the U.S. government's decision to send troops to Somalia to assist in providing famine relief.[3]

However, it is not enough merely to bring the issue to the attention of policymakers through the media. You must get the issue onto the institutional agenda. This is accomplished by winning support for the issue among policy subgovernments. Some political scientists have called **policy subgovernments** the "iron triangles," because they basically control the policy process. Iron triangles refer to three powerful participants in the policy-making process: interest groups, congressional committees or subcommittees, and administrative agencies. The policy subgovernments are not formal, recognized units of government, but they often exert enormous control over the policy-making process. The policy subgovernments consist of anyone interested in policy issues and outcomes, such as government administrators, members of Congress and their staffs, bureau chiefs, interest groups, professionals (e.g., dietitians, physicians, bankers,

Policy subgovernments Although not formal units of government, these "iron triangles" have a powerful influence on policy and agenda setting.

real estate agents), university faculty members, governors, and members of state and local governments.

2. **Policy formulation.** In this stage of the policy cycle, an issue placed on the policy agenda is further defined, additional information about the problem is collected and discussed, alternative solutions are considered, and a preferred choice of action is decided upon. **Policy formulation** has been described as a difficult game to play, "because any number of people can play and there are few rules."[4] In the process of fashioning a solution to a problem, such factors as the efficiency, economy, and cost-effectiveness of the proposed solution are evaluated before a decision is reached. The process of policy formulation may be molded by self-interest groups that use their powers of bargaining and persuasion to influence the outcome. Just as often, the habits, long-standing traditions, and standard operating procedures of government bodies and agencies influence the policy decision.

   As Table 3-2 shows, policy in the United States is formulated by the legislative, executive, and judicial branches of the government at the national, state, and local levels. How policies are formulated is not well understood and is the subject of much study by policy analysts.

3. **Policy implementation.** In the "boil the ocean syndrome" story at the beginning of this chapter, the solution proposed by the operations researcher did not consider how the policy would be implemented, or even whether it *could* be implemented. The act of making policy was uncoupled from the process of implementing it—an unworkable situation in real life. Implementation refers to the process of putting a policy into action to accomplish a public good. The implementors of public policy in the United States number literally in the millions. Employees of federal, state, and local governments work with private organizations, interest groups, and other parties to carry out government policy.

Policy formulation The development of a mechanism for solving a public problem.

LEVEL OF GOVERNMENT	LEGISLATIVE	EXECUTIVE	JUDICIAL
National	U.S. Congress	President and cabinet	U.S. Supreme Court, federal district courts, and other federal courts
State	Fifty state legislatures	State governors and state administrative agencies	State appellate courts
Local	Numerous county commissions, city councils, and township councils	County commissioners and departments, city mayors, managers, and administrative agencies	County courts, magistrate courts

TABLE

3-2

Public Agencies Involved in Policy Formulation
Source: Excerpts from PUBLIC POLICY IN AMERICA: GOVERNMENT IN ACTION by Dennis J. Palumbo, copyright © 1988 by Harcourt Brace & Company, reproduced by permission of the publisher.

4. **Policy evaluation.** As soon as public policies move into the agenda-setting stage, the evaluation process begins. The purpose of policy evaluation is to determine whether a program is achieving its stated goals and reaching its intended audience, what the program is actually accomplishing, and who is benefiting from it.

   From almost the moment of their conception, public policies undergo both formal and informal evaluations by citizens, legislators, administrative agencies, the news media, academicians, research firms, auditors, and interest groups. Ideally, public policies should be evaluated *after* they have been implemented, using the best available research methods and according to a systematic plan. In the real world, policy evaluation seldom works this way. Because evaluation is part of the policy-making cycle, it is both a political and a technical matter. It is political because those people who support a policy or program are likely to believe that it has succeeded, whereas those who are ideologically opposed are likely to conclude that the program failed. It is technical because it involves a formal, institutionalized process that draws on scientific principles and both qualitative and quantitative research methods to help policymakers make good decisions about programs and policies.

5. **Policy termination.** A policy or program may be terminated for any of several reasons: the public need was met, the nature of the problem changed, government no longer had a mandate in the area, the policy lost political support, private agencies relieved the need, a political system or subgovernment ceased to function, or the policy was too costly. Just as identifying a public problem in the first place is somewhat subjective, so is determining that a policy should be or has been terminated. At what point do you decide that the public's need has been met? What measures do you use to conclude that the problem has been solved? Typically, policy termination represents a process of adjustment in which the policymakers shift their focus to other policy concerns. While some policy systems go out of existence, others survive and expand, bringing the policy cycle full circle to a redefinition of the public problem.[5]

The People Who Make Policy

The stages of the policy cycle outlined in Figure 3-1 do not correspond directly to the agencies and institutions involved in making government policy. We tend to assume that policy is formulated by legislatures and implemented by administrative agencies, such as the Public Health Service or the Health Care Financing Administration, to name only two government agencies involved in public health. In point of fact, however, administrative agencies sometimes formulate policy, and legislatures become involved in policy implementation.

This leads us to ask, "Who makes policy?" Although it is true that "policymakers"—that is, the members of Congress and state legislatures and the senior administrators of official government agencies—make policy, so do **street-level bureaucrats**: welfare workers, public health nurses, police officers, schoolteachers, sanitation workers, housing authority managers, judges, and the many other people working in government agencies. In the course of carrying out their jobs, these street-level bureaucrats daily make policy decisions by interpreting government laws and regulations for citizens. As a community nutritionist, you may find yourself making policy when you decide to tailor a program to meet a particular client's needs.

Street-level bureaucrats
Individuals within government who have direct contact with citizens.

Legitimating Policy

Once it has been decided that a policy should be put into effect, a choice must be made about *how* it will be implemented. This is not a trivial decision. Consider, for example, the decision by the Food and Drug Administration (FDA) to allow food product labels to carry health claims. Some consumers, scientists, and food companies objected to this policy, while others believed it would help the public make healthful food choices. Thus, a policy may be perceived as benefiting some citizens and working to the detriment of others. Because achieving universal agreement on a policy and its effects is impossible, careful attention must be given to the process by which policy decisions are made. This is the point at which legitimating policy is important.

Legitimacy is "the belief on the part of citizens that the current government represents a proper form of government and a willingness on the part of those citizens to accept the decrees of that government as legal and authoritative."[6] In this sense, legitimacy is mainly in the mind, for it depends on a majority of the population accepting that the government has the right to govern. In the case of the FDA's health claim policy, the appearance of health claims on food labels indicates that consumers and food companies accept the FDA's *authority* to allow this action. In contrast, the protests and student demonstrations against the war in Vietnam were a challenge to legitimacy.

Government, then, must somehow legitimate each policy choice. Several mechanisms exist for legitimating policies: the legislative process; the regulatory process; the court system; and various procedures for direct democracy, such as referenda, which put sensitive issues directly before the people. The next section will explore the legislative and regulatory processes in greater detail, as most policies in the areas of health, food, and nutrition arise through these mechanisms.*

*The use of the court system for legitimating policy in the nutrition arena is not discussed in detail in this chapter, although it is important in formulating food and nutrition policy. Regulations *are* challenged through the court system. When the FDA issued a final rule establishing nutrition labeling regulations in 1973, a portion of the regulations dealing with special dietary foods was challenged in the courts by the National Nutritional Foods Association (see *National Nutritional Foods Association v. FDA* and *National Nutritional Foods Association v. Kennedy* as cited in the *Federal Register* 1990 [July 19]: 29476–77).

The Legislative and Regulatory Process

Governments can use any number of instruments to influence the lives of their citizens: taxes and tax incentives, services such as defense and education, price supports for commodities, unemployment benefits, and laws, to name only a few. Laws are a unique tool of government. In the United States, we traditionally associate law making with Congress, the primary legislative body. It is Congress that sets policy and supplies the basic legislation that governs our lives.

◆ LAWS AND REGULATIONS

The laws passed by Congress tend to be somewhat vague. A law defines the broad scope of the policy intended by Congress. For example, the Special Supplemental Food Program for Women, Infants, and Children (WIC) was authorized by Public Law 92–433 and approved on September 26, 1972. This law authorized a two-year, $20 million pilot program for each of the fiscal years 1973 and 1974. It gave the secretary of agriculture the authority to make cash grants to state health departments or comparable agencies to provide supplemental foods to pregnant and lactating women, infants, and children up to four years of age who were considered at "nutritional risk" by competent professionals. As written, this law was too vague to implement. It did not define or specify which professionals would determine the eligibility of clients. It did not define the concept of "nutritional risk" and other eligibility requirements, the method by which clients would obtain food products, or other aspects of the proposed program. Sorting out these details was left to the U.S Department of Agriculture (USDA).

Thus, once a law is passed, it is up to the administrative bodies such as the USDA to interpret the law and provide the detailed regulations or rules that put the policy into effect. These regulations are sometimes called "secondary legislation." The total volume of this activity is enormous, as seen by the size of the *Federal Register,* a weekly publication that contains all regulations and proposed regulations, and the *Code of Federal Regulations (CFR),* a compendium of all regulations currently in force. When the WIC program was started, the details of the regulations were not published in the *Federal Register* until July 11, 1973, nearly nine months after Congress passed the law. Over time, new laws and amendments to the existing law were enacted to increase the amount of money allocated for the WIC program, specify the means by which the program should be implemented, and authorize the continuation of the program for additional budget years.[7] (A detailed discussion of the WIC program appears in Chapter 12.)

◆ HOW AN IDEA BECOMES LAW

All levels of government pass laws. (At the local level, laws are sometimes called ordinances or bylaws.) The process by which an idea becomes law is complicated and cumbersome. It may take many months, or even years, for an idea or issue to work its way onto the policy agenda. Then, once it reaches the legislative body empowered to act on it, the formal rules and procedures of that body can delay

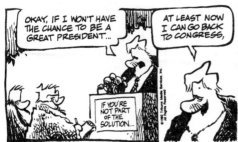
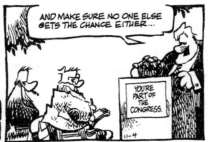

decision making on a proposed bill or scuttle it altogether. A heavy workload combined with infighting and vote trading can thwart the law-making process, especially at the end of legislative sessions when logjams are common. Lewis Carroll, writing in *Alice in Wonderland,* could have been speaking of the U.S. Congress when he wrote: "I don't think they play at all fairly, and they quarrel so dreadfully one can't hear oneself speak—and they don't seem to have any rules in particular: at least, if there are, nobody attends to them—and you've no idea how confusing it is."[8]

The general process by which laws are made is outlined in Figure 3-2, which shows the path a bill would take on its way through Congress. The process is much the same for bills introduced into state legislatures. Remember, the process begins when a concerned citizen, group of citizens, or organization brings an issue to the attention of a legislative representative at either the local, state, or national level. Typically, the issue is presented to private attorneys or the staff of the legislative counsel, who draft the bill in the proper language and style. A bill is introduced by sending it to the clerk's desk, where it is numbered and printed. It must have a member as its sponsor. Simple bills are designated as either "H.R." or "S." depending upon the house of origin. Note in Figure 3-3 that the Nutrition Labeling and Education Act was designated "H.R. 3562," indicating that the bill was introduced into the House of Representatives. There is no limit on the number of bills a member can introduce, although the informal "rules of the game" mandate that a member not introduce "too many." When the bill is introduced, the bill's title is entered in the *Congressional Journal* and printed in the *Congressional Record.*[9]

In the next step, the bill is sent to the appropriate committee or subcommittee, where it is examined closely. There are many committees and subcommittees. The House, for example, has 21 standing (permanent) committees and about 150 subcommittees. The committee or subcommittee to which the bill is assigned reviews the bill's merits and alters the original bill as deemed necessary. Generally, committees and subcommittees can make one of the following decisions about a bill:[10]

"There are two things in the world you do not want to watch being made—sausages and laws."
—cited in T. R. Dye, *Politics in States and Communities*

◆ Report the bill out of committee
◆ Report out the bill with amendments

FIGURE
3-2

How an Idea Becomes Law

Source: J. H. Ferguson and D. E. McHenry, *The American System of Government,* p. 344. Copyright 1973 by McGraw-Hill, Inc. Reproduced with permission of McGraw-Hill, Inc.

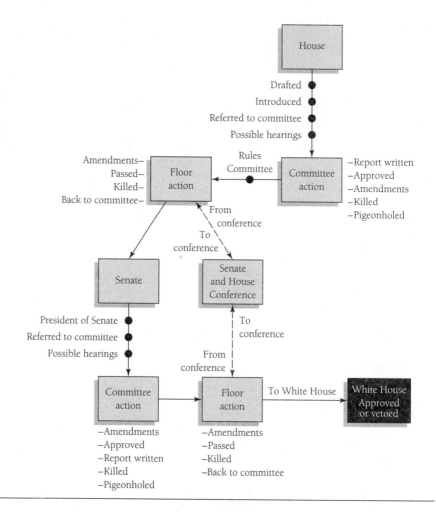

◆ Report out a substitute to the bill originally introduced

◆ Give the bill an unfavorable review (i.e., "kill it")

When the bill is reported out of a committee, it is sent to the Rules Committee, which evaluates the bill further and determines whether it should be sent to the floor for consideration by the entire House. In the process of evaluating a bill, a committee may hold public hearings and seek the testimony of interested persons or experts before deciding whether to move the bill forward. Bills moved out of committee onto the floor of the House are debated and voted on. After a bill is passed by the House, it is sent to the Senate where a similar process takes place.

If the bill approved by the Senate is identical to the one passed by the House, it is sent to the president to be signed. If the two versions differ, a joint House-Senate conference committee is formed to modify the bill by mutual agreement. Once both houses agree on the compromise bill, it is sent to the president, who

CONGRESSIONAL RECORD—HOUSE

NUTRITION LABELING AND EDUCATION ACT OF 1990

Mr. WAXMAN. Mr. Speaker, I move to suspend the rules and pass the bill (H.R. 3562) to amend the Federal Food, Drug, and Cosmetic Act to prescribe nutrition labeling for foods, and for other purposes, as amended. The Clerk read as follows:

H.R. 3562

Be it enacted by the Senate and House of Representatives of the United States of America in Congress assembled,

SECTION 1. SHORT TITLE, REFERENCE.

(a) Short Title.—This Act may be cited as the "Nutrition Labeling and Education Act of 1990".

(b) Reference.—Whenever in this Act an amendment or repeal is expressed in terms of an amendment to, or repeal of, a section or other provision, the reference shall be considered to be made to a section or other provision of the Federal Food, Drug, and Cosmetic Act.

SEC. 2. NUTRITION LABELING.

(a) Nutrition Information.—Section 403 (21 U.S.C. 343) is amended by adding at the end the following new paragraph:

"(q)(1) Except as provided in subparagraphs (3), (4), and (5), if it is a food intended for human consumption and is offered for sale, unless its label or labeling bears nutrition information that provides—

"(A)(i) the serving size which is an amount customarily consumed and which is expressed in a common household measure that is appropriate to the food, or

"(ii) if the use of the food is not typically expressed in a serving size, the common household unit of measure that expresses the serving size of the food,

"(B) the number of servings or other units of measure per container,

"(C) the total number of calories—

"(i) derived from any source, and

"(ii) derived from the total fat, in each serving size or other unit of measure of the food, and

"(D) the amount of the following nutrients: Total fat, saturated fat, cholesterol, sodium, total carbohydrates, complex carbohydrates, sugars, dietary fiber, and total protein contained in each serving size or other unit of measure.

by subparagraph (1)(C) or (1)(D) or clause (A) of this subparagraph to be included in the label or labeling of food is not necessary to assist consumers in maintaining healthy dietary practices, the Secretary may by regulation remove information relating to such nutrient from such requirement.

"(3) For food that is received in bulk containers at a retail establishment, the Secretary shall, by regulation, provide that the nutrition information required by subparagraphs (1) and (2) may be displayed at the location in the retail establishment at which the food is offered for sale.

FIGURE

3-3

A Portion of the Nutrition Labeling and Education Act Published in the *Congressional Record,* July 30, 1990, p. II 5836.

---

may sign it into law, allow it to become law without his signature, or veto it. When Congress overrides the president's veto by a two-thirds majority vote in both houses, the bill becomes law without the president's signature.[11] (In state legislatures, of course, the bill would be sent to the governor.) When the bill is signed into law by the president, it becomes an *act* and is given the designation "P.L.," which stands for Public Law, and a number: the first two or three digits indicate the number of the congressional session in which the law was enacted, and the remaining digits represent the number of the bill. Recall that the bill authorizing the WIC supplemental feeding program became Public Law 92–433 (i.e., bill number 433, enacted by the 92nd Congress).

Before a law enacted by Congress goes into effect, it is reviewed by the appropriate federal agency, which is responsible for issuing guidelines or regulations that detail how the law will be implemented and any penalties that may be imposed if the law is violated. These regulations are published in the *Federal Register*. Because federal law requires that the public have the opportunity to comment on an agency's proposed guidelines, the agency first issues "proposed regulations." During the comment period that follows the publication of proposed regulations, the general public, experts, companies, and interested organizations submit their written comments and, in some cases, present their views at public hearings. From 30 to 90 days are allowed for comment, depending upon the type and complexity of the regulations. At the end of the comment period, the agency reviews all comments, both positive and negative, before issuing its final regulations, which are incorporated into the *CFR*. The *CFR* and the *Federal Register* are available at most local libraries and county courthouses.

Examine the proposed rule shown in Figure 3-4. Notice that it summarizes the main points of the proposed regulations, indicates when written comments are due and the address to which they should be sent, and provides the name of a contact person within the agency should an interested party have additional questions. It outlines relevant background information and then gives the details of the agency's proposed rules (this information is not shown in the figure). As a community nutritionist responding to this proposed rule, you would outline

---

FIGURE

3-4

A Portion of a Proposed Rule Published by the Food and Drug Administration in the *Federal Register*

Federal Register / Vol. 55, No. 139 / Thursday, July 19, 1990 / Proposed Rules

21 CFR PART 101

[Docket No. 90N-0165]

RIN 0905-AD08

Food Labeling; Serving Sizes
AGENCY: Food and Drug Administration, HHS.
ACTION: Proposed rule.

SUMMARY: The Food and Drug Administration (FDA) is proposing to amend its nutrition labeling regulations (1) To define serving and portion size on the basis of the amount of food commonly consumed per eating occasion by persons 4 years of age or older, by infants, or by children under 4 years of age (toddlers); (2) to require the use of both U.S. and metric measures to declare serving size; (3) to permit the declaration of serving (portion) size in familiar household measures; (4) to permit the optional declaration of nutrient content per 100 grams (or 100 milliliters); and (5) to define a "single serving container" as that which contains 150 percent or less of the standard serving size for the food product. FDA also is proposing to establish standard serving sizes for 159 food product categories to assure reasonable and uniform serving sizes upon which consumers can make nutrition comparisons among food products.
DATES: Written comments by November 16, 1990. The agency is proposing that any final rule that may issue based upon this proposal become effective 1 year following its publication in the Federal Register.
ADDRESSES: Written comments to the Dockets Management Branch (HFA–305), Food and Drug Administration, rm. 4–62, 5600 Fishers Lane, Rockville, MD 20857, 301–443–4874.
FOR FURTHER INFORMATION CONTACT: Youngmee K. Park, Center for Food Safety and Applied Nutrition (HFF–265), Food and Drug Administration, 200 C Street SW., Washington, DC 20204, 202–485–0089.

your particular concerns about the proposed regulations and offer specific alternative actions or policies in a letter mailed to the Dockets Management Branch at the FDA.

Finally, laws and regulations will have no effect unless there are funds to enforce them. Congress must enact appropriations bills to fund the programs and services mandated by federal legislation. The federal budget process has been described as "fractured, contentious, and chaotic."[12] Even so, Congress is usually able to push through a budget resolution detailing how much money is available to federal agencies to spend on their programs.

◆ THE POLITICAL PROCESS

It is sometimes difficult to appreciate the challenges and complexities of the legislative and policy-making process or the years required to reach a critical mass in public support for a policy change. As a case in point, consider that until 1906 no *federal* legislation regulated the nation's food supply and protected consumers against food adulteration, mislabeling, and false advertising. Even then, more than 25 years of persistent pressure from consumers and the agricultural community had been required to achieve this legislative milestone.[13] Check the boxed insert for a description of the imperfect process leading to the passage of the Food and Drugs Act.[13]

A more recent example of the political process relates to food and nutrition labeling policy. The type and format of nutrition information provided on packaged food labels were governed by regulations adopted by the FDA in 1973 under the authority of the Federal Food, Drug, and Cosmetic Act (FD&C Act). These regulations applied only to retail packaged foods other than meat and poultry products, which were, and still are, regulated by the USDA. By the late 1980s, an estimated half of all packaged foods did *not* bear nutrition labeling. Moreover, nutrition labeling information was not required on or in conjunction with the sale of fresh and frozen meats, poultry, seafood, and eggs; fruits and vegetables; foods prepared and sold for immediate consumption by take-home food bars, restaurants, and supermarkets; and foods sold in institutional settings.

With the publication of the Surgeon General's report and the National Research Council's *Diet and Health* report, the call for uniform labeling grew. Many consumers and some industry groups believed that existing labels were incomplete, confusing, and too complex for most people to understand and use.[14] Congress concurred and considered three food labeling bills, including the Waxman Bill (H.R. 3562) introduced by Representative Henry A. Waxman (D, California). The bill proposed requiring food labels to carry more useful information and be easier to understand.[15]

The first major overhaul of food and nutrition labeling in nearly 20 years occurred on November 8, 1990, when President George Bush signed into law H.R. 3562 (P.L. 101–535), the Nutrition Labeling and Education Act (NLEA), which amended the FD&C Act. The NLEA called for nationally uniform food labels and mandatory nutrition labeling information on nearly all foods marketed to U.S. consumers. Its specific provisions are shown on the next pages.[16]

The Legislative Process in Real Life

Between 1880 and 1906, nearly two hundred bills designed to protect consumers against food adulteration, misbranding, and false advertising were introduced into Congress without success. One such bill was submitted to the House and passed in 1904; the Senate began debating and eventually passed a similar bill, with amendments, in 1906. During the debates on this bill, Dr. Harvey W. Wiley, who was the chief chemist of the Department of Agriculture, testified about adulterated foods, bringing examples to show before Congress. At his urging, women who were concerned about food safety also lobbied Congress to pass the bill. When the bill went to the conference committee to iron out differences between the two houses, tensions were high. At one point, President Theodore Roosevelt felt compelled to lean upon Congress and express his support for the pure foods bill. Finally, the bill passed both the House and Senate on June 27, 1906, and was signed into law by President Roosevelt on June 30, 1906. The Food and Drugs Act became law effective January 1, 1907.

Unfortunately, the law was defective. In the beginning, Congress failed to pass appropriation bills to provide the funds to enforce the law. Congress also failed to authorize the development of standards of food composition and quality, an omission that made it difficult for authorities to prove in court that a food was an imitation and not the genuine food product. Thus, because the Food and Drugs Act lacked teeth, food adulteration remained a threat to public health. Attempts to strengthen the law failed until 1938, when Congress passed the Federal Food, Drug, and Cosmetic Act, which was signed into law by President Franklin D. Roosevelt in 1938. It became effective one year later and is the primary legislation by which our food supply is regulated today.*

*__Source:__ Adapted from H. W. Schultz, *Food Law Handbook* (Westport, Conn.: Avi Publishing Company, 1981), pp. 3–21.

1. Mandatory nutrition labeling for most foods under the jurisdiction of the FDA; meat and poultry products come under the jurisdiction of the USDA. The nutrition label must include

   ◆ the serving size in an amount customarily consumed and expressed in common household measures;

   ◆ the number of servings per container or unit;

   ◆ the total number of calories per serving and the number of calories derived from fat; and

   ◆ the amount of the following nutrients per serving: total fat, saturated fat, cholesterol, sodium, total carbohydrates, complex carbohydrates, sugars, dietary fiber, and total protein.

2. *Voluntary* nutrition guidelines for raw agricultural commodities (fruits and vegetables) and fish.[17]

3. Exemptions from labeling requirements for foods sold in restaurants or similar establishments, infant formula, and medical foods, or if a food contains insignificant amounts of the nutrients required to be listed on the label.

4. Activities to educate consumers about nutrition labeling so that they can comprehend the information and understand how it can be used to select a healthful daily diet.

5. Authorization for certain label claims concerning nutrients and their relationship to health and disease. The secretary will issue regulations to determine whether claims should be permitted for the following nutrients and conditions: calcium and osteoporosis, dietary fiber and cancer, lipids and cardiovascular disease, lipids and cancer, sodium and hypertension, and dietary fiber and cardiovascular disease. The act requires that certain terms commonly used on labels, such as "light," "lite," and "low salt," have consistent meanings.

6. Development of a system for evaluating the validity of health claims for dietary supplements.

7. Federal preemption for nutrient labeling and health claims, meaning that federal law supersedes any state laws on these topics.

Following the passage of the NLEA, the FDA had 24 months in which to develop proposed rules, allow the public to comment on them, and publish final regulations. After reviewing hundreds of comments, the FDA published final rules related to food and nutrition labeling on January 6, 1993 (58 FR 2066–2964).[18]*

Like other legislation, the provisions of the NLEA have not pleased everyone. Some states, for example, have voiced concern that the imposition of nationally uniform nutrition labeling by the federal government has impinged on states' rights. Some local officials and consumer groups have questioned whether the FDA has the resources and personnel to enforce the law and whether local officials might be better positioned to make decisions regarding locally grown foods. At the other end of the spectrum, most food companies have voiced support for uniform labeling requirements, citing the managerial and production costs associated with nonstandardized labels.[19] On balance, the NLEA provided for mechanisms to address the concerns raised by states and consumers, while moving the nation toward a single, comprehensive national labeling system.

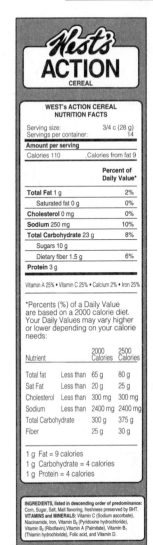

Consult Appendix B for information about government agencies and health organizations with a nutrition focus.

◆ EMERGING POLICY ISSUES

In this chapter, we have seen that laws and regulations are the means by which public problems are addressed. We have also come to appreciate that laws are not static. They are dynamic, changing as conditions, circumstances, and issues change. In the food and nutrition arena, existing laws are constantly being challenged by market forces, scientific knowledge, and consumer practices and attitudes. The following issues have the potential to change current policies:

◆ **The Delaney Clause.** The 1958 Food Additives Amendment to the FD&C Act contains the Delaney Clause, which prohibits the use in food of any additive shown to cause cancer in humans or animals. This has become a

*The designation "58 FR 2066–2964" refers to Volume 58 of the *Federal Register,* pages 2006 through 2964.

thorny issue for regulatory agencies, policymakers, scientists, and consumers who face the same question today about the safety of food components as did policymakers in 1958. What is meant by safety? What food components should be regulated? How rigorously should the law be enforced? How compelling is the scientific evidence that shapes the law? One of the major problems with enforcing the Delaney Clause in the 1990s is that scientists have made enormous technical strides in detecting and measuring food components. High-performance liquid chromatography, mass spectrometry, and other methods allow scientists to quantify compounds on the level of parts per trillion or quadrillion—a considerable advance since 1958. The problem is complicated by the fact that naturally occurring compounds with carcinogenic properties are found in many foodstuffs. The challenge, then, for policymakers and scientists is to achieve a public policy that will allow for an evaluation of both the risks and benefits of chemical compounds in an environment in which the complete absence of risk is not attainable.[20]

◆ **Biotechnology**. Biotechnology is "the utilization of biologically derived molecules, structures, cells, or organisms to carry out a specific process."[21] Biotechnology is not new; it has been practiced for more than 8000 years. Early applications of food biotechnology include the production of vinegar, alcoholic beverages, sourdough, and cheese. Today, biotechnology has many applications in the dairy, baking, meat, enzyme, and fermentation industries.[22] Because biotechnology uses DNA recombinant technology to custom design protein molecules and other compounds of great purity,[23] there have been questions about the safety of foods produced by this method. To address these questions, in May 1992, the FDA published regulations to guide industry in its use of this relatively new technology. According to the new policy, most products of biotechnology, such as proteins, carbohydrates, and fats, will not raise new safety issues, because they resemble existing approved food additives or GRAS (Generally Recognized As Safe) substances. The FDA recognizes, however, that some substances produced by this method *will* require premarket approval, just like any other food additive, because they have no history of safe use.[24] Although the FDA's new policy maps a regulatory path for food companies that develop new foods using biotechnology, new advances in this area will continue to challenge existing regulations.

◆ **Medical foods**. The term *medical foods* refers to enteral formulas used to feed hospitalized patients or foods for people with rare diseases.[25] These formulas and foods are designed to provide complete or partial nutrition support to individuals who have special physiological or nutritional needs or who cannot ingest food in a conventional form. From a regulatory standpoint, medical foods lie at the interface of foods and drugs. They were initially classified as prescription drugs under the FD&C Act to ensure that their use would be supervised by physicians and to prevent abuse by consumers. In 1972, the FDA changed their regulatory status from drugs to "special dietary foods" to enhance further development in this area. However, the problem of how to label medical foods remained. In 1984, the FDA drafted a specific medical food regulation, which was never published, leaving unanswered certain questions about their conditions of use and labeling. With the enactment of the NLEA, a definition for medical foods was proposed, although it exempted these products from the requirements for nutrition labeling. Specific labeling regulations for medical foods will be developed at a future date.

♦ **Nutraceuticals.** The term *nutraceutical* is a newly minted name for food products created by new technologies and scientific developments. A proposed definition for nutraceutical is "any substance that may be considered a food or part of a food and provides medical or health benefits, including the prevention and treatment of disease." Under this definition, nutraceuticals would include nutrients, dietary supplements, herbal products, genetically engineered "designer" foods, and some processed foods. The Foundation for Innovation in Medicine, a nonprofit educational organization, has proposed a system for government review and approval of foods with potential or proven medical and health benefits. The foundation's 40-page white paper outlining its proposal has been sent to members of Congress, U.S. regulatory agencies, scientists, and food and drug companies.[26] This is another area where the FDA and other agencies may need to develop standards and guidelines for industry.

Policies in the food and nutrition arena will continue to evolve as our knowledge of foods and their relationship to health expands and the issues of public concern change. The broad scope of food and nutrition policy provides ample opportunity for you to become involved in the policy process.

Other policy issues in nutrition are discussed in Chapters 4 and 5.

Policy Making and the Community Nutritionist

You may not think of yourself as a political beast. You may think of politics as being confined to committee meetings, public hearings, and the inner workings of massive government buildings. However, if you've ever lobbied your parents for late-night privileges, your best friend to let you borrow his car, or a professor to allow you to take an exam at a later date, then *you* have walked onto the political stage. You have tried to get something you want by presenting compelling reasons why an existing policy should be changed in your favor. Your forays into the political arena in community nutrition may differ only slightly from the "politicking" you do in your personal life.

As in other disciplines, the policy-making process in community nutrition tends to be formal, ritualized, and rooted in tradition. Whether the issue is food legislation, health care reform, licensure of registered dietitians, or funding for the School Lunch Program, you will be able to influence the policy-making process in one of two ways: by becoming directly involved in politics or by joining an interest group. Both approaches, together with specific tactics for influencing the political system, are described in greater detail in the next sections.

◆ DIRECT INVOLVEMENT

When you choose direct involvement, *you* become a political actor and run for political office, sponsor a referendum, or initiate a campaign to achieve a common goal. You might decide, for example, to seek an elected position within your state or the national dietetic association as one means of influencing the practice of dietetics, or you may choose to participate on a local advisory board that is in a position to directly influence the political process in your community. You might organize the collection of signatures for a petition to be sent to your state legislature or city council, or you may work to elect a candidate to political office. Getting involved directly in the political process can be rewarding, but it requires a commitment of time and energy.

◆ INTEREST GROUPS

Interest group A body of people acting in an organized manner to advance shared political interests.

You may choose to join an interest group. **Interest groups** are pressure groups that try to influence public policy in ways that are favorable to their members. They consist of people who work together in an organized manner to advance a shared political interest.[27] Interest groups may exert pressure by persuading government agencies and elected officials to reach a particular decision, by supporting or opposing certain political candidates or incumbents, through litigation, or by trying to shape public opinion (another means of getting an issue onto the policy agenda). While interest groups are sometimes accused of being bureaucratic and power-hungry and of not always representing their constituents fairly, they do contribute to the political process. Among other things, they encourage political participation and strengthen the link between the public and the government. In addition, they provide government officials with valuable technical and policy information that may not be readily obtained elsewhere.[28]

There are different types of interest groups. Business, for example, is well represented on Capitol Hill by lobbyists from particular companies, such as Kellogg's, Procter & Gamble, and the Coca-Cola Company, or from trade associations, such as the American Meat Institute, the Sugar Association, and the National Soft Drink Association. Professional groups, such as the American Dietetic Association and the American Medical Association, also have particular interests and policy concerns. "Public interest" groups are a special category, in that they work to achieve goals that do not directly benefit their membership. The Sierra Club and Common Cause are two well-known public interest groups. Still other interest groups may represent particular segments of the population, such as blacks (e.g., the National Association for the Advancement of Colored People) and women (e.g., the National Organization for Women). Activities to influence the political process even occur within the government itself—that is, government lobbying government. The National Governors' Association and the Hall of the States, for example, have been active in trying to set and direct the policy agenda.

◆ TACTICS FOR INFLUENCING THE POLITICAL PROCESS

Interest groups and their memberships employ a number of tactics to influence the political process. Litigation is increasingly being used to change policy through the court system. Filing a class action suit in court on behalf of all persons who might benefit from a court action is one example. Another tactic is the public relations campaign, in which interest groups try to influence public opinion favorably. Three other common tactics are political campaign activities, lobbying, and building coalitions.

Political Action Committees (PACs)   A political action committee or PAC is the political arm of an interest group. It has the legal authority to raise funds from its members or employees in support of candidates or political parties. The purpose of a PAC is to help elect candidates whose views are favorably aligned with the group's mission or goals. PACs also work to keep the lines of communication open between policymakers and the interest group's membership.[29] Some PACs, such as that of the American Medical Association, have a powerful influence on the policy-making process and its outcome.

Lobbying   Lobbying is often the method of choice when trying to influence the political system. "It is probably the oldest weapon, and certainly one of the most criticized."[30] Lobbying has acquired a negative connotation of cigar-smoking, back-slapping professional supplicants who bend the political process through large campaign contributions. While this image may be appropriate to some situations, it doesn't apply to all lobbyists. Remember, **lobbying** means talking to public officials and legislators to persuade them to consider the information you provide on an issue you believe is important.[31] Lobbyists' experience, knowledge of the legal system, and political skills make them an important part of the political process. They provide technical information to policymakers, help draft laws, testify before committees, and help speed (or slow) the passage of bills.

Lobbying Providing information to elected officials.

When employing this tactic, three issues are important: deciding how to lobby, knowing whom to lobby, and determining when to lobby. One of your first decisions is whether to lobby directly or hire a registered lobbyist. In some cases, you or your organization may not need a registered lobbyist to achieve your objective; in other situations, you may not be successful without the knowledge of the political machine and its players that a registered lobbyist will offer.

Knowing whom to lobby and when are also critical decisions. To do this, identify the politicians or elected officials who are in a position to act on your concern by studying the formal government structure and its agencies, reading the newsletters of interest groups, and talking with policymakers who share your concern. Sometimes, reporters who cover certain events can help you identify the proper authority figures. Once you know whom to lobby, choose the right time. You will accomplish little if you lobby a legislator when a bill is up for the final reading instead of when it was being considered in subcommittee. Use a triggering event to bring an issue to a politician's attention. If possible, turn the triggering event into an opportunity for placing the issue on the policy agenda. The release of a national report on the AIDS epidemic and the growing need of AIDS patients for nutritional home care may improve your lobbying efforts to obtain third-party reimbursement of nutritional services in your state. Above all, remember that you will have to lobby for as long as it takes, even if the process requires years. Establishing rapport and building recognition for your concern among elected officials take time.

Having determined where and when to lobby, you must consider how to do it most effectively. Four points are helpful when trying to influence public officials:

1. Show that you are concerned about the official's image. You want to make it easy for the politician to give you what you want, and *at the same time,* you want to make the politician look good. You must not appear to be applying force directly. Instead, provide a compelling rationale for the politician to support your proposal.

2. Accept the constraints under which elected officials work. Politicians must deal daily with many pressing issues and diverse groups, including their constituents and staff, lobbyists, party politics, committee leadership, fund raising, campaigning, and the media. All of these place demands on the official's time. Effective lobbyists recognize the cross pressures politicians face and, when possible, develop strategies for reducing those pressures.

3. Consider reaching elected officials indirectly. Politicians can be influenced through their staff, campaign workers, former colleagues, financial contributors, business associates, and friends. Approaching someone among these groups may speed your ability to refine your proposal and avoid creating a problem for the politician.

4. Provide information for the official through letters, phone calls, and meetings. Ralph Nader, the consumer advocate, once remarked: "Talking frequently to legislators is the best way to persuade them of your position; the importance of this simple method cannot be overstated."[32]

Building Coalitions   In some situations, an organization is too small or isolated to influence the political system effectively. It can better achieve policy changes by working with other organizations toward a common goal. Depending on the scope or depth of the cooperative effort, the joint venture may be a formal coalition or a more informal network or alliance. Formal coalitions tend to arise in geographical areas where problems affect many people across different communities. Coalitions may bring together social service organizations, church groups, professional associations, neighborhood groups, and business organizations to develop a long-term, joint commitment to solving problems. The challenge, of course, is getting such diverse groups to agree on which problems deserve immediate attention.

Networks tend to arise when different organizations across the country share a variety of problems. A network may support a permanent staff in one location and have a common training and information system, but individual members of the network may pursue different problems. In general, network members share a common philosophy about how to mobilize people for action. ACORN (Associations of Community Organizations for Reform Now) and Citizen Action are examples of networks. Alliances, by comparison, tend to bring together organizations that are dispersed geographically to address one specific problem. The level of participation in alliance activities tends to wax and wane according to the urgency of the issue.

Coalitions, networks, and alliances are usually formed to increase the pressure on the political system. By joining forces, organizations can launch more effective public information and media campaigns to mobilize public support for an issue and bring it to the attention of policymakers. The American Dietetic Association (ADA), for example, reported that it has more than 150 partners in government, industry, and health care. For example, the ADA is spearheading the Food Label Education Dialogue Group, a coalition of more than 20 leading health organizations and government agencies. Plus, it formed an alliance with McDonald's to develop a National Nutrition Month program called "FOOD FUNdamentals."[33] The ADA also formed a partnership with the American Institute of Wine and Food to promote healthful food as both good-looking and great-tasting.[34] These activities enhance the ADA's efforts to educate the public about healthful eating practices.

◆ POLITICAL ACTION IN COMMUNITY NUTRITION

Community nutritionists are increasingly being asked to become a part of the political process and to help support the initiatives of the national dietetic office or other health organizations. Here are a few things to keep in mind when attempting to influence the political environment.

Write Effective Letters   A personal letter to an elected official from a constituent can be a powerful instrument for change. Consider the following points when writing to your elected official:[35]

- ◆ Limit your letter to one page. Letters should be typed or handwritten legibly.
- ◆ Write about a single issue.
- ◆ Refer to the legislation by bill number and name. Note the names of sponsors and refer to hearings that have been held.
- ◆ Explain how a legislative issue will affect your work, your organization, or your community.
- ◆ Use logical rather than emotional arguments in support of your position. Let the facts speak for themselves.
- ◆ Ask direct questions and request a reply.
- ◆ Be cooperative. Offer to provide further information. Do not seek confrontation but don't hesitate to ask for your legislator's position on the issue.
- ◆ Follow up. Congratulate your legislator for a positive action or express concern again if the legislator acted contrary to your view on the issue.
- ◆ Write as an individual rather than as a member of the American Dietetic Association (although you should identify yourself as a registered dietitian).

Make Effective Telephone Calls   Getting through to a legislator or other elected official can be difficult. When the opportunity presents itself, remember the points shown on the next page when phoning an elected official.

◆ Write down the points you wish to make, your arguments supporting them, and the action you want the legislator to take.

◆ Don't expect to speak directly with the legislator. Contact the staff person responsible for the issue you want to discuss.

◆ Request a written response so that you have a record of the legislator's position on the subject.

Learn to Handle Public Forums   Public meetings and hearings have a tone and decorum all their own. Formal and informal rules of order and conduct facilitate the decision-making process. Learning how to present your arguments in public forums will provide benefits in both your personal and professional life. Consider these points when speaking in public meetings and hearings:

◆ Prepare ahead of time. Analyze administrative records to determine the history of the issue placed before the legislative body.

◆ Know what you want to say and keep your comments brief.

◆ Identify yourself and your affiliations.

◆ Avoid a public fight with opponents. Be authoritative and courteous in refuting any arguments raised by your opponents. It never helps to make an opponent lose face.

Political Realities

Go back and reread the quotations at the beginning of this chapter. Together they highlight two of the most important aspects of policy making: (1) policies change

TABLE
3-3

Political Realities

Source: C. O. Jones, *An Introduction to the Study of Public Policy*, p. 9. Copyright 1970 Wadsworth Publishing Company. Used with permission.

◆ Events in society are interpreted in different ways by different people at different times.
◆ Many "problems" may result from the same event.
◆ People have varying degrees of access to the policy process in government.
◆ Not all public problems are acted on in government.
◆ Many private problems are acted on in government.
◆ Most problems aren't "solved" by government, though many are acted on there.
◆ Most decision making is based on very little information and poor communication.
◆ Problems and demands are constantly being defined and redefined in the policy process.
◆ Policymakers sometimes define problems for people who have not defined problems for themselves.
◆ Much policy is made without ever clearly defining the problem.
◆ All policy systems have a bias.
◆ No ideal policy system exists apart from the preferences of the architect of that system.

as circumstances and events change, and (2) moving an issue onto the policy agenda can be the most difficult aspect of achieving change.

Getting involved in the policy-making process is one way to strengthen your connections with other people and with your community. It can be frustrating and chaotic at times, but knowing that your effort as an individual improved your community or helped it achieve a common goal can also provide great personal satisfaction. The next time you have the opportunity to become a part of the policy-making process, reflect on the points in Table 3-3, but do not allow these political realities to stop you. Your success as a policy changer can be enhanced by understanding the policy-making process, knowing how to be heard, and relying on persistence and patience.

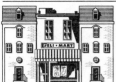 **COMMUNITY LEARNING ACTIVITY**

This Community Learning Activity is designed to help you become acquainted with the policy-making process in foods and nutrition. Go back to the Introduction to this chapter, and choose one of the issues outlined there (for example, "Are dietary guidelines developed for adults appropriate for children?"). Assume that your organization has been asked to respond to legislation on this topic. Carry out the following activities:

1. Briefly outline your position on this issue giving at least two reasons in support of it.
2. List the individuals and organizations in your community that you would contact to build a coalition on the issue. Why are these particular people important to your effort?
3. Draft a letter to your representative in Congress outlining your concerns about the issue and your position on the policy.
4. How would you go about getting the media involved in this issue?
5. Gather and evaluate the positions of your classmates on the particular issue you selected. Provided that at least one opinion differs from your own, was your position on the issue influenced or changed by your classmate's position? What does this tell you about the process of formulating a position on a particular issue?

The Benefits of Mentoring

Mentoring is a skill with the potential to increase your level of job satisfaction and help you achieve your personal and professional goals.

Derived from Greek mythology—Mentor was the wise and trusted guardian, teacher, and friend to whom the adventurer Odysseus entrusted the education of his son—mentoring refers to the deliberate pairing of a "young adult and an older, more experienced adult [in a relationship] that helps the younger individual learn to navigate in the adult world and the world of work. A mentor supports, guides, and counsels the young adult as he or she accomplishes this important task."[1] Although the Greeks were among the first to actively facilitate mentoring, the tradition of apprenticing a young person to a master continued through the Middle Ages. In today's industrial society, the master/apprentice relationship has been transformed into the mentor/protégé relationship. Many examples of mentoring exist in business, the arts, and medicine. Pop rock star Michael Jackson, for example, has often spoken of singer Diana Ross as his mentor.

Roles of the Mentor and the Protégé

A mentor has been described variously as a coach, senior adviser, counselor, experience leader, trainer, master, guide, role model, sponsor, luminary, leader, and boss. One essential ingredient of the mentor/protégé relationship is that each knows what is expected of the other. Mentors may agree to perform one or more of the following functions for protégés:[2]

- ◆ Serve as a source of information about the mission and goals of the organization
- ◆ Provide insight into the organization's management style and philosophy of human development
- ◆ Tutor skill development, effective behavior, and how to perform and function well within the organization
- ◆ Give feedback on performance
- ◆ Assist in career advancement by sponsoring the protégé for promotions and by giving the protégé exposure and access to senior executives
- ◆ Protect the protégé from unjust criticism when necessary
- ◆ Agree to a conclusion of the mentoring relationship when the time is right
- ◆ Maintain the integrity of the mentor/protégé relationship

The protégé likewise has responsibilities to the mentor and to the relationship:

- ◆ Assume responsibility for personal growth and development
- ◆ Endeavor to perform well in more than one area
- ◆ Seek challenging assignments and new responsibilities
- ◆ Be receptive to feedback and coaching
- ◆ Agree to end the relationship when the time is right
- ◆ Maintain the integrity of the mentor/protégé relationship

The mentor/protégé relationship benefits both parties. The mentor has the opportunity to share the insights and wisdom gleaned from years of personal experience, while the

Continued

protégé develops confidence and competence and enjoys new professional challenges. In the words of the actor Tom Berenger, "In the theater, you often learn without knowing where or how it happened. A good mentor helps you to know when you've got it right and, more importantly, helps you know how to do it again."

Benefits of Mentoring

Getting ahead in an organization can be difficult and risky. Mentors help their protégés overcome the internal barriers that may block advancement.[3] Securing a mentor has been shown to offer many advantages. Protégés tend to have higher performance and productivity ratings, to be paid more, and to have greater job satisfaction than nonprotégés. They also have a good working knowledge of the organization and all aspects of its business.

The organization benefits as well. Employees participating in a formal mentoring program have been found to be more productive than nonprotégés. Mentoring programs can be cost-effective, improve long-range planning by increasing the pool of highly qualified employees, and enhance communication channels throughout the organization.

Gender Differences in Mentoring

While mentoring relationships are important for men, they may be essential for women. Compared with male managers, female managers face greater individual, interpersonal, and organizational barriers to recognition and advancement.[4] Mentors serve to protect the female manager from both covert and overt forms of discrimination. A mentor confers legitimacy on a woman's performance, affirms her as an individual, and helps alter coworkers' stereotypic perceptions of female managers. Through "reflected power," mentors signal others within the organization that the female protégé has their backing and approval.[5]

Unfortunately, women tend to be less likely than men to develop these relationships, possibly because they fail to recognize the importance of gaining a sponsor and naively believe that only competence is required for advancement. Another reason may be that women have difficulty accessing suitable mentors. Some male mentors may not be comfortable selecting a female protégé because they perceive her as being a greater "investment" risk than her male counterparts. In addition, male mentors may avoid sponsoring female protégés because they fear potential sexual involvements. In one study, about one-quarter of the 381 professional women surveyed indicated that they had sex with their mentors.[6] The political fallout from such an entanglement can have serious consequences for both parties.[7] When both the mentor and the protégé in a cross-gender relationship work to maintain the integrity of their relationship, the possibility that a romance will develop between them is diminished.

How to Make Mentoring Work for You

The mentoring relationship can be extremely satisfying for both parties. Keep these points in mind when you select a mentor to facilitate your professional and personal growth:

1. Know yourself and what you have to offer your mentor.
2. Be realistic about what you can expect your mentor to help you accomplish.
3. Look for a person who both talks and listens, who has an extensive network of friends and colleagues, who is respected by peers, and who says, "Give it a try!"

Continued

4. Accept that the mentor/protégé relationship may not last a lifetime. Some mentoring relationships may last a year or two, while others persist for decades. Knowing when to end a mentoring relationship is as important as knowing when to search for one.

Over the course of your career, you will probably have several mentors and different types of mentoring relationships, some being more formal than others. Each will be unique, but each will serve to help you figure out who you are and what you can do well. As you mature in your career, find time to mentor others. Mentoring will help ensure that enthusiastic and qualified professionals are recruited and retained for community service in nutrition and dietetics.[8]

1. K. E. Kram, *Mentoring at Work: Developmental Relationships in Organizational Life* (Glenview, Ill.: Scott, Foresman, 1985), p. 2.
2. The section describing the roles of mentors and protégés was adapted from Kram, *Mentoring at Work,* pp. 1–46, and M. Murray, *Beyond the Myths and Magic of Mentoring* (San Francisco: Jossey-Bass, 1991), pp. 1–40.
3. The Ross Professional Development Series, *Linking Strategies for Dietitians: Networking, Liaison Building, and Mentoring* (Columbus, Ohio: Ross Laboratories, 1989), pp. 33–42.
4. S. C. Goh, Sex differences in perceptions of interpersonal work style, career emphasis, supervisory mentoring behavior, and job satisfaction, *Sex Roles* 24 (1991): 701–10.
5. B. R. Ragins, Barriers to mentoring: The female manager's dilemma, *Human Relations* 42 (1989): 1–22.
6. Ibid., p. 9.
7. H. S. Baum, Mentoring: Narcissistic fantasies and Oedipal realities, *Human Relations* 45 (1992): 223–45.
8. B. G. Wenberg, Use of mentor programs in dietetic education, *Journal of the American Dietetic Association* 92 (1992): 71–73.

NOTES

1. This story, the discussion of the policy cycle, and the margin definitions were adapted from D. J. Palumbo, *Public Policy in America—Government in Action* (San Diego: Harcourt Brace Jovanovich, 1988), pp. 1–155.
2. Ibid, p. 8.
3. Landscape of death, *Time* 140 (December 14, 1992): 44.
4. This quotation and portions of the discussion of policy were adapted from B. G. Peters, *American Public Policy—Process and Performance* (New York: Franklin Watts, 1982), pp. 3–85.
5. C. O. Jones, *An Introduction to the Study of Public Policy* (Belmont, Calif.: Wadsworth, 1970), pp. 1–15.
6. Peters, *American Public Policy,* p. 69.
7. J. E. Austin and C. Hitt, *Nutrition Intervention in the United States* (Cambridge, Mass.: Ballinger, 1979), pp. 39–41.
8. L. Carroll, *Alice in Wonderland* (New York: Washington Square Press, 1951).
9. The discussion of how a bill is introduced into Congress was adapted from T. R. Dye, *Politics in States and Communities,* 7th ed. (Englewood Cliffs, N.J.: Prentice-Hall, 1991), pp. 156–75.
10. Society for Nutrition Education, *Influencing Food and Nutrition Policy—A Public Policy Handbook* (Oakland, Calif.: Society for Nutrition Education, 1987), pp. 1–16.
11. *How Congress Works,* 2d ed. (Washington, D.C.: Congressional Quarterly, 1991), p. 140.
12. Society for Nutrition Education, *Influencing Food and Nutrition Policy—A Public Policy Handbook,* p. 5.
13. H. W. Schultz, *Food Law Handbook* (Westport, Conn.: Avi Publishing Company, 1981), pp. 3–21.
14. Committee on the Nutrition Components of Food Labeling, Food and Nutrition Board, Institute of Medicine, National Academy of Sciences, *Nutrition Labeling—Issues and Directions for the 1990s*

(Washington, D.C.: National Academy Press, 1990), pp. 55–73.

15. N. H. Mermelstein, The status of food labeling, *Food Technology* 44 (1990): 86–91.

16. Provisions of the Nutrition Labeling and Education Act of 1990 as cited in *The Congressional Record—House,* July 30, 1990, pp. II 5836–40, and Legislative Highlights, Wrap-up of ADA's issues in the 101st Congress, *Journal of the American Dietetic Association* 90 (1990): 1653–55.

17. Legislative Highlights, Update: The Nutrition Labeling and Education Act of 1990, *Journal of the American Dietetic Association* 91 (1991): 1054.

18. Department of Health and Human Services, Food and Drug Administration, Food labeling; general provisions; nutrition labeling; label format; nutrient content claims; health claims; ingredient labeling; state and local requirements; and exemptions; final rules, *Federal Register* 58 (1993): 2066–2964.

19. Committee on State Food Labeling, Food and Nutrition Board, Institute of Medicine, *Food Labeling—Toward National Uniformity* (Washington, D.C.: National Academy Press, 1992), pp. 141–61.

20. The discussion of the Delaney Clause was adapted from Schultz, *Food Law Handbook,* pp. 171–85, and S. A. Miller and K. Skinner, Science and the law: The basis for new food safety legislation, in *Environmental Aspects of Cancer: The Role of Macro and Micro Components of Foods,* ed. E. L. Wynder, G. A. Leveille, J. H. Weisburger, and G. E. Livingston (Westport, Conn.: Food & Nutrition Press, 1983), pp. 230–37.

21. Expert Panel on Food Safety & Nutrition, Scientific Status Summary, Food biotechnology, *Food Technology* 42 (1988): 133–46.

22. D. Knorr and A. J. Sinskey, Biotechnology in food production and processing, *Science* 229 (1985): 1224–29.

23. S. Harlander, Food biotechnology: Yesterday, today, and tomorrow, *Food Technology* 43 (1989): 196–206.

24. D. A. Kessler, Reinvigorating the Food and Drug Administration, *Food Technology* 46 (1992): 20, 22, 24, 27, 30.

25. The discussion of medical foods was adapted from the Scientific Status Summary of the Expert Panel on Food Safety and Nutrition, Medical foods, *Food Technology* 46 (1992): 87–96.

26. D. E. Pszczola, Highlights of "The nutraceutical initiative: A proposal for economic and regulatory reform," *Food Technology* 46 (1992): 77–79.

27. E. C. Ladd, *The American Polity—The People and Their Government* (New York: W. W. Norton, 1985), p. 351.

28. G. Starling, *Understanding American Politics* (Homewood, Ill.: Dorsey, 1982), pp. 184–85.

29. J. M. Burns, J. W. Peltason, and T. E. Cronin, *Government by the People,* 12th ed. (Englewood Cliffs, N.J.: Prentice-Hall, 1984), pp. 167–68.

30. Ibid., p. 169.

31. H. J. Rubin and I. S. Rubin, *Community Organizing and Development* (New York: Macmillan, 1992), pp. 274–95.

32. Ibid., p. 282.

33. McDonald's Corporation, FOOD FUNdamentals Partnership Kit, 1993.

34. S. C. Finn and B. Bajus, President's Page: Partnerships forge opportunity, innovation, and action, *Journal of the American Dietetic Association* 93 (1993): 195.

35. The description of how to communicate effectively with elected officials was taken from the *Journal of the American Dietetic Association* 92 (1992): 296.

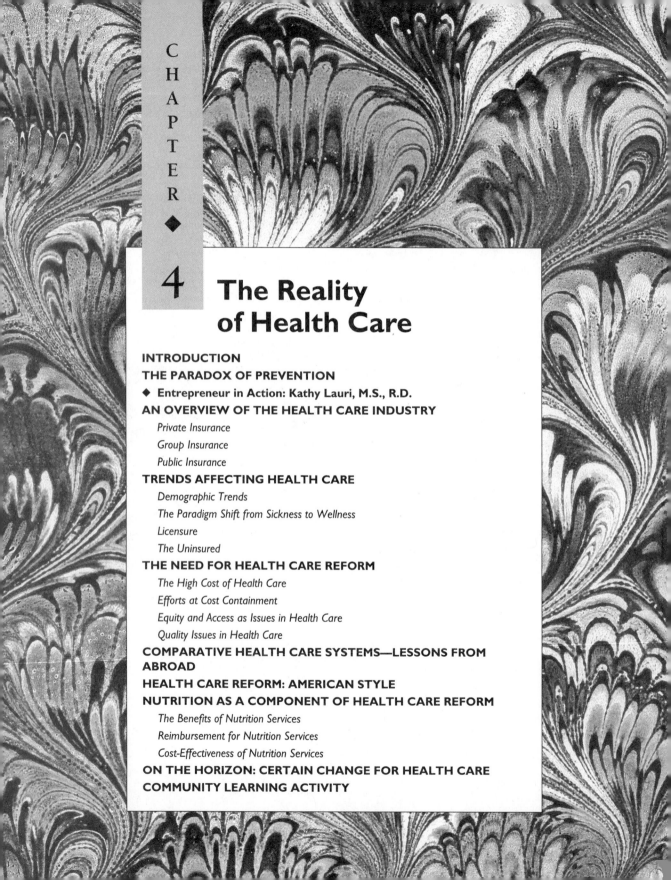

C H A P T E R ◆

4

The Reality of Health Care

Something to Think About . . .

The enjoyment of the highest attainable standard of health is one of the fundamental rights of every human being without distinction of race, religion, political
belief, economic or social condition. . . . Governments have a responsibility for the
health of their peoples which can be fulfilled only by the provision of adequate
health and social measures.
>   —Preamble to the Constitution of the World Health Organization

Introduction

The U.S. health care system is approaching a breaking point. In 1992, Americans
spent more than $839 billion for health care—more than $3160 per person.[1] This
hefty sum represents over 13 percent of the gross national product (GNP)—up
from 9 percent in 1980.[2] Health care expenditures continue to increase at a rate
two to three times greater than inflation. Indeed, federal budget estimates predict
that a quarter to a third of our GNP growth in the next few years will come from
increases in health care spending.

The United States spends more money and a larger percentage of its GNP on
health care than any other nation in the world. In spite of these expenditures,
however, internationally the United States ranks 20th in infant mortality and
17th in life expectancy.[3] Consequently, many are asking, "Are we getting value
for our dollars?"

In 1992, diet-related disease consumed a major portion of the nation's health
costs. Consider the following list:[4]

- ◆ $136 billion spent for coronary heart disease in direct health expenditures
  alone.
- ◆ More than $11 billion spent for stroke health care.
- ◆ More than $72 billion spent for cancer treatment including lost productivity.
- ◆ Between $3.5 and $7.5 billion spent annually on low birth weight infants.
  Medicaid paid almost $19,000 per delivery of a low birth weight infant
  versus $3500 per delivery of a normal weight infant.
- ◆ $288 billion, or 36 percent of health care costs, spent for older citizens,
  while Medicare spent just $97.2 billion on older citizens in 1992.
- ◆ $20 billion spent annually on diabetes treatment.
- ◆ Another $33 billion spent annually on illusionary "quick fix" weight-loss
  solutions by 65 million Americans.

Note the large sums of money spent on preventable diseases. Health promotion and disease prevention can readily reduce the proportion of our health care dollar spent treating such conditions. Federal publications such as *The Surgeon General's Report on Nutrition and Health* (1988), the *Diet and Health Report* (1989), and *Healthy People 2000: National Health Promotion and Disease Prevention Objectives* (1990) have clearly documented the relationship between diet and health. *The Surgeon General's Report* points out that eating and drinking habits contribute to heart disease, cancers, strokes, diabetes mellitus, obesity, and other killing diseases.[5] *Healthy People 2000* states that good health comes from improving one's quality of life and decreasing unnecessary illness and premature death and disability.[6] These documents were to be the catalyst for ushering in a new era of prevention. Nevertheless, in spite of the current evidence linking diet to disease, the United States spends only 4 percent of its health care dollars on disease prevention.[7]

Current nutrition recommendations are discussed in Chapter 5.

The challenge today is not in determining appropriate nutrition recommendations to offer the public, but rather in providing the public with the opportunity to benefit from appropriate nutrition services. Today's consumers need information and guidance to make the wisest health choices, and nutrition plays a daily role in those choices.[8]

The Paradox of Prevention

To a greater extent than most of us are willing to accept, today's disorders of overweight, heart disease, cancer, blood pressure, and diabetes are by and large preventable. In this light, true health insurance is not what one carries on a plastic card, but what one does for oneself.
—L. Power in G. Edlin and E. Golanty, Health and Wellness, 3d ed.

A paradox exists today in health care in the United States. As Louis Sullivan, the former secretary of health and human services observed, prevention "must become a national obsession."[9] He went on to say: Health promotion and disease prevention comprise perhaps our best opportunity to reduce the ever-increasing portion of our resources that we spend to treat preventable illness and functional impairment. . . .

Yet the Medicaid and Medicare systems and the Health Care Financing Administration provide almost no reimbursement for prevention activities and/or procedures. In addition, major third-party payers offer limited reimbursement for preventive procedures.[10]

In 1974, a landmark Canadian document—*The Lalonde Report: A New Perspective on the Health of Canadians*—was the first modern government document to acknowledge that our emphasis upon a biomedical health care system is wrong. It stressed that we must look beyond the traditional health care (sick care) system if we wish to improve the public's health. The report was followed by similar reports in Great Britain, Sweden, and the United States.

Public policy in the 1990s is now attempting to direct our medical system toward health promotion, disease prevention, and the efficient use of scarce resources. The American Dietetic Association (ADA) is among the organizations involved in formulating a reform policy that assures access to appropriate and affordable health care for all.[12] The ADA's position paper states that quality health care should be available, accessible, and affordable to all Americans.

◆ ENTREPRENEUR IN ACTION

Introducing Kathy Lauri, M.S., R.D.

◆ HER BACKGROUND . . .

Kathy Lauri began her career as a hospital-based clinical dietitian providing diet instruction to patients with heart disease and their families. She is currently Account Supervisor at Porter/Novelli, a public relations firm based in New York City, where her clients include pharmaceutical companies and medical trade associations. Through direct education programs and the media, she educates health care professionals and consumers about health issues. She is currently working on a program that addresses the problem of undertreatment of pain and the need for appropriate pain management in people with cancer and AIDS. Lauri is an intrapreneur—that is, someone who develops creative ideas and programs within the framework of an organization.

◆ SHE HAS THIS TO SAY ABOUT ENTREPRENEURSHIP . . .

"An entrepreneur is one who undertakes a project that is especially difficult, complicated, or risky. For me, leaving my job as a clinical dietitian and entering the field of public relations *was* risky, simply because I was entering the unknown. But I soon learned that I was well-suited for the skills required in this area. What I have learned in this job is that public relations is really the business of education through communication."

Lauri can appreciate the risk that goes with a new venture, for she had the opportunity to be in on the ground-floor development of the first comprehensive nutrition guidelines for people with AIDS. "In 1987, when I first began wearing my public relations hat," she says, "little was discussed or done about the wasting syndrome or the eating difficulties experienced by people with AIDS. Although the value of proper nutrition in AIDS treatment was clearly accepted by physicians, in practice, nutrition assessment and counseling were not routinely implemented in the clinical setting. My colleagues and I found that many people with AIDS were following unsound dietary practices that could jeopardize their already compromised health."

With this in mind, Lauri and her colleagues developed a program to address this issue. Their first step was to form a task force, the Task Force on Nutrition Support in AIDS, whose charge was to formulate nutrition guidelines for people with AIDS. The 11-member task force was comprised of researchers and practitioners who specialized in nutrition and AIDS treatment.

"The guidelines," indicates Lauri, "addressed the issue of appropriate nutrition intervention over the course of the disease, but they were intended for physicians, not patients. So we developed a patient pamphlet—printed in both English and Spanish—to provide practical advice about a variety of problems such as G.I. distress, mouth sores, and weight loss. Eventually, the guidelines and patient pamphlets were made available to physicians, dietitians, and other caregivers involved in the management of AIDS patients."

Lauri found the project very satisfying from a career perspective. "This project taught me about working as part of a team, helped me to think more creatively, and enabled me to build relationships with nutrition 'thought leaders.' As a dietitian, I was able to reach millions of people with information that was truly critical to their well-being and quality of life. I made a difference!"

Quality health care is defined to include nutrition services that are integral to meeting the *preventive* and therapeutic health care needs of all segments of the population.[13]

Many studies show that early detection and intervention, immunization, and behavior change could significantly reduce many of the leading causes of death and disability.[14] By investing in health maintenance through health promotion and disease prevention, we can avoid the much greater economic and social costs of disease and injury. As Louis Sullivan has pointed out, we can preserve good health *and* reduce costs if we concentrate on the "front end" rather than waiting to devote substantial resources to illness and disability after they strike.[15]

This chapter introduces you to the challenges facing health care in the 1990s. One question, for example, is how we can balance the physician/medical model of health care with a wellness/preventive medicine model. Other issues include resource allocation and cost containment, social justice and adequate access to health care resources, program accountability and quality in health care, and funding for health promotion and disease prevention. We hope you will become an advocate for health care reform and, specifically, for a model of health care that includes nutrition services as a valuable and reimbursable component. Before we talk about changing our present system of health care, however, we must first understand how that system works.

An Overview of the Health Care Industry

Our pluralistic system of health care includes many parts: private insurance, group insurance, Medicare, Medicaid, Workers' Compensation, the Veterans' Administration medical care system, the Department of Defense hospitals and clinics, the Public Health Service's Native American Health Service, state and local public health programs, and the Department of Justice's Federal Bureau of Prisons. One other piece is missing from the system: the uninsured. Currently, the system is structured around the provision of health insurance.

There are three general categories of **health insurance** in the United States: traditional private, prepaid, **fee-for-service** insurance; private, prepaid **group contract** insurance; and public health insurance.[16] Fee-for-service plans can be either individual or group policies. Group policies make up over 70 percent of all policies and are usually employer based and offered as a fringe benefit.

◆ PRIVATE INSURANCE

Private insurance is provided by both commercial insurance companies and not-for-profit organizations such as Blue Cross and Blue Shield and independent employee health plans. Approximately 147 million Americans have health insurance coverage through an employer-sponsored plan.[17] The traditional fee-for-service plans of the 1980s account for only 16 percent of insurance coverage today. Critics of fee-for-service plans claim that they encourage physicians to provide more services than are necessary.[18]

Health insurance Protection against the financial burdens associated with health care services and assurance of access to the health care system.

Fee-for-service A billing system in which the provider of care charges a fee for each service rendered.

Group contract A health insurance contract that is made with an employer or other entity and covers a group of persons identified as individuals by reference to their relationship to the entity.

◆ GROUP INSURANCE

Currently, the health care financing system is undergoing a transition from the unmanaged fee-for-service system to a more **managed-care system**, represented by the **health maintenance organizations (HMOs)** and **preferred provider organizations (PPOs)**. Both are prepaid group practice plans that offer health care services through groups of medical practitioners.

Congress provided an impetus for the growth of HMOs when it passed the Health Maintenance Organization Act of 1973 in an effort to contain utilization, control escalating medical costs, and improve the quality of health care. The law requires employers with 25 or more employees to offer their employees HMO membership as an alternative to traditional health insurance plans.

In HMOs, physicians practice as a group, sharing facilities and medical records. The physicians may either be salaried or provide contractual services. There are four general models of HMOs:

◆ **Staff HMO.** A model in which the HMO owns and operates its own facility, is equipped for laboratory, pharmacy, and X-ray services, and hires its own physicians and other health care providers.

◆ **Group practice HMO.** A model in which the HMO contracts with a multi-specialty group practice to provide health care services to its members. A predetermined payment is made to the group for each HMO enrollee.

◆ **Network HMO.** A model in which the HMO contracts with multiple group practices, hospitals, and other providers to provide services to its members.

◆ **Independent practice association (IPA).** A model in which physicians work in their own offices and serve both HMO and non-HMO patients.

The HMO idea—a fixed cost to the consumer, with health care insurer and health care provider as one and the same—is viewed as a more cost-effective way of practicing medicine than the fee-for-service systems. Because HMOs make money by keeping you healthy, they have a greater stake in your wellness than most fee-for-service doctors.[19]

Prepaid group health plans emphasize health promotion, since they provide health care services at a preset cost. By keeping people healthy, HMOs avoid lengthy hospitalizations and costly services. Enrollees of HMOs are hospitalized less frequently than patients of fee-for-service physicians.[20]

◆ PUBLIC INSURANCE

The two major public health insurance plans in the United States are **Medicare** and **Medicaid**. A comparison of their features is provided in Table 4-1. Medicare is a federal health insurance program for people 65 years of age or older, people of any age with permanent kidney failure that requires dialysis or a kidney replacement, and certain people with disabilities under 65 years. It is administered by the Health Care Financing Administration (HCFA, pronounced *hic-fa*) of the Department of Health and Human Services. The Social Security Administration provides information about the program and handles enrollment.[21]

Managed care An approach to paying for health care in which insurers try to limit the use of health services, reduce costs, or both. The term typically refers to HMOs and PPOs. Managed care aims to prevent unnecessary treatment by requiring enrollees to obtain approval for nonemergency hospital care and denying payment for wasteful treatment.

Health maintenance organization (HMO) A prepaid plan that both finances and delivers health care. Enrollees do not pay deductibles or file claims. Checkups and other forms of preventive care typically are covered. Enrollees generally must use the plan's providers or face financial penalties. In many HMOs, providers are paid a fixed sum, eliminating the financial incentive to overtreat.

Preferred provider organization (PPO) A group of providers, usually hospitals and doctors, who agree to provide health care to subscribers for a negotiated fee, which is usually discounted. PPOs are subject to peer review and strict use controls in exchange for a consistent volume of patients and speedy turnaround on claim payments.

Medicare A health insurance program for (1) people who are 65 years of age or over and eligible for Social Security benefits; (2) qualified railroad retirement beneficiaries; (3) people eligible for Social Security disability; (4) certain workers with end-stage renal disease; and (5) merchant seamen.

TABLE

4-1

A Comparison of Medicare and Medicaid Services

Source: Adapted from U.S. Department of Health and Human Services, *1992 Guide to Health Insurance for People with Medicare* (Washington, D.C.: U.S. Department of Health and Human Services, 1992), pp. 1–19; H. J. Cornacchia and S. Barrett, *Consumer Health: A Guide to Intelligent Decisions,* 4th ed. (St. Louis: Times Mirror/Mosby, 1989), pp. 488–89.

	MEDICARE	MEDICAID
Administration	Social Security Office Federal Insurance Program	Local welfare office Federal-state partnership assistance program
Financing	Trust funds from Social Security; contributions from insured	Taxes from federal, state, and local sources
Eligibility	People 65 years of age and older, people with end-stage renal disease, people eligible for Social Security disability programs for more than 2 years	Needy and low-income people, people 65 or older, the blind, persons with disabilities, members of families with dependent children, all pregnant women and infants with family incomes below 133% of poverty level, possibly others
Benefits	Same in all states **Hospital insurance (Part A)** *helps* pay for inpatient hospital care, skilled nursing facility care, home health care, hospice care.	Varies from state to state **Hospital services:** inpatient and outpatient hospital services, other laboratory and X-ray services, physician services, screening, diagnosis, and treatment of children, home health care services
	Medical insurance (Part B) *helps* pay for physicians' services, outpatient hospital services, home health visits, diagnostic X-ray, laboratory, and other tests; necessary ambulance services, other medical services and supplies, and outpatient physical therapy and speech pathology.	**Medical services:** many states pay for dental care, health clinic services, eyecare and glasses, prescribed medications, other diagnostic, rehabilitative, and preventive services, including nutrition services
	Exclusions: regular dental care and dentures, routine physical exams and related tests, preventive services, eyeglasses, hearing aids and examinations to prescribe and fit them, prescription drugs, nursing home care (except skilled nursing care), custodial care, immunizations (except for pneumonia), cosmetic surgery	Varies from state to state
Premium Costs	Part A: none if eligible, or $192/month Part B: $31.80/month	None (federal government contributes 50% to 80% to states to cover eligible persons)

Medicaid A federally aided, state-administered program that provides medical benefits for certain low-income persons in need of health and medical care.

Medicare consists of two separate parts: hospital insurance (Part A) and medical insurance (Part B). No monthly premium is required for Medicare Part A if a person or his or her spouse is entitled to benefits under either Social Security or the Railroad Retirement System or has worked a sufficient period of time in federal, state, or local government to be insured. Those not meeting these qualifications may purchase Part A coverage if they are at least age 65 years of age and meet certain requirements.

Part A provides hospital insurance benefits that include up to 90 days of inpatient care annually with a 20 percent **coinsurance** fee for hospital charges. Hospital inpatient charges are reimbursed according to a **prospective payment system** known as **diagnosis-related groups (DRGs)**—discussed in detail later in the chapter. Since 1983, the government has shifted a larger portion of health care costs to Medicare beneficiaries through larger **deductibles**, greater use of services with coinsurance, and use of services not covered by Medicare.

Medicare Part B is an optional insurance program financed through premiums paid by enrollees and contributions from federal funds; it provides medical insurance benefits (see Table 4-1). The two most notable gaps in Medicare coverage are prescription drugs and long-term institutional care.[22] Prescription drugs are not covered at all under the Medicare program. Only 100 days of long-term care are covered annually. Thereafter, patients or their families must either pay the costs themselves or "spend down" to be eligible for Medicaid long-term care coverage. Medicare enrollees often purchase **supplemental insurance** policies from private insurance companies to help pay the deductible, coinsurance fees, and prescription drug costs.

Medicaid was established as a joint state and federal program, with the latter paying 50 percent or more of the costs depending on a state's per capita income. Medicaid currently covers less than half of those below the poverty line.[23] To be eligible, one must meet three criteria: income, categorical, and resource. Those eligible for Aid to Families with Dependent Children (AFDC) and Supplemental Security Income (SSI) are automatically eligible for Medicaid. For example, an elderly couple in 1988 had to have a combined income of less than $472 a month to be eligible for Medicaid. In 1989, the average income threshold for a family of three to qualify for Medicaid was $4942, approximately 49 percent of the federal poverty level of $10,080.[24]

To meet the categorical requirements, one must be a member of a family with dependent children or be aged, blind, or a person with a disability. To pass the resource test, the maximum liquid resources a family could have in 1986 were $1000, a house, and a motor vehicle valued at no more than $1500.[25] Income and asset eligibility standards vary widely among the 50 states.

Trends Affecting Health Care

The future of health care in the United States will be shaped by current trends in society at large and in the field of health care, as well as by the choices we make for health care reform. Some of the trends and issues that will shape the future of health care are described in the next sections.

◆ DEMOGRAPHIC TRENDS

Between 1946 and 1964, 76.4 million babies were born in the United States; these individuals now make up one-third of the population.[26] By the year 2030, the

Coinsurance A cost-sharing requirement that provides that the insured will assume a portion of the costs of covered services.

Prospective payment system (PPS) A payment system under which hospitals are paid a fixed sum per case according to a schedule of diagnosis-related groups.

Diagnosis-related groups (DRGs) A method of classifying patients' illnesses according to principal diagnosis and treatment requirements for the purpose of establishing payment rates. Under Medicare each DRG has its own payment rate, which a hospital is paid regardless of the actual cost of treatment. The rate is payment in full, nonnegotiable, and not subject to appeal.

Deductible The amount of loss or expense that must be incurred by a person who is insured before an insurer will assume any liability for all or part of the remaining cost of covered services. Deductibles may be fixed dollar amounts or the value of specified services (e.g., two days of hospital care or one visit to a physician).

Supplemental health insurance Insurance that covers medical expenses not covered by separate health insurance held by the insured.

A recent Senate bill—the Long-Term Care Family Security Act—if passed, would make every American eligible for government-sponsored home services and community-based or short-stay nursing home care. If extended nursing home care is needed, the bill would make it possible for nondisabled spouses to retain their own income, $30,000–$60,000 in assets, and the family home.

baby boom will become a senior boom, with 21 percent of the population—30 million more Americans than today—over 65 years of age.[27]

Not only will the elderly be greater in number, but they will potentially require care for a greater number of years, placing a heavier burden on the long-term care system (see Figure 4-1). Since older Americans consume a disproportionate amount of medical care, the demand for such care, including pharmaceutical products and services, can be expected to rise.[28]

Racial and geographic factors in the population are also important to the shape of the future. In some parts of the United States, particularly the Southwest, the Hispanic population will dramatically increase. To the extent that such a population may exhibit differing utilization patterns for medical services or pharmaceuticals, such changes may significantly affect the marketplace. Geographic factors will also be important, especially if the population drift from the Northeast to the Southwest and the Sun Belt continues.[29]

◆ THE PARADIGM SHIFT FROM SICKNESS TO WELLNESS

For several decades, the dominant paradigm has been the medical model. During the 1970s, people were guided by the philosophy that the health care system would do everything possible in terms of curative and treatment services to make them well. In the 1980s, people began to view wellness as a function of prevention and to accept responsibility for their own health. The focus on the pursuit of health during the 1980s, marked by an increased interest in nutrition, fitness, and health promotion, was reflected in the growth of corporate "wellness" programs and a widening choice of health care practitioners.

Our health care system still contains a number of barriers to focusing on prevention of poor health habits, however. The biomedical approach to illness under-

FIGURE

4-1

Number of Elderly Needing Long-term Care, 1990 and 2030

Source: *A Call for Action: Final Report of the Pepper Commission* (Washington, D.C.: U.S. Government Printing Office, 1990).

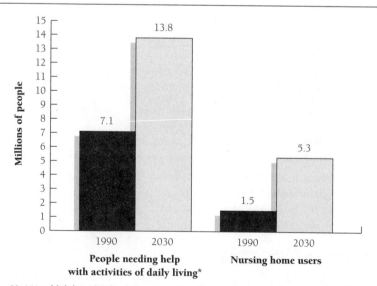

*Activities of daily living (ADL) include activities such as bathing, dressing, toileting, continence, and feeding.

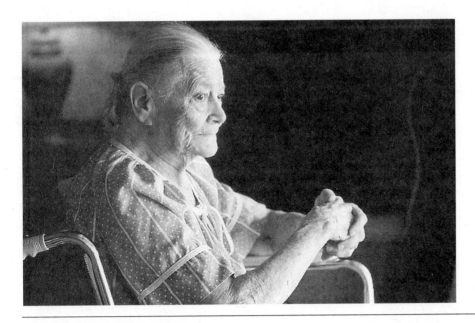

By the year 2030, the number of elderly needing nursing home care will triple.

estimates and underemphasizes behavioral or lifestyle influences on disease. Physicians think in terms of treating or correcting conditions rather than preventing them. Also, both formal diagnostic processes and systematic reimbursement for prevention are lacking. Consider, for example, that Medicare Part A will reimburse for enormous hospital bills, but Part B won't reimburse for prevention.

The challenge for the 1990s is to change the United States's approach to health care from a system based on treatment of acute conditions to one based on disease prevention and health promotion. Physicians, public health workers, registered dietitians and other health practitioners, health educators, and community health organizations have joined ranks to emphasize health promotion and disease prevention as a more economical route to good health than the more costly procedures necessitated by sickness and disease.[30]

◆ LICENSURE

Licensure protects the public from the fraudulent and unqualified practitioners of various alternative health care therapies that have made inroads into the health care marketplace. Licensure of physicians has been the principal social mechanism for quality control in health care. In the past two decades, increasing numbers of *licensed,* nonphysician health care providers, such as nurse practitioners, physician assistants, midwives, physical therapists, and dental hygienists, have appeared. They provide at a lower cost many services formerly reserved for doctors.[31]

The Professional Focus in Chapter 5 discusses nutrition and health fraud and offers tips on spotting quackery.

◆ THE UNINSURED

In theory, health care coverage is available to virtually all U.S. citizens through one of four routes: Medicare for the elderly and people with disabilities, Medicaid for

Licensure of Nutrition Professionals

In medicine, the educational standards for the medical degree (M.D.) are governed by law. Unfortunately, in many states, the term *nutritionist* is not legally defined at present, and as a result, the public can be the hapless prey of anyone who wishes to use this title. Some "nutritionists" obtain their diplomas and titles without the rigorous training required for a legitimate nutrition degree. Due to lax state laws, it is even possible for an irresponsible "correspondence school"—a diploma mill—to pass out degrees to anyone who pays a fee.

Licensure of qualified nutritionists protects consumers from unqualified practitioners, particularly those who have no training in nutrition but nevertheless refer to themselves as "nutritionists." Licensure is designed to protect the public, control malpractice, and ensure minimum standards of practice.

Today, better consumer protection with respect to nutrition services is evident in many states. As of 1991, 29 states had enacted some form of licensure law. Several states have passed legislation restricting the fraudulent use of the title "dietitian." In Alabama, self-styled nutritionists with diploma mill degrees are now forbidden to use the nutritionist title. Several other states have passed legislation to prohibit people from calling themselves nutritionists without a license that requires a background in dietetics.

The advantages of licensure are clear. Americans are accustomed to identifying *licensed* health professionals. The initials L.D. (licensed dietitian) after a person's name assure consumers, health professionals, and insurance companies that the person providing the nutrition services meets the specific professional standards established by the state's Department of Professional Regulation.*

*S. J. Gillespie, Statement of cost benefits, *Reimbursement and Insurance Coverage for Nutrition Services* (Chicago: American Dietetic Association, 1991), p. 107.

low-income women and children and some low-income men and people with certain disabilities, employer-subsidized coverage at the workplace, or self-purchased coverage for those ineligible for the previous three.[32] Efforts to control health care costs, however, have led to an estimated 37 million people with no insurance coverage at all, and to perhaps an even larger number whose coverage is inadequate for any major illness.[33]

Who, then, are the uninsured? Statistics show that they are not the elderly, who have Medicare, or the very poor, who have Medicaid. Instead, those who lack coverage are primarily people in the middle—for example, the working poor and people who work for small businesses. They include the self-employed, those who work part-time, seasonal workers, the unemployed, and full-time workers whose employers offer unaffordable insurance or none at all.[34] These persons are classified further as the employed uninsured, the nonworking uninsured, and the medically uninsurable. Included among the uninsured are 10 to 12 million children.[35]

The employed uninsured number 15 million and, with their dependents, represent 70 percent of all uninsured persons. The second group, the nonworking uninsured, number about 9 million; they include the homeless, some deinstitutionalized mentally ill patients, and low-income people who do not qualify for

Medicaid because they are not categorically eligible or because their income is above the cutoff level for their state. Finally, a small but growing group of 1 million people are unable to obtain insurance because of a preexisting medical condition.[36] For example, some AIDS patients and persons infected with HIV are not able to obtain insurance.

When those without health insurance do get sick, they often wind up using the most expensive treatment available—hospital emergency-room care—or they delay getting treatment and later require more expensive and prolonged medical services. These costs are shifted to the people who are insured.

The Need for Health Care Reform

To determine the rating of a particular health care system, one must examine three crucial variables: cost, quality, and access.[37] At the zero end of the scale is no health care system. As already discussed, millions of Americans cannot afford to buy into or gain meaningful, ongoing access to any health care at all. At the other end of the scale is high-quality, reasonably priced, accessible health care. On such a scale, how does the U.S. health care system rate? Before you respond, consider the following scenario:[38]

> Imagine you are the decision maker in a large corporation and I come in to you and try to sell you a product. I say that I want to sell you a key piece of equipment that meets the following specifications:
>
> ◆ It will cost you $3200 per employee per year.
>
> ◆ It will consume up to half of each profit dollar and will rise in price by 15–30 percent annually.
>
> ◆ There is a tremendous unexplained variation in this product depending on who uses it.
>
> ◆ There is no way to measure its quality in terms of appropriateness, reliability, or outcome.
>
> ◆ And, you'll just have to take my word for it when I tell you that we adhere to the highest professional standards.

Would you buy this product? Many believe the current U.S. health care system fits this description. Not only is it expensive, but we don't necessarily know what we're paying for, or if what we're paying for is worth it.[39]

Health care reform refers to the efforts undertaken to ensure that everyone in the United States has access to quality health care at an affordable price. Among the challenges for health care reform are how to make health care accessible to everyone, contain costs, provide nursing home care to those who need it, and ensure that Medicare and Medicaid can serve all who are eligible.[40]

As you will see, cost, access, and quality are interrelated; manipulating one has an astounding impact on the others. For example, some people argue that we should abandon free enterprise and turn the system over to the government, as has been done in other countries, including Canada. Critics of government-run

The computerized axial tomography (CAT) scan is a noninvasive procedure used to visualize internal organs and structure, such as tumors.

health care systems say they appear promising at first but soon bog down in bureaucracy, unable to keep pace with advances in medical technology. Some point to the Canadians who come south to the United States to purchase treatment out of their own pockets rather than wait in queues. Consider the CAT scanner: this diagnostic tool is commonplace in the United States, but the Canadian province of Alberta (four times as large as Florida) has only two scanners for its population of 2.4 million.[41] The question arises, How can the scope of the system be extended without sacrificing quality?

Health care policymakers are studying alternative models of delivery and financing in hopes of applying other nations' successes to the United States. The quest for a new health care strategy is particularly pressing because public sentiment for health care reform is at unprecedented levels.[42] The U.S. health care system appears to have both higher costs (see Figure 4-2) and less access than the systems of other industrialized nations. During the 1980s, U.S. health care trends differed from those in other nations in a variety of ways, most notably, rising

FIGURE

4-2

Total Health Expenditures as a Percentage of Gross Domestic Product (GDP),* 1970–1989

Source: Organization of Economic Cooperation and Development, Paris, 1991. Reprinted from *Hospitals*, Vol. 65, No. 10, by permission, May 20, 1991, Copyright 1991, American Hospital Publishing, Inc.

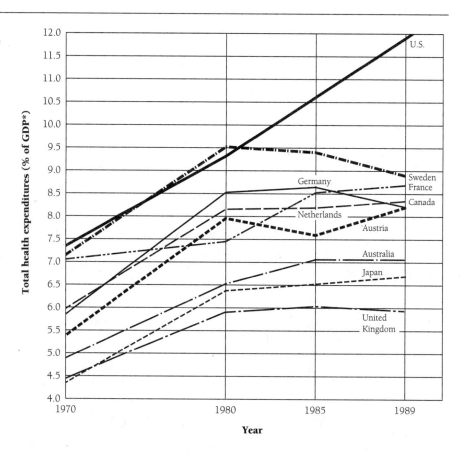

*Gross domestic product (GDP) represents the total value of a nation's output, income or expenditures produced within its borders. GDP is more specific than gross national product (GNP), the total retail market value of all goods and services.

costs, eroding access, and quality in health care service delivery. The following
sections consider each of these in turn.

◆ THE HIGH COST OF HEALTH CARE

Health care inflation is well established. Figure 4-3 tracks the rise in U.S. health
care costs since 1960. Since that year, health care expenditures have increased
over 800 percent. The level of health care activity is expected to grow as a result
of various factors, including an aging population, increased demand (fostered in
part by more consumer awareness of health issues), and continuing advances in
medicine, which make it possible to do more for people than ever before.[43]

A major contributor to health care expenditures in the United States is the
cost of the insurance process itself. Figure 4-4 shows the trends in administrative
costs in both Canada and the United States since 1960. Note that 30 years ago,
when the U.S. system was still dominated by not-for-profit insurers reimbursing
private medical practitioners and not-for-profit hospitals, the overhead costs were
proportionally lower—similar to Canada's. Since then, administrative costs have
increased, while coverage has decreased.[44]

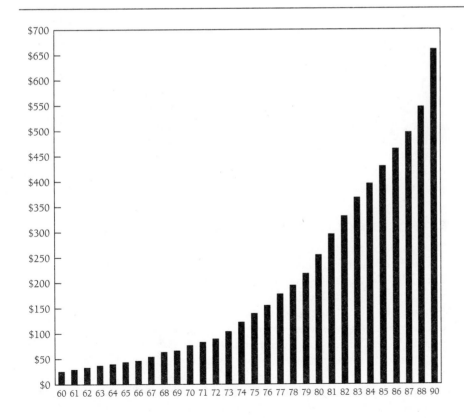

FIGURE

4-3

**National Health
Expenditures (billions of
dollars), 1960–1990**
Source: Adapted from *Source Book
of Health Insurance Data*
(Washington, D.C.: Health Insurance
Association of America, 1992), p. 49.

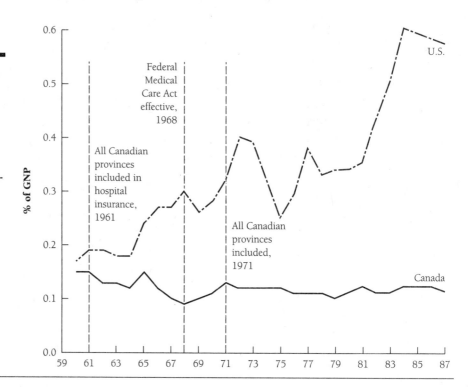

FIGURE

4-4

Costs of Insurance and Administration as a Share of GNP, Canada and the United States, 1960–1987

Source: R. G. Evans, Tension, compression, and shear: Directions, stresses, and outcomes of health care cost control, *Journal of Health Politics, Policy, and Law* 15: 1. Copyright Duke University Press, 1990. Reprinted with permission.

Yet another factor contributing to the cost of our health care is the practice of defensive medicine and the associated phenomenon of ever-rising professional-liability costs. Some say that we have become a litigious society. At present a neurosurgeon in New York City pays more than $70,000 for malpractice insurance.[45] The cost of health care would be dramatically reduced if physicians did not feel forced to practice defensive medicine.

Copayment The portion of the charge that the patient must pay.

Third-party reimbursement involves three parties in the process of paying for medical services: The first party (patient or client) receives a service from the second party (physician, hospital, other health care provider). The third party (insurance company, government) pays the bill. The first party may also pay 20 percent or less as coinsurance of the second party's fee.

◆ EFFORTS AT COST CONTAINMENT

Efforts to curb soaring health care costs cover a broad spectrum: slowing hospital construction, modifying hospital and physician reimbursement mechanisms, reducing the length of hospital stays, increasing **copayments** and deductibles for insured employees and Medicare recipients, changing eligibility requirements for Medicaid, reducing unnecessary surgery by requiring patients to obtain second opinions, restricting the access of new technology, encouraging alternative delivery systems, and emphasizing prevention.[46]

The recent cost-containment effort in the United States is actually a fierce competition among *third-party* payers (government, insurance companies, employers) to control their own costs. This effort has been characterized by three trends listed on the next page.[47]

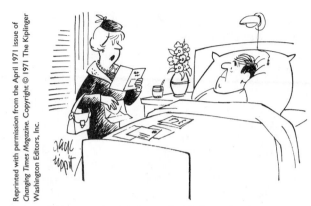

"It's a get-well card from your hospitalization insurance company."

1. There is a movement away from traditional fee-for-service health care to newer models of managed care, evident in the increasing enrollments in HMOs and PPOs.

2. As more and more of their profits are siphoned off into health care coverage, companies are increasingly attempting to manage the health care of their employees themselves to reduce expenditures. In an effort to avoid **cost shifting,** many businesses are **self-insuring** their health plans, thereby assuming the risks involved.

3. The payers (government, insurance companies, employers) are actively setting **reimbursement** restrictions and limitations.

The largest components of national health care expenditures are hospital care (39 percent) and physician services (21 percent).[48] Therefore, efforts to contain costs have largely been aimed at these providers. One example of cost containment is the prospective payment system (PPS) that the federal government implemented as a result of the 1983 Social Security Act Amendments. The purpose of the PPS was to change the behavior of health care providers by changing incentives under which care is provided and reimbursed.[49] Prospective payment means knowing the amount of payment in advance. The PPS uses diagnosis-related groups (DRGs) as a basis for reimbursement. Patients are classified according to their **principal diagnosis,** secondary diagnosis, sex, age, and surgical procedures.

The DRG approach is based on a system of classifying hospital admissions. The system begins with the ninth edition of *International Classification of Diseases—Clinical Modifications,* abbreviated **ICD-9-CM,** which contains approximately 10,000 possible reasons for a hospital admission, organized into 23 major categories. The 23 categories are subdivided into 490 DRGs. Tables compute average cost per discharge by state, region (rural or urban), hospital bed size, and other factors.[50] All DRGs have been assigned a *relative weight* that reflects the cost of caring for a patient in the particular category. Table 4-2 shows a sample payment based on DRGs. Note that a patient with a complication or comorbidity (for example, with malnutrition) is assigned a higher relative weight, reflecting the need for more intensive services.

Self-insured employer An employer that pays medical costs directly rather than through an insurance company.

Cost shifting A much criticized aspect of the existing health care system in which hospitals and other providers bill indemnity insurers higher rates to recover the costs of charity care and to make up for discounts given to HMOs, PPOs, Medicare, and Medicaid.

Reimbursement Payment made by a third party (e.g., government or private or commercial insurance).

Principal diagnosis The condition that is chiefly responsible for the patient's need for health care services. The principal diagnosis determines the payment the hospital receives for Medicare.

TABLE 4-2		Sample Payment Based on DRGs, with and without Complication/Comorbid Condition					
NAME OF DRG	DRG NO.	1991 MEDICARE RELATIVE WEIGHT		BASE RATE		PAYMENT AMOUNT
Respiratory infections and inflammations without complication/comorbid condition	080	1.0404	×	$4000	=	$4162
Respiratory infections and inflammations with complication/comorbid condition	079	1.8144	×	$4000	=	$7258

Source: D. D'Abate Cicenas, Increasing Medicare reimbursement through improved DRG coding, *Reimbursement and Insurance Coverage for Nutrition Services* (Chicago: American Dietetic Association, 1991), p. 53. Used with permission of Ross Products Division, Abbott Laboratories, Columbus, OH 43216, © 1990 Ross Products Division, Abbott Laboratories.

*Secondary diagnoses are also referred to as **comorbidities**. A comorbid condition is present at the time of admission to the hospital but is not the primary reason for treating that patient. For example, if a patient is admitted for a chole-cystectomy and has diabetes melli-tus, diabetes mellitus is a comorbid condition.*

ICD-9-CM (International Classification of Diseases—Clinical Modifications, 9th edition) Codes used by health care providers on billing forms to classify diseases/diagnoses.

One consequence of the PPS has been an increased focus on outpatient services as opposed to more costly inpatient care. For dietetics, the trend has brought increased consultation in outpatient settings, such as hospital nutrition clinics, home health agencies, private-practice counseling, HMOs, community health centers and clinics, and group patient education classes.[51]

◆ EQUITY AND ACCESS AS ISSUES IN HEALTH CARE

Is health care a basic right? Most people in the United States would answer affirmatively. Public opinion polls show that a large majority of people in the United States believe that all citizens are entitled to access to health care.[52] In reality, as deVise has observed, health care may be more of a privilege than a right:

> If you are either very poor, blind, disabled, over 65, male, female, white, or live in a middle- or upper-class neighborhood in a large urban center, you belong to a privileged class of health care recipients, and your chances of survival are good. . . . But, if you are none of these, if you are only average poor, under 65, female, black, or live in a low-income urban neighborhood, small town, or rural area, you are a disenfranchised citizen as far as health care rights go, and your chances of survival are not good.[53]

In 1983, a presidential commission studying ethical issues in medicine stated, "Society has a moral obligation to ensure that everyone has access to adequate [health] care without being subjected to excessive burdens."[54] Proponents of this view argue that just as the federal government provides for defense, postal delivery, and certain other services, it should provide at least a *minimal* amount of basic health care.[55]

This debate leads to another question, access to what? What *is* an acceptable level of health care? The states that have considered or passed health care plans for their uninsured have aimed at providing "basic" or "minimum" health care benefits unlike the "comprehensive benefits" offered through the national health plans of other industrialized countries.

Comprehensive benefits, of course, do not necessarily mean unlimited care. The right to health care in Britain, Germany, and Canada does not mean the right to all treatments. Although most services provided in these countries are covered, the extent to which services are offered varies substantially across countries. Equity in health care in reality means a commitment to providing some common, adequate level of care. As yet, however, no country has explicitly determined what this level is.[56]

In countries with universal access, referral systems tend to restrict access to high-technology services while maintaining comprehensive coverage of services. This is different from the U.S. approach of providing open access to technological services but restricting the type and quantity of services that are covered under the various insurance plans.[57]

◆ QUALITY ISSUES IN HEALTH CARE

Unfortunately, spending the most dollars on health care hasn't made us the healthiest. On the basis of crude outcome measures such as infant mortality and life expectancy as well as access to care, the United States is below many other industrialized countries. Canada, which culturally most resembles the United States, has an infant mortality rate 25 percent lower. The rate of heart disease in Canada is 20 percent lower than in the United States. Canadians' average life span—77.1 years—is almost two years longer than that of persons in the United States.[58]

In an effort to enhance the quality, efficiency, and effectiveness of the health care system, policymakers are urging physicians and health professionals to develop **practice guidelines** that clearly specify appropriate care and acceptable limits of care for each disease state or condition. Care delivered according to a **protocol** has been linked with positive **outcomes** for the patient or client.[59] The ADA has begun to develop practice guidelines and encourages all its practitioners to document the **cost-effectiveness** of nutrition services.

Practice guidelines
Guidelines to be used by doctors, hospitals, and other health professionals for treating various conditions to ensure the most effective care.

Protocol Detailed guidelines for care that are specific to the disease or condition and type of patient.

Comparative Health Care Systems—Lessons from Abroad

Practically all industrialized countries except the United States have national health care programs.[60] Coverage is generally universal (everyone is eligible regardless of health status) and uniform (everyone is entitled to the same benefits). Costs are paid entirely from tax revenues or by some combination of individual and employer premiums and government subsidization.

Some countries, such as Sweden, have a single, uniform program administered at the national level. Others, such as Canada, set minimum benefits at the national level but allow programs to vary as they are administered by individual provinces or states. Some attribute the success of the Canadian system to Canada's parliamentary system, which is less vulnerable than the U.S. system to

Outcome An end result of the health care process; a measurable change in the patient's state of health or functioning.

Cost-effectiveness analysis An approach to evaluation that takes into account both costs and outcomes of intervention for a specific purpose. The analysis is especially useful for comparing alternative methods of intervention.

pressures by special interests; its strong tradition of civil service; and the smaller size and cultural homogeneity of Canadian provinces compared with many of the larger U.S. states.[61]

Yet another model is the German system, which permits qualifying, nongovernmental programs to operate at the local level through nonprofit sickness funds and medical associations. In general, Germans appear to be very happy with their system. The *Harvard Community Health Plan Annual Report 1990*, which surveyed health care consumers in six countries, found that the Germans were the second most satisfied overall with their system, behind the Canadians but ahead of the Britons, Swedes, Japanese, and persons in the United States.[62]

There is a growing interest in how other countries are coping with the problems of costs, quality, and access. Table 4-3 provides a summary of the costs, availability, and quality of health care services in six countries. As the table reveals, financing and organization are much different in the United States than in these other countries. Keep in mind, however, that comparing data across countries is not a simple task because the accuracy of the data varies and controlling for social, medical, cultural, demographic, economic, and policy differences among countries is difficult.[63]

Experts say that no health care system is perfect and that every system is a compromise among the competing goals of equity, access, cost, and quality of care. For example, a system is not necessarily better than another simply because it costs less. One must look at specific interventions and specific diseases—for example, heart disease—and see if people do better in the United States than in Canada, Germany, or Japan.

Health Care Reform: American Style

The concept of government-sponsored comprehensive health care is not new to the United States.[64] In 1934, President Franklin D. Roosevelt strongly supported national health insurance (NHI) and almost pushed to have it included with old age and unemployment insurance in the Social Security Act of 1935. Fearing that NHI might jeopardize passage of the Social Security Act, however, he decided to drop the proposal. As a result of World War II and the passage of the Hill-Burton Act of 1946, federal monies were diverted away from NHI and used for construction of new hospitals. Two decades later, the nation shifted its focus from NHI to providing for those without private insurance. Consequently, through the efforts of Presidents John F. Kennedy and Lyndon B. Johnson, Congress enacted the Social Security Amendments of 1965, which created Medicare (Title XVIII) and Medicaid (Title XIX).

The Hill-Burton Act (Hospital Survey and Construction Act) made federal funds available for the first time for hospital construction, expansion, or improvement.

Now, almost 30 years later, President Bill Clinton has made health care reform a top priority of his administration. Early in his presidency, he appointed the first lady, Hillary Rodham Clinton, to head the administration's Task Force on National Health Care Reform. The task force was charged with developing recommendations for a plan for national health care reform.

Health care reform for the United States raises a formidable list of issues including overall cost containment, universal access, emphasis on prevention, and reduction in administrative superstructure and costs.[65] These issues require difficult decisions. Consider the following questions:[66]

♦ Who should be covered?

♦ How can coverage be increased to reach all people?

♦ What services should be considered in basic health care packages?

♦ Should health care cover both acute problems and prevention?

♦ Who should decide what constitutes preventive services?

♦ Who will pay for this coverage—consumers, employers, government?

♦ Where will government get the money to pay for it?

♦ How can health care costs be reduced or contained?

♦ What are the advantages and disadvantages of the play-or-pay and single-payer systems?

Although much attention has been focused on the Canadian system and, to a lesser extent, the British system, most analysts believe that political and practical considerations will prevent the wholesale adoption of a Canadian or British plan in the United States.[67] Both are government-run systems offering minimal choice outside the main delivery network. Because costs are sometimes controlled by limiting the availability of technology, there can be long waits to receive care. Some question whether people in the United States would accept queues. For these reasons, some predict that the U.S. system will evolve into one similar to the German system, where the bulk of policy making is left to the private sector. The German government closely regulates this private sector to achieve national goals, however.

People in the United States are undecided on what kind of health care system they want or how to pay for it. Polls find the public split into thirds on the issue of health care reform: one-third favors a single-payer system, one-third favors strengthening employer-based coverage, and one-third favors no governmental action stronger than tax credits.[68] For general information about these three plans, see Table 4-4. The question now is, Which plan shall we choose?

Two of the main proposals being considered are the **play-or-pay** and **single-payer** systems.[69] Play or pay is an employer-based system where the employer must either offer health insurance or pay a new federal payroll tax. The single-payer system is a **national health insurance** system that would tax Americans at a rate that would cover all health benefits regardless of the individual's employment status.

A third proposal being considered is **managed competition**. The theory of managed competition holds that the quality and cost of health care delivery will improve if independent provider groups compete for consumers.[70] Embraced favorably by the Clinton administration, managed competition is based on two assumptions listed on pages 110 and 111.[71]

Play-or-pay plans A system of paying for health care in which employers must either provide coverage for employees or pay a tax to finance a public insurance plan covering the uninsured.

Single-payer plan A system of paying for health care in which the government or some other entity is the sole payer, financed through a combination of payroll, corporate, and income taxes. Proponents say this approach saves billions of dollars because providers need not deal with hundreds of insurance companies, verify eligibility, and incur collection expenses.

National health insurance A system in which a person is guaranteed coverage merely by being a citizen of the country or resident of the state involved.

Managed competition The creation of large groups of insurance purchasers to give them the bargaining power needed to create strong incentives for providers to supply the highest-quality service for the lowest possible cost.

| TABLE 4-3 | Comparison of National Health Care Systems | | |

COUNTRY	ACCESS	COSTS	FINANCE
Canada	Canada provides health care for all its citizens through a national health insurance program operated by the provincial governments. Primary care providers are evenly distributed and specialists are concentrated in "centers of excellence."	Canada spends about 8.6% of GNP* on health care. Doctors are paid on a fee-for-service basis with rates negotiated annually with the provincial government. Hospitals have global annual budgets set by the provincial government.	The Canadian federal and provincial governments share the financing of health costs. The federal share comes primarily from income taxes, as does the provincial share.
Great Britain	Great Britain provides health care for all its citizens through a government-operated national health service.	Great Britain spends 6.1% of GNP on health care. The government operates the hospitals and employs hospital-based doctors with a budget based on allocations by Parliament. General practitioners are paid based on government-set rates.	89% of the financing of health care in Great Britain is from general federal revenues. 9% is from an employee/employer contribution fund. The final 2% is from direct patient payment.
Germany*	Germany provides all its citizens with ready access to health care through a century-old system of social insurance that represents a middle ground in the spectrum of approaches Western countries have adopted to protect their populations from the economic consequences of illness.	Germany spends an average of 8.5% of GNP on health care. A formal price-fixing mechanism exists for physician fees and hospital rates. Fee increases are negotiated by not-for-profit insurance organizations and regional "doctors" payment organizations.	90% of citizens receive care coverage by a system of "sickness funds" into which employees and employers are mandated by law to make matching contributions based on a fixed percentage of income (average 12.8%). Most other citizens purchase comprehensive private insurance.
Japan	Japan provides access to health care for all its workers and their families through an employer-mandated health insurance program. All other citizens are covered through a national health insurance program.	Japan spends 6.7% of GNP on health care. The Health Ministry sets rates for private and public providers on a fee-for-service basis. It operates a utilization review system. Providers can, in some cases, charge more than the government rate, but this overcharge must be paid out-of-pocket.	About 60% of health costs in Japan come from the employment-based health program that is financed through an 8–9% payroll tax split by the employee-employer. 30% comes from local taxes, with the final 10% from direct patient payment.
Sweden	Sweden provides access to health care for all its citizens through an almost completely government-operated national health service program.	Sweden spends 9% of GNP on health care. 95% of doctors are employed by county councils that operate the health system locally. Hospitals are run by either local or area agencies with budgets based on the medical needs of the area.	60% of the financing for Sweden's health system is from a proportional wage tax of 13.5%. 35% of costs are covered by general federal revenues. The final 4% is paid for through direct patient fees.
United States	Access to health care is not a right in the U.S. Medicaid covers 17 million low-income people. Medicare covers 30 million seniors and 2 million people with disabilities. Private insurance, usually employment based, covers 137 million people. 37 million Americans are uninsured.	The U.S. spends over 12% of GNP on health care. Most providers are private with little rate setting (Medicaid, Medicare for hospital services, and a few private insurance companies). Hospital care consumes about $1/2$ of health costs, with doctor services another $1/4$.	Private insurance pays 31% of health costs. Medicare, financed through a 3.5% payroll tax and premiums, pays 17% of health costs. Medicaid pays 10% and is funded jointly by federal and state taxes. Other government programs pay 14%. Direct patient payments pay 25%. Private sources pay the remaining 3%.

Continued

TABLE
4-3

Comparison of National Health Care Systems—*Continued*

COUNTRY	ADMINISTRATION	BENEFITS	QUALITY
Canada	The Federal Ministry of Health sets standards for provincial government annual plans. Providers are mostly private, but provincial governments negotiate rates with doctors. The government sets global hospital budgets.	The same benefits are provided as in Sweden (Sweden has the most comprehensive benefits package and is used as the standard for comparison) except that eye care is not covered and dental care is limited.	Infant mortality rate improved from 13.5 deaths/1000 births in 1975 to 7.9 in 1986, ranking Canada 3rd in this chart. Life expectancy rose from 74.3 years in 1975 to 75.0 in 1986, ranking Canada in a tie for 3rd in this chart.
Great Britain	The Secretary for Social Services oversees the health system. It sets fees for private physicians. It sets hospital budgets and employs hospital doctors. Input comes from regional, district, and community boards.	The same benefits are provided as in Sweden except dental care is limited.	Infant mortality rate improved from 14.3 deaths/1000 births in 1975 to 8.8 in 1986, ranking Great Britain 4th in this study. Life expectancy rose from 73.4 in 1975 to 75.0 in 1986, ranking Great Britain in a tie for 3rd in this study.
Germany*	The German government sets limits on overall health spending by parliamentary edict, leaving all operational details to insurers, hospitals, and physicians. Insurance organizations known as sickness funds establish and collect contributions from employers and workers.	All of Germany's citizens have access to a comprehensive set of benefits as in Sweden (comprehensive dental coverage is included; preventive services include visits to spas) with free choice of physicians and hospitals and virtually immediate access to all services.	Infant mortality rate was 10.2 deaths/1000 live births in 1986, ranking Germany 5th in this comparison. Life expectancy was 75.0 in 1986, ranking Germany in a three-way tie for 3rd in this study.
Japan	The Minister of Health oversees both the employer-mandated health program ($^2/_3$ of population) and the National Health Insurance program (all others). It sets fees for hospitals, clinics, and their doctors.	The same benefits are provided as in Sweden except paramedical treatment, eye care, and psychiatric care are not covered and dental care is limited.	Infant mortality rate improved from 9.3 deaths/1000 births in 1975 to 5.2 in 1986, ranking Japan 1st in this study. Life expectancy rose from 75.5 in 1975 to 76.0 in 1986, ranking Japan 2nd in this study.
Sweden	The Ministry of Health and Social Affairs oversees 23 county councils and three municipal boards, elected every three years, that employ doctors and operate hospitals and clinics. Six medical regions operate specialized facilities.	Sweden covers hospital services (tests, lab work, nonelective surgery), physician services, preventive care, home care and nursing home care, prescription drugs, dental care, eye care, paramedical services, and psychiatric care.	Infant mortality rate improved from 8.3 deaths/1000 births in 1975 to 5.9 in 1986, ranking Sweden 2nd in this study. Life expectancy rose from 75.5 in 1975 to 77.0 in 1986, ranking Sweden 1st in this study.
United States	The federal government sets hospital rates and standards for Medicare. States set rates and regulate Medicaid. Over 1500 private insurers set their own regulations. Doctors are mostly private. Only 5% of hospitals are public.	Private plans vary but few compare to Sweden. Medicare does not cover dental, eye and preventive care, or paramedical services and limits psychiatric, drug, and long-term care. Medicaid can have fuller coverage, but few states offer all options.	Infant mortality rate improved from 16.1 deaths/1000 births in 1975 to 10.4 in 1986, ranking the U.S. 6th, or last, in this study. Life expectancy rose from 73.5 in 1975 to 74.0 in 1987, ranking the U.S. 4th or last, in this study.

*GNP: gross national product
*Germany refers to the former West Germany. A formidable challenge facing the recently unified Germany is the transformation of East Germany's national health service into the market-oriented social insurance model of West Germany.

Source: Adapted from Comparison of national health care systems, *Nursing and Health Care* 13 (1992): 202–3. Reprinted by permission from the advocacy group, Citizen Action, 1120 19th Street, NW, Washington, D.C. 20036.

TABLE 4-4	Three Approaches to Health Care Reform		
	MANAGED COMPETITION APPROACH	**SINGLE-PAYER APPROACH**	**PLAY-OR-PAY APPROACH**
Financing	◆ Gives tax subsidies to individuals who buy health insurance. ◆ Gives vouchers to low-income taxpayers.. ◆ Does not detail how plan would be paid for.	◆ Government pays for all health care with revenues from payroll and/or income taxes, replacing insurance premiums and subsuming existing public programs. ◆ Most likely would require modest copayments and deductibles.	◆ Requires employers to offer their employees a minimum health plan (play) or contribute to a government-subsidized plan through payroll taxes (pay). ◆ Additional taxes would be needed to cover low-income workers and the unemployed in the public plan. Supplants Medicaid but retains a separate Medicare program for the elderly.
Delivery	◆ Individuals would be able to choose among private health plans, with an emphasis on managed care. ◆ A maximum premium and/or a minimum benefits package would be defined.	◆ Individuals allowed to choose private doctors and hospitals. ◆ Some versions encourage the use of HMOs and other managed-care plans.	◆ Individuals covered by employer-sponsored insurance plans would be unaffected. ◆ Uninsured individuals would be covered by some form of government-sponsored plan.
Cost containment	◆ Competition among health care plans would force providers to keep prices down and become more efficient.	◆ Government at the federal and state levels would set spending targets or caps, negotiate fees for doctors and budgets for hospitals, and monitor the use of high-tech equipment and procedures.	◆ Government would set spending targets for health care and negotiate fees for doctors and hospitals. ◆ Encourages use of HMOs and managed-care plans.
Pros	◆ Covers the uninsured by giving substantial subsidies to the poor. ◆ Although it would increase government spending considerably, other plans would cost more.	◆ Guarantees universal coverage. ◆ Eliminates high administrative and marketing costs of competing private insurance plans. ◆ Eliminates incentives for cost shifting.	◆ Guarantees universal coverage. ◆ Retains current employer-based system and puts much of the burden of new subsidies on business, not individual taxpayers.
Cons	◆ Does not guarantee coverage for everyone. ◆ Does not completely end cost shifting. ◆ Individuals who use managed care or HMOs are likely to find their choices restricted.	◆ Likely to cost more initially than current system as it extends coverage to those who are uninsured. ◆ Tax financing means a major redistribution of cost.	◆ Small businesses would be faced with larger share of existing costs. ◆ Requires raising taxes to subsidize low-wage employees, the unemployed and uninsured, and former Medicaid recipients. ◆ Does not reduce administrative costs as effectively as single-payer plan.

Source: Adapted from *ADA Courier* 31 (May 1992): 3.

◆ The free-market approach to health care reform is unworkable because of the imbalance of power between sellers (insurance companies and providers) and purchasers (businesses and individuals).

◆ Consumers have no incentive to shop among health plans because employer-based insurance is deductible by employers and nontaxable for employees.

Under managed competition, physicians and hospitals would be divided into competing economic units called **accountable health partnerships** (AHPs), which would contract with **health insurance purchasing cooperatives** (HIPCs) to provide health care to consumers.[72] Unlike the fee-for-service system, providers would offer standardized packages of health care benefits for fixed per capita rates. Since Medicare may be used as the model for a basic benefits package, the ADA has urged that Title XVIII of the Social Security Act be amended so that nutrition services will be included in the Medicare package of covered benefits.[73]

On the 200th anniversary of the convening of the nation's first Congress, Howard Nemerov, the poet laureate of the United States, read a poem to a joint session of Congress. It concluded with the following lines:

> Praise without end the go-ahead zeal
> of whoever it was invented the wheel;
> But never a word for the poor soul's sake
> that thought ahead and invented the brake.

The poet has clearly identified two essential elements of any future U.S. health care system: "we must think ahead and we must invent (and apply) a brake."[74]

Accountable health partnerships/plans (AHPs) The plans that current managed-care plans (HMOs, PPOs) are encouraged to become under managed competition. AHPs must offer, at minimum, the federally mandated standard benefits package. AHPs are not allowed to exclude persons with preexisting medical conditions.

Health insurance purchasing cooperatives (HIPCs) The heart of managed competition, HIPCs act as purchasing agents for large groups of consumers. They would offer a range of plans to consumers.

Nutrition as a Component of Health Care Reform

During the summer of 1992, the House Select Committee on Aging held a hearing on "Adequate Nutrition: The Difference between Sickness and Health for the Elderly." The purpose of the hearing was "to examine the critical role that nutrition plays in the lives of the American elderly population, and to determine how we can optimize the delivery of nutrition services, which include screening, assessment, counseling, and therapy, to this population."[75]

As a result of this hearing, its sponsor, Congressman Edward Roybal stated:

> Now I am even more convinced that nutrition services play a vital role in maintaining the health, independence, and quality of life of older Americans. Nutrition services must become an integral part of the health care services provided to not only the elderly, but every citizen of the United States. The benefits of proper nutrition have been shown time and time again. Nutrition screening, assessment, and counseling save money. When an older person is malnourished, he/she is at risk for disease and other health problems. Eighty-five percent of all older persons have one or more chronic diseases, such as diabetes, osteoporosis, atherosclerosis, hypertension, and cancer. Nutrition is linked to prevention and treatment of these diseases. . . . We must change the system so that nutrition services are specifically reimbursable and not just included in administrative funds. Nutrition services must be made available to elderly Americans in preventive, acute, long-term care, and home health settings. Nutrition

Nutrition services include the following:

Nutrition assessment The evaluation of the nutrition needs of individuals based upon appropriate biochemical, anthropometric, physical, and dietary data to determine nutrient needs and recommend appropriate nutrition intake.

Nutrition screening The process of discovering characteristics known to be associated with dietary or nutritional problems. Its purpose is to identify individuals who are at high risk of nutritional problems or who have unrecognized malnutrition.

Intervention A purposefully planned action designed to achieve a defined outcome (e.g., nutrition counseling over a 12-week period to enable the patient to decrease caloric consumption and thereby reduce weight).

Nutrition treatment Intervention and counseling of individuals on appropriate nutrition intake by integrating information from the nutrition assessment with information on food and other sources of nutrients and meal preparation consistent with the client's cultural background and socioeconomic status.

screening to identify those at risk can be a cost-effective prevention measure. . . . Nutritional care should be considered specialized care and should be reimbursed just as respiratory, occupational, and physical therapies are.[76]

Many believe that **nutrition services** are the cornerstone of cost-effective prevention and are essential to halting the spiraling cost of health care. The ADA has urged that provision of nutrition services be included in any health care reform legislation.[77]

In addition, health care reform legislation needs to recognize the registered dietitian as the nutrition expert of the health care team with a scope of practice that includes the following:[78]

◆ *Nutrition assessment* for the purpose of determining individual and community needs and recommendation of appropriate nutrient intake to maintain, recover, or improve health.

◆ *Nutrition counseling and education* of individuals, families, community groups, and health professionals.

◆ *Research and development* of appropriate nutrition practice guidelines.

◆ *Administration* through *management* of time, finances, personnel, protocols, and programs.

◆ *Consultation* with patients, clients, and other health professionals.

◆ *Evaluation* of the effectiveness of nutrition counseling/education and community nutrition programs.

◆ THE BENEFITS OF NUTRITION SERVICES

One cannot have good health without proper nutrition. Conversely, poor nutrition contributes substantially to infant mortality, retarded growth and development of children, premature death, illness, and disability in adults, and frailty in the elderly, causing unnecessary pain and suffering, reduced productivity in the workplace, and increased health care costs.[79]

The contribution of nutrition to preventing disease, prolonging life, and promoting health is well recognized. Accumulated evidence shows that when nutrition services are integrated into health care, diet and nutrition status change with the following results:[80]

◆ The birth weight distribution of infants born to high-risk mothers improves.

◆ The prevalence of iron-deficiency anemia is reduced.

◆ Weight reduction and long-term weight maintenance are achieved.

◆ The rate of dental caries declines.

◆ Serum cholesterol and the risk of heart attacks are reduced.

◆ Glucose tolerance in persons with diabetes improves.

◆ Blood pressure in hypertensive patients is lowered.

The benefits of providing nutrition services far outweigh the costs of providing those services.[81] A 1992 U.S. General Accounting Office estimate of the Special Supplemental Food Program for Women, Infants, and Children (WIC) found that every dollar invested in WIC for pregnant women yielded up to $4.21 in Medicaid savings.

◆ REIMBURSEMENT FOR NUTRITION SERVICES

Nutrition services are not routinely covered in public programs (except WIC and, in some states, Medicaid) and only sporadically reimbursed by private health insurance. Some insurance companies will pay for outpatient nutrition counseling when it is ordered by a physician and provided by a registered dietitian.

The ADA believes that reimbursement for nutrition services through both Medicare and Medicaid is wholly inadequate. Often, the elderly choose not to seek appropriate nutrition services because Medicare's coverage is limited and they are unable to pay for the services themselves.[82] The **Nutrition Screening Initiative** recommends that nutrition screening for the elderly be included in the U.S. health care system and that Medicare cover and reimburse nutrition assessment and treatment for those found to be at nutritional risk. Such action is crucial to lowering health care costs, since malnourished persons have longer hospital stays and higher hospital costs than persons without malnutrition.[83]

In arguing for reimbursable nutrition services, say, to an HMO benefits coordinator or local legislator, consider highlighting the following list of benefits:[84]

> **Nutrition Screening Initiative** A program of the American Academy of Family Physicians, the ADA, and the National Council on Aging, formed in 1990 as a five-year multifaceted effort to promote nutrition and improved nutrition care for the elderly in the U.S. health care system.

- ◆ Nutrition services are attractive, progressive health benefits that are relatively inexpensive compared to other types of benefits.
- ◆ Nutrition services benefits enhance the insurance product (employee benefit package).
- ◆ Nutrition services have a preventive medicine component (they help keep employees healthy).
- ◆ Nutrition services benefits attract healthy subscribers.
- ◆ Nutrition services are manageable—they can be easily documented.
- ◆ Nutrition services help patients become more self-reliant by helping them fight disease, avoid hospitalization, and reduce the use of other, more expensive medical therapies.
- ◆ Nutrition care speeds recovery.

◆ COST-EFFECTIVENESS OF NUTRITION SERVICES

Community nutritionists need to compete successfully for a fair share of the health care dollar. To do so, they must document the demand for and effectiveness of nutrition services so they can market those services to health care officials, providers, payers, and the public.

Obviously, no payer in the health care system wants additional costs. For a new technology or service, including nutrition services, to be a reimbursable benefit, it must prove its cost-effectiveness. Only services that have a proven impact on the quality of patient care will be funded. As Simko and Conklin have said, no expenditure of resources is justified for a service that fails to achieve its intended outcome.[85]

Cost-effectiveness studies compare the costs of providing health care against a desirable change in patient health outcomes (for example, a reduction in serum cholesterol in a patient with hypercholesterolemia).[86] Figure 4-5 shows a model for testing the costs and benefits of nutrition services. As this model shows, effective nutrition counseling can produce economic benefits as a result of altered food habits and risk factors.

Developing standardized protocols of care (practice guidelines) for nutrition intervention, as mentioned earlier in the chapter, is considered a must for achieving payment for nutrition services and expanding current levels of third-party reimbursement.[87] An example of standardized practice guidelines developed by the National Cholesterol Education Program (NCEP) is shown in Figure 4-6. Note the orchestrated steps for identifying persons at risk for heart disease and establishing goals for dietary intervention.

Documentation of specific *outcomes* of nutrition intervention—clinical data, laboratory measures, anthropometric measures, and dietary intake data—is also necessary. Figure 4-7 shows examples of outcome measures of nutrition intervention in burn injury, prenatal care, diabetes, and obesity.[88] When determining the

---

FIGURE

4-5

Benefits of Nutrition Intervention

Source: Adapted from M. Mason and coauthors, Requisites of advocacy: Philosophy, research, documentation. Phase II of the costs and benefits of nutritional care, *Journal of the American Dietetic Association* 80 (1982): 213.

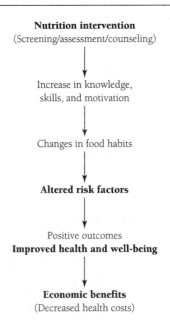

Nutrition intervention
(Screening/assessment/counseling)

↓

Increase in knowledge,
skills, and motivation

↓

Changes in food habits

↓

Altered risk factors

↓

Positive outcomes
Improved health and well-being

↓

Economic benefits
(Decreased health costs)

FIGURE 4-6   National Cholesterol Education Program Guidelines for Dietary Treatment

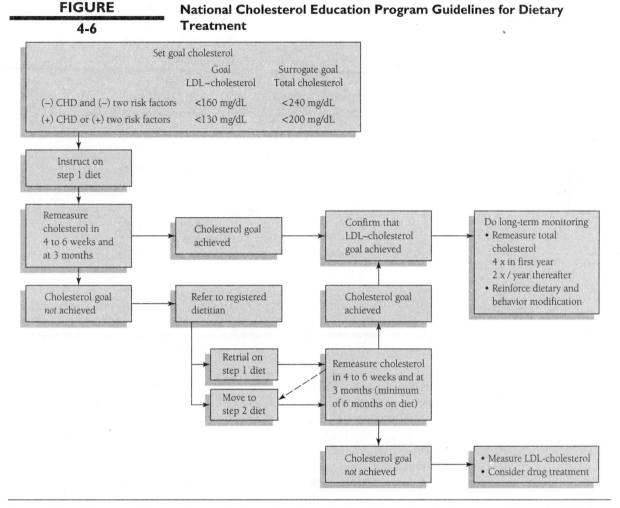

Source: National Cholesterol Education Program, *Highlights of the Report of the Expert Panel on Detection, Evaluation, and Treatment of High Blood Cholesterol in Adults* (Washington, D.C.: U.S. Department of Health and Human Services, 1987).

outcomes of a given intervention, remember to ask the following questions: (1) Does the nutrition intervention make a difference in terms of disease-specific indicators? (2) Is the nutrition intervention worth the cost? Table 4-5 offers steps for developing protocols that enhance the effectiveness of nutrition services and make it easier to evaluate their quality and effectiveness.[89]

The collection of cost-effectiveness data for nutrition services provided by dietetic practitioners is crucial to ADA's health care reform activities. The *Pepper Commission* report, upon which several health care reform proposals are based, recommends coverage only for preventive services that have been proven cost-effective.

The U.S. Bipartisan Commission on Comprehensive Health Care (called the Pepper Commission after its first chairman, Congressman Claude Pepper) is primarily concerned with access to comprehensive care by the elderly and people with disabilities. The commission recommends legislation that will ensure all Americans coverage for health care and long-term care.

FIGURE

4-7

Measurable Outcomes of Nutrition Intervention
Source: R. Gould, The next rung on the ladder: Achieving and expanding reimbursement for nutrition services. © The American Dietetic Association. Reprinted by permission from *Journal of the American Dietetic Association* 91 (1991): 1383.

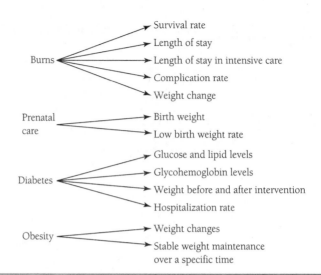

On the Horizon: Certain Change for Health Care

The future offers much that is positive for the profession of dietetics. The public's thinking about health and nutrition has matured, interest in positive health is growing steadily, and demand for health promotion products and services is increasing. Yet to be achieved, however, are the effective provision and allocation of resources such as nutrition services as part of preventive care. To accomplish this, a coordinated strategy for health care, political will, and active collaboration of both health care professionals and consumers of health care services will be required.

As we noted earlier, health care reform is a difficult undertaking. It involves more than cost containment and universal access. Community nutritionists need to educate the payers of health care about the inherent value of including nutrition services in their policies.[90] At the same time, consumers need to demand reimbursement for nutrition services from *their* insurance companies.

As this book went to press, health care reform for the United States seemed certain, but the exact nature of the reform was yet to be decided. Undoubtedly, the health care system will change slowly over time. Nevertheless, the health care reform process stands to have a major impact—for better or worse—on our profession. It is imperative that you keep up-to-date with both national and local developments in health care reform.

Remember that change at the federal level begins with local advocacy. Remember, too, that the prescription for success is persistence. We need to maintain the pressure to achieve meaningful legislation in health care reform. The Community Learning Activity that follows asks you, as a consumer of health care services, to explore both current legislation concerning health care reform and your own health care coverage benefits.

1. Define the patient population:
   ◆ Select a prevalent problem (diagnosis).
   ◆ Select a population or problem for which evidence (in the literature or your own experience) indicates that nutrition intervention can produce clinical outcomes.
   ◆ Define the population as specifically as possible, based on medical diagnosis, state of diagnosis if relevant (e.g., new diagnosis versus long-standing diagnosis of diabetes), and other relevant factors (medication, age, other medical conditions). Example: hypercholesterolemic patients (cholesterol $\geq$ 200 mg/dL) who are either newly diagnosed or first-time referrals.
2. Define the treatment:
   ◆ Base standards for treatment on accepted methods of nutritional management (e.g., the National Cholesterol Education Program guidelines; National Institutes of Health Consensus Panel recommendations on diabetes management).
   ◆ Emphasize individualization of specific dietary patterns within limits of treatment standards.
   ◆ Specify expected length of treatment (e.g., three-month trial of diet) and expected minimum number of visits.
   ◆ Specify expected length of each visit as well as length of time between visits.
   ◆ Outline specific activities or topics to be addressed during the course of treatment and provide appropriate educational materials and tools.
3. Identify expected outcomes:
   ◆ Include as appropriate:
   Anthropometric measurements (weight, body mass index, skinfolds, etc.)
   Lab values (fasting blood sugar, hemoglobin A_{1c}, cholesterol, lipid profile, etc.)
   Clinical data (medication change, blood pressure change, etc.)
   Dietary intake
   ◆ Specify appropriate points in time when outcomes should be measured.
   ◆ If possible, specify expected magnitude of change and associated timeline.
   ◆ Identify expected and measurable intermediate outcomes (e.g., positive changes in knowledge, behavior, decision making, involvement in self-care).

TABLE

4-5

Development of Patient Care Protocols

Source: M. K. Fox, Defining appropriate nutrition care. © 1991, The American Dietetic Association. Reprinted by permission from *Reimbursement and Insurance Coverage for Nutrition Services,* 1991, p. 93.

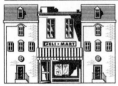

COMMUNITY LEARNING ACTIVITY

1. A good place to start pursuing health care reform is in your own backyard. Does your own health care insurance plan (or that of your family) include reimbursement for services rendered by a registered dietitian or for nutritional products? If the answer is "no," plan a strategy to have nutrition services become part of the insurer's policy. Write a practice letter to the insurer's benefits coordinator. Start by outlining the potential benefits of nutrition services.

2. Most state insurance commissioner's offices track the top 10 insurers for their population. Try to obtain a copy of this list for the class. Next, obtain a sample policy from as many of these companies as possible and compare their benefits and exclusions. Are nutrition services covered? If the answer is "no," proceed as in step 1.

3. Grassroots lobbying is an effective way for people to influence legislation that may affect them in one way or another. Lobbying, as discussed in Chapter 3,

can take many forms—personal meetings with a legislator or a legislator's aide, a letter, or a phone call. Legislators and their aides are sensitive to public opinion on issues. We ask that you get to know your congressperson's position on health care reform. What legislation is he or she supporting? Does he or she have his or her own bill or support positions of reform such as prevention? You can call your congressperson's local district office to obtain copies of bills and testimony. The phone number can be found in the federal government section (usually blue pages) of your telephone book.

The following House subcommittees have jurisdiction over health issues:

◆ House Ways and Means Committee/Subcommittee on Health

◆ Energy and Commerce Committee/Subcommittee on Health

The following Senate committees are also involved with health care reform:

◆ Committee on Labor and Human Resources

◆ Committee on Finance

Does your congressperson or senator serve on one of these committees? If you need to learn a legislator's name or find out what committees he or she serves on, you can contact the League of Women Voters in your area.

NOTES

1. *Washington Post,* January 4, 1993.
2. C. Tokarski, 1980s prove uncertainty of instant cures, *Modern Healthcare,* January 8, 1990, p. 51.
3. *A Call for Action: Final Report of the Pepper Commission* (Washington, D.C.: U.S. Government Printing Office, 1990).
4. The list of diet-related diseases is from *Executive Summary of the Legislative Platform of the American Dietetic Association: Economic Benefits of Nutrition Services* (Chicago: American Dietetic Association, October 1992), p. 3.
5. U.S. Department of Health and Human Services, Public Health Service, *The Surgeon General's Report on Nutrition and Health* (Washington, D.C.: U.S. Government Printing Office, 1988), as cited in *Economic Benefits of Nutrition Services,* p. 6.
6. U.S. Department of Health and Human Services, Public Health Service, *Healthy People 2000: National Health Promotion and Disease Prevention Objectives* (Washington, D.C.: U.S. Government Printing Office, 1990), as cited in *Economic Benefits of Nutrition Services,* p. 6.
7. W. O. Wiener, Year 2000 objectives: Altering the medical model, *Medicine and Health Perspectives,* October 23, 1989, p. 3.
8. *Economic Benefits of Nutrition Services,* p. 6.
9. President's Column, A new era for prevention, *The Nation's Health* (January 1990): 2.
10. G. E. A. Dever, *Community Health Analysis,* 2nd ed. (Gaithersburg, Md.: Aspen Publishers, 1991), p. xiii.
11. T. Hancock, Beyond health care: Creating a healthy future, *The Futurist* 16 (1982): 4.
12. Position of the American Dietetic Association: Affordable and accessible health care services, *Journal of the American Dietetic Association* 92 (1992): 746.
13. Ibid.
14. L. W. Sullivan, *Healthy People 2000:* Promoting health and building a culture of character, *American Journal of Health Promotion* 5 (1990): 5–6.
15. Ibid, p. 6.
16. The margin definitions throughout this section are from *Reimbursement and Insurance Coverage for Nutrition Services* (Chicago: American Dietetic Association, 1991), pp. 121–25.
17. Health Insurance Institute, *Sourcebook of Health Insurance Data* (New York: Health Insurance Institute, 1989).
18. R. S. Stern, A comparison of length of stay and costs for health maintenance organizations and fee-for-service patients, *Archives of Internal Medicine* 149 (1989): 1185–88.
19. S. Wolfe, Handling your health care, *Buyer's Market* 1 (1985): 2.

20. Stern, A comparison of length of stay and costs.
21. The discussion of the public health plans was adapted from J. S. Ahluwalia, Health care in the United States: Our dynamic jigsaw puzzle, *Archives of Internal Medicine* 150 (1990): 256–58; U.S. Department of Health and Human Services, Social Security Administration, *Understanding Social Security* (Washington, D.C.: U.S. Government Printing Office, 1991), pp. 1–40; and National Association of Insurance Commissioners and the Health Care Financing Administration of the U.S. Department of Health and Human Services, Guide to Health Insurance for People with Medicare (Washington, D.C.: U.S. Government Printing Office, 1992), pp. 1–20.
22. Health care reform: A post election guide, *Harvard Health Letter* (January 1993): 11.
23. Health care reform, *The American Dietetic Association's Legislative Newsletter* (October 1991): 1–3.
24. State Medicaid Information (July 1989); available from the National Governors' Association, Washington, D.C.
25. T. Gup, Health care: Beyond bromides, *Time*, October 31, 1988, pp. 21–22.
26. Dever, *Community Health Analysis*, p. 13.
27. Legislative Highlights: Finn offers testimony on nutrition and the elderly, *Journal of the American Dietetic Association* 92 (1992): 1064–65.
28. R. Carlson, Healthy people, *Canadian Journal of Public Health* 76 (1985): 27–32.
29. Ibid., p. 29.
30. L. W. Sullivan, Partners in prevention: A mobilization plan for implementing *Healthy People 2000, American Journal of Health Promotion* 5 (1991): 291–97.
31. C. Bezold, Health care in the U.S.: Four alternative futures, *The Futurist* 16 (1982): 14–18.
32. E. Friedman, The uninsured: From dilemma to crisis, *Journal of the American Medical Association* 265 (1991): 2491–95.
33. Library of Congress, Congressional Research Service, *Health Insurance and the Uninsured: Background Data Analysis* (Washington, D.C.: U.S. Government Printing Office, 1988).
34. B. Harvey, A proposal to provide health insurance to all children and all pregnant women, *New England Journal of Medicine* 323 (1990): 1216–20.
35. Ibid., p. 1216.
36. Ahluwalia, Health care in the United States, p. 258.
37. Wolfe, Handling your health care, p. 2.
38. J. Galley, Editorial, *Boston Globe*, September 1991, as quoted by M. K. Fox, Reimbursement practices and trends, presented at the American Dietetic Association's annual meeting in Dallas, Texas, October 1991.
39. Ibid.
40. Harvard Health Letter, 1993, p. 9.
41. The discussion of bureaucracy in government-run health care was adapted from E. Brodsky, Government-run health care isn't worth the wait, *Health and You* (Spring 1992): 2.
42. As stated by J. Neel, Healthcare: U.S. looks to German model, *Nature* 351 (1992): 433.
43. K. Hogue, C. Jensen, and K. M. Wiljanen, *The Complete Guide to Health Insurance* (New York: Avon Books, 1989); S. Finn and G. Martin, This shifting balance of power: A new decade of decision for dietitians, *Dietetic Currents* 18 (1991): 1–6; as cited in M. K. Fox, Overview of third-party reimbursement, in *Reimbursement and Insurance Coverage for Nutrition Services*, pp. 3–5.
44. R. Evans, Tension, compression, and shear: Directions, stresses, and outcomes of health care cost control, *Journal of Health Politics, Policy, and Law* 15 (1990): 101–28.
45. E. Ginzberg, The monetarization of medical care, *New England Journal of Medicine* 310 (1984): 1162–65.
46. The margin definitions throughout this section are from *Reimbursement and Insurance Coverage for Nutrition Services*, pp. 121–25.
47. The discussion of cost-containment trends was adapted from Fox, Overview of third-party reimbursement, pp. 3–5.
48. S. W. Letsch, K. R. Levit, and D. R. Waldo, National health expenditures, 1987 health care financing trends, *Health Care Financing Review* 10 (1988): 109–29.
49. P. Stanfill and G. E. Soper, The economic realities of health care, *Health Administration Today* 1 (1988): 8–11.
50. D. Beck, The hospital's financial future, *The Health Care Supervisor* (January 1985): 1–10.
51. L. Bell and M. M. Fairchild, Development of a productivity index to increase accountability of ambulatory nutrition services, *Journal of the American Dietetic Association* 89 (1989): 517–19.
52. Harvey, A proposal to provide health insurance, p. 1216.
53. P. deVise, *Misuses and Misplaced Hospitals and Doctors: A Locational Analysis of the Urban Health Care Crisis*, Resource Paper no. 2 (Commission on College Geography, 1973), p. 1.
54. *Report: The Ethical Implications of Differences in the Availability of Health Services* (Washington, D.C.: President's Commission for the Study of Ethical Problems in Medical and Biomedical and Behavioral Research, 1983), p. 22.
55. Ahluwalia, Health care in the United States, p. 256.
56. C. Grogan, A comparison of Canada, Britain, Germany, and the United States, *Journal of Health Politics, Policy,*

and Law 17 (1992): 213–32.

57. Ibid., p. 226.

58. A. Schmitz, Health assurance, *In Health* (January/February 1991): 39–47.

59. American College of Physicians, Access to health care, *Annals of Internal Medicine* 112 (1990): 641–61.

60. The discussion of national health coverage was adapted from American College of Physicians, Access to health care, pp. 641–61.

61. A. Enthoven and R. Kronick, A consumer-choice health plan for the 1990s: Universal health insurance in a system designed to promote quality and economy, *New England Journal of Medicine* 320 (1989): 94–101.

62. M. M. Hagland, Looking abroad for changes to the U.S. health care system, *Hospitals* 65 (1991): 32.

63. The discussion of comparative health care systems was adapted from Organization for Economic Cooperation and Development, *Financing and Delivering Health Care: A Comparative Analysis of OECD Countries* (Paris: Social Policies Studies, 1987), pp. 9–23; Hagland, Looking abroad for changes, pp. 30–35; R. Collins-Nakai, H. A. Huysmans, and H. E. Scully, Task Force 5: Access to cardiovascular care: An international comparison, *Journal of the American College of Cardiology* 19 (1992): 1477–85; and J. K. Iglehart, Health Policy Report: Germany's health care system, *New England Journal of Medicine* 324 (1991): 503–8.

64. The discussion of U.S. history was adapted from Ahluwalia, Health care in the United States, pp. 256–58.

65. G. S. Omenn, Challenges facing public health policy, *Journal of the American Dietetic Association* 93 (1993): 643.

66. Division of Government Affairs, Health care reform, *Legislative Newsletter* (October 1991): 2.

67. The discussion of the Canadian system was adapted from Hagland, Looking abroad for changes, pp. 30–35.

68. Closing session offers frank talk of health care reform prospects, *The Nation's Health* (December 1992): 14.

69. The margin definitions throughout this section are from *Insuring the Uninsured: A Guide to the Proposals and the Players* (Washington, D.C.: Faulkner & Gray, 1991).

70. R. Kronick and coauthors, The marketplace in health care reform: The demographic limitations of managed competition, *New England Journal of Medicine* 328 (1993): 148–52.

71. Managed competition: Wonder drug or snake oil? *The Nation's Health* (March 1993): 1, 9–10.

72. The discussion of managed competition was adapted in part from J. K. Iglehart, Managed competition, *New England Journal of Medicine* 328 (1993): 1208–12. The margin definitions of managed competition and related

terms are from Managed competition, *The Nation's Health*, p. 9.

73. M. Tate, Health care reform, in *Public Health Nutrition Practice Group: The Digest* (Chicago: American Dietetic Association, Spring 1993), p. 3.

74. This quotation and comment are from *New York Times*, March 3, 1989, p. 10, and N. E. Davies and L. H. Felder, Applying brakes to the runaway American health care system, *Journal of the American Medical Association* 263 (1990): 73–76.

75. Legislative Highlights: Finn offers testimony, pp. 1064–65.

76. E. Roybal, Support for nutrition services for the elderly, *Congressional Record—House,* August 12, 1992, p. 119.

77. Economic benefits of nutrition services, October 1992. The margin definitions are from "A guide to some terms used in the discussion of health care reform," provided by the ADA's Division of Government Affairs, October 1992.

78. Position of the American Dietetic Association: Nutrition services in health maintenance organizations and alternative delivery systems, *Journal of the American Dietetic Association* 87 (1987): 1391–1393.

79. The Florida Dietetic Association Public Policy Statement, *The Orange Blossom* 40 (1989): 11.

80. The list of benefits is from Nutrition services in state and local public health agencies, *Public Health Reports* 98 (1983): 7–20.

81. Ibid., p. 10.

82. Legislative Highlights: Finn offers testimony, 1064–65.

83. G. Robinson, M. Goldstein, and G. M. Levine, Impact of nutritional status on DRG length of stay, *Journal of Parenteral and Enteral Nutrition* 12 (1988): 587–91.

84. The list of benefits is from K. Smith, How to argue for nutrition services, *DBC Dimensions* (Fall 1992): 7.

85. M. D. Simko and M. T. Conklin, Focusing on the effectiveness side of the cost-effectiveness equation, *Journal of the American Dietetic Association* 89 (1989): 485–87.

86. Ibid., p. 486.

87. R. Gould, The next rung on the ladder: Achieving and expanding reimbursement for nutrition services, *Journal of the American Dietetic Association* 91 (1991): 1383–84.

88. P. Splett, Effectiveness and cost effectiveness of nutrition care: A critical analysis with recommendations, *Journal of the American Dietetic Association* 91 (1991): S1–S50.

89. M. K. Fox, Defining appropriate nutrition care, in *Reimbursement and Insurance Coverage for Nutrition Services,* pp. 89–95.

90. President's Page: The Midas touch, *Journal of the American Dietetic Association* 90 (1990): 1278–81.

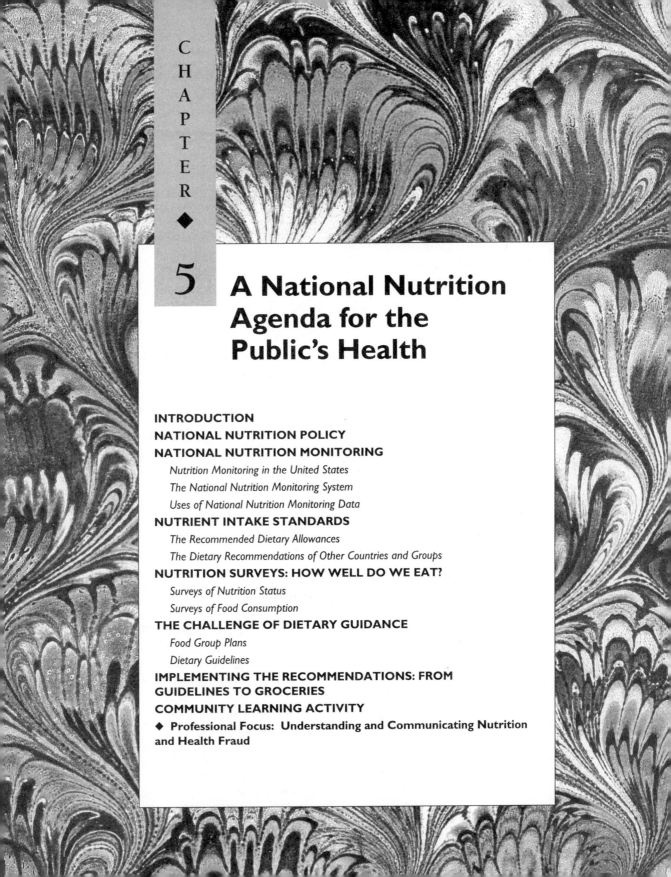

A National Nutrition Agenda for the Public's Health

Something to Think About . . .

If you are among the two out of three Americans who do not smoke or drink excessively, your choice of diet can influence your long-term health prospects more than any other action you might take.

Eight out of the ten leading causes of death, including heart disease, strokes, some types of cancer, and diabetes, are related to diet.

—The Surgeon General's Report on Nutrition and Health

Introduction

Time was when scientists investigating the role diet plays in health zeroed in on the consequences of getting too little of one nutrient or another. Until the end of World War II, in fact, nutrition researchers concentrated on eliminating deficiency diseases such as goiter and pellagra.

These days, however, the focus is just the opposite. While an abundant food supply and the practice of fortifying foods with essential nutrients have virtually eliminated deficiency diseases in the United States, diseases related to dietary excess and imbalance are widespread. As mentioned in Chapter 1, five of the ten leading causes of death, namely, heart disease, cancer, stroke, diabetes, and atherosclerosis, have been linked to diet. Another three are associated with excessive alcohol consumption: liver disease, accidents, and suicides. Together these eight problems account for more than 70 percent of the two million deaths that occur each year, not to mention hospitalizations, time lost on the job, and poor quality of life among many people in the United States. Dietary excesses and imbalances contribute to other ills as well, including high blood pressure, dental disease, and osteoporosis.[1]

That's not to say that diet is the sole culprit responsible for those conditions. A number of environmental, behavioral, social, and genetic factors work together to determine a person's likelihood of falling victim to a disease, as was illustrated in Table 1-3 in Chapter 1. Diet notwithstanding, someone who smokes, doesn't exercise regularly, and has a parent who suffered a heart attack, for example, is more likely to end up with heart disease than a nonsmoker who is physically active and does not have a close relative with heart disease. The way to alter disease risk is to concentrate on changing the day-to-day habits that can be controlled. The results can be significant.

Consider that when researchers examined the habits of a group of nearly 7000 Californians, they were able to pinpoint six common lifestyle elements among those who were particularly healthy for their age. The effects of these factors were cumulative; that is, the more of the six positive health practices the adults followed, the better their health, regardless of their age in calendar years. In fact, the physical well-being of those who reported adhering to all six positive health practices was consistently about the same as that of people *30 years younger* who followed few or none of them.[2] The six health practices that affected the adults' **physiological age** were as follows:

1. Get adequate sleep. People who typically sleep about eight hours a night are physiologically younger.
2. Eat regular meals. People who don't skip meals are physiologically younger.
3. Maintain desirable weight. People who maintain their body weight close to the average for their height and sex are physiologically younger.
4. Do not smoke. People who never take up the habit are physiologically younger.
5. Drink alcohol moderately or not at all. People who abstain or imbibe modest amounts are physiologically younger.
6. Exercise regularly. People who work out regularly are physiologically younger.

> **Physiological age** Age as estimated from the body's health and probable life expectancy. (Age as measured in years from birth is chronological age.)

These findings illustrate that although you cannot alter the year of your birth, you can change the probable length and quality of your life. Nutrition is involved in at least half of the lifestyle behaviors listed above, leaving no doubt that it plays a key role in maintaining good health. Yet, as indicated earlier, malnutrition related to dietary excesses and imbalances is common within the U.S. population, suggesting that large numbers of people have not adopted the behaviors that lead to optimum nutrition and good health. How do we know that dietary imbalances exist in the United States and that certain population subgroups are at risk of malnutrition? And having determined who is malnourished, what guidelines exist to help community nutritionists and other health professionals address the nutritional needs of malnourished groups? The answers to these questions are found in the policy arena, for nutrition policy dictates the strategies used to determine who is malnourished and outlines the appropriate dietary guidance to improve nutritional intake.

National Nutrition Policy

Let's begin with a simple question: Does the United States have a national nutrition policy? The answer is both "yes" and "no." The answer is "no" in the sense that there is no one federal body or agency whose sole mandate is to establish, implement, and evaluate national nutrition policy. This deficiency in national policy making and planning was recognized nearly 20 years ago, when Senator George McGovern, the chairman of the Senate Select Committee on Nutrition and Human Needs (the so-called McGovern Committee), called for the formation of such a body as noted in the quote that follows.

> We need a Federal Nutrition Office. The White House Conference on Food, Nutrition and Health recommended such an Office more than five years ago. Events since the 1969 meeting strongly reaffirm the importance of institutionalizing responsibility for nutrition policy . . . . We cannot continue to operate on the assumption that the increasingly complex threads affecting nutrition policy will automatically weave themselves together into a coherent plan.[3]

McGovern went on to say that the policy in existence at that time (in 1975) lacked focus, direction, and coordination, all of which contributed to growing conflicts within the administration over program priorities. The Panel on Nutrition and Government had offered a similar recommendation at the National Nutrition Policy Study Hearings in 1974: There should be an independent office, operating outside all existing agencies, whose function would be to coordinate and direct federal nutrition policy. This federal nutrition office would follow through on the commitments made by federal agencies in implementing a national nutrition plan, help develop surveillance systems to monitor the population's overall health and nutrition status, and guarantee that any secondary nutritional implications of major policy decisions would be recognized and published in a "nutrition impact statement."[4]

Twenty years later, there is no Federal Nutrition Office, and nutrition policy in the United States is still fragmented. The problem with formalizing federal policy decisions in the nutrition arena lies in determining which agency should be the "power center" responsible for final decisions. This task is both complex and politically sensitive, because nutrition policy cuts across several policy areas, including agriculture, exports, imports, commerce, foreign relations, public health, and even national defense. No one federal agency can claim exclusive jurisdiction over nutrition issues. It is interesting that the comments made by McGovern in 1975 are still relevant in today's health care and policy environment:

> Nutrition is treated as a neglected stepchild of income maintenance programs which themselves are woefully inadequate. This narrow conception virtually denies the nutrition dimension in comprehensive health care, or even that nutrition is a health issue. This parochial view ignores disturbing questions about misleading food advertising and other issues totally unrelated to income inequality. It fails to grapple with the reality that even wealthy Americans are often nutritionally illiterate, and that arteriosclerosis and other diseases associated with the aging process affect more than the poor. These and other issues germane to the health and well-being of the American people go far beyond the perils of poverty, and require a much broader Federal conception of the nation's nutritional policy requirements.[5]

Even though no Federal Nutrition Office currently exists, the United States can still be said to have a national nutrition policy, however fragmented and disjointed it may be. Recall D. J. Palumbo's comment in Chapter 3 that "we can assume that no matter what was intended by government action, what is accomplished *is* policy."[6] Thus, we can point to the Department of Agriculture and the Department of Health and Human Services and their policies and programs as components of U.S. nutrition policy. National nutrition policy in the United States manifests itself in food assistance programs, regulations to safeguard the food supply and ensure the proper labeling of food products, dietary guidance systems such as the Dietary Guidelines and the Food Guide Pyramid, monitoring and surveillance programs, and other activities in the nutrition arena. These activities form the basis of the nation's nutrition agenda to improve the public's health. Some aspects of national nutrition policy, such as food assistance programs, are discussed in later chapters; this chapter focuses on two elements of U.S. nutrition policy, namely, national monitoring and surveillance activities and dietary guidance systems.

National Nutrition Monitoring

Most nations monitor the health and nutrition status of their populations as a means of deciding how to allocate scarce resources, enhance the quality of life, and improve productivity. National nutrition policies are typically guided by the outcomes of health surveys designed to obtain data on the distribution of foodstuffs, the extent to which people consume food of sufficient quality and quantity, the effects of infectious and chronic diseases, and the ways these factors relate to human health. Such information can be derived by any of several methods, including **nutrition assessment, nutrition monitoring, nutrition surveillance,** and **nutrition screening.**[7] These methods are sometimes treated together under the rubrik "nutrition monitoring." Such activities provide regular information about nutrition in populations and all the factors that influence food consumption and nutrition status. The objectives of any national nutrition monitoring system, as outlined by the United Nations Expert Committee Report, are shown in Table 5-1.[8]

Nutrition assessment The measurement of indicators of dietary status and nutrition-related health status to identify the possible occurrence, nature, and extent of impaired nutrition status (ranging from deficiency to toxicity).

Nutrition monitoring The assessment of dietary or nutrition status at intermittent times with the aim of detecting changes in the dietary or nutrition status of a population.

◆ NUTRITION MONITORING IN THE UNITED STATES

The U.S. federal government has been involved in tracking certain elements of the food supply and food consumption for more than eight decades, beginning with the U.S. Department of Agriculture's (USDA's) Food Supply Series undertaken in 1909. In the 1930s, the first USDA Household Food Consumption

◆ To describe the health and nutrition status of a population, with particular reference to defined subgroups who may be at risk

◆ To monitor changes in health and nutrition status over time

◆ To provide information that will contribute to the analysis of causes and associated factors and permit selection of preventive measures, which may or may not be nutritional (for example, smoking)

◆ To provide information on the interrelationship of health and nutrition variables within population subgroups

◆ To estimate the prevalence of diseases, risk factors, and health conditions and of changes over time, which will assist in the formulation of policy

◆ To monitor nutrition programs and evaluate their effectiveness in order to determine met and unmet needs related to target conditions under study

TABLE

5-1

Objectives of a National Nutrition Monitoring and Surveillance System
Source: G. B. Mason and coauthors, *Nutritional Surveillance* (Geneva: World Health Organization, 1984). Used with permission.

Nutrition surveillance The continuous assessment of nutrition status for the purpose of detecting changes in trend or distribution so that corrective measures can be taken; "to watch over nutrition in order to make decisions which will lead to improvements in nutrition in populations."

Nutrition screening A system that identifies specific individuals for nutrition or public health intervention, often at the community level.

See Appendix C for a list of the surveys that form part of the National Monitoring and Surveillance System, together with details of their design, the agency responsible for conducting the survey, and Appendix B for information on ordering data tapes.

Survey was conducted (in 1965 this survey became known as the Nationwide Food Consumption Survey). In the late 1960s, concerns about the "shocking" nutrition status of Mississippi schoolchildren and widespread chronic hunger and malnutrition led to the nation's first comprehensive nutrition survey, the Ten-State Nutrition Survey, conducted between 1968 and 1970 in 10 states: California, Kentucky, Louisiana, Massachusetts, Michigan, New York, South Carolina, Texas, Washington, and West Virginia.[9] In the 1970s, other surveys, such as the National Health and Nutrition Examination Surveys (NHANES I and II) and the Pediatric Nutrition Surveillance System, were added to the roster of methods used to obtain information about the nutrition status of the population.

Beginning in the 1980s, the Joint Nutrition Monitoring Evaluation Committee was set up as a federal advisory committee, jointly sponsored by the USDA and the Department of Health and Human Services (DHHS), to develop reports on the nutrition status of the U.S. population; these reports were to be submitted jointly to Congress at three-year intervals. The first report was published in 1986; the second, in 1989.[10] The survey activities of these two federal departments were conjoined to form the National Nutrition Monitoring System (NNMS). The NNMS is designed to systematically generate data on the dietary status and nutritional health of the U.S. population and to detect and track favorable and unfavorable trends in the American diet.[11] Although the Nationwide Food Consumption Survey, conducted by the USDA, and the NHANES programs, conducted by the DHHS, form the basis of the NNMS, the total system extends beyond these two surveys. With the passage of the National Nutrition Monitoring and Related Research Act (P.L. 101–445) in October 1990, the federal commitment to a national nutrition monitoring system was strengthened.[12]

◆ THE NATIONAL NUTRITION MONITORING SYSTEM

National Nutrition Monitoring System (NNMS) An assortment of activities that provides regular information about the contributions that diet and nutrition status make to the health of the U.S. population and about the factors affecting diet and nutrition status.

The NNMS includes all data collection and analysis activities of the federal government related to (1) measuring the health and nutrition status, food consumption, dietary knowledge, and attitudes about diet and health of the U.S. population and (2) measuring food composition and the quality of the food supply.[13] Overall, the NNMS has the following goals:[14] *to ensure adequate nutrition [math sure]*

- ◆ Provide the scientific foundation for the maintenance and improvement of the nutrition status of the U.S. population and the nutritional quality and healthfulness of the national food supply.

- ◆ Collect, analyze, and disseminate timely data on the nutrition and dietary status of the U.S. population, the nutritional quality of the food supply, food consumption patterns, and consumer knowledge and attitudes concerning nutrition.

- ◆ Identify high-risk groups and geographic areas, as well as nutrition-related problems and trends, in order to facilitate prompt implementation of nutrition intervention activities.

- ◆ Establish national baseline data and develop and improve uniform standards, methods, criteria, policies, and procedures for nutrition monitoring.

◆ Provide data for evaluating the implications of changes in agricultural policy related to food production, processing, and distribution that may affect the nutritional quality and healthfulness of the U.S. food supply.

The NNMS surveys can be grouped into five areas: health status measurements, food consumption measurements, food composition measurements, dietary knowledge and attitudes, and food supply determinations. The next sections, which describe the major surveys in each area, are based on the directory of federal nutrition monitoring activities compiled by the Interagency Committee on Nutrition Monitoring.[15] Consult Figure 5-1 to clarify how the various surveys are used to obtain information about the relationship of food to health.

FIGURE 5-1   **A Conceptual Model of the Relationships of Food to Health**

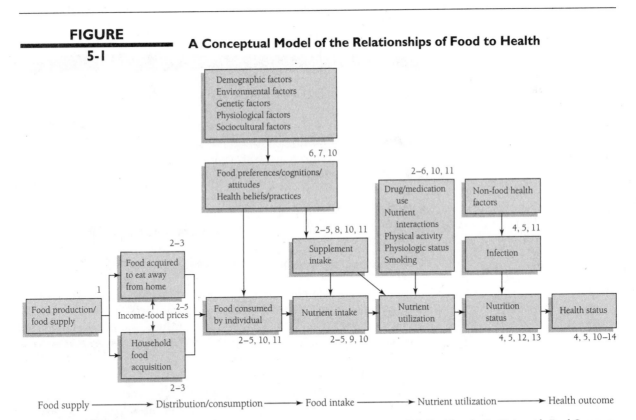

Identification of data sources from the National Nutrition Monitoring System. Data source: 1 = U.S. Food Supply; 2 = Nationwide Food Consumption Survey; 3 = Continuing Survey of Food Intakes by Individuals; 4 = National Health and Nutrition Examination Survey; 5 = Hispanic Health and Nutrition Examination Survey; 6 = Behavioral Risk Factors Surveillance System; 7 = Health and Diet Study; 8 = Vitamin/Mineral Supplement Intake Survey; 9 = Total Diet Study; 10 = National Health Interview Survey; 11 = NHANES I Epidemiologic Followup Study; 12 = Pediatric Nutrition Surveillance System; 13 = Pregnancy Nutrition Surveillance System; 14 = Vital Statistics.

Source: Adapted from the Second National Nutrition Monitoring Report of the Expert Panel (July 1989), by C. E. Woteki and M. T. Fanelli-Kuczmarski, The National Nutrition Monitoring System, in *Present Knowledge in Nutrition*, 6th ed. (Washington, D.C.: International Life Sciences Institute/Nutrition Foundation, 1990), p. 416. Reprinted with permission from International Life Sciences Institute.

Health and Nutrition Status Measurements The surveys that form the basis of the health and nutrition status component of the NNMS target a variety of specific population groups, including noninstitutionalized civilians over the age of 55 years, children aged 2 to 6 years, women of reproductive age, and individuals residing in nursing homes. The surveys collect data on diverse issues, such as family structures, community services, risk factors associated with cancer, aspects of family planning and fertility, and the causes of low birth weight among infants. The NHANES and the Coordinated State Surveillance System (CSSS) are included in this component. The CSSS is a surveillance program that monitors the nutrition status of low-income pediatric and pregnant populations at high risk for nutrition-related problems through the collection of measurements such as height, weight, hemoglobin, and hematocrit. In addition, findings are reported on anemia, abnormal weight changes, fetal survival, birth weight of the child, and whether breast or bottle feeding was used and for how long. Examples of the types of data collected in the NHANES and CSSS are shown in Table 5-2. The NHANES includes four programs:

♦ **National Health and Nutrition Examination Survey (NHANES I).** Conducted in 1971–1974, the NHANES I, like the other NHANES programs, was designed to collect and disseminate data that could be obtained best or only by direct physical examination, laboratory and clinical tests, and related measurements. The target population was civilian noninstitutionalized persons aged 1 through 74 years. The measures included dietary interviews, body composition measurements, hematologic tests, urine tests, X rays of the hand and wrist, dental examinations, and other measurements.

♦ **NHANES II.** Conducted in 1976–1980, this program targeted civilian noninstitutionalized persons aged 6 months through 74 years. It collected the same types of data as the NHANES I.

♦ **Hispanic Health and Nutrition Examination Survey (HHANES).** This survey, conducted in 1982–1984, was designed to collect and disseminate data obtained from physical examinations, diagnostic tests, anthropometric measurements, laboratory analyses, and personal interviews of Mexican Americans, Puerto Ricans, and Cubans. The target population consisted of "eligible" Hispanics aged 6 months through 74 years. "Eligible" Hispanics were limited to Mexican Americans living in five southwestern states; Cubans living in Dade County, Florida; and Puerto Ricans living in New York, New Jersey, and Connecticut.

♦ **NHANES III.** The NHANES III was conducted in 1988–1994. Its target population was civilian noninstitutionalized persons aged 2 months and over. The hematologic, biochemical, and examination components of NHANES III are shown in Table 5-3.

Food Consumption Measurements These surveys collect data on food consumption behavior. The Vitamin and Mineral Intake Survey, for example, assesses quantitatively the nutrient intake from vitamin and mineral supplements and the characteristics of supplement users. The Survey of Infant Feeding Practices

INDICATOR	NATIONAL HEALTH AND NUTRITION EXAMINATION SURVEY		COORDINATED STATE SURVEILLANCE SYSTEM	
	I[a]	II[b]	Pediatric	Pregnant
Height	Yes	Yes	Yes	...
Weight	Yes	Yes	Yes	...
Skinfold thickness:				
Triceps	Yes	Yes	...	...
Subscapular	Yes	Yes	...	...
Head circumference	...	Yes	Yes	...
Hemoglobin	Yes	Yes	Yes	Yes
Hematocrit	Yes	Yes	Yes	Yes
Red blood cell count	...	Yes	...	...
White blood cell count	Yes	Yes	...	...
Mean corpuscular volume	...	Yes	...	...
Mean corpuscular hemoglobin concentration	...	Yes	...	...
Red blood cell protoporphyrin	...	Yes	...	...
Serum iron	Yes	Yes	...	...
Serum total iron-binding capacity	Yes	Yes	...	...
Transferrin saturation	Yes	3–74 years	...	...
Ferritin	...	(c)	...	...
Serum zinc	...	3–74 years	...	...
Serum copper	...	3–74 years	...	...
Serum vitamin C	...	3–74 years	...	...
Serum albumin	...	3–74 years	...	...
Serum vitamin A	...	3–11 years	...	...
Red blood cell folate	...	(c)	...	...
Serum folate	...	(c)	...	...
Serum cholesterol	Yes	20–74 years	...	...
Serum triglycerides	...	20–74 years	...	...
High-density lipoprotein	...	20–74 years	...	...
Serum vitamin B$_{12}$	...	(c)	...	...
Breastfeeding	...	(c)	...	Yes
Low birth weight	...	...	Yes	Yes

[a]Ages surveyed are 1–74 years.
[b]Unless otherwise specified, ages surveyed are 6 months–74 years.
[c]Performed on a subsample of persons ages 3–74 years.

TABLE

5-2

Sources of Data on Indicators of Nutrition Status

Source: C. E. Woteki, Appendix VIII: Measuring dietary patterns in surveys, in Department of Health and Human Services, *Vital and Health Statistics: Dietary Methodology Workshop for the Third National Health and Nutrition Examination Survey* (Washington, D.C.: U.S. Government Printing Office, 1992), p. 102.

obtains data on the transition between breast and bottle feeding, the introduction of cow's milk, and the type and timing of the introduction of solid foods. The following are the other major surveys of this NNMS component:

◆ **Nationwide Food Consumption Survey (NFCS).** Conducted every 10 years (most recently, in 1987–1988) by the Human Nutrition Information Service of the USDA, the NFCS collects data that are used to describe food consumption behavior and to evaluate the nutritional content of diets for their implications for food policies, marketing, food safety, food assis-

Consult Appendix C for a list of specific data elements from the Nationwide Food Consumption Survey.

| TABLE 5-3 | Hematologic, Biochemical, and Examination Components for the NHANES III |

HEMATOLOGIC AND BIO-CHEMICAL ASSESSMENTS FOR THE NHANES III NUTRITIONAL COMPONENT[a]	EXAMINATION COMPONENTS FOR NHANES III BY AGE GROUP			
	2–11 Months	1–4 Years	5–19 Years	20 Years +
CBC[b]	Physician exam	Physician exam	Physician exam	Physician exam
Red cell distribution width (RCDW)	Body measurements	Body measurements	Body measurements	Body measurements
Iron and total iron-binding capacity	Tympanic impedance	Tympanic impedance	Tympanic impedance	Dietary interview
Ferritin	Dietary interview	Dietary interview	Dietary interview	Dental exam
Folate, serum and red cell		Dental exam (2+)[d]	Dental exam	Venipuncture
Protoporphyrin		Venipuncture	Venipuncture	Urine
Retinol and retinyl ester			Audiometry (6+)	Allergy skin test
Vitamin E			Urine	Spirometry
Carotenoids, total and individual			Cognitive test (5–17)	Bioelectrical impedance
Vitamin C			Allergy skin test (6+)	Hand and knee X-rays (60+)
25-hydroxyvitamin D			Spirometry (8+)	Electro-cardiogram
Calcium, serum and ionized				Oral glucose tolerance test
Selenium				Ultrasound exam
Cholesterol, total and HDL[c]				Bone densitometry
Triglycerides				
Apolipoproteins A_1 and B				
Lead				
Cadmium				

[a]This list includes analyses of most direct interest to nutritionists. Additional analyses planned for selected age groups are: herpes, hepatitis, *Chlamydia* and HIV serologies; cotinine; selected immunoglobulins; fibrinogen; creatinine, uric acid, glucose, alkaline phosphatase and others.
[b]The complete blood count includes the number of white blood cells (WBC) and red blood cells (RBC), the mean corpuscular volume (MCV), the mean corpuscular hemoglobin concentration (MCHC), hematocrit, and hemoglobin.
[c]HDL = high density lipoprotein
[d]The number given in parentheses (2+) indicates the age of subjects in years for which the examination component is recommended.

Source: C. E. Woteki and coauthors, National Health and Nutrition Survey—NHANES: Plans for NHANES III, *Nutrition Today* (January/February 1988): 26. © Williams & Wilkins. Used with permission.

tance, and nutrition education. The target population consists of private households of all incomes. The measures include the food used from home food supplies during one week by the entire household and the food ingested by individual household members both at home and away from home over a three-day period. The nutrient databases from the 1977–1978 and 1987 surveys are shown in Table 5-4.

1977–1978 DATABASE	1987 DATABASE
Food energy	Food energy
Protein	Protein
Total fat	Total fat
Carbohydrate	Carbohydrate
Vitamin A (IU)	Vitamin A (IU)
Vitamin C	Vitamin C
Thiamin	Thiamin
Riboflavin	Riboflavin
Niacin	Niacin
Vitamin B_6	Vitamin B_6
Vitamin B_{12}	Vitamin B_{12}
Calcium	Calcium
Phosphorus	Phosphorus
Magnesium	Magnesium
Iron	Iron
	Saturated fatty acids
	Monounsaturated fatty acids
	Polyunsaturated fatty acids
	Cholesterol
	Dietary fiber
	Vitamin A (RE)
	Carotenes
	Vitamin E
	Folate
	Zinc
	Copper
	Sodium
	Potassium

TABLE

5-4

USDA Nutrient Database for the Nationwide Food Consumption Surveys
Source: B. Peterkin, R. Rizek, and K. Tippett, Nationwide Food Consumption Survey, 1987, *Nutrition Today* (January/February 1988): 19. © Williams & Wilkins. Used with permission.

◆ **Continuing Survey of Food Intakes by Individuals (CSFII), 1985 and 1986.** The CSFII was designed to provide timely data on U.S. diets in general, the diets of high-risk population subgroups, and changes in dietary patterns over time. The target population was persons of selected sex and age in private households with incomes at any level (basic survey) and at or below 130 percent of the poverty guidelines (low-income survey). The 1985 survey focused on women and men aged 19–50 years and children aged 1–5 years. The 1986 survey focused on women and children and did not include men. Dietary measures included food intakes from multiple 24-hour recalls collected by interview.

◆ **Continuing Survey of Food Intakes by Individuals (CSFII), 1989–1996.** This survey resembles the CSFII series conducted in 1985 and 1986. The target population is men, women, and children of all ages. The dietary component includes the kinds and amounts of food ingested both at home and away from home by individual household members for three consecutive days as measured by a 24-hour recall (obtained by personal interview) and a two-day food diary.

Consult Appendix C for an at-a-glance summary of the sources of data on nutrients and other food constituents obtained from several NNMS surveys.

◆ **Total Diet Study (TDS).** This survey, conducted annually by the FDA, is designed to assess the levels of various nutritional components and organic and elemental contaminants of the U.S. food supply. The Selected Minerals in Food Survey, a component of the TDS, estimates the level of 11 essential minerals in representative diets. The target population is eight age-sex groups: infants, young children, male and female teenagers, male and female adults, and male and female older persons. The design includes collecting 234 foods from retail markets in urban areas, preparing them for consumption, and analyzing them for nutritional elements and contaminants four times a year.

Food Composition Measurements Information about the nutrient content of foods is provided by four different activities. The FDA's Total Diet Study estimates the daily intake of nutrients, pesticides, and contaminants. The Food Label and Package Survey (FLAPS), also undertaken by the FDA, is designed to monitor the labeling practices of U.S. food manufacturers; it analyzes about 300 foods to check the accuracy of nutrient values on food labels. Other activities include the following:

◆ **National Nutrient Data Bank.** This continuous activity of the Human Nutrition Information Service of the USDA compiles and disseminates data on the nutrient composition of foods. Sources of nutrient data include government-funded university research, scientific publications, food processors and trade groups, and the results of food analyses by the Nutrient Composition Laboratory.

◆ **Nutrient Composition Laboratory.** This research program of the nutrient composition laboratory, conducted by the USDA's Agricultural Research Service, is designed to develop new and/or improved methods for analyzing nutrients in foods and to transfer these methods and new technologies to the government, academic, and industrial sectors worldwide.

Dietary Knowledge and Attitude Assessment Surveys in this component of the NNMS gather data on weight-loss practices; the general public's knowledge about the relationship of diet to health problems such as hypertension, coronary heart disease, and cancer; awareness among the general public, physicians, nurses, and dietitians of the risk factors of high blood cholesterol and coronary heart disease; and knowledge and attitudes about cancer prevention and lifestyle risk factors. For example, the Diet-Health Knowledge Survey (DHKS) was initiated in 1989 by the USDA as a follow-up to the CSFII. It measures consumers' awareness, understanding, and attitudes about diet-health relationships and dietary guidance.

Food Supply Determinations Food available for consumption by the U.S. civilian population is determined by the USDA through its Food and Nutrition Supply Series surveys. These food supply or disappearance data have been available annually since 1909. The nutrient content of the available food supply is determined using food composition data and then used to estimate the nutrient content of the food supply on a per capita basis.

◆ USES OF NATIONAL NUTRITION MONITORING DATA

The primary purpose of national nutrition monitoring activities is to obtain the information needed to ensure a population's adequate nutrition. The collected data are used in health planning, program management and evaluation, and timely warning and intervention efforts to prevent acute food shortages.[16] A schematic representation of the relationship of nutrition monitoring to nutrition policy and research is shown in Figure 5-2. Data related to the population's nutrition status and dietary practices, obtained through national nutrition monitoring activities, are then used in directing research activities and making a variety of policy decisions involving food assistance programs, nutrition labeling, and education. Specific uses of a single survey, the Nationwide Food Consumption Survey, are listed in Table 5-5.

Congress, in particular, needs the data from nutrition monitoring activities to formulate nutrition and health policies and programs, assess the consequences of such policies, oversee the efficacy of federal food and nutrition assistance programs, and evaluate the extent to which federal programs result in a consistent

FIGURE	**Relationships Among Nutrition Research, Monitoring, and Policy Making**
5-2	

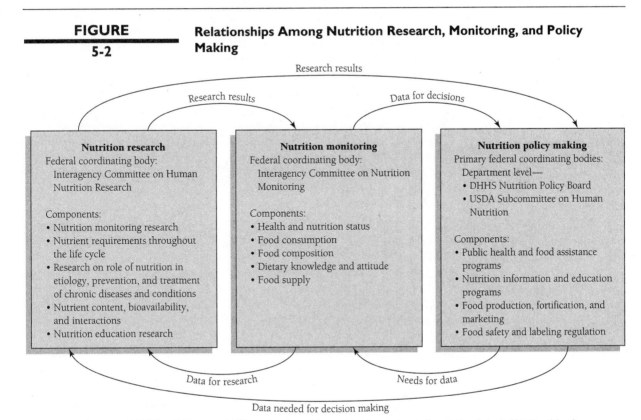

Source: C. Woteki and M. T. Fanelli-Kuczmarski, The national nutrition monitoring system, in *Present Knowledge in Nutrition,* 6th ed. (Washington, D.C.: International Life Sciences Institute/Nutrition Foundation, 1990), p. 416. Reprinted with permission from International Life Sciences Institute.

TABLE

5-5

Uses of Data from the Nationwide Food Consumption Surveys
Source: B. Peterkin, R. Rizek, and K. Tippett, Nationwide Food Consumption Survey, 1987, *Nutrition Today* (January/February 1988): 21. © Williams & Wilkins. Used with permission.

Assessment of Dietary Intake

◆ Provide detailed benchmark data on food and nutrient intake of the population
◆ Monitor the nutritional quality of diets
◆ Determine the size and nature of populations at risk
◆ Identify the intervention (food assistance, fortification, or education) most appropriate for populations at risk
◆ Identify socioeconomic factors associated with diets

Economics of Food Consumption

◆ Assess demand for agricultural products, marketing facilities, and services
◆ Determine the effects of socioeconomic factors on the demand and expenditure for food
◆ Determine the importance of home food production
◆ Determine the demand for food away from home and its effects on the nutritional quality of diets

Food Programs and Guidance

◆ Identify factors affecting participation in some large food programs and estimate the effect of participation on food expenditures and diet quality
◆ Estimate the effect of food programs on demand for food
◆ Identify populations that might benefit from intervention programs
◆ Identify changes in food and nutrient consumption that would reduce risk
◆ Develop food guides and plans that reflect food consumption practices and meet nutritional and cost criteria (e.g., Thrifty Food Plan used as a basis for allotment for the Food Stamp Program)
◆ Determine suitable amounts of foods to offer in food distribution programs

Food Safety Considerations

◆ Identify patterns of use of foods and food components in the diets of a population
◆ Estimate intake of incidental contaminants, food additives, and naturally occurring toxic substances
◆ Identify extreme and unusual patterns of intakes of foods or food ingredients, including additives
◆ Predict food items in which a food additive can safely be permitted in specified amounts
◆ Determine the need to modify regulations in response to changes in consumption
◆ Identify size and nature of population at risk from use of particular foods and food products

Historical Trends

◆ Correlate food consumption and dietary status with incidence of disease over time
◆ Follow food consumption through the life cycle
◆ Predict changes in food consumption and dietary status as they may be influenced by economic, technological, and other developments

and coordinated effort (a significant activity considering that no Federal Nutrition Office exists at the present time).[17] The data collected through the NNMS activities can be analyzed in several ways, as you will see in the Community Learning Activity later in this chapter.[18]

Nutrient Intake Standards

Merely collecting data on a population's nutrient intake and eating habits is not enough. Such data are meaningless on their own; to be valuable, they must be compared with some national standard related to nutrient needs. In the United States, two national committees are engaged in defining recommended nutrient intakes that best support health: the Committee on Diet and Health and the Committee on Dietary Allowances. Both are funded by the federal government and come under the auspices of the National Research Council of the National Academy of Sciences (NAS/NRC). The Committee on Diet and Health pays particular attention to reducing the risk of chronic disease and makes recommendations regarding certain dietary inadequacies and excesses, as shown in Table 5-6. These recommendations are intended to be used together with the Recommended Dietary Allowances (RDA) in planning optimal diets.

◆ THE RECOMMENDED DIETARY ALLOWANCES

The RDA are recommendations for nutrient intakes published by the Committee on Dietary Allowances, which focuses on energy and nutrient needs and the maintenance of health (see the inside front cover of this book for a table of the RDA). Periodically, the committee reexamines and revises these recommenda-

RDA The amounts of energy, protein and other selected nutrients (11 vitamins and seven minerals) considered adequate to meet the nutrient needs of practically all healthy people.

◆ Reduce total *fat* intake to 30% or less of calories. Reduce saturated fatty acid intake to less than 10% of calories, and the intake of cholesterol to less than 300 mg daily.[a]

◆ Increase intake of starches and other *complex carbohydrates*.[b]

◆ Maintain *protein* intake at moderate levels.[c]

◆ Balance food intake and physical activity to maintain appropriate *body weight*.

◆ For those who drink *alcoholic beverages*, the committee recommends limiting consumption to the equivalent of less than 1 oz of pure alcohol in a single day.[d] Pregnant women should avoid alcoholic beverages.

◆ Limit total daily intake of *salt* (sodium chloride) to 6 g or less.[e]

◆ Maintain adequate *calcium* intake.

◆ Avoid taking dietary *supplements* in excess of the RDA in any one day.

◆ Maintain an optimal intake of *fluoride*, particularly during the years of primary and secondary tooth formation and growth.

[a]The intake of fat and cholesterol can be reduced by substituting fish, poultry without skin, lean meats, and low- or nonfat dairy products for fatty meats and whole-milk products; by choosing more vegetables, fruits, cereals, and legumes; and by limiting oils, fats, egg yolks, and fried and other fatty foods.
[b]Every day eat five or more servings of a combination of vegetables and fruits, especially green and yellow vegetables and citrus fruits and six or more daily servings of a combination of breads, cereals, and legumes.
[c]Meet at least the RDA for protein; do not exceed twice the RDA.
[d]The committee does not recommend alcohol consumption. One ounce of pure alcohol is the equivalent of two cans of beer, two small glasses of wine, or two average cocktails.
[e]Limit the use of salt in cooking and avoid adding it to food at the table. Salty, highly processed salty, salt-preserved, and salt-pickled foods should be consumed sparingly.

TABLE

5-6

The National Research Council's Nutrition Recommendations

Source: Adapted with permission from the National Academy of Sciences report, *Diet and Health: Implications for Reducing Chronic Disease Risk,* which was produced by the Committee on Diet and Health of the Food and Nutrition Board of the National Research Council. Copyright 1989 by the National Academy of Sciences. Courtesy of the National Academy Press, Washington, D.C.

tions on the basis of new evidence regarding the nutrient needs of Americans. It then publishes an updated set of RDA. The most recent set was published in 1989. The following factors offer a perspective on the RDA:

◆ The RDA are based on available scientific research.

◆ The RDA are recommendations, not requirements, and certainly not minimal requirements. They include a substantial margin of safety.

◆ The RDA take into account differences among individuals and define a range within which most healthy people's intakes of nutrients probably should fall. Individuals whose nutrient needs are higher than the average are included within this range.

◆ The RDA are tools best suited for evaluating the nutrient intakes of populations or groups. They are less useful—but still often used—for estimating an individual's nutrition status. Ideally, when comparing an individual's dietary intake to the RDA, the individual's typical intake should be determined as an average derived from several days' intakes.

◆ THE DIETARY RECOMMENDATIONS OF OTHER COUNTRIES AND GROUPS

The Canadian RNI, Food Guide, and Guidelines for Healthy Eating are given in Appendix D.

Various nations and international groups have published different sets of standards similar to the RDA. The Canadian recommendations—the RNI (Recommended Nutrient Intakes)—differ from the RDA in some respects, partly due to differences in interpreting the data from which they were derived.[19]

Among the most widely used recommendations are those of the Food and Agriculture Organization (FAO) and the World Health Organization (WHO). The FAO/WHO recommendations are considered sufficient for the maintenance of health in nearly all people. They differ from the RDA because they are based on slightly different judgment factors and serve different purposes. The FAO/WHO recommendations, for example, assume a protein quality lower than that commonly consumed in the United States and so recommend a higher intake of this nutrient. They also take into consideration that people worldwide are generally smaller and more physically active than the U.S. population. For the most part, the various recommendations all fall within the same general range.

Nutrition Surveys: How Well Do We Eat?

When the results of national surveys are compared to standards such as the RDA, what do they tell us about the nutrition status and dietary patterns of Americans? How well do we eat? The answer to these questions has been mixed from the beginning. Although we are well nourished, we are also generally overfat, under-exercised, and beset to some extent with nutrient deficiencies. The picture has also been changing. People today eat out much more often than they did 50 years ago. They eat far more processed and convenience foods and fewer whole, farm-type foods. The following section reviews the major survey findings from the past 60 years. Later in the chapter, the nation's recommended strategies for obtaining optimal nutrition are presented.

◆ SURVEYS OF NUTRITION STATUS

Before World War II, a food consumption survey suggested that as many as a third of the U.S. population might be poorly fed.[20] During the 1940s, 1950s, and 1960s, other surveys confirmed this impression. Nutrients found lacking in subgroups of the population included calcium, iron, thiamin, riboflavin, vitamin A, and occasionally vitamin C. Most vulnerable to nutrient deficiencies were girls, women, and elderly men; no group was without some cases of iron deficiency. Other nutrients now known to be important in human nutrition, such as vitamin B_6, folate, magnesium, and zinc, were not studied in the early surveys.

During the 1970s, hunger and malnutrition in the United States came to the public's awareness through the Ten-State Survey, which included measures of dietary intake (by means of diet histories), physical examinations, and laboratory tests of nutrition status. The physical examinations revealed few severe deficiencies, but the findings included the following:

◆ Iron nutrition was a problem in all groups, especially among African Americans.

◆ Vitamin A status was a major concern among teenagers and Hispanics.

◆ Riboflavin deficiency appeared to be a potential problem, especially among African Americans, Hispanics, and young people of all ethnic groups.

◆ Protein deficiency was not widespread but was seen among people with low incomes.

◆ Pregnant and lactating women had lower protein intakes and lower blood levels of protein than most other groups.

Indicators of nutrient deficiencies among participants in the Ten-State Survey tended to cluster together. A person deficient in iron was likely to lack vitamin A as well. Generally, African Americans and Hispanics had a higher incidence of multiple deficiencies; a higher incidence also occurred in the low-income states. An important finding was that more multiple low values occurred in families where the homemaker had completed fewer years of school. Importantly, trends observed among the children were also found in adults in the same families.

Anthropometric measures revealed that people who were less economically deprived had greater height, weight, fatness, skeletal weight, and other indicators of earlier and greater physical development. Obesity was more prominent in adult women, especially in black women. Sugar intakes were high in most groups, and high sugar intakes were often accompanied by dental caries, especially in adolescents. Dental decay was associated with low income in all groups.

The Ten-State Survey had a built-in bias; it oversampled among the poor. Still, it provided a disturbing answer to the question, How well do we eat? Clearly, not as well as might be expected in one of the most prosperous nations

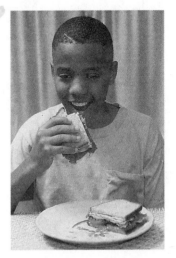

National surveys report that dietary patterns observed among children resemble those of their parents.

in the world. The concerns raised by the survey led to the design and implementation of another population-based survey, the NHANES I, conducted among 20,000 people at 65 sampling sites in the United States. NHANES I avoided the bias of the Ten-State Survey by adjusting for the effects of oversampling among vulnerable groups. Careful efforts were also made to evaluate protein and energy intakes in relation to height, sex, and age on an individual basis.

The NHANES investigators studied intakes of the same seven nutrients as in the Ten-State Survey and niacin and food energy intakes as well. Nutrient deficiencies were found for protein, calcium, vitamin A, and iron. As expected, these were more extensive among people below the poverty line than among those above, and they were generally more extensive in African Americans than in whites. Among the generalizations that emerged were the following:

- ◆ Calcium intakes were low for adult black women of all income groups.
- ◆ Vitamin A intakes were low for adolescent black girls of all income groups.
- ◆ Iron intakes were low for all women and for infant boys regardless of income.

The NHANES II, conducted as a follow-up to NHANES I, likewise found malnutrition within the sample population:

- ◆ Low blood values for protein and vitamin A in up to 3 percent of subjects
- ◆ Low blood values for thiamin in up to 14 percent of white and 29 percent of black subjects
- ◆ Low blood values for riboflavin in up to 3 percent of white and 8 percent of black subjects
- ◆ Low blood iron values, by three measures, in 5–15 percent of white and 18–27 percent of black subjects

Not everyone with low intakes of a nutrient had low laboratory values, and the investigators suggested that some of those with low intakes were at the very beginning stages of deficiency—"at risk" for malnutrition. In measuring the heights and weights of people, the NHANES researchers observed a continuing trend toward higher amounts of body fat among Americans.

Caution must be exercised in interpreting the NHANES data. On the one hand, when average nutrient intakes are examined, severe deficiencies in individuals can be missed. On the other hand, findings based on a single day's intake—as the NHANES findings were—can overestimate the extent of undernutrition. The survey's principal usefulness lies in its ability to identify the population subgroups most at risk of deficiency and the nutrients most in need of attention.

◆ SURVEYS OF FOOD CONSUMPTION

The Nationwide Food Consumption Survey (NFCS) was conducted in 1977–1978 to see how much and what kind of food people were eating at home and outside the home. The NFCS, like the Ten-State Survey, found that dietary adequacy was related to income. Table 5-7 shows the results for six nutrients. People with lower

NUTRIENT	INCOME TO $6,000	INCOME OF $6,000 TO $9,999	INCOME OF $10,000 TO $15,999	INCOME OF $16,000 AND OVER
Vitamin A	36%	33%	32%	29%
Vitamin B$_6$[a]	59	51	49	48
Vitamin C	30	29	27	23
Calcium	49	43	39	39
Iron[b]	29	31	33	33
Magnesium	48	40	36	35

Data indicate the percentage of persons in each income group with intakes at or below 70% of the RDA. For example: 36% of all those surveyed whose incomes were at or below $6000 per year had vitamin A intakes at or below 70% of the RDA.

[a]Vitamin B$_6$ intakes may not be as deficient as they appear. People who get along on minimal protein intakes need less than the RDA of vitamin B$_6$ to handle the amount of protein they consume.
[b]Notice that with the exception of iron, as income increases, the incidence of inadequate nutrient intakes diminishes.

TABLE

5-7

Nationwide Food Consumption Survey Findings
Source: U.S. Department of Agriculture, Nationwide Food Consumption Survey, NFCS 1977–1978.

incomes had lower intakes of five of them. Folate and zinc intakes were not assessed in the NFCS; insufficient data were available at the time on food contents of these nutrients and on the factors in food that affect their assimilation and use by the body. Some of the survey findings included the following:

◆ Very few of those surveyed had fat intakes below the recommended maximum of 30 percent of total calories.

◆ Sugar constituted 10 to 15 percent of the calorie intakes of most children.

◆ Cholesterol intakes ranged up to 450 to 500 milligrams per day in boys and men.

Data from the 1987 NFCS reveal that the diets of most adults do not conform to current dietary guidelines.[21] The survey results suggest that as the nutritional adequacy of the diet rises, the percentage of calories from fat also tends to rise.[22] Indeed, despite the media attention to nutrition over the past decade, the nation's food intake changed little between the two surveys.

Information is still accumulating from ongoing analyses of the data from the most recent surveys, but a general trend has emerged. People are overconsuming calories, underexpending energy, or both. The majority are adequately nourished with respect to most individual nutrients, but deficiencies and marginal intakes of nutrients do exist.[23]

The Challenge of Dietary Guidance

If nutrition monitoring activities reveal that a population is malnourished in some capacity, then what steps can be taken to improve the population's overall nutritional intake? Several approaches can be used to remedy the situation (refer to Figure 5-2). Research into the role of diet in health and disease can be undertaken to provide data on nutrient needs, lifestyle factors, and aspects of the disease process; policy decisions can be made about the distribution of foodstuffs; and existing food assistance programs can be evaluated for their effectiveness in meeting food and nutritional needs, to name a few. The development and dissemination of dietary guidance systems is another approach, a type of educational effort to improve the public's knowledge about healthful eating. In his report to the American Society for Clinical Nutrition on "The Evidence Relating Six Dietary Factors to the Nation's Health," former assistant Secretary for Health and Surgeon General Julius Richmond commented: "Individuals have the right to make informed choices and the government has the responsibility to provide the best data for making good dietary decisions."[24] Dietary guidance systems, such as food group plans and dietary guidelines, are methods by which the federal government helps the American people make prudent dietary decisions.

◆ FOOD GROUP PLANS

Food group plan A diet-planning tool that sorts foods of similar origin and nutrient content into groups and then specifies that a person eat a certain number of foods from each group.

Dietary guidance in the form of **food group plans** has been provided to the U.S. population since the turn of the century. The early forms of dietary recommendations tended to focus on the consumption of adequate amounts of the foods needed to provide nutrients and energy intake for good health.[25] The USDA, for example, published its first dietary guidance plan in 1916. At that time, human nutrient requirements were classified into five food groups: protein sources (milk, eggs, meat, fish, poultry, and meat alternatives), vegetables and fruits, breads and cereals, butter and other fats, and simple sugars (see Table 5-8 for a comparison of U.S. food guides).

TABLE

5-8

A Comparison of Early U.S. Food Group Plans

FIVE FOOD GROUPS (1916)	BASIC SEVEN (1943)	BASIC FOUR (1956)[a]
Protein foods Milk, eggs, meat, poultry, fish, and meat alternatives	Milk and milk products (2)[b] Meat, poultry, fish, etc. (2), eggs (4/week)	Milk and milk products (2) Meat, poultry, fish, eggs, and meat alternatives (2)
Vegetables and fruits	Green and yellow vegetables (1)	Fruits and vegetables (4)
	Citrus fruits and cabbage (1) Potatoes, other fruits and vegetables (2)	
Bread and cereal foods	Bread, flour, cereal (enriched or whole grain) (3)	Bread, flour, cereal (enriched or whole grain) (4)
Butter and other fats	Equivalent of 2 tablespoons of butter or fortified margarine	
Simple sugars		

[a]The Harvard School of Public Health developed the original version of the Basic Four Food Groups in 1955; the USDA published a similar version in 1956.
[b]The number of recommended servings appears in parentheses.

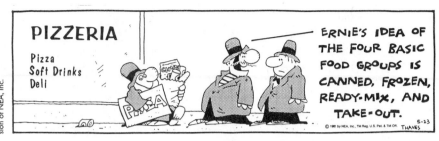

Between 1916 and the late 1940s, a variety of food group plans, featuring anywhere from 5 to 12 food groups, were published by federal agencies and voluntary health organizations. All had as a common theme the advice to eat a balanced diet providing nutrient-dense foods in the right proportion and containing an adequate energy level.[26] In 1943, the Bureau of Home Economics published a food guide that promoted seven food groups as part of the USDA's National Wartime Nutrition Program. The Basic Seven guide served as the basis of virtually all nutrition education programs for more than a decade. Then, in 1955, the Department of Nutrition at the Harvard School of Public Health published a recommendation that the food groups be collapsed into four groups: fruits and vegetables, cereals, milk and dairy products, and meat and meat alternatives.[27]

The Four Food Group plan, as it came to be called, has been promoted as an educational tool by the USDA since 1956. The Basic Four Food Groups highlighted intakes of protective or nutrient-bearing foods and ensured adequate intakes of the 1953 recommended levels of protein, vitamins A and C, and calcium. Meal plans based on the Basic Four were also generally adequate in thiamin, riboflavin, and niacin and in iron for men. The USDA added a fifth group (fats, sweets, and alcohol) to the plan in 1979 to draw attention to foods targeted for moderation but did not offer specific limitations for the fifth group.

Since the publication of the Basic Four Food Groups, however, the emphasis of nutritional guidance has expanded from just meeting nutrient needs to also eating a diet low in saturated fat and cholesterol and generous in fiber. With the publication of the *Surgeon General's Report on Nutrition and Health* in 1988, the overconsumption of certain dietary constituents became a major concern. For this reason, the Food Guide Pyramid was introduced to reinforce our understanding of the nutrient composition of foods, human nutrient needs, and the relationship of diet to health. The Food Guide Pyramid, shown in Figure 5-3, conveys five of the essential components of a healthful daily diet: adequacy, balance, moderation, calorie control, and variety. It can also be used to implement the Dietary Guidelines (described in the next section).

The Food Guide Pyramid differs from the Basic Four Food Groups in that it provides guidance for a total rather than a foundation diet. The framework of food groups, illustrated as a pyramid, is supplemented by additional information about food energy, total fat, types of fat, sodium, sweeteners, and cholesterol. The nutrition goals of the Food Guide Pyramid are to help consumers select diets that

FIGURE

5-3

The Daily Food Guide and Food Guide Pyramid
Source: *The Food Guide Pyramid* (Hyattsville, Md.: USDA, 1992), Home and Garden Bulletin No. 252.

The Daily Food Guide

Breads, Cereals, and Other Grain Products

These foods are notable for their contributions of complex carbohydrates, riboflavin, thiamin, niacin, iron, protein, magnesium, and fiber.

6 to 11 servings per day.

Serving = 1 slice bread; $^1/_2$ c cooked cereal, rice, or pasta; 1 oz ready-to-eat cereal; $^1/_2$ bun, bagel, or English muffin; 1 small roll, biscuit or muffin; 3 to 4 small or 2 large crackers.

◆ Whole grains (wheat, oats, barley, millet, rye, bulgur), enriched breads, rolls, tortillas, cereals, bagels, rice, pastas (macaroni, spaghetti), air-popped corn.

◆ Pancakes, muffins, cornbread, crackers, low-fat cookies, biscuits, presweetened cereals.

◆ Croissants, doughnuts, granola.

Vegetables

These foods are notable for their contributions of vitamin A, vitamin C, folate, potassium, magnesium, and fiber, and for their lack of fat and cholesterol.

3 to 5 servings per day (use dark green, leafy vegetables and legumes several times a week).

Serving = $^1/_2$ c cooked or raw vegetables; 1 c leafy raw vegetables; $^1/_2$ c cooked legumes; $^3/_4$ c vegetable juice.

◆ Bean sprouts, broccoli, brussels sprouts, cabbage, carrots, cauliflower, cucumbers, green beans, green peas, leafy greens (spinach, mustard, and collard greens), legumes, lettuce, mushrooms, tomatoes, winter squash.

◆ Corn, potatoes, sweet potatoes.

◆ French fries, potato salad.

Fruits

These foods are notable for their contributions of vitamin A, vitamin C, potassium, and fiber, and for their lack of sodium, fat, and cholesterol.

2 to 4 servings per day.

Serving = typical portion (such as 1 medium apple, banana, or orange; $^1/_2$ grapefruit, 1 melon wedge); $^3/_4$ c juice; $^1/_2$ c berries; $^1/_2$ c diced, cooked, or canned fruit; $^1/_4$ c dried fruit.

◆ Apricots, cantaloupe, grapefruit, oranges, orange juice, peaches, strawberries, apples, bananas, pears.

◆ Canned fruit.

◆ Dried fruit, coconut.

Meat, Poultry, Fish, and Alternatives

These foods are notable for their contributions of protein, phosphorus, vitamin B_6, vitamin B_{12}, zinc, magnesium, iron, niacin, and thiamin.

2 to 3 servings per day.

Servings = 2 to 3 oz lean, cooked meat, poultry, or fish (total 5 to 7 oz per day); count 1 egg, $^1/_2$ c cooked legumes, or 2 tbsp peanut butter as 1 oz meat (or about $^1/_3$ serving).

◆ Poultry, fish, lean meat (beef, lamb, pork, veal), legumes, egg whites.

◆ Fat-trimmed beef, lamb, pork; refried beans; egg yolks.

◆ Hot dogs, luncheon meats, peanut butter, nuts.

Key:
◆ Foods generally highest in nutrient density.
◆ Foods moderate in nutrient density.
◆ Foods lowest in nutrient density.

Continued

Milk, Cheese, and Yogurt

These foods are notable for their contributions of calcium, riboflavin, protein, vitamin B_{12}, and, when fortified, vitamin D and vitamin A.

2 servings per day.

3 servings per day for teenagers and young adults, pregnant/lactating women.

4 servings per day for pregnant/lactating teenagers.

Serving = 1 c milk or yogurt; 2 oz process cheese food; 1 $^1/_2$ oz cheese.

◆ Nonfat and 1% low-fat milk (and nonfat products such as buttermilk, cottage cheese, cheese, yogurt); fortified soy-milk.

◆ 2% low-fat milk (and low-fat products such as yogurt, cheese, cottage cheese); frozen yogurt; ice milk.

◆ Whole milk (and whole-milk products such as cheese, yogurt, cottage cheese); cream; sour cream; cream cheese; custard; milk shakes; pudding; ice cream.

Fats, Sweets, and Alcoholic Beverages

These foods are notable for their contributions of sugar, fat, alcohol, and food energy. These foods are not in the pattern because they provide few nutrients. Note that some of the following items could be placed in more than one group or in a combination group. For example, doughnuts are high in both sugar and fat.

◆ Foods high in fat include margarine, salad dressings, oils, mayonnaise, cream, cream cheese, butter, gravy, and sauces.

◆ Foods high in sugar include cake, pie, cookies, doughnuts, sweet rolls, candy, soft drinks, fruit drinks, jelly, syrup, gelatin, desserts, sugar, and honey.

◆ Alcoholic beverages include wine, beer, and liquor.

Note: Serve children at least the lower number of servings from each group, but in smaller amounts (for example, $^1/_4$ to $^1/_3$ cup rice). Children should receive the equivalent of 2 cups of milk each day, but again in smaller quantities per serving (for example, 4 half-cup portions). Pregnant women may require additional servings of fruits, vegetables, meats, and breads to meet their higher needs for energy, vitamins, and minerals.

FIGURE

5-3

The Daily Food Guide and Food Guide Pyramid—Continued

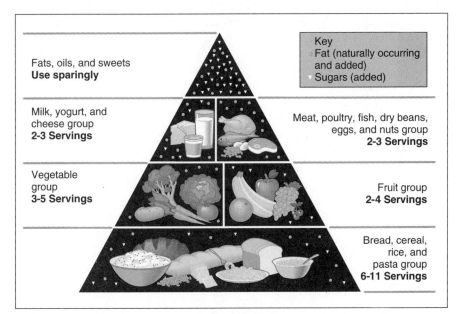

Food Guide Pyramid

A Guide to Daily Food Choices

The breadth of the base shows that grains (breads, cereals, rice, and pasta) deserve most emphasis in the diet. The tip is smallest: use fats, oils, and sweets sparingly.

provide an appropriate amount of energy to maintain a healthful weight; meet the RDA for all nutrients without depending on supplements or a few highly fortified foods; are varied in types of fat and moderate in total fat, caloric sweeteners, sodium, cholesterol, and alcohol; and are adequate in complex carbohydrates and fiber.

◆ DIETARY GUIDELINES

Food group plans focus on recommended levels of food consumption. Dietary guidelines are typically broader than food group plans and focus on goal statements related to overall nutrient intake and daily eating patterns. The first attempt to formulate national dietary guidelines was undertaken in 1977, with the publication of the "Dietary Goals for the United States," a report of the U.S. Senate Select Committee on Nutrition and Human Needs. In the 1980s, so many dietary guidelines were published that consumers were overwhelmed by the dietary advice, not knowing which group to listen to. In this section, we describe the major dietary guidelines published by both government and nongovernment organizations.

Government Guidelines   Although the federal government's decision to promote a set of dietary goals or guidelines to improve the public's health would seem to be a straightforward matter of setting national nutrition policy, in fact, there has been much discussion about whether the government *should* establish such guidelines for the entire population. Concerns have focused on whether scientists could achieve a consensus on research outcomes and the relationship of diet to disease processes. Other questions also arose: What obligation do nutrition scientists and educators have to the general public to explain study outcomes and the differences that sometimes arise in interpreting study results? Who decides when research results are firm enough to warrant incorporating them into dietary guidance systems for the public? Is it appropriate to make general dietary recommendations for the *entire* population, when only a portion may be at risk for a specific disease condition? In what ways will the availability of national dietary guidelines—or the lack of them—affect the delivery of health care and educational efforts in the public health arena?[28]

Consider the comments made by Marc LaLonde, Canada's former minister of National Health and Welfare, in 1974:

> Even such a simple question as whether one should severely limit his consumption of butter and eggs can be a subject of endless scientific debate.
>
> Faced with conflicting scientific opinions of this kind, it would be easy for health educators and promoters to sit on their hands; it certainly makes it easy for those who abuse their health to find a real "scientific" excuse.
>
> But many of Canada's health problems are sufficiently pressing that action has to be taken even if all scientific evidence is not in.[29]

These words are relevant today in both Canada and the United States. Keep these comments and issues in mind as you read the following descriptions of various dietary guidelines.

◆ **U.S. Dietary Goals.** The U.S. Dietary Goals were designed to serve as "a practical guide to promote good eating habits" and as a catalyst for both government and industry action to help the public meet the recommended dietary goals.[30] The goals arose from a widespread concern among nutritionists, scientists, and policymakers that malnutrition—both underconsumption and overconsumption—was widespread in the United States, largely because the U.S. diet had changed since the turn of the century. Whereas the U.S. diet had consisted largely of complex carbohydrates, with only small amounts of fat and sugar, it had shifted by the 1970s to a diet in which fat and sugar comprised at least 60 percent of total caloric intake. Concerns about the link between fat- and calorie-rich diets and the risk of diseases such as coronary heart disease, cancer, hypertension, diabetes, and obesity led to the formulation of population-wide dietary goals to encourage the consumption of the most healthful foods (see Table 5-9).

The Dietary Goals met with much discussion and disagreement. Some nutritionists argued that the general public urgently needed dietary guidance, considering the complexity of our diets, nutrient needs, and disease processes and patterns. They argued that "it is the responsibility of a government to provide guidelines and to have a well-reasoned and consistent food and nutrition policy."[31] Others argued that some disease conditions were not exclusively nutrition problems and hence population-wide dietary goals were not appropriate. These opponents were concerned about how dietary goals might influence the dietary patterns of children, whether such goals could be expected to deliver the promised benefits, and how nutrition education practices would change if dietary goals were widely adopted.[32] There has never been complete agreement on the appropriateness of the Dietary Goals as an instrument of national nutrition policy, and they have stimulated much controversy and debate.

TABLE
5-9

1. To avoid overweight, consume only as much energy (calories) as is expended; if overweight, decrease energy intake and increase energy expenditure.
2. Increase the consumption of complex carbohydrates and "naturally occurring" sugars from about 28% of energy intake to about 48% of energy intake.
3. Reduce the consumption of refined and processed sugars by about 45% to account for about 10% of total energy intake.
4. Reduce overall fat consumption from approximately 40% to about 30% of energy intake.
5. Reduce saturated fat consumption to account for about 10% of total energy intake; and balance that with polyunsaturated and monounsaturated fats, which should account for about 10% of energy intake each.
6. Reduce cholesterol consumption to about 300 mg a day.
7. Limit the intake of sodium by reducing the intake of salt to about 5 g a day.

The U.S. Dietary Goals
Source: U.S. Senate, Select Committee on Nutrition and Human Needs, *Dietary Goals for the United States,* 2nd ed. (Washington, D.C.: Government Printing Office, 1977).

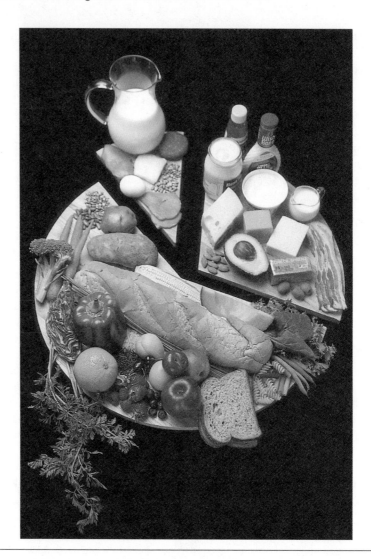

The *U.S. Dietary Goals* recommend a balanced diet composed of 12% protein from animal or vegetable sources, 58% carbohydrate from fruits, vegetables, legumes, and whole grains, and no more than 30% of total calories from fat, including the fat from meats and dairy products.

◆ **Dietary Guidelines for Americans.** The third edition of the *Dietary Guidelines for Americans* was published jointly by the USDA and the DHHS in 1990 (earlier editions had been published in 1980 and 1985). The principles of healthful eating promoted by the 1990 edition of the Dietary Guidelines, illustrated in Figure 5-4, grew out of reports such as the *Surgeon General's Report on Nutrition and Health,* the National Research Council's report on *Diet and Health,* and the National Cholesterol Education Program's *Report of the Expert Panel on Detection, Evaluation, and Treatment of High Blood Cholesterol in Adults.*[33] These reports all pointed to the need to change and improve the eating patterns of the U.S. population.

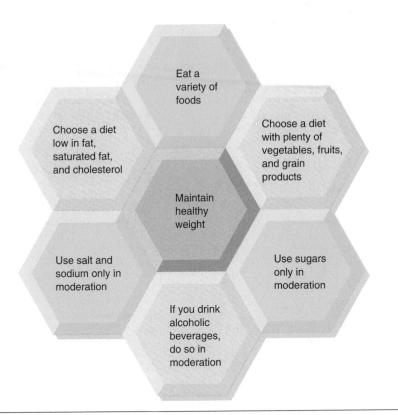

FIGURE

5-4

The Dietary Guidelines
Consumers are urged to use the seven guidelines together in choosing a healthful and enjoyable diet.

Thus, the Dietary Guidelines were designed to be consistent with these reports and the recommendations of other government and voluntary health organizations. They emphasize moderation and the avoidance of over- and underconsuming foods. They apply to the diet as consumed over several days, not to a single meal or food. The key guideline is to consume a variety of foods providing adequate amounts of nutrients and a calorie level that maintains a reasonable body weight.[34] Figure 5-5 shows how the Food Guide Pyramid serves as a mechanism for implementing the Dietary Guidelines.

◆ **Other U.S. government dietary guidelines.** A variety of government agencies, including the Surgeon General's office, the National Cancer Institute, and the National Heart, Lung, and Blood Institute, issued dietary guidelines during the 1980s. Some of these recommendations are quite general, while others contain very specific recommended intakes of certain dietary components, such as saturated fat, polyunsaturated fat, and fiber. Consult Table 5-10 for a comparison of dietary recommendations by these and other groups.

Nongovernment Dietary Recommendations During the 1980s, dietary recommendations were also issued by a variety of voluntary health organizations,

The nutrition recommendations for Canadians and those promoted by the World Health Organization are shown in the boxed insert on page 149.

FIGURE
5-5
The USDA/DHHS Food Guide Graphic as a Mechanism for Putting the Dietary Guidelines into Action

Dietary Guidelines for Americans, 1990	Key Concepts of the USDA Food Guide	Graphic Requirements
• Eat a variety of foods.	**Variety**—Eating a selection of foods of various types that together meet nutritional needs.	**Variety**—The graphic must present six categories of food.
• Choose a diet with plenty of vegetables, fruits, and grain products.	**Proportionality**—Eating appropriate amounts of various types of foods to meet nutritional needs.	**Proportionality**—The graphic must present the relative amounts of the various food groups to eat daily and the range in the number of servings to eat within food groups.
• Maintain healthy weight. • Choose a diet low in fat, saturated fat, and cholesterol. • Use sugars only in moderation. • Use salt and sodium only in moderation.	**Moderation**—Avoiding too much of food components in the total diet that have been linked to disesases.	**Moderation**—The graphic must indicate moderation of fat and added sugars in the total diet. Foods in the fats, oils, and sweets group should be identified as concentrated sources of fat and/or added sugars, but other food group sources should be identified as well.
• If you drink alcoholic beverages, do so in moderation.	**Usability**—The food guide must be practical and flexible enough to meet the needs and preferences of healthy Americans over the age of 2 years.	**Usability**—The key concepts listed above must be understandable and memorable.

Source: S. Welsh, C. Davis, and A. Shaw, Development of the Food Guide Pyramid, *Nutrition Today* 27 (1992): 16. © Williams & Wilkins. Used with permission.

such as the American Heart Association, American Cancer Society, and American Institute for Cancer Research. These groups were motivated to provide dietary guidance for the public by the growing scientific evidence linking certain dietary patterns with increased risk for heart disease and some types of cancer. The main dietary recommendations of these groups are given in Table 5-10. These recommendations represent attempts to create broad, noncontroversial recommendations for dietary habits in the United States.

The ten leading causes of death in the United States were shown in Chapter 1 (see page 9). In all, eight of them have been linked to our diet, as mentioned earlier. The various sets of guidelines are proposed in order to reduce the risks associated with diet. A sedentary life-style and overconsumption of foods high in calories, salt, sugar, fat, cholesterol, and alcohol have been associated with obesity, high blood pressure, heart attacks, strokes, diabetes, dental caries, liver disease, and some forms of cancer—the so-called **life-style diseases**. To alter these trends, the recommendations suggest a general increase in the consumption of complex carbohydrates such as fruits, vegetables, and whole grains, and a decrease in the consumption of meats and foods high in fat, sugar, and salt.

Life-style diseases Conditions that may be aggravated by modern life-styles that include too much eating, drinking, and smoking, and too little exercise.

Other Nutrition Recommendations

Nutrition Recommendations for Canadians

Like the *Diet and Health* report, the Nutrition Recommendations for Canadians examines the relationships linking nutrition and disease. The intent is to make recommendations that will supply enough nutrients, while reducing the risk of chronic disease. The Scientific Review Committee adopted the following key statements as the Nutrition Recommendations for Canadians.

- ◆ The Canadian diet should provide energy consistent with the maintenance of body weight within the recommended range.
- ◆ The Canadian diet should include essential nutrients in amounts recommended in the RNI (see Appendix D).
- ◆ The Canadian diet should include no more than 30 percent of energy as fat and no more than 10 percent as saturated fat.
- ◆ The Canadian diet should provide 55 percent of energy as carbohydrate from a variety of sources.
- ◆ The sodium content of the Canadian diet should be reduced.
- ◆ The Canadian diet should include no more than 5 percent of total energy as alcohol, or two drinks daily, whichever is less.
- ◆ The Canadian diet should contain no more caffeine than the equivalent of four regular cups of coffee per day.
- ◆ Community water supplies containing less than 1 milligram per liter should be fluoridated to that level.

Nutrition Recommendations from WHO

WHO has also assessed the relationships between diet and the development of chronic diseases. Its recommendations are expressed in average daily ranges that represent the lower and upper limits:

- ◆ Total energy: sufficient to support normal growth, physical activity, and body weight.
- ◆ Total fat: 15 to 30 percent of total energy.
  - ◆ Saturated fatty acids: 0 to 10 percent of total energy.
  - ◆ Polyunsaturated fatty acids: 3 to 7 percent of total energy.
  - ◆ Dietary cholesterol: 0 to 300 milligrams per day.
- ◆ Total carbohydrate: 55 to 75 percent of total energy.
  - ◆ Complex carbohydrates: 50 to 75 percent of total energy.
  - ◆ Dietary fiber: 27 to 40 grams per day.
  - ◆ Refined sugars: 0 to 10 percent of total energy.
- ◆ Protein: 10 to 15 percent of total energy.
- ◆ Salt: upper limit of 6 grams/day (no lower limit set).

Source: Adapted from Scientific Review Committee and the Communications/Implementation Committe, *Nutrition Recommendations: A Call for Action* (Ottawa: Canadian Government Publishing Centre, 1989); *Diet, Nutrition, and the Prevention of Chronic Diseases. Report of a WHO Study Group* (Geneva: World Health Organization, WHO Technical Report Series, No. 797, 1990), p. 108.

TABLE 5-10   **Dietary Recommendations for Healthy Americans (1982–Present)**

TITLE AND ORGAN-IZATION	PURPOSE OF REPORT	ENSURE NUTRIENT ADEQUACY/ VARIETY IN DIET	MAINTAIN DESIRABLE BODY WEIGHT	REDUCE TOTAL FAT (% kcal)	REDUCE SATURATED FAT (% kcal)	POLY UNSATU-RATED FAT (% kcal)
REDUCE CANCER RISK						
Diet, Nutrition and Cancer, 1982. National Research Council	Scientific review for the scientific community with interim guidelines for the public	—	—	To 30%	Yes	Reduce
Nutrition and Cancer: Cause and Prevention—A Special Report, 1984. American Cancer Society	Referenced report for health professionals	—	Yes	Yes	—	—
Planning Meals That Lower Cancer Risk: A Reference Guide, 1984. American Institute for Cancer Research	A food guide for health professionals	—	—	To 30% or less	—	—
NCI Dietary Guidelines: Rationale, 1988. National Cancer Institute, U.S. Dept. of Health and Human Services	Referenced statement for health professionals	—	Yes	To 30% or less	—	—
Recommended Dietary Allowances, 1989. National Research Council	Basis for evaluating the nutrient adequacy of diets for population groups by health professionals	Yes	—	To 30% or less	< 10%	Up to 10%
REDUCE HEART DISEASE RISK						
Dietary Guidelines For Healthy American Adults, 1988. American Heart Association	Referenced statement for health professionals	Yes	Yes	< 30%	< 10%	Up to 10%

Continued

TABLE
5-10

**TABLE
5-10**

Dietary Recommendations for Healthy Americans (1982–Present)—
Continued

LIMIT CHOLES-TEROL (mg/day)	INCREASE COMPLEX CARBO-HYDRATES	INCREASE FIBER	LIMIT REFINED SUGARS	REDUCE SODIUM (mg/day)	LIMIT ALCOHOL	RECOMMEN-DATIONS/ COMMENTS
—	Implied	Implied	—	—	Yes	Increase consumption of fruits, vegetables, and whole grains. Minimize salt-cured, pickled, and smoked foods.
—	Implied	Eat more high-fiber foods	—	—	Yes	Minimize salt-cured, salt-pickled, and smoked foods.
—	Implied	—	—	—	Yes	Increase consumption of fruits, vegetables, and whole-grain cereals. Minimize consumption of salt-cured, smoked, or charcoal-broiled foods.
—	Implied	To 20–30 g/day with an upper limit of 35 g	—	—	Yes	Include a variety of fruits and vegetables in the daily diet. Minimize salt-cured, salt-pickled, or smoked foods.
< 300	Yes	Yes	Yes	Yes	—	To be used in conjunction with recommendations in *Diet and Health*, 1989.
< 300	To 50% or more	—	—	< 3000	To 1–2 oz per day	Protein intake of 15% kcal

Continued

TABLE
5-10

Dietary Recommendations for Healthy Americans (1982–Present)—
Continued

TITLE AND ORGANIZATION	PURPOSE OF REPORT	ENSURE NUTRIENT ADEQUACY/ VARIETY IN DIET	MAINTAIN DESIRABLE BODY WEIGHT	REDUCE TOTAL FAT (% kcal)	REDUCE SATURATED FAT (% kcal)	POLY UNSATURATED FAT (% kcal)
Report of the Expert Panel on Population Strategies for Blood Cholesterol Reduction, 1990. National Cholesterol Education Program, National Heart, Lung, and Blood Institute	Referenced rationale for health professionals with implementation strategies	—	Yes	Average of 30% or less	< 10%	—
GENERAL HEALTH MAINTENANCE						
Nutrition and Your Health: Dietary Guidelines for Americans, 3rd ed., 1990. USDA and DHHS	Publication for the general public and basis for nutrition education programs	Eat a variety of foods	Maintain healthy body weight	30% or less	< 10%	—
The Surgeon General's Report on Nutrition and Health, 1988. DHHS	Scientific resource document to develop national nutrition policy	Implied	Yes	Yes	Yes	—
Diet and Health, 1989. National Research Council	Scientific consensus for recommendations and basis for future research direction	Implied	Yes	To 30% or less	< 10%	Up to 10%

Continued

| TABLE 5-10 | Dietary Recommendations for Healthy Americans (1982–Present)— *Continued* |

LIMIT CHOLES- TEROL (mg/day)	INCREASE COMPLEX CARBO- HYDRATES	INCREASE FIBER	LIMIT REFINED SUGARS	REDUCE SODIUM (mg/day)	LIMIT ALCOHOL	RECOMMEN- DATIONS/ COMMENTS
< 300	Implied	—	—	—	—	
Yes	Choose a diet with plenty of vegetables, fruits, and grain products	Choose a diet with plenty of vegetables, fruits, and grain products	Use in moderation	Use in modera- tion	Yes	Get blood choles- terol and blood pressure checked
Yes	Yes	Yes	Yes	Yes	Yes	For some groups: Increase calcium and iron con- sumption. Adequate fluoride.
< 300	To at least 55% kcal	Yes	Yes	< 2400 or ≤ 6 g salt/day	To < 1 oz or 2 drinks/day	Eat more than 5 daily servings of vegetables and fruit. Eat more than 6 daily serv- ings of breads, legumes. Maintain ade- quate calcium and moderate protein intakes.

Source: Adapted from R. Mathews, A review of dietary guidelines and their implications, *Oat Fiber Factor* (Chicago: Quaker Oats Company, Fall 1990), p. 4. Used with permission.

Implementing the Recommendations: From Guidelines to Groceries

The challenge for the 1990s is to help consumers put the wide assortment of dietary recommendations into practice. As the old saying goes, "Food is not food until it is eaten." Consider the words of one commentator: "If cars crashed *hourly* at an intersection, we'd re-design the intersection, rather than blame all the drivers that came upon the intersection. Yet we tend to view the eating problems of countless Americans as signs of personal weakness, rather than that something is awry with the broader situation."[35]

The problem alluded to here is that the dietary recommendations in Table 5-10 are broad-based guidelines for promoting healthful diets. To be useful to the public, however, the recommendations must be translated into food-specific guides that consumers can implement in their homes, at the grocery store, or in restaurants.[36] For example, consider the dietary guideline: *Choose a diet low in fat, saturated fat, and cholesterol.* This broad guideline must first be translated into food-specific behaviors for the consumer. For example:[37]

◆ Eat more fresh fruits and vegetables, whole-grain breads and cereals, potatoes, rice, noodles, dried beans, peas, and lentils.

◆ Choose low-fat dairy products, including nonfat, 1 percent, and 2 percent milk, low-fat cheeses, and low-fat or nonfat yogurt.

◆ Choose lean meats, fish, chicken, and turkey.

The process of breaking down a dietary guideline into specific behaviors can be carried a step further. The guideline can be translated into an actual eating pattern, as shown in Table 5-11.

The task of identifying successful approaches to improving the diets of Americans was undertaken by a 20-member committee of the Institute of Medicine of the National Academy of Sciences (IOM/NAS).[38] Table 5-12 presents a guide designed by the committee for meeting the dietary recommendations. The committee identified a number of individuals and groups with responsibility for getting this information to consumers: the food industry, government, health care professionals, the media, advertisers, and educators. Three strategies for achieving the recommended dietary changes have been identified:[39]

◆ Increase involvement of government and health professionals as policymakers, role models, and agenda setters in implementing recommendations.

◆ Increase the public's knowledge of nutrition and their opportunities to adopt healthy behaviors.

◆ Increase the availability of health-promoting foods.

How do we get more people to eat a nutritious diet? A number of efforts are underway to help consumers implement the dietary guidelines, decrease risk of chronic disease, and enjoy optimal health. These include the following:[40]

MEALS	GRAMS FAT
Breakfast	
fruit, 1 serving	0
whole wheat bread, 1 serving	2
cereal, 1 serving	2
1 tsp margarine	5
1 c 2% milk	5
2 tsp jelly	0
Lunch	
whole wheat bread, 2 servings	4
2 to 3 oz lean meat, poultry, fish, or low-fat cheese	8
vegetable, 1 serving	1
1 tsp margarine or sandwich spread	5
1 c 1% milk	2
Snack	
fruit, 1 serving	0
whole wheat bread or crackers	2
Dinner	
2 to 3 oz lean meat, fish, poultry, or low-fat cheese	9
starchy vegetable, 1 serving	1
vegetable, 1 serving	0
salad, 1 serving	0
1 tbsp salad dressing	5
whole wheat bread, 1 serving	2
1 $\frac{1}{2}$ tsp margarine	8
fruit, 1 serving	0
dessert	5

*Adapted from menus in USDA Food 1, Home and Garden Bulletin No. 228.

TABLE

5-11

Eating Pattern for a 2000-Calorie Diet with 30 Percent of Calories from Fat*

Source: R. Mullis and coauthors, Developing nutrient criteria for food-specific dietary guidelines for the general public. Copyright The American Dietetic Association. Reprinted by permission from *Journal of the American Dietetic Association* 90 (1990): 848.

◆ Government and industry have cooperated to make nutrition labeling more useful to consumers. The new nutrition panel not only includes information about the absolute amounts of fat, saturated fat, cholesterol, sodium, total carbohydrate, sugars, dietary fiber, and protein in a serving of the food, but also relates the nutrient content of the food to a day's ideal total for these nutrients based on an average daily energy intake.

◆ Voluntary health organizations have undertaken education campaigns to promote positive dietary changes.

◆ The food industry has used nutrition messages and introduced a variety of new healthful food products.

◆ Federal efforts—such as the National Cholesterol Education Program— have helped raise consumer awareness of the diet-health connection.

◆ Dietetic associations across the nation have become more visible as a result of their nutrition awareness campaigns (i.e., National Nutrition Month activities).

TABLE

5-12

Guide to Meeting Dietary Recommendations*

Source: Reprinted with permission from *Improving America's Diet and Health: From Recommendations to Action.* Copyright 1991 by the National Academy of Sciences. Courtesy of the National Academy Press, Washington, D.C.

FOOD GROUP	RECOMMENDED NUMBER OF SERVINGS
Grains and legumes	At least six servings per day; consume grains in their whole form as often as possible. A serving is equivalent to one slice of bread or one small roll; $1/2$ bun, bagel, or muffin; $1/2$ c of cooked cereal, rice, or pasta; 1 oz of ready-to-eat cereal; or $1/2$ c of cooked legumes.
Vegetables and fruits	At least five servings per day, with an emphasis on a variety of green and yellow vegetables (e.g., broccoli, kale, sweet potatoes, and carrots) and citrus fruits (e.g., oranges and grapefruits). A serving is equivalent to $1/2$ c of fresh or cooked vegetables or fruits, 1 medium fresh fruit or vegetable, 1 c of leafy raw vegetables, 6 oz of juice, or $1/4$ c of dried fruit.
Dairy products	Two servings per day for children, three to four servings per day from ages 11 to 25 and for pregnant and lactating women, and two to three servings per day from age 25. A serving is equivalent to 8 oz (1 c) of milk or yogurt, $1\frac{1}{2}$ oz of natural cheese, and 2 oz of processed cheese.
Meat, poultry, fish, and alternatives (eggs, legumes, nuts, and seeds)	Two servings per day. A serving is equivalent to approximately 3 oz (cooked weight) (4 oz raw) of lean meat, fish, or poultry. Count 1 egg, $1/2$ c of cooked legumes, or 2 tbsp of peanut butter as 1 oz of meat. Limit egg yolks to no more than three to four per week; there are no limits on egg whites.
Other foods (fats, sweets, and alcohol)	Limit use of foods that are high in oil, fat, or simple sugars; limit use of these items in food preparation. For those who drink alcoholic beverages, limit consumption to less than 1 oz of pure alcohol per day.

*This guide has been constructed from the following sources: *Healthy People 2000* (DHHS, 1990); *Diet and Health* (NRC, 1989), and *Dietary Guidelines and Your Diet* (USDA, 1990). Modest differences exist among these sources in the way foods are grouped (e.g., in the placement of legumes) and in the recommended number of servings from each group (e.g., should there be a minimum recommended number of servings for both vegetables and fruits?). Nevertheless, they are very similar in the general type of eating pattern recommended.

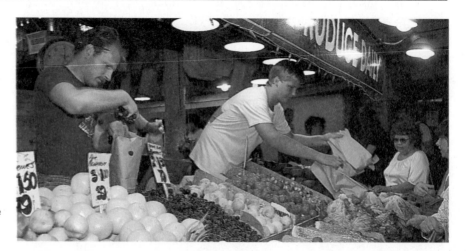

The National Cancer Institute's *National 5 A Day for Better Health* program urges consumers to eat five or more servings of fruits and vegetables every day for better health.

The task of formulating a national nutrition agenda is daunting. Government must make a commitment to develop and promote a coordinated plan to improve the nation's nutrition and health status, scientists must reach a consensus on the interpretation of scientific findings and appropriate dietary advice for all Americans, and sufficient financial resources must be allocated to implement the policy. The Institute of Medicine captured the essence of the task in its report, *Improving America's Diet and Health—From Recommendations to Action:* "The main challenge no longer is to determine what eating patterns to recommend to the public (although, admittedly, there is more to be learned), but also how to inform and encourage an entire population to eat so as to improve its chance for a healthier life.[41]

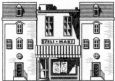 # COMMUNITY LEARNING ACTIVITY

1. As discussed in the chapter, the data from the National Nutrition Monitoring System can be used in many different ways. This activity asks you to search the scientific nutrition literature for articles that have cited or otherwise utilized data from the various surveys and surveillance activities discussed in this chapter. Search through at least three different publications for at least three articles using NNMS data. Examples of journals include the *Journal of the American Dietetic Association, American Journal of Clinical Nutrition, American Journal of Public Health,* and *Journal of Nutrition Education.*

2. Once you have located your articles, determine how the data were used:

   a. Were the data used to give prevalence estimates for certain conditions—anemia, for example?

   b. Were the data used to evaluate interrelationships among diet, nutrition status, demographic factors, environmental factors, and health? For example, the NHANES data have been analyzed to determine whether there is a relationship between calcium intake and hypertension.

   c. Were the data used to monitor a trend in a particular subgroup of the population (e.g., a trend of generalized improvement in blood cholesterol levels in men)?

   d. Note any other uses you find for the NNMS data in the articles you read.

3. Finally, search the current lay literature for examples of articles offering consumer advice for implementing one or more of the nutrition recommendations mentioned in this chapter. Identify at least three such articles and the recommendation(s) made by the author.

Understanding and Communicating Nutrition and Health Fraud

At the same time that science has shown that to some extent we really are what we eat, many consumers are more confused than ever about how to translate the steady stream of new findings about nutrition into healthful eating.[1] Each additional nugget of nutrition news that comes along raises new concerns: Is caffeine bad for me? Does oat bran reduce cholesterol? Should I take vitamin supplements? Will diet pills work? Can a sports drink improve my performance? Do pesticides pose a hazard? As a community nutritionist, you will find that many consumers turn to you as the resident expert on these questions and more.

Some manufacturers of food and nutrition-related products, as well as many members of the media, feed into the confusion by offering a myriad of unreliable products and misleading dietary advice targeted to health-conscious consumers. Unfortunately many consumers fall prey to this vast array of information. Americans spend some $25 billion annually on medical and nutritional health fraud and quackery, up from $1 billion to $2 billion in the early 1960s.[2] The problem is so widespread that the Food and Drug Administration (FDA) ranked false nutritional schemes and food products such as bee pollen, over-the-counter herbal remedies, and wheat germ capsules among its list of top 10 health frauds. In addition, weight-loss gimmicks—skin patches, herbal capsules, grapefruit diet pills, and magic weight-loss earrings—made the FDA's list, leaving no doubt that nutrition-related quackery is big business.[3] Even more disturbing is that such misinformation can be harmful. One survey of 29,000 claims, treatments, and theories for losing weight found fewer than 6 percent of them effective—and 13 percent dangerous.[4] The sale of weight-loss programs and products—not all of them sound—has become a $32 billion industry.[5] This Professional Focus provides a sieve with which you can help consumers separate valid from bogus nutrition information.

Money down the drain is just one of the problems stemming from misleading dietary information. While some fraudulent claims about nutrition are harmless and make for a good laugh, others can have tragic consequences. Swallowing false claims about nutritional products has been known to bring about malnutrition, birth defects, mental retardation, and even death in extreme cases. Negative effects can happen in two ways. One is that the product in question causes direct harm. Even a seemingly innocuous substance such as vitamin A, for instance, can cause severe liver damage over time if taken in large enough doses. The other problem is that spurious nutritional remedies build false hope and may keep a consumer from obtaining sound, scientifically tested medical treatment. A person who relies on a so-called anticancer diet as a cure, for example, might forgo possible life-saving interventions such as surgery or chemotherapy.

Part of the confusion consumers experience stems from the way the media choose to interpret the findings of scientific research. The oat bran story is a good case in point. In the late 1980s, a nutritional "star" was born. Shortly after publication of a study showing that including oat bran as part of a low-fat diet could reduce blood cholesterol levels,

Continued

spending on the once lowly grain reached $100 million. Unlikely foods such as potato chips, pretzels, and beer made with oat bran showed up on store shelves.[6] Consumer surveys reportedly indicated that people would buy Life Savers with oat bran added.[7]

In 1990, however, a flurry of headlines such as "Is It Still the Right Thing to Do?" and "The Rise and Fallacies of Oat Bran" threatened to pull the rug out from under the grain's pedestal.[8] A study published in the *New England Journal of Medicine* found that Cream of Wheat was just as effective as oat bran at reducing blood cholesterol levels.[9] In other words, it implied that the oat bran brouhaha had been for naught.

But the oat bran story illustrates how news stories based on one study alone can leave the public with the impression that scientists can't make up their minds. First, oat bran is hailed as the "magic bullet" that will lower Americans' blood cholesterol. One study and several news reports later, oat bran is virtually dismissed as just another fad. However, the truth of the matter is that even those experts who believe that oat bran does have an effect on blood cholesterol levels never suggested that oat bran will do so when it is included in a high-fat diet or put in high-fat muffins or potato chips. Most health professionals advise eating oatmeal or oat bran as part of a low-fat diet in place of high-fat foods such as fried eggs or bacon.

Contrary to what some headlines imply, reputable scientists do not base dietary recommendations for the public on the findings of just one or two studies. In the case of oat bran, scientists are still conducting experiments to determine if and when the substance does, in fact, help lower blood cholesterol. Other factors, however, sometimes confound the matter at hand. In the case of the oat bran study, some critics charged that, among other things, the scientists who conducted it did not carefully control the amount of fat in the oat eaters' diets, a factor that may have considerably altered the outcome of the experiment, as other studies have shown that a high-fat diet raises blood cholesterol levels.[10] Moreover, even if an experiment is carefully designed and carried out, its findings cannot be considered definitive until they have been confirmed by other research. Testing and retesting reduce the possibility that the outcome was simply the result of chance or an error or oversight on the part of the experimenter. When making dietary recommendations for the public, experts pool the results of different types of studies and consider all of them before coming to any conclusions. The dietary guidelines spelled out in the 1300-page *Diet and Health* report are based on the results of hundreds of studies. Thus, if a story in the paper or on television advises making a dramatic change in your diet based on just one study, exercise a little caution and a lot of common sense. The study may make a good story, but it may not be strong enough evidence for a radical diet or lifestyle change.

Consumers sometimes ask why the government doesn't prevent the media from delivering misleading nutrition information, but the government lacks the power to do so. The First Amendment guarantees freedom of the press, which means that people may express whatever views they like in the media, whether sound, unsound, or even dangerous. By law writers cannot be punished for publishing misinformation unless it can be proved in court that the information has caused a reader bodily harm.

Fortunately, most professional health groups maintain committees to combat the spread of health and nutrition misinformation. A list of organizations that provide reliable

Continued

scientific information appears in Appendix B of this book, and any of them can serve as sources for your inquiries about the authenticity of scientific information in their areas.*

Unlike journalists, purveyors of products are bound by law to make only true statements about their wares. The FDA has the authority to prosecute companies that display false nutrition information on product labels or in advertising materials. Combating health fraud, however, is an overwhelming task requiring enormous amounts of time and money. As one FDA official put it, "Quack promoters have learned to stay one step ahead of the laws either by moving from state to state or by changing their corporate names." Indeed, the FDA estimates that 38 million consumers have used a fraudulent health product during the last year.

It's not always easy to separate the nutrition wheat from the chaff, given that many misleading claims are supposedly backed by scientific-sounding statements, but you can offer your clients some tips to help them tell whether a product is bogus. The following red flags can help you spot a quack:

◆ *The promoter claims that the medical establishment is against him or her, and that the government won't accept this new "alternative" treatment.*

If the government or medical community cannot accept a treatment, it is because the treatment has not been proved to work. Reputable professionals do not suppress knowledge about fighting disease. On the contrary, they welcome new remedies for illness, provided the treatments have been carefully tested.

◆ *The promoter uses testimonials and anecdotes from satisfied customers to support claims.*

Valid nutrition information comes from careful experimental research, not from random tales. A few persons' reports that the product in question "works every time" are never acceptable as sound scientific evidence.

◆ *The promoter uses a computer-scored questionnaire for diagnosing "nutrient deficiencies."*

Those programs are designed to show that just about everyone has a deficiency that can be reversed with the supplements the promoter just happens to be selling, regardless of the consumer's symptoms or health.

◆ *The promoter claims that the product will make weight loss easy.*

Unfortunately, there is no simple way to lose weight. In other words, if a claim sounds too good to be true, it probably is.

◆ *The promoter promises that the product is made with a "secret formula" available only from this one company.*

* If you have questions about a medical book, product, or service, write to the American Medical Association; about an anticancer book, product, or service, to the American Cancer Society; about a heart disease preventive, to the American Heart Association; about a diet or nutrient supplement, to the American Dietetic Association; and so forth. Many of the professional organizations have also banded together to form the National Council Against Health Fraud (NCAHF), which has branches in many states. The NCAHF monitors radio, television, and other advertising; investigates complaints; and publishes a bimonthly newsletter to keep consumers informed on the latest health misinformation. You can write to the NCAHF at P.O. Box 1276, Loma Linda, CA 92354.

Continued

◆ PROFESSIONAL FOCUS—*Continued*

Legitimate health professionals share their knowledge of proven treatments so that others can benefit from it.

◆ *The treatment is provided only in the back pages of magazines, over the phone, or by mail-order ads in the form of news stories or 30-minute commercials (known as infomercials) in talk-show format.*

Results of studies on credible treatments are reported first in medical journals and administered through a physician or other health professional. If information about a treatment only appears elsewhere, it probably cannot withstand scientific scrutiny.[†]

[†] If you or your client think you have been duped by a quack, write the FDA, Consumer Affairs and Information, 5600 Fishers Lane, HFC-110, Rockville, MD 20857; your state Attorney General's office; the Federal Trade Commission, Correspondence Branch, Room 692, Sixth and Pennsylvania Avenues, N.W., Washington, D.C. 20580; and/or the newspaper, magazine, TV or radio station running the ad. If you ordered the product by mail, alert the U.S. Postal Service, Chief Postal Inspector, 475 L'Enfant Plaza, Washington, D.C. 20260. If you want to take legal action and need help finding an experienced lawyer, write or call the National Council Against Health Fraud's Task Force on Victim Redress at P.O. Box 33008, Kansas City, MO 64114; (816) 444-8615.

1. This discussion was adapted from M. A. Boyle and G. Zyla, *Personal Nutrition,* 2nd ed. (St. Paul, Minn.: West Publishing Company, 1992), Chapter 1.
2. Position of the American Dietetic Association, Identifying food and nutrition misinformation, *Journal of the American Dietetic Association* 88 (1988): 1589–91.
3. Top 10 health frauds, *FDA Consumer* (October 1989): 29–31.
4. M. Simonton, An overview—advances in research and treatment of obesity, *Food and Nutrition News* (March/April 1982).
5. Remarks of R. Wyden in *Deception and Fraud in the Diet Industry—Part 1: Hearing before the House of Representatives, Subcommittee on Regulation, Business Opportunities, and Energy, Committee on Small Business* (Washington, D.C.: U.S. Government Printing Office, March 26, 1990), p. 1.
6. Oat bran's last gasp? *The Lempert Report,* January 24, 1990, p. 1.
7. A. Miller and coauthors, Oat-bran heartburn, *Newsweek,* January 29, 1990, p. 50.
8. J. Seligmann, Is it still the right thing to do? *Newsweek,* January 29, 1990, p. 52; C. Sugarman, The rise and fallacies of oat bran, *Washington Post,* January 31, 1990, p. E1.
9. F. W. Swain and coauthors, Comparison of the effects of oat bran and low-fiber wheat on serum lipoprotein levels and blood pressure, *New England Journal of Medicine* 322 (1990): 147–52.
10. Statement from Dr. James Anderson, University of Kentucky, in response to the *New England Journal of Medicine's* article entitled "Comparison of the effects of oat bran . . .," issued January 17, 1990.

NOTES

1. U.S. Department of Health and Human Services, Public Health Service, *The Surgeon General's Report on Nutrition and Health: Summary and Recommendations* (Washington, D.C.: U.S. Government Printing Office, 1988), pp. 2–4.
2. N. B. Belloc and L. Breslow, Relationship of physical health status and health practices, *Preventive Medicine* 1 (1972): 409–21.
3. J. E. Austin and C. Hitt, *Nutrition Intervention in the United States* (Cambridge, Mass.: Ballinger, 1979), p. 355.
4. Ibid., pp. 357–85.
5. Quoted in ibid., p. 356.
6. D. J. Palumbo, *Public Policy in America—Government in Action* (San Diego: Harcourt Brace Jovanovich, 1988), p. 17.
7. U.S. Department of Health and Human Services, U.S. Department of Agriculture, *Nutrition Monitoring in the United States: An Update Report on Nutrition Monitoring* (Washington, D.C.: U.S. Government Printing Office, DHHS [PHS] Pub. No. 89–1255, 1989); G. B. Mason and coauthors, *Nutrition Surveillance* (Geneva: World

Health Organization, 1984); the discussion of the five types of data collection and end-use activities was adapted from E. Yetley, A. Beloian, and C. Lewis, Dietary methodologies for food and nutrition monitoring, in U.S. Department of Health and Human Services, *Vital and Health Statistics: Dietary Methodology Workshop for the Third National Health and Nutrition Examination Survey* (Washington, D.C.: U.S. Government Printing Office, 1992), pp. 58–67.

8. Mason and coauthors, *Nutrition Surveillance,* and R. R. Briefel and C. T. Sempos, Introduction, in Department of Health and Human Services, *Vital and Health Statistics,* pp. 1–2.

9. G. Ostenso, National Nutrition Monitoring System: A historical perspective, *Journal of the American Dietetic Association* 84 (1984): 1181–85.

10. U.S. Department of Health and Human Services, U.S. Department of Agriculture, *Nutrition Monitoring in the United States* (Washington, D.C.: U.S. Government Printing Office, 1986), and *Nutrition Monitoring in the United States: An Update Report.*

11. *Nutrition Monitoring in the United States, 1986.*

12. ADA timely statement on implementation of National Nutrition Monitoring and Related Research Act, *Journal of the American Dietetic Association* 91 (1991): 482.

13. The margin definition of the NNMS was adapted from C. E. Woteki and M. T. Fanelli-Kuczmarski, The national nutrition monitoring system, in *Present Knowledge in Nutrition,* 6th ed. (Washington, D.C.: International Life Sciences Institute/Nutrition Foundation, 1990), pp. 415–29.

14. *Nutrition Monitoring in the United States: An Update Report,* pp. 2–3.

15. The section that follows was taken from *Nutrition Monitoring in the United States: The Directory of Federal Nutrition Monitoring Activities* (Washington, D.C.: Department of Health and Human Services, U.S. Department of Agriculture, 1989), pp. 1–64.

16. Mason and coauthors, *Nutrition Surveillance,* p. 12.

17. G. E. Brown, Jr., National Nutrition Monitoring System: A congressional perspective, *Journal of the American Dietetic Association* 84 (1984): 1185.

18. C. E. Woteki and F. L. Wong, Interpretation and utilization of data from the National Nutrition Monitoring System, in *Research: Successful Approaches,* ed. E. R. Monsen (Chicago: American Dietetic Association, 1992), pp. 204–19.

19. T. K. Murray and J. L. Beare-Rogers, Nutrition recommendations, 1990, *Journal of the Canadian Dietetic Association* 50 (1990): 391–95.

20. The discussion of survey findings was adapted from E. N. Whitney, E. M. N. Hamilton, and M. A. Boyle, *Understanding Nutrition,* 4th ed. (St. Paul, Minn.: West Publishing Company, 1987), pp. 452–56.

21. S. Murphy and coauthors, Demographic and economic factors associated with dietary quality for adults in the 1987–1988 Nationwide Food Consumption Survey, *Journal of the American Dietetic Association* 92 (1992): 1352–57.

22. Ibid., p. 1357.

23. A. M. Stephan and N. J. Wald, Trends in individual consumption of dietary fat in the United States, 1920–1984, *American Journal of Clinical Nutrition* 52 (1990): 457–69; G. Block, W. F. Rosenberger, and B. H. Patterson, Calories, fat, and cholesterol: Intake patterns in the U.S. population by race, sex, and age, *American Journal of Public Health* 78 (1988): 1150–55.

24. J. B. Richmond, Forward, *American Journal of Clinical Nutrition* 32 (1979): 2621–22.

25. P. M. Behlen and F. J. Cronin, Dietary recommendations for healthy Americans summarized, *Family Economics Review* 3 (1985): 17–24.

26. L. Light and F. J. Cronin, Food guidance revisited, *Journal of Nutrition Education* 13 (1981): 57–62.

27. O. Hayes, M. F. Trulson, and F. J. Stare, Suggested revision of the basic 7, *Journal of the American Dietetic Association* 31 (1955): 1103–7.

28. K. W. McNutt, An analysis of the Dietary Goals for the United States, second edition, *Journal of Nutrition Education* 10 (1978): 61–62.

29. The Report of the U.S. Senate Select Committee on Nutrition and Human Needs, Dietary Goals for the United States, *Nutrition Today* (September/October 1977): 22.

30. Ibid., pp. 20–30.

31. M. C. Latham and L. S. Stephenson, U.S. Dietary Goals, *Journal of Nutrition Education* 9 (1977): 152–54.

32. A. E. Harper, U.S. Dietary Goals—against, *Journal of Nutrition Education* 9 (1977): 154–56, plus letters to the editor, pp. 156–57.

33. U.S. Department of Health and Human Services, Public Health Service, *The Surgeon General's Report;* Committee on Diet and Health, National Research Council, *Diet and Health: Implications for Reducing Chronic Disease Risk— Executive Summary* (Washington, D.C.: U.S. Government Printing Office, 1989); The Expert Panel, Report of the Expert Panel on Detection, Evaluation, and Treatment of High Blood Cholesterol in Adults, *Archives of Internal Medicine* 148 (1988): 36–69.

34. *Nutrition and Your Health: Dietary Guidelines for*

Americans (Washington, D.C.: U.S. Department of Agriculture, U.S. Department of Health and Human Services, Home and Garden Bulletin No. 232, 1990).

35. Editorial by E. N. Brandt, as quoted by P. R. Thomas at the annual American Dietetic Association meeting in Dallas, October 1991.

36. R. M. Mullis and coauthors, Developing nutrient criteria for food-specific dietary guidelines for the general public, *Journal of the American Dietetic Association* 90 (1990): 847.

37. The list of food suggestions is from ibid., p. 849.

38. Committee on Dietary Guidelines Implementation, Food and Nutrition Board, Institute of Medicine, *Improving America's Diet and Health: From Recommendations to Action* (Washington, D.C.: National Academy Press, 1991).

39. The list of strategies is from Dietary Guidance: A changing environment, *Dairy Council Digest: An Interpretative Review of Recent Nutrition Research* 62 (1991): 1–6.

40. P. Crawford, The nutrition connection: Why doesn't the public know? *American Journal of Public Health* 78 (1988): 1147–48.

41. Committee on Dietary Guidelines Implementation, *Improving America's Diet,* p. 1.

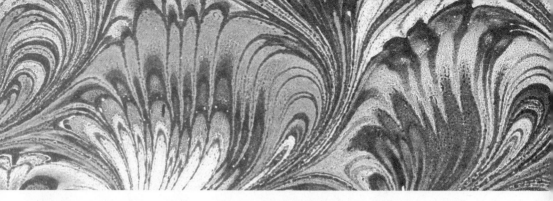

Using the Tools: Designing and Implementing Community Nutrition Programs

Open any handbook on wiring, plumbing, or masonry and you will find a section on tools. The tool kit for plumbing emergencies, for example, might include a basin wrench, an auger, a seat dresser, solder, emery cloth, and a tube bender. Each tool has a specific purpose. Together, they help you repair and maintain your home's plumbing system.

Tools are important to the practice of community nutrition as well. A community nutrition tool kit might contain models of consumer behavior, goals and objectives, a strate-

gic plan, a program plan, a budget, marketing strategies, logos and bylines, educational materials, and survey instruments. These and other topics form the basis of our discussion of how to develop, implement, and evaluate community-based nutrition programs.

This section is designed to help you become familiar with the tools used by community nutritionists. We encourage you to master these tools, for they have many applications in diverse situations.

Program Planning and Management

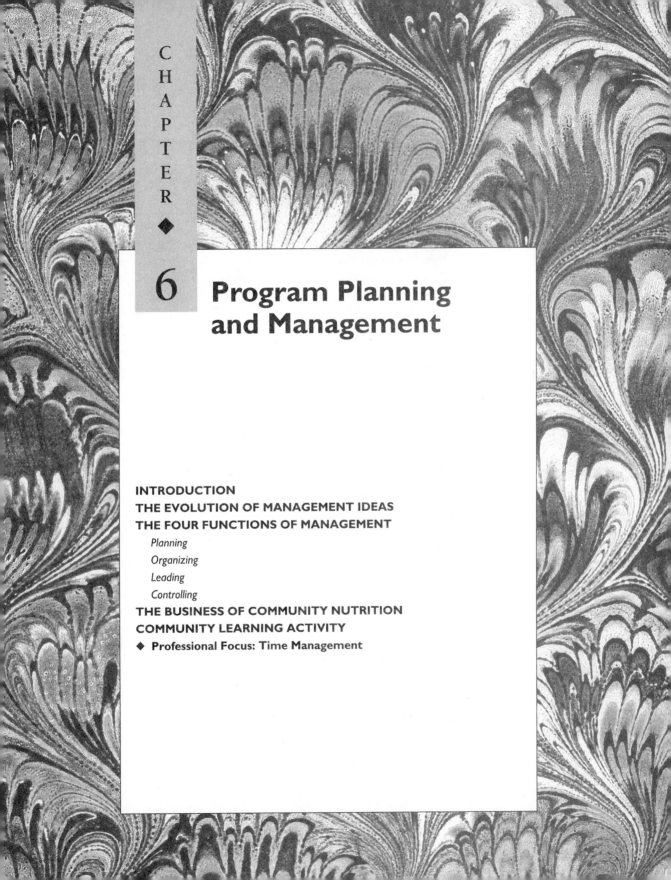

Do you want to be a positive influence in the world? First, get your own life in order. Ground yourself in the single principle so that your behavior is wholesome and effective. If you do that, you will earn respect and be a powerful influence. Your behavior influences others through a ripple effect. A ripple effect works because everyone influences everyone else. Powerful people are powerful influences.

   If your life works, you influence your family.
   If your family works, your family influences the community.
   If your community works, your community influences the nation.
   If your nation works, your nation influences the world.
   If your world works, the ripple effect spreads throughout the cosmos.
                                    —Lao Tzu, *Tao Te Ching (The Tao of Leadership)*

Introduction

Community nutritionists must be good planners and managers. One of the past presidents of the American Dietetic Association (ADA), Judith L. Dodd, said this about dietitians' need for management expertise: ". . . it's not enough to have technical knowledge. Other skills are necessary, whether you want to call them leadership skills or communication skills or simply survival skills. We must know how to communicate, how to negotiate, how to persuade, and how to work with various groups within any of our market environments."[1] In other words, community nutritionists charged with implementing programs to improve the public's health must have good management skills.

Management The process of achieving organizational goals through engaging in the four major functions of planning, organizing, leading, and controlling.

   Management refers to the process of achieving organizational goals through planning, organizing, leading and controlling.[2] In this chapter we examine the functions of management and consider how they are used by community nutritionists. We begin by reviewing a few pioneering ideas in management, many of which continue to mold management practice today.

The Evolution of Management Ideas

The seeds of management science were planted during the industrial revolution of the early 1800s.[3] As workers moved from the fields into factories, managers began looking for ways to run factories more efficiently and increase production. Early innovators, like the British entrepreneur Robert Owen, tried to improve working conditions in factories, limit employment to workers over the age of 10 years, and reduce the workday to 10½ hours. Later in the century, the concept of scientific management of workers emerged. Scientific management emphasized the formal, scientific study of work methods as a means of improving worker efficiency. Two advocates of this approach were Frank and Lillian Gilbreth, who studied motion and its relation to efficiency. The Gilbreth family included 12 children, two of whom wrote a popular book, *Cheaper by the Dozen*, describing life with their innovative parents.[4] The French industrialist Henri Fayol also contributed many ideas in this area. He believed that it is possible to develop management theories that can be taught to managers, and he described several functions of management: planning, organizing, leading, and controlling. Many of Fayol's ideas form the basis for management practice today.

In the early 1900s, managers began to study how the job environment influences productivity. The famous Hawthorne studies, conducted at the Hawthorne plant of the Western Electric Company during the late 1920s and 1930s, were designed to determine how working conditions such as lighting, special privileges, free lunches, rest periods, and amount of supervision contributed to productivity. In one Hawthorne study, two groups of workers were assigned to different lighting conditions: no changes in lighting were made for one group (the comparison group), while the lighting was decreased over a period of time for the other (the experimental group). The researchers found that performance increased steadily among workers in the experimental group up to the point at which the lighting was so dim that they could hardly see! These and other results led the researchers to describe the "Hawthorne effect," the possibility that individuals singled out for a study show an improvement in performance simply because they are receiving special attention, rather than because of any specific intervention effect being tested.[5]

Although the design of the Hawthorne studies was severely flawed, they were pioneering in many respects. They led eventually to a focus on human behavior within organizations and the development of the human relations movement. Two major theorists of this movement were Abraham Maslow, whose theory of the hierarchy of human needs is described in Chapter 8, and Douglas McGregor, who developed Theory X and Theory Y to describe the possible assumptions managers make when dealing with their workers. Theory X managers tend to assume that workers dislike their work and try to avoid it; they believe workers must be controlled, coerced, and threatened with punishment to get them to work toward the organization's goals. Theory Y managers tend to assume workers do not inherently dislike work, will exercise self-control, and can be creative and innovative in solving work-related problems. McGregor believed that managers organize and motivate their workers according to their own personal assumptions about their workers' nature. Both Maslow's theory and McGregor's are used widely today to help managers understand and motivate their employees.

Other theories and methods have gained prominence in recent years. Systems theory is a management approach based on the idea that organizations can be conceptualized as systems, much like the major organ systems of the human body. A public health department, for example, can view itself as a system, with resources such as personnel, equipment, and finances (the inputs) grouped into one area and products and services such as educational materials and telephone hotlines (the outputs) grouped into another. Systems theory helps managers evaluate how well the inputs and outputs work together.

Contingency theory is an approach that argues that there is no one best way for a manager to act, because circumstances change constantly. The decision that is appropriate to one situation is not appropriate to another. Many aspects of contingency theory can be applied to such areas as organizational design, leadership, technology, and problem solving.

The science and practice of management continue to change. North American managers, for example, are studying the Japanese style of management to gain new insights into how management styles and philosophy influence employee behavior.[6] The ideas that grow out of management research provide new ways of motivating employees to perform at their best.

The Four Functions of Management

Although managers have many tasks, their main activities and responsibilities can be grouped into four areas or functions, as shown in Figure 6-1. *Planning* is the forward-looking aspect of a manager's job; it involves setting goals and objectives and deciding how best to achieve them. *Organizing* focuses on distributing and arranging human and nonhuman resources so that plans can be carried out successfully. *Leading* involves influencing others to carry out the work required to reach the organization's goals. *Controlling* is the function that regulates certain organizational activities to ensure that they meet established standards and goals. This section describes each management function.

FIGURE

6-1

The Four Functions of Management

Source: K. M. Bartol and D. C. Martin, *Management,* p. 7. Copyright 1991 by McGraw-Hill, Inc. Used with permission of McGraw-Hill, Inc.

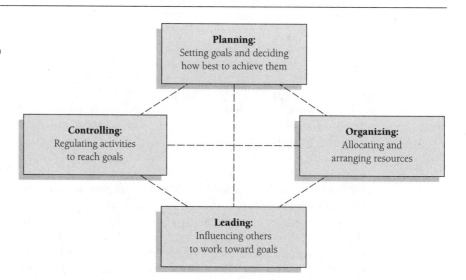

Planning:
Setting goals and deciding how best to achieve them

Controlling:
Regulating activities to reach goals

Organizing:
Allocating and arranging resources

Leading:
Influencing others to work toward goals

◆ PLANNING

A colossal marketing blunder made headlines around the world in the spring of 1993. Hoover, a subsidiary of the Maytag Corporation, launched a promotional campaign in Ireland and Britain in which consumers who purchased any of its household appliances (worth at least $150 US) were offered two free return plane tickets to Europe or the United States (valued at about $500 US). Hoover's aim was to stimulate interest in its products, a feat it readily achieved. For reasons not entirely clear, Hoover's management failed to anticipate the number of customers who would accept the promotion's restrictions and demand the promised air tickets. The result was a $30 million loss, the firing of three top executives, and a place in management textbooks as "one of the great marketing gaffes of all time."[7]

What is the lesson in this story for community nutritionists? In two words: *plan ahead.* To those of us standing outside the Hoover snafu, it seems incredible that no one foresaw the shortfall between anticipated revenues and actual expenses. What happened on the inside may never be fully known. Regardless, the magnitude of the event suggests a glitch in the planning process, a failure of managers to calculate accurately the direct and indirect costs associated with the promotional campaign and anticipate the unexpected.

For the individual manager or managerial team, **planning** involves deciding what to do and when, where, and how to do it. It focuses on future events and finding solutions to problems. Planning is ongoing. It involves performing a number of activities in a generally logical, predetermined sequence and considering a variety of solutions before a plan of action is chosen.[8]

Planning A process that helps find solutions to problems; the basis for good management and the key to success.

Types of Planning   There are different types of planning and varying time frames for the planning process. **Strategic planning** is broad in scope and addresses the organization's overall goals. Strategic planning occurs over a period of several years and is usually undertaken by the organization's senior managers. The focus of strategic planning is on formulating objectives; assessing past, current, and future conditions and events; evaluating the organization's strengths and weaknesses; and making decisions about the appropriate course of action. Table 6-1 outlines the ADA's strategic plan, *Achieving Competitive Advantage.* The product of 15 months of hard work, the plan has a single objective: "to ensure the success of the dietetics professional in an increasingly competitive marketplace."[9] The plan grew out of the organization's mission statement and targets four market segments that represent current and potential career environments for dietitians.

Strategic planning Long-term planning that addresses an organization's overall goals.

The strategic plan guides the development of operational plans. **Operational planning** is short term and typically is done by mid-level managers. It deals with specific actions, expenditures, and controls and with the timing of these activities in a formal, structured process.[10] Consider the first initiative outlined in the ADA's strategic plan under the market segment "Consumer Education": maximize media exposure. Managers responsible for implementing the ADA's strategic plan must develop a plan for achieving this initiative. Specific activities for maximizing media exposure might include mailing press releases to leading health and science writers and publishing the ADA's consumer information telephone num-

Operational planning Short-term planning that focuses on the activities and actions required to meet the organization's goals.

| TABLE 6-1 | The American Dietetic Association's Strategic Plan, *Achieving Competitive Advantage* |

MISSION STATEMENT

The American Dietetic Association is the advocate of the dietetics profession serving the public through the promotion of optimal nutrition, health and well-being.

MARKET SEGMENTS, KEY LINKAGES, AND STRATEGIC INITIATIVES

Consumer Education	Foodservice	Health Care, Acute and Long-term Care	Health Care, Prevention and Wellness
Media/Communications Industry ◆ Maximize media exposure. ◆ Promote and expand NCND* hotline as a public resource for nutrition information. ◆ Expand media training. ◆ Position advanced-degree members as sources for nutrition information.	**Commercial Foodservice** ◆ Form strategic alliances to advocate nutritional quality of commercially prepared foods. ◆ Expand services based on industry assessment. ◆ Enhance education in commercial foodservice. ◆ Establish career paths in commercial food industry.	**Physicians** ◆ Establish a leadership institute to enhance professional skills. ◆ Collaborate with allied groups to provide educational programming. ◆ Promote reimbursement for nutrition services. ◆ Communicate through medical media.	**Federal Government** ◆ Influence health care reform legislation. ◆ Obtain federal requirement for dietetic licensure. ◆ Encourage member involvement in political process. ◆ Promote national nutrition policy that mandates nutrition care for every American.
Food, Health, and Pharmaceutical Industries ◆ Collaborate with industry groups to establish food labeling standards. ◆ Share ADA knowledge with industry groups. ◆ Market consulting expertise to foodservice manufacturers. ◆ Seek partners for cooperative advertising of nutrition information.	**Allied Foodservice Groups** ◆ Collaborate with industry groups to set foodservice standards. ◆ Develop partnerships with employer groups and industry leaders. ◆ Participate in mutually beneficial projects. ◆ Collaborate with industry to develop training programs.	**Health Care Payers** ◆ Research payer market. ◆ Educate members on payment methods, criteria, and regulations. ◆ Explore self-insurance for RD malpractice. ◆ Collaborate with allied groups seeking reimbursement.	**Media/Communications Industry** ◆ Position NCND as premiere health information resource. ◆ Promote establishment of a President's Council on Nutrition. ◆ Expand ADA's influence through targeted nutrition messages. ◆ Expand media training.

*NCND = National Center for Nutrition and Dietetics, the public education arm of the American Dietetic Association.

Source: How the new strategic plan works—for you. Copyright The American Dietetic Association. Reprinted by permission from *Journal of the American Dietetic Association,* Vol. 92: 1992, pp. 1070–71.

ber in national women's magazines. After developing the action plan, the managers must specify the costs related to these activities and the time frame for implementing them.

The Program Planning Process   Ideally, the process of developing, implementing, and evaluating a nutrition program proceeds step-by-step from start to finish in an orderly fashion. In real life, however, the planning process is not always rational and orderly. An organization's plans to launch a community-wide nutrition program may not proceed in a logical order; some portions of the process may be repeated or may occur out of sequence. Programs may be started without a full understanding of the problem, or a shift in the political or social environment may force the planners to change their goals.

In many respects, program planning is a shape-shifter much like policy making, and it is just as changeable and complex. Even so, it can be viewed as a sequence of events, as shown in Figure 6-2. Not all steps in the sequence are described in this chapter. Needs assessment, behavior change strategies (an element of program design), marketing, and evaluation are discussed in Chapters 7–10. This chapter focuses on planning to achieve goals, managing people, and using control systems such as budgets. The discussion beginning on page 172 provides an overview of the program planning process.

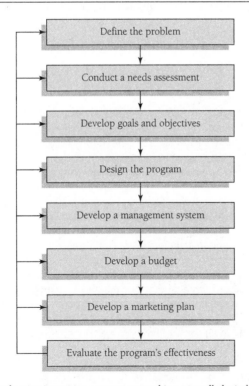

FIGURE

6-2

The Program Planning Process
Source: Adapted from P. M. Kettner, R. M. Moroney, and L. L. Martin, *Designing and Managing Programs* (Newbury Park, Calif.: Sage Publications, 1990), pp. 13–27.

The steps involved in planning a nutrition program proceed in a generally logical fashion, beginning with defining the community's nutritional problem. Note that evaluation occurs on a continuous basis. The program's goals, objectives, and overall design may change as managers consider the personnel, financial, and marketing resources available to implement the program.

1. **Define the problem.** Most nutrition programs are developed to address a specific nutritional problem within the community and to meet the needs of particular clients. The extent to which the community's or clients' nutritional needs are met becomes the gauge for measuring the program's effectiveness. Thus, the first step in the program planning process is to develop a picture of the type, size, and scope of the nutritional problem. This task is a fact-finding mission where one begins by asking a few basic questions, such as those in Table 6-2.[11] Whether the nutritional problem is a lack of food among homeless people, inadequate growth among infants in foster care, or a high prevalence of overweight within the community, you must think about the problem before looking for solutions. Your view of the problem will be shaped by the outcome of the needs assessment undertaken in the next step.

2. **Conduct a needs assessment.** Once a problem has been identified and defined, it must be translated into needs, which will eventually be translated into services. What is a need? The Title XX Amendments to the Social Security Act define a **need** as "any identifiable condition which limits a person or individual, or a family member in meeting his or her full potential."[12] After managers identify the nutritional problem within the community, a needs assessment is required. The purpose of the needs assessment is to gather information about the social, political, economic, and environmental factors that influence the need and the population at

A problem that is inadequately defined is not likely to be solved.
—P. M. Kettner, R. M. Moroney, and L. L. Martin in Designing and Managing Programs

TABLE

6-2

Questions to Ask When Defining a Community's Nutritional Problem
Source: Adapted from P. M. Kettner, R. M. Moroney, and L. L. Martin, *Designing and Managing Programs* (Newbury Park, Calif.: Sage Publications, 1990), pp. 37–41.

- **What is the nature of the nutritional condition or situation?** Different perspectives on the problem are gathered from community leaders, health professionals, and the general public.
- **How are the terms being defined?** Managers agree upon the definition of the nutritional problem (e.g., obesity, poor eating habits).
- **What are the characteristics of those experiencing the nutritional problem or condition?** The sociocultural, environmental, and individual factors contributing to the problem are identified.
- **What are the scale and distribution of the condition?** Answering this question involves estimating (1) the number of people experiencing the problem, a figure that helps managers determine the level of intervention effort required; and (2) how the condition is spread throughout the community or population (its distribution), a figure that may provide managers with a direction for the intervention.
- **How widely recognized is the condition?** Problems with a high degree of community awareness are more likely to receive support than those that are relatively unknown to the community. If awareness is low, strategies to enhance awareness are needed.
- **What is the cause of the problem?** The techniques described in the chapter on epidemiology can be used to describe the etiology of the nutritional condition.
- **Are there gender and ethnic considerations?** Managers strive to develop specific interventions that focus on the health and nutritional problems of special populations.

risk. Managers must then decide the level of financial and personnel resources to be allocated to meeting the need.[13]

For example, homeless women and their children who live in hotels and shelters without kitchen facilities tend to have poor quality diets. Such families *need* stoves and refrigerators, hot plates, small appliances, and storage areas to ensure an adequate food and nutrient intake. A community trying to provide adequate food to homeless families must determine the availability of kitchen facilities in local hotels and shelters, the number of homeless families without kitchen facilities, how soup kitchens and food pantries can provide food for homeless families with this need, and how food assistance programs can provide counseling and financial assistance to these families to ensure an adequate food intake.[14]

The steps involved in evaluating a community's nutrition status and setting priorities among nutritional needs are discussed in Chapter 7.

3. **Establish goals and objectives.** The development of goals and objectives is the framework for action in program planning. The first step is to consider the organization's **mission statement**, which describes the organization's overall purpose, the reason why it exists. An agency's mission statement might read "to promote and protect the public's health" or "to provide nutrition education activities that help people develop the skills required to choose healthful diets." The ADA's mission statement is given in Table 6-1.

Mission statement A statement of the purposes for which the organization exists.

With the mission statement in mind, the managers proceed to develop **goal statements**, which provide programmatic direction. Goals do not need to be achievable or measurable, but they should reflect long-range accomplishments toward which the program efforts are targeted. Generally, goals do not specify a time frame for action. Recall the three goals of the *Healthy People 2000* initiative listed in Chapter 1 on page 11.[15]

Goal statements Statements of expected outcomes for the problem that the program is designed to prevent, eradicate, or ameliorate.

Once the goals are in place, the managers develop **objectives** for the program that reflect the strategies they will use to address the problem. Two types of objectives are usually developed: (1) *outcome objectives* establish the results that the program is expected to achieve, and (2) *process objectives* specify the manner in which the outcome objectives will be achieved.

Objectives Statements of the results the organization wishes to obtain or of how the results will be achieved.

Whether an objective deals with outcomes or processes, it should be clear, specific in terms of the results to be achieved, measurable, limited in time, and realistic; it should also specify who has responsibility for achieving the objectives. Managers consider five specific elements in writing objectives:[16]

◆ Time frame

◆ Target of the change

◆ Results to be achieved

◆ Criteria by which results will be documented, monitored, or measured

◆ Responsibility for implementing and measuring the achievement of the objective

Table 6-3 shows the *Healthy People 2000* nutrition objective that deals with reducing the prevalence of overweight.[17] Note that it specifies the

TABLE

6-3

One Nutrition Objective from *Healthy People 2000* **Source:** U.S. Department of Health and Human Services, Public Health Service, *Healthy People 2000: National Health Promotion and Disease Prevention Objectives* (Washington, D.C.: U.S. Government Printing Office, 1990), pp. 114–15.

Reduce overweight to a prevalence of no more than 20% among people aged 20 and older and no more than 15% among adolescents aged 12 through 19. (Baseline: 26% for people aged 20 through 74 in 1976–1980, 24% for men and 27% for women; 15% for adolescents aged 12 through 19 in 1976–1980)

SPECIAL POPULATION TARGETS

Overweight Prevalence	2000 Target Percentage Decrease
Low-income women aged 20 and older	25%
Black women aged 20 and older	30%
Hispanic women aged 20 and older	25%
American Indians/Alaska Natives	30%
People with disabilities	25%
Women with high blood pressure	41%
Men with high blood pressure	35%

Note: For people aged 20 and older, overweight is defined as body mass index (BMI) equal to or greater than 27.8 for men and 27.3 for women. For adolescents, overweight is defined as BMI equal to or greater than 23.0 for males aged 12 through 14, 24.3 for males aged 15 through 17, 25.8 for males aged 18 through 19, 23.4 for females aged 12 through 14, 24.8 for females aged 15 through 17, and 25.7 for females aged 18 through 19. The values for adolescents are the age- and gender-specific 85th percentile values of the 1976–1980 National Health and Nutrition Examination Survey (NHANES II), corrected for sample variation. BMI is calculated by dividing weight in kilograms by the square of height in meters. The cut points used to define overweight approximate the 120% of desirable body weight definition used in the 1990 objectives.

time frame for achieving the goal (by the year 2000), the target population (adults over the age of 20 years and adolescents between the ages of 12 and 19 years), and the desired outcome (a reduction in the prevalence of overweight from a baseline rate). The criterion for documenting the change is the body mass index (BMI) obtained from population surveys such as the National Health and Nutrition Examination Survey (NHANES). Responsibility for achieving this objective is specified in supporting documentation and through other objectives related to physical activity, dietary patterns, and food labeling.

Refer to Table 6-4 for examples of outcome and process objectives developed for the ABC Fitness Program, a worksite-based program developed and implemented by a hypothetical company called Nutrition in Action, which specializes in nutrition education and fitness programs. The objectives for the fitness program were drawn from the company's mission statement: To promote good nutrition and an active lifestyle among people of all ages.

4. **Design the program.** Using the goals and objectives as a guide, the managers design the program, taking into consideration a variety of factors such as the number of clients expected to use the program; the staff, equipment, and material resources required to administer the program; and the facilities available. The managers plan how the program will work after asking many questions: What criteria determine a client's eligibility? How is a client "processed" once he walks in the door? What federal, state, or local regulations must be considered in administering the pro-

Program Goal

Improve the fitness level and eating habits of employees in participating worksites.

Outcome Objectives

1. Improve the fitness level of 75% of the employees participating in the 6-month program as determined by a Nutrition in Action dietitian using the Rockport Walking Test.*
2. Reduce the fat intake to less than 30% of total calories among more than 75% of the employees participating in the 6-month program as determined by a Nutrition in Action dietitian using a 24-hour recall.

Process Objectives

1. Provide two nutrition lectures per month to groups of participants over the course of the 6-month program.
2. Provide each participant with one individual nutrition counseling session and an individual dietary plan at the beginning of the 6-month program.
3. Obtain an estimate of each participant's dietary fat intake using a 24-hour recall taken at the beginning and end of the program.
4. Obtain an estimate of each participant's cardiovascular fitness level using the Rockport Walking Test, one to be taken at the beginning and the other at the end of the program.

*The Rockport Fitness Walking Test can be used to evaluate cardiovascular health. The test was developed by the Rockport Walking Institute, Marlboro, MA.

gram? What educational materials are needed to convey important nutrition messages? What provisions should be made for follow-up? What marketing tools will best reach the intended audience? Who will be responsible for implementing the program and determining its effectiveness? How much money is required to administer the program? Well-designed programs are scrutinized before the first client ever sets foot in the door.

The program's format is dictated partly by the goals and objectives. The nutrition outcome objective for the ABC Fitness Program shown in Table 6-4 focuses on dietary fat. Thus, the program might be designed around 8 short classes on food composition and two demonstrations of low-fat cooking. The type of educational instruction chosen to fulfill the objective is influenced by the staff and funding available for the program.

Information about choosing behavior change strategies and influencing consumer behavior is given in Chapter 8.

5. **Develop a management system.** In this context, *management* refers to two types of structures needed to implement the program: personnel and data systems. The personnel structure refers to the employees responsible for overseeing the program and determining whether it meets its objectives. The structure of the data management system refers to the manner in which data about the clients, their use of the program, and the outcome measures are recorded and analyzed. These concepts are discussed later in this chapter.

6. **Develop a budget.** An important part of program planning is calculating the "management" costs of the program. Both direct costs, such as the

salaries and wages of program personnel, materials needed, travel expenses, and equipment, and indirect costs, such as office space rental, utilities, and janitorial services, must be determined to identify the true cost of a program. More detail on budgeting is given later in the chapter.

7. **Develop a marketing plan.** A key element of a successful nutrition program is its marketing strategy. A marketing plan doesn't have to be elaborate and costly, but it should let clients know about the service. Basic marketing concepts are described in Chapter 9.

8. **Evaluate the program and its components.** Stephen Covey's advice for highly effective people is to "begin with the end in mind."[18] An effective program meets your client's needs *and* your organization's mandate. Determining whether a program does this requires the same level of planning as any other aspect of program development. Note in Figure 6-2 that evaluation does not occur only at the end of the planning process. Rather, evaluation occurs on a continuous basis at all stages of program planning. Chapter 10 provides detailed information about the purposes and types of program evaluation.

◆ ORGANIZING

Organizing is the process by which carefully formulated plans are carried out. Managers must arrange and group human and nonhuman resources into workable units to achieve organizational goals. To do this, certain structures must be in place to guide employees in their activities and decision making. Imagine the confusion that would result if you had a problem and didn't know who your supervisor was! In this section, we describe organization structures and how people are managed as part of the process of organizing.

Organization Structures   Just as a building's layout—the arrangement of offices, windows, hallways, restrooms, and stairwells—affects the way people work, so does an organization's structure.[19] The **organization structure** is the formal pattern of interactions and activities designed by management to link the tasks of employees to achieve the organization's goals. The word *formal* is used intentionally here to denote management's official operating structure in contrast to the informal patterns of interaction that exist in all organizations.[20] In developing the organization structure, managers consider how to assign tasks and responsibilities, how to define jobs, how to group individual employees to carry out certain tasks, and how to institute mechanisms for reporting on progress.

Organization structure The formal pattern of interactions designed by management to link the tasks of individuals and groups to achieve organizational goals.

Organization chart A line diagram that depicts the broad outlines of an organization's structure.

In organizing their employees, managers may find an **organization chart** helpful. You are already familiar with this concept, as the organization charts for the Departments of Health and Human Services and Agriculture have already been given (see Figures 1-2 and 1-3). Organization charts give employees information about the major functions of departments, relationships among departments, channels of supervision, lines of authority, and certain position titles within units.[21] According to the organization chart for a typical public health department (shown in Appendix A), the community nutritionist who coordinates the maternal, infant, and child care programs reports to the department manager, the director of nutrition, who in turn reports to the medical health officer.

Nontraditional organization charts also exist. Figure 6-3 shows a different structure for organizing employees and their reporting relationships using our hypothetical company Nutrition in Action. The "web" format has the advantage of promoting teamwork and consensual decision making, but it can create confusion over authority and responsibility. This design is more likely to work well in small companies than in large organizations.

Although organization charts can be useful for establishing lines of communication and procedures, they do not depict rigid systems. An organization's informal structure, depicted humorously in Figure 6-4, is often quite powerful and sometimes represents a more realistic picture of how the organization actually works. The informal structure arises spontaneously from our interactions, brief alliances, and friendships with coworkers throughout the organization.[22]

Another essential dimension of organization structure is departmentalization or the manner in which employees are clustered into units, units into departments, and departments into divisions or other larger categories. Departmentalization directly influences how managers carry out their duties, supervise their employees, and monitor group dynamics and perspectives. An important aspect of departmentalization is the **span of management** or **span of control**, which refers to the number of subordinates who report directly to a specific manager.[23] Deciding how many employees should report to a single manager is not a trivial decision. When a manager must supervise a large number of employees directly, she may feel overwhelmed and have difficulty coordinating tasks and keeping on schedule; with too few employees to supervise, she may feel underutilized and disaffected. The ideal span of management has not been

Span of management or **span of control** The number of subordinates who report directly to a specific manager.

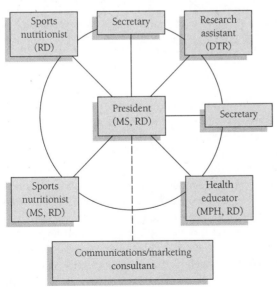

FIGURE

6-3

Nontraditional Organization Chart for Nutrition in Action

In this nontraditional organization structure, employees have roughly the same rank, and there is no strict hierarchy of authority.

FIGURE
6-4

The Typical Organization Chart on Paper and in Practice

Source: Reprinted with the permission of Macmillan College Publishing Company from ORGANIZATIONAL BEHAVIOR: CONCEPTS AND APPLICATIONS by Jerry L. Gray and Frederick A. Starke. Copyright © 1988 by Macmillan College Publishing Company, Inc.

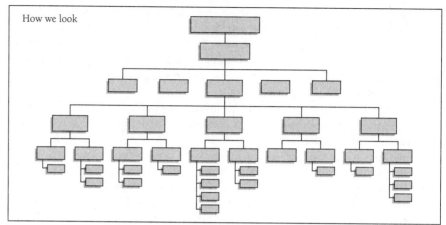

How we look

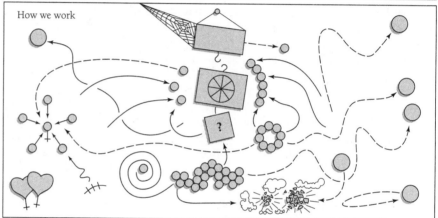

How we work

How an organization looks on paper differs from how it really works. Whereas the formal organization structure shows the lines of authority and how communications should travel, the informal organization reveals the actual patterns of social interaction between employees in different units of the organization.

identified precisely. Some researchers argue that the range is about 5 to 25 employees, depending upon the level of organization; theoretically, lower-level managers can supervise more employees directly than managers higher in the hierarchy. Napoleon once remarked: "No man can command more than five distinct bodies in the same theater of war." Most management experts now recommend that only three to seven subordinates be supervised directly.[24]

Another method of coordinating an organization's activities is through **delegation** or the assignment of part of a manager's work to others. "Everyone knows about delegating, but not too many people do it, and fewer still do it well."[25] The inability to delegate work to others has felled many a fast-track manager.[26] Some people do the work themselves because they don't realize they can delegate it, don't know how to get the most out of a computer, or don't appreciate how delegating work makes *them* work more efficiently. Table 6-5 gives tips on how managers can delegate some activities to their employees.

Delegation The assignment of part of a manager's work, along with both the responsibility and the authority necessary to achieve the expected results, to others.

TABLE

6-5

Tips for Delegating Your Work to Others
Source: Adapted from L. Baum, Delegating your way to job survival, *Business Week*, November 2, 1987, p. 206.

◆ The first step to take when delegating your work to subordinates is to evaluate their skill levels and the difficulty of the task. The trick is to select the employee with the appropriate skills who will find the task challenging but not frustrating.

◆ Once you have chosen the best employee, give him or her all the information needed to do the job well. Be honest about the work; if it's drudgery, say so.

◆ Do these three things to ensure success:
  1. Give the employee *responsibility* for completing the project or task.
  2. Hold the employee *accountable* for the results.
  3. Provide the employee with the *authority* to make needed decisions, direct others to help with the project, and carry out actions as required.

◆ Make sure the employee has the necessary materials, equipment, time, and funds to complete the project.

◆ Evaluate the employee's progress periodically and be prepared to accept a less-than-perfect result.

Line and staff relationships also help clarify an organization's structure. A person in a **line position** has direct responsibility for achieving the organization's goals and objectives. The term *staff* is commonly used to refer to the groups of employees who work in a particular unit or department—for example, the director of nutrition in a public health department is said to supervise the nutrition staff. In management practice, however, *staff* has a particular meaning. An employee in a **staff position** assists those in line positions. To some extent, the concept of line and staff positions is a holdover from eighteenth- and nineteenth-century management theory, but the terms are still used today in many organizations to help employees identify individuals with the authority and responsibility for fulfilling the organization's mandate.

Line position A position with the authority and responsibility for achieving the organization's main goals and objectives.

Staff position A position whose primary purpose is to assist those in line positions.

Job Design and Analysis   Managers in community nutrition are responsible for **job design**, that is, determining the various duties associated with each job in their area. They sometimes need to conduct a **job analysis** to determine the purpose of a job, the skill set and educational background required to carry it out, and the manner in which the employee holding that job interacts with others. The formal outcome of a job analysis is the preparation of a job description.[27]

A job description helps employees understand what is expected of them and to whom they report. Although there is no standard format, most job descriptions include the items shown in Table 6-6.[28] The job description serves as a basis for rating and classifying jobs, setting wages and salaries, and conducting a performance appraisal (described later). It helps organizations comply with the accrediting, contractual, legal, and regulatory directives of the government or other institutions, and it provides a basis for decisions about promotions and training. In addition, it can be adapted for use in recruiting and hiring prospective employees. For example, the text of a position announcement to be published in a newspaper or journal can be taken from the job description. A sample job description for a nutrition officer with the Food and Agriculture Organization is given in Figure 6-5.

Job design The specification of tasks and activities associated with a particular job.

Job analysis The systematic collection and recording of information about a job's purpose, its major duties, the conditions under which it is performed, and the knowledge, skills, and abilities needed to perform the job effectively.

TABLE
6-6

Components of a Job Description

Source: Adapted from J. G. Liebler and coauthors, *Management Principles for Health Professionals,* 2nd ed. (Gaithersburg, Md.: Aspen Publishers, 1992), pp. 181–82.

◆ **Job title.** The job title clarifies the position and its skill level (for example, *director, supervisor, assistant,* or *secretary*).

◆ **Immediate supervisor.** The job description states the position and title of the immediate supervisor.

◆ **Job summary.** The job summary is a short statement of the purpose of the job and its major tasks and activities.

◆ **Job duties.** This section of the job description is a detailed statement of the specific duties of the job and how these duties are carried out.

◆ **Job specifications.** This is a list of minimum hiring requirements, usually derived from the job analysis; it includes the skill requirements for the job, such as educational level, licensure requirements, and experience (usually expressed in years), and any specific knowledge, advanced training, manual skills, and communication skills (both oral and written) required to do the job. The physical demands of the job, if any, including working conditions and job hazards, are included here.

Affirmative action Any activity undertaken by employers to increase equal employment opportunities for groups protected by federal equal employment opportunity (EEO) laws and regulations.

Human Resource Management   Paying attention to the people who produce a product or service is what human resource management is all about. Community nutritionists report being involved in several aspects of managing people, including recruiting people for the organization and evaluating the performance of their employees.[29] Both these activities are described in the next paragraphs.

◆ **Staffing.** Staffing is the set of human resource activities designed to recruit individuals to help meet the organization's goals and objectives. Recruitment has two distinct phases: (1) attracting applicants and (2) hiring candidates.[30] Both direct and indirect recruiting strategies are often used to attract applicants. Direct methods include media-based advertising in newspapers and journals, mailing personalized letters to potential applicants, and participating in job recruitment fairs. Indirect methods are activities that keep the organization's name in the public's eye such as collaborative projects with other institutions and training sessions for professionals.

An important aspect of recruiting is **affirmative action,** which includes all activities designed to ensure and increase equal employment opportunities for groups protected by federal laws and regulations. A significant law in this area is Title VII of the Civil Rights Act of 1964, which forbids employment discrimination on the basis of sex, race, color, religion, or national origin. Most organizations have some type of affirmative action plan that details its goals and policies related to hiring, training, and promoting protected groups. In fact, organizations with federal contracts exceeding $50,000 and with 50 or more employees *must* file an affirmative action plan with the Department of Labor's Office of Federal Contract Compliance Programs; others may develop such plans on a voluntary basis.[31]

The hiring process involves conducting job interviews with potential candidates, screening applicants, selecting the best candidate, checking

POSITION TITLE: Nutrition Officer (Nutrition Information)
RESPONSIBLE TO: Senior Officer (Nutrition Assessment)
LEVEL (GRADE):   P–4

RESPONSIBILITIES:

Under the general direction of the Chief of the Nutrition Planning, Assessment and Evaluation Service, Food Policy and Nutrition Division, and the supervision of the Senior Officer (Nutrition Assessment), this specialist is responsible for the development of activities aimed at improving information necessary for assessing and analyzing nutrition status of populations at global, national and local levels, especially in the drought-prone African countries.

JOB DUTIES:

In accordance with departmental policies and procedures, this specialist carries out the following duties and responsibilities:

◆ Assists member countries in the design and implementation of data collection and analysis activities to meet the needs of policymakers and planners concerned with food and nutrition issues;

◆ In cooperation with other organization units, strengthens the skills and technical capacity of member countries, particularly within the agricultural sector, to assess, analyze, and monitor the food and nutrition situation of their own population;

◆ Provides data and background information for Expert Committees and Councils;

◆ Provides consultations on energy and nutrient requirements, dietary assessment methodology, and foodways;

◆ Prepares relevant reports for the organization and its committees; and

◆ Performs other related duties.

QUALIFICATIONS AND EXPERIENCE—ESSENTIAL

The specialist should have the following educational qualifications and experience:

◆ A university degree in Nutrition or Biological Science with postgraduate qualification in Nutrition.

◆ Seven years of progressively responsible professional experience, including the planning and implementation of nutrition data collection, processing, and analysis.

◆ Experience in the management and analysis of nutrition-related data using advanced statistical applications on microcomputers.

QUALIFICATIONS AND EXPERIENCE—DESIRABLE

◆ Experience in international work and research.

◆ Relevant work experience in Africa.

◆ Experience in the organization of seminars, training courses, or conferences.

SKILLS

◆ Working knowledge of English and French (level C).

◆ Demonstrated ability to write related technical reports. Familiarity with project design techniques.

◆ Courtesy, tact, and ability to establish and maintain effective work relationships with people of different national and cultural backgrounds.

◆ Experience using word-processing equipment and software.

DATE:
REVISIONS:

FIGURE

6-5

Sample Job Description
Source: Adapted from Vacancy Announcement (No. 130–ESN), 1992, of the Food and Agriculture Organization of the United Nations. Used with permission.

references, and, finally, offering the position. In some cases, two or three suitable candidates will be invited back for interviews with key managers in other departments or divisions before a final candidate is chosen.

◆ **Evaluating job performance.** Providing feedback to employees about their performance is essential to maintaining good working relationships and can occur informally at any time. In the daily course of solving unexpected problems and reviewing the progress on a project, managers in community nutrition have ample opportunity to update their employees about their performance. In fact, the best managers spend up to 40 percent of their time in face-to-face interactions with their employees that allow time for performance feedback.[32]

Performance appraisal A manager's formal review of an employee's performance on the job.

The **performance appraisal** is a formal method of providing feedback to an employee. It is designed to influence the employee in a positive, constructive manner and involves defining the organization's expectations for employee performance and measuring, evaluating, and recording the performance compared with those expectations. The performance appraisal is used to help define future performance goals, determine training needs and merit pay increases, and assess the employee's potential for advancement. Because employees are often uneasy about the review process, managers must take care to be objective in their rating of performance. One way to reduce employees' discomfort is to let them know in advance how the process works and what to expect during the performance appraisal interview. Employees are most likely to have a favorable impression of the process when they are aware of the evaluation criteria used, have the opportunity to participate in the process, and are able to discuss their career development.[33]

The performance appraisal interview is a good time for reviewing and changing both organizational and personal goals. Managers who spend time helping subordinates develop their personal goals are more likely to achieve their organization's goals, since setting challenging personal goals is linked strongly with performance.[34]

Employees want to hear from management, and they want management to listen to them.
—D. Keith Denton

The key to conducting a good performance appraisal interview is to start with clear objectives, focus on observable behavior, and avoid vague, subjective statements of a personal nature. Consult Table 6-7 for a list of questions that can be used in talking about performance and giving constructive criticism.[35]

◆ LEADING

Leading is the management function that involves influencing others to achieve the organization's goals and objectives. Supreme Court Justice Potter Stewart once said about obscenity: "I cannot define it for you, but I know it when I see it."[36] The same might be said about leadership and management. Fortunately, the wealth of research in this area in recent years has helped define the behaviors and attitudes of good managers and leaders.

Leading versus Managing Leading and managing are separate, distinct skills. The difference between the two has been described by Warren Bennis, an interna-

TABLE
6-7

How to Provide Constructive Criticism
Source: J. G. Goodale, Seven ways to improve performance appraisals, *HRMagazine* 38 (1993): 79. Reprinted with the permission of HRMagazine (formerly Personnel Administrator) published by the Society for Human Resource Management, Alexandria, VA.

Use the process outlined here to offer constructive criticism to your employees without making them defensive. While these questions can be used in a performance appraisal interview, they lend themselves to many other job-related discussions. Most people questioned in this manner make specific suggestions to improve their performance.

♦ **Initiate.** "How would you rate your performance during the last six months?" or "How do you feel about your performance during the last quarter?"

♦ **Listen.** If you get a general response like "fine," or "pretty good," or "8 on a 10-point scale," follow up with a more focused question: "What in particular comes to mind?" or "What have you been particularly pleased with?" Your objective is to discuss a positive topic raised by the employee.

♦ **Focus.** "You mentioned that you were particularly satisfied with . . . . Let's talk further about that aspect of your job."

♦ **"How" probe.** "How did you approach . . . ?" or "What method did you use?"

♦ **"Why" probe.** "How did you happen to choose that approach?" or "What was your rationale for that method?"

♦ **"Results" probe.** "How has it worked out for you?" or "What results have you achieved?"

♦ **Plan.** "Knowing what you know now, what would you have done differently?" or "What changes would you make if you worked on this again?"

tionally recognized consultant, writer, and researcher on leadership: "Leaders are people who do the right thing; managers are people who do things right. Both roles are crucial, but they differ profoundly."[37] In general, managers crunch numbers, orchestrate activities, and control supplies, projects, and data. Leaders fertilize and catalyze; they enhance people, allowing them to stretch and grow. Where managers push and direct, leaders pull and expect.[38] Other differences between managers and leaders are listed in Table 6-8.

What exactly is leadership? **Leadership** is "the process of influencing others toward the achievement of organizational goals."[39] Leaders understand how an organization works (or doesn't work, as the case may be) and how people work—that is, what motivates them to be top performers. Leaders value and respect diversity in people and recognize the importance of involving many different people in the collective process of reaching a goal.[40] The traits of successful leaders number more than a hundred according to recent studies, although not all experts agree on the importance of every trait.[41] Some of the attributes commonly ascribed to leaders include intelligence, credibility, energy, sociability, discipline, courage, generosity, and accountability. Warren Bennis reminds us that leaders come in all shapes, sizes, and temperaments, but he believes they all have a guiding vision, passion, integrity, curiosity, and daring.[42] Check the boxed insert for a description of the principles of leadership outlined by General H. Norman Schwarzkopf, who guided U.S. troops to victory in the Gulf War.

Leadership The process of influencing others toward the achievement of organizational goals.

Motivating Employees   Organizations need strong leaders *and* good managers. One of the most important functions of managers is to motivate their employees to "get the job done." Barcy Fox, a vice president with Maritz Performance

TABLE

6-8

Differences between Leaders and Managers

Source: *On Becoming a Leader* (pg. 45), © 1990 by Warren Bennis, Inc. Reprinted by permission of Addison-Wesley Publishing Company, Inc.

◆ The manager administers; the leader innovates.

◆ The manager is a copy; the leader is an original.

◆ The manager maintains; the leader develops.

◆ The manager focuses on systems and structure; the leader focuses on people.

◆ The manager relies on control; the leader inspires trust.

◆ The manager has a short-range view; the leader has a long-range perspective.

◆ The manager asks how and when; the leader asks what and why.

◆ The manager has her eye on the bottom line; the leader has her eye on the horizon.

◆ The manager imitates; the leader originates.

◆ The manager accepts the status quo; the leader challenges it.

◆ The manager is the classic good soldier; the leader is his own person.

Improvement Company, comments: "Your employees aren't you. What works for you won't work for them. What motivates you to pursue a goal won't motivate them. Until you grasp that, you won't set attainable goals for your workers."[43] There is no single strategy for motivating employees to perform, and opinions differ on exactly what managers need to do to stimulate motivation. Peter Drucker, cited in our discussion of entrepreneurship in Chapter 1, argues that managers can do four things to obtain peak performance from their employees:[44]

◆ Set high standards and stick to them. Employees become demoralized when managers do not hold themselves to the same high standards set for other workers in the organization. Employees are stimulated to work hard with a manager who expects a lot of herself, believes in excellence, and sets a good example.

◆ Put the right person in the right job. Employees take pride in meeting a challenge and doing a job well. Their sense of accomplishment enhances their performance. Underutilizing employees' skills destroys their motivation. As Wess Roberts notes in *Leadership Secrets of Attila the Hun,* "a wise chieftain always gives tough assignments to Huns who can rise to the occasion."[45]

◆ Keep employees informed about their performance. Employees should be able to control, measure, and evaluate their own performance. To do this, they need to know and understand the standard against which their performance is being compared. The job description and performance appraisal interview help keep employees informed about what managers expect of them. Keep in mind the unwritten rule of managing people: Put praise in writing. When you must reprimand an employee, do so verbally and in private.

◆ Allow employees to be a part of the process. One means of motivating employees is to give them a managerial vision, a sense of how their work contributes to the success of the project, program, or organization. In a sense, a manager cannot "give" his own vision to his employees, but he

---

Leadership Views of General H. Norman Schwarzkopf

◆ **You must have clear goals.** Having specific goals and articulating them clearly makes it easy for everyone involved to understand the mission.

◆ **Give yourself a clear agenda.** First thing in the morning, write down the five most important things you need to accomplish that day. Whatever else you do, get those five things done.

◆ **Let people know where they stand.** You do a great disservice to an employee or student when you give high marks for mediocre work. The grades you give the people who report to you must reflect reality.

◆ **What's broken, fix now.** If it's broken, fix it now. Problems that aren't dealt with lead to other problems, and in the meantime, something else breaks and needs fixing.

◆ **No repainting the flagpole.** Make sure that all the work your people are doing is essential to the organization and its goals.

◆ **Set high standards.** Too often we don't ask enough of people. People generally won't perform above your expectations, so it is important to expect a lot.

◆ **Lead, and then get out of the way.** Yes, you must put the right people in the right place to get the job done, but then step back. Allow them to own their work.

◆ **People come to work to succeed.** Nobody comes to work to fail. Why do so many organizations operate on the principle that if people aren't watched and supervised, they'll bungle the job?

◆ **Never lie. Ever.** Lying undermines your credibility. Be straightforward in your thinking and actions.

◆ **When in charge, take command.** Leaders are often called upon to make decisions without adequate information. It is usually a mistake to put off making a decision until all the data are in. The best policy is to decide, monitor the results, and change course if necessary.

◆ **Do what's right.** "The truth of the matter," said Schwarzkopf, "is that you *always* know the right thing to do. The hard part is doing it."

Source: Schwarzkopf on leadership, *Inc.* 14 (1992): 11. Reprinted with permission, *Inc.* magazine, January, 1992. Copyright 1992 by Goldhirsh Group, Inc., 38 Commercial Wharf, Boston, MA 02110.

---

can allow them to help mold and shape the vision, thereby making it theirs as well as his.

Being able to influence people successfully is one of the most important determinants of a manager's effectiveness. Keeping employees' morale and productivity high requires a variety of tactics. But which ones work best? According to one study, the most effective tactic was the inspirational appeal—a request that aroused enthusiasm or appealed to the employee's value system or aspirations. Consultation, or engaging the employee's assistance and support for undertaking an activity or changing procedures, was also an effective method. The least effective tactics included demands, threats, and frequent checking of an employee's work; claiming authority over workers; and coalition, or seeking the aid of other workers in influencing a worker to do what the manager wants. These "hard" tactics do not motivate employees, gain their cooperation, or enhance their commitment to the team process and the organization.[46]

Communicating with Employees   Communicating is a critical managerial activity that can take many forms. Verbal communication is the written or oral use of words to communicate messages. Written communications can take the form of reports, résumés, telephone messages, memorandums, procedure manuals, policy manuals, and letters. Oral communications, or the spoken word, usually take place in forums such as telephone conversations, committee meetings, and formal presentations. Good managers are skilled in both of these areas (review the Professional Focuses for Chapters 11 and 12). Nonverbal communication in the form of gestures, facial expressions, and so-called body language is also important. Tone of voice—the *way* something is said as opposed to *what* is said—sometimes relays information more effectively than the actual words. Even the placement of office furniture communicates certain elements of attitude and style. Reportedly, nonverbal communication accounts for between 65 and 93 percent of what actually gets communicated.[47]

Becoming a good communicator means paying attention to people and events, observing the nuances of nonverbal and verbal communication, and becoming a good listener. Open communication in an organization does not occur by accident. It results from the daily use of certain techniques and skills that promote communication. Merck, the pharmaceutical company, uses an approach called Face-To-Face communication. The four rules upon which this communication is built are listed in Table 6-9.[48] Communicating effectively with

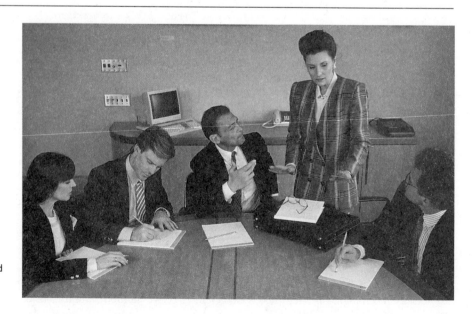

Leaders are open to new experiences, accept lifestyles and values that differ from their own, are good listeners, and can laugh at themselves.

◆ **Be candid.** Any questions or comments that arise during face-to-face interactions (be they performance appraisal interviews or committee meetings) should be addressed truthfully. If appropriate, indicate that you cannot answer the question because of its confidential nature. If you do not know the answer to a question, say so.

◆ **Be prepared.** Ask participants to submit questions or topics for discussion several weeks or days before the meeting is scheduled to occur. Organize an agenda, preferably a written one. This strategy has the advantage of ensuring that topics of interest to you and your employees are covered. If you develop a written agenda, distribute it to the participants before the meeting so that they can arrive prepared.

◆ **Encourage participation.** Conduct the face-to-face meeting in a relaxed and friendly atmosphere where people feel comfortable expressing their ideas.

◆ **Focus on listening, not judging.** When sensitive topics arise, try not to appear upset or judgmental. Listen carefully to questions and the discussion they prompt. Pay attention to nonverbal cues and group dynamics. The bottom line for good communications is simple: Treat others with respect.

TABLE

6-9

Four Rules of Face-to-Face Communication
Source: Adapted from Merck's Face-To-Face Communication, in D. K. Denton, *Recruitment, Retention, and Employee Relations* (Westport, Conn.: Quorum Books, 1992), pp. 158–59.

coworkers is a skill that, like other skills described in this book, can be acquired with practice and determination.

Handling Conflict   To help foster teamwork, managers must be able to deal with conflict, a by-product of how people interact in groups. Conflict often has a negative connotation and typically is viewed as a signal that something is wrong. Most people try to avoid conflict at all costs. Yet, conflict is inevitable in all relationships. "For Huns, conflict is a natural state," writes Wess Roberts.[49] It can arise from competition among workers for scarce resources, questions about authority relationships, pressures arising outside the organization, or even from solutions developed for dealing with previous conflicts. The problem in most organizations and work groups is that conflicts are avoided and left unresolved. When this occurs, employees are likely to be defensive and hostile and to feel that they can't trust one another.[50]

To handle conflict positively, managers should begin by remembering that conflict usually emerges because of differences in values, attitudes, beliefs, and feelings. Appreciating and being sensitive to such differences helps establish a climate of cooperation. Next, managers work to pinpoint the underlying cause of the conflict. Finally, they resolve the differences through open negotiation. If necessary, rules and procedures are changed to address the underlying problem. At all times, managers work to ensure that employees feel that their complaints and concerns are perceived as legitimate and that management listens to them.[51]

◆ CONTROLLING

Controlling is the management function concerned with regulating organizational activities so that actual performance meets accepted organizational standards and goals.[52] The controlling function involves determining which activities need control, establishing standards, measuring performance, and correcting deviations. Managers set up control systems or mechanisms for ensuring that resources, quality of products and services, client satisfaction, and other activities are regulated properly. Such controls help managers cope with the uncertainties that arise when plans go awry. An unforeseen reduction in the public health department's budget, for example, forces the manager of the nutrition division to reallocate personnel and institute tighter spending controls.

Community nutritionists often have responsibility for program and departmental budgets and managing information. The ADA's role delineation study determined that managers in community or public health programs were responsible for preparing financial analyses and reports, controlling program costs, monitoring a program's financial performance, documenting a program's operations, and making decisions about capital expenditures.[53] Strong management skills enable community nutritionists to detect irregularities in client service or cost overruns and handle complex projects and programs. Two aspects of the control process are described in the next paragraphs.

Financial and Budgetary Control The primary tools of financial control are the two types of financial statements: balance sheets and income statements. The **balance sheet** lists the organization's assets and liabilities. Assets include cash, accounts receivable (sales of a product or service for which payment has not yet been received), inventories, and items such as buildings, machinery, and equipment. Liabilities include accounts payable (bills that must be paid to outside suppliers and the like), short- and long-term loans, and shareholders' equity such as common stock. (Government agencies and most small, independent companies do not have shareholders' equity.) The **income statement** summarizes the organization's operations over a specific time period, such as a quarter or a year. It generally lists revenues (the assets derived from selling goods and services) and expenses (the costs incurred in producing the revenue). The difference between revenues and expenses is the organization's profit or loss—sometimes called the "bottom line."

Financial control is typically managed through a budget, which is "a plan for the accomplishment of programs related to objectives and goals within a definite time period, including an estimate of resources required, together with an estimate of the resources available."[54] Budgets can be planned for the organization as

Balance sheet A financial statement that depicts an organization's assets and claims against those assets (liabilities) at a given time.

Income statement A financial statement that summarizes the organization's financial position over a specified period, such as a quarter or a year.

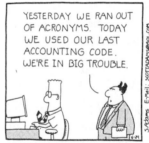
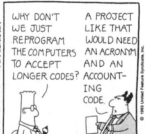
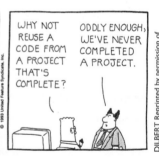

DILBERT Reprinted by permission of USS, Inc.

a whole or for subunits such as divisions, departments, and programs. **Budgeting** is closely linked to planning. It is the process of stating in quantitative terms (usually dollars) the planned organizational activities for a given period of time. Although the terms *budgeting* and *accounting* are sometimes used interchangeably, they are not the same thing. Accounting is a purely financial activity, while budgeting is both a financial and a program planning activity.

Organizations typically have a master budget that helps maintain budgetary control. A master budget consists of three types of budgets: the capital expenditures, financial, and operating budgets. The capital expenditures budget is a plan for acquiring or selling major fixed assets such as land, buildings, or equipment like office furniture, computers, and file cabinets. The financial budget specifies how the organization is going to acquire and use its cash. It helps managers determine whether they have the funds on hand to carry out certain projects or activities. The operating budget is most important for our purposes. It is a statement of the financial plan for each program or department that outlines the revenues and expenses related to its operation. A sample operating budget for Nutrition in Action appears in Table 6-10.

Classifying expenses uniformly is an important aspect of the budgeting process. Having a uniform code of accounts, such as the one published by the American Hospital Association and the American Association of Hospital Accountants, helps ensure that expenses are assigned to the proper category for budgetary purposes. Nutrition in Action might use the following account codes:

Budgeting The process of stating in quantitative terms, usually dollars, the planned organizational activities for a given period of time.

Account Code	Account Name
200	Furniture
210	Capital equipment
520	Equipment rental
530	Equipment maintenance and service contracts
580	Purchased services—communications/marketing consultant
600	Travel
610	Dues and subscriptions
720	Office supplies

These categories can be broken down further to give detailed information about specific expenditures within each account code. The expenditures for dues and subscriptions for Nutrition in Action might be broken down as follows:

Account Code	Account Name: Dues and Subscriptions	
610.1	ADA dues ($150.00 × 4 RDs)	$600.00
	ADA dues ($87.50 × 1 DTR)	87.50
610.2	ADA registration fee ($25.00 × 5)	125.00
610.3	Harvard Health Letter	35.00
	U of C at Berkeley Wellness Letter	24.00
610.5	Int'l Journal of Sports Nutrition	36.00
	American Journal of Clinical Nutrition	65.00
	Annual Review of Nutrition	38.00

TABLE

6-10

Sample Operating Budget for Nutrition in Action, July 1, 1993, through June 30, 1994

Revenue and income	
Fitness at Work Program	$ 82,500
Counseling	128,000
Sales—merchandise	50,000
Honoraria	20,000
Executive seminars	2,500
Total revenue	$283,000
Expenses	
Direct expenses	
Salaries	$163,500
Consultant services	4,000
Telephone	8,000
Furniture	1,250
Equipment	6,000
Equipment rental	800
Equipment maintenance and service contracts	1,800
Travel	8,000
Office supplies	6,200
Postage	3,500
Advertising	1,000
Dues and subscriptions	1,000
Total direct expenses	$205,050
Indirect expenses	
Benefits (29%)	$ 47,415
Rent	7,800
Utilities	1,000
Equipment depreciation	7,200
Maintenance and repairs	2,000
Janitorial services	4,300
Total indirect expenses	$ 69,715
Total expenses	$274,765
Net profit or loss	$ 8,235

Since all expenses of an organization—everything from pencils and paper clips to salaries and benefits—must be accounted for, the budgeting process requires considerable planning and managing. Some organizations use "top-down budgeting," in which top management outlines the overall figures that managers in middle and lower levels use in their planning. This approach allows top managers to keep track of resources and progress toward organizational goals. Other organizations use "bottom-up budgeting," in which middle- and lower-level managers specify their budgetary needs, and top management strives to accommodate their requests. This approach uses the knowledge base of managers "in the trenches" to keep the organization on track in meeting its goals and objectives.[55]

In addition to these two structural approaches to budgeting, there are two procedural approaches. In **incremental budgeting**, the budget database is increased by a flat rate. For example, the personnel portion may be increased by 5 percent, while the supplies budget is increased by 2 percent. Incremental budgeting provides a certain degree of consistency and efficiency, but it does not allow for flexibility in handling unexpected problems or responding to unforeseen mar-

Incremental budgeting A budget process whereby previously budgeted amounts are increased by a flat rate.

ket conditions. With the other approach, outputs are evaluated, resources are allocated, and funds are made available to meet a program's goals. This process is sometimes called **zero-based budgeting.** Managers using zero-based budgeting must continually justify their activities in terms of the organization's goals and objectives; this requires efficient feedback mechanisms to track resources, funds, and overall project progress. Zero-based budgeting became popular during the 1960s when it was mandated in the Department of Defense. It has been used by large companies such as Xerox and Texas Instruments and by some state and local governments. It seems to work best in organizations that have fairly long reporting periods for the budgeting process and a large budgeting staff.

The budgeting process is cyclic. It usually begins with a review of the previous budget period and then proceeds to the development of a new budget. Most programs and projects receive a monthly budgetary review. The primary areas to be examined include total project funding, expenditures to date, current estimated cost to complete the project, anticipated profit or loss, and an explanation of any deviations from the planned budget expenditure. Periodic status summaries help managers control resources and keep to the planning schedule.[56] The internal approval process for a new budget can involve bargaining, compromise, and outright competition for scarce resources. Managers who can justify their budget requests are more likely to be successful in appropriating funds for their program's projects and activities.

Information Control   In the course of your community work, you will need to collect, organize, retrieve, and analyze many types of data and information. You need to know about the health and nutrition status of the population in your district, the demographic profile of your client base, how people in your community use your organization's programs and services, how cost-effective your programs are, and the expenses incurred by your staff in carrying out their program activities, to name only a few. At this point, a distinction must be made between "data" and "information." **Data** are unanalyzed facts and figures. For example, a survey of infants in your community shows that over the past 12 months 36 of 478 infants had birth weights less than 2500 grams. These data don't mean much on their own; to be meaningful, they must be transformed into **information.** By processing the data further (for example, converting the data into a percentage or calculating the mean weights), the manager can compare these figures with those from previous reporting years. A change in the figures may signal the need to reassess program goals and reallocate resources to prevent low birth weight.

The primary purpose of information is to help managers make decisions. Information is a decision support tool in that it helps managers answer these questions: What do we want to do? How do we do it? Did we do what we said we were going to do? The first question addresses the planning function of management; the second, the organizing function; and the third, the controlling function. Managers begin the decision-making process by organizing the data into usable information. They then identify the means by which the data are to be analyzed. This process involves sorting, formatting, extracting, and transforming the data, usually following certain statistical methods. Finally, managers interpret the output and prepare reports that summarize the information. Decisions are then

Zero-based budgeting A budget process whereby managers start with zero in preparing their budget requests and must justify their activities in terms of future goals.

Data Unanalyzed facts and figures.

Information Data that have been analyzed or processed into a form that is meaningful for decision makers.

based on the figures in the reports.[57] Of course, managers' decisions are only as good as their information. Constant vigilance is required to prevent the GIGO (garbage in/garbage out) syndrome.

With the advent of computers, processing information has become both simpler and more complex. It is simpler because many aspects of data analysis are carried out on computers and not by hand. It is more complex because one can choose from hundreds of computer systems and software programs. Because computers can produce reams of data very quickly, managers are apt to become overwhelmed by the magnitude and diversity of the data available to them. To be useful, information must be:[58]

1. **Relevant.** The information must be relevant to the problem or issue at hand. Although it is sometimes difficult to know precisely what information is needed, managers should try to identify the information most germane to the decision-making process.

2. **Accurate.** If information is inaccurate or incorrect, the quality of the decision will certainly be questionable.

3. **Timely.** Information must be available when it is needed.

4. **Complete.** Information must cover all of the areas important to the decision-making process.

5. **Concise.** Information should be concise, providing a summary of the items central to the decision.

The Business of Community Nutrition

Whether you work in the public or private sector, you need strong management skills. You must be able to set a direction for your business or program; define goals and objectives; organize the delivery of your product or service; motivate people to help your organization reach its goals; allocate materials, equipment, personnel, and funds to your operations; control data systems; and provide leadership. More than ever before, management and leadership skills are needed to gain a competitive edge in what has become an increasingly competitive health care environment. As you move into the community with your ideas, products, and nutrition services, keep these four strategies for success in mind:[59]

◆ Continually assess the competitive environment.
◆ Continually assess your strengths.
◆ Build organizational skills.
◆ Build managerial (people and process) skills.

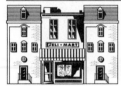

COMMUNITY LEARNING ACTIVITY

Beginning with this Community Learning Activity and continuing throughout Section II, you will be working as part of a team to develop, market, and evaluate your own community nutrition program. Your team should choose *one* of the following scenarios and complete the activities that follow. The scenario you choose will be the basis for the remaining Community Learning Activities in this section.

◆ **Scenario 1.** You have been asked to develop a breastfeeding program for pregnant adolescents. The request for this program comes from an administrator in a nonprofit health organization who has received $27,500 from a local community fund to develop and test the program. Clients will be referred to the program from area hospitals and clinics, social workers, and physicians in private practice.

◆ **Scenario 2.** You have been asked to develop a program for HIV-positive children aged 2 to 10 years and their families or caretakers. The request for this new program comes from a local coalition of hospital administrators, health educators, researchers, and AIDS groups who have obtained $112,000 from the government to develop and test a program over a period of one year. Although the local hospital has an in-patient program for HIV-positive infants, currently no community program addresses the needs of HIV-positive children in their homes. The program would target the families or caretakers of HIV-positive children, many of whom were born to women with AIDS. A few of these women can provide some care for their HIV-positive children; most of the children, however, have lost their mothers and are being cared for by foster families or relatives.

1. Define the problem presented in your scenario using the questions in Table 6-2 as a guide. Which questions are difficult to answer because you have not completed a nutrition assessment of your community?

2. Develop goals and objectives for your program. Specify both outcome and process objectives.

3. How many people are needed to administer and implement the program? How was your decision influenced by the amount of funding available for the program?

Time Management

Time is a nonrenewable resource, a precious commodity. "Time is life," wrote Alan Lakein in his best-selling book, *How to Get Control of Your Time and Your Life*.[1] "It is irreversible and irreplaceable. To waste your time is to waste your life, but to master your time is to master your life and make the most of it."

Many of us have difficulty deciding how to spend our time. Every day we must choose among dozens of activities and duties, all competing for our time and attention: family, friends, work, school, shopping, sports, television, movies, hobbies. The list is endless. Given that we all have a limited amount of time available each day, how can we choose from the multitude of jobs around us? The key to effective time management, argues Lakein, is *control*.

◆ CONTROL IS ESSENTIAL

Control means recognizing that it is easy to become overwhelmed by the number of decisions we face about how we spend our time. The secret to controlling time effectively is making conscious decisions about which activities deserve our attention and effort—and which don't. Taking control of your time means *planning* how you will spend your time. Planning starts with deciding what your priorities are.

◆ QUADRANT II IS WHERE THE ACTION SHOULD BE

Stephen Covey, author of *The 7 Habits of Highly Effective People*, writes that the essence of good time management can be summarized in the following phrase: Organize and execute (in other words, *plan*) around priorities. Covey developed a time management matrix, shown in Figure 6-6, to demonstrate how most people spend their time.[2]

Covey defines activities as either "urgent" or "important." Urgent activities demand immediate attention. Important activities have to do with results; they require a more proactive approach than urgent activities. Look at the time management matrix. Quadrant I activities are both urgent and important. These activities are called "crises" or "problems." All of us have Quadrant I activities in our lives. The problem with focusing on Quadrant I activities, though, is that they tend to lead to stress, burnout, and a sense that we are always putting out brushfires.

Some people spend quite a bit of their time in Quadrant III, thinking that they are in Quadrant I. They are reacting to things that are urgent and appear important, but that actually yield short-term results. People who spend their time in Quadrant III are likely to feel out of control. Covey believes that people who devote most of their time to Quadrant III and IV activities lead irresponsible lives, because they do not manage themselves and their actions.

Highly effective people spend their time with Quadrant II activities. It is through these activities that we accomplish the truly important things in life.

◆ IT'S AS EASY AS ABC

The first step in taking control of your time is setting priorities—determining those things that are most important to you. Lakein calls this process the ABC Priority System. "A" activities have a high value; "B" items, a medium value; and "C" items, a low value.

Continued

◆ **PROFESSIONAL FOCUS**—*Continued*

	Urgent	Not urgent
Important	**Quadrant I** Activities: 　Crises 　Pressing problems 　Deadline-driven projects	**Quadrant II** Activities: 　Prevention 　Relationship building 　Recognizing new opportunities 　Planning, recreation
Not important	**Quadrant III** Activities: 　Interruptions, some calls 　Some mail, some reports 　Some meetings 　Proximate, pressing matters 　Popular activities	**Quadrant IV** Activities: 　Trivia, busy work 　Some mail 　Some phone calls 　Time wasters 　Pleasant activities

FIGURE 6-6

Time Management Matrix

Source: Excerpted chapters from *The Seven Habits of Highly Effective People,* p. 151, by Stephen R. Covey. Copyright © 1989 by Stephen R. Covey. Reprinted by permission of Simon & Schuster, Inc., and Covey Leadership Center, 1-800-331-7716.

Take three minutes to write down all of the things you should or would like to accomplish in the next three months. These activities probably fall into several categories: personal, family, community, social, school, career, financial, and spiritual goals. Don't hesitate to include some things that are off-the-wall. Now, for each item, assign a value of A, B, or C. Remember, the A activities are those with the highest value in your life. In addition, rank each activity within each category: A-1, A-2, and so forth.

Your A activities are top priorities, the items you want to find time for. The key to finding time for them lies not in prioritizing the activities on your schedule, but in scheduling your priorities. In other words, if your A-1 activity is learning Japanese, then schedule time for it, even if you can spend only 10 or 15 minutes a day.

Keep three things in mind as you carry out this task. First, only you can decide what your priorities are. No one else can do this for you. Secondly, your A list will probably change over time and should be reviewed periodically. What is important to you now may not be important to you in six months. Finally, because planning in advance is the best thing you can do for yourself, write down your priorities. "A daily plan, in writing, is *the* single most effective time management strategy, yet not one person in ten does it. The other nine will always go home muttering to themselves, 'Where did the day go?'"[3]

◆ THE TOP 10 TIME WASTERS

People from different jobs and disciplines have similar problems with managing time. A survey of 40 sales representatives and 50 engineering managers from 14 countries identified the following activities as the top time wasters:[4]

- ◆ Telephone interruptions
- ◆ Drop-in visitors
- ◆ Meetings (scheduled and unscheduled)
- ◆ Crises

Continued

- ◆ Lack of objectives, priorities, and deadlines
- ◆ Cluttered desk and personal disorganization
- ◆ Ineffective delegation
- ◆ Attempting too much at once
- ◆ Indecision and procrastination
- ◆ Lack of self-discipline

These are not the only time bandits by any means. Paper work, inadequate staffing, too much socializing, and travel all undermine our ability to manage time well. The key to managing these time wasters is to take control of them. Schedule your telephone calls for certain periods of the day and do not accept telephone interruptions during "quiet" times, unless there is an emergency. Minimize interruptions from colleagues and visitors. Attend only meetings directly related to your work.

◆ LEARN TO SAY "NO"

When you set your priorities—that is, when you say "yes" to one thing—you must say "no" to something else. You will *always* be saying "no" to something. You can never do everything that you want to do, or everything everyone else wants you to do! The key to managing your time effectively is to learn to say "no" firmly, politely, and courteously. Sometimes this can be difficult, for a task that is a B- or C-priority for you may be an A-priority for someone important to you. When this happens, take a moment to consider the consequences to you, the other person, and your mutual relationship if you say "no." In many cases, you can reach a compromise and maintain goodwill by deciding together how to rank an activity.

◆ WORK SMARTER, NOT HARDER

It is a myth that the harder you work, the more you accomplish. Many workaholics fall into this trap. They are more attuned to time spent working than quality time spent working. Avoid the trap of thinking that time spent working is automatically time spent valuably. "If it is not quality time and quality work, you are wasting time."[5]

Mastering the principles of good time management can take several months or even years. If you experience difficulty wresting control of your time, don't give up. Keep working at it. Although your progress may seem slow, you are further along than if you had never done it at all.

1. The description of the ABC Priority System was adapted from A. Lakein, *How to Get Control of Your Time and Your Life* (New York: Penguin Books, 1973).
2. S. R. Covey, *The 7 Habits of Highly Effective People* (New York: Simon & Schuster, 1989), p. 151.
3. The quotation is from A. Mackenzie, *The Time Trap* (New York: AMACOM, 1990), p. 41.
4. M. LeBoeuf, Managing time means managing yourself, in *The Management of Time,* ed. A. D. Timpe (New York: Facts on File Publications, 1987), pp. 31–36.
5. The quotation is from J. C. Levinson, *The Ninety-Minute Hour* (New York: E. P. Dutton, 1990), p. 168.

NOTES

1. How the new strategic plan works—for you, *Journal of the American Dietetic Association* 92 (1992): 1070.

2. The definition of management was taken from K. M. Bartol and D. C. Martin, *Management* (New York: McGraw-Hill, 1991), p. 6. Other definitions appearing in this chapter were also taken or adapted from this textbook.

3. The discussion of management ideas and viewpoints was adapted from Bartol and Martin, *Management*, pp. 41–70.

4. F. B. Gilbreth, Jr., and E. G. Carey, *Cheaper by the Dozen* (New York: Bantam Books, 1948).

5. R. G. Greenwood and C. D. Wrege, The Hawthorne studies, in *Papers Dedicated to the Development of Modern Management*, ed. D. A. Wren and J. A. Pearce II (New York: Academy of Management, 1986), pp. 24–35.

6. K. R. Mehtabdin, *Comparative Management—Business Styles in Japan and the United States*, vol. 1 (Lewiston/Queenston: Edwin Mellen Press, 1986), pp. 1–11.

7. Hoover: It sucks, *The Economist* 327 (1993): 66.

8. J. S. Rakich, B. B. Longest, Jr., and K. Darr, *Managing Health Services Organizations* (Philadelphia: W. B. Saunders, 1985), pp. 213–41.

9. How the new strategic plan works—for you, *Journal of the American Dietetic Association*, p. 1069.

10. K. G. Hardy, The three crimes of strategic planning, *Business Quarterly* 57 (1992): 71–74.

11. P. M. Kettner, R. M. Moroney, and L. L. Martin, *Designing and Managing Programs* (Newbury Park, Calif.: Sage Publications, 1990), pp. 31–41.

12. Ibid., p. 44.

13. J. Rothman and L. M. Gant, Approaches and models of community intervention, in *Needs Assessment: Theory and Methods*, ed. D. E. Johnson, et al. (Ames, Iowa: Iowa State University Press, 1987), pp. 35–44.

14. J. L. Wiecha and coauthors, Nutritional and economic advantages for homeless families in shelters providing kitchen facilities and food, *Journal of the American Dietetic Association* 93 (1993): 777–83.

15. U.S. Department of Health and Human Services, Public Health Service, *Healthy People 2000: National Health Promotion and Disease Prevention Objectives* (Washington, D.C.: U.S. Government Printing Office, 1990), p. 6.

16. Kettner and coauthors, *Designing and Managing Programs*, pp. 101–2.

17. U.S. Department of Health and Human Services, *Healthy People 2000*, p. 114.

18. S. R. Covey, *The 7 Habits of Highly Effective People* (New York: Simon & Schuster, 1989), pp. 96–99.

19. D. R. Dalton and coauthors, Organization structure and performance: A critical review, *Academy of Management Review* 5 (1980): 49–64.

20. J. L. Gray and F. A. Starke, *Organizational Behavior—Concepts and Applications*, 4th ed. (Columbus, Ohio: Merrill Publishing Company, 1988), pp. 426–27.

21. J. G. Liebler and coauthors, *Management Principles for Health Professionals*, 2nd ed. (Gaithersburg, Md.: Aspen Publishers, 1992), pp. 160–97.

22. Gray and Starke, *Organizational Behavior*, pp. 424–57.

23. Bartol and Martin, *Management,* p. 348.

24. D. D. Van Fleet and A. G. Bedeian, A history of the span of management, *Academy of Management Review* 2 (1977): 356–72.

25. J. C. Levinson, *The Ninety-Minute Hour* (New York: E. P. Dutton, 1990), p. 51.

26. M. W. McCall, Jr., and M. M. Lombardo, What makes a top executive? *Psychology Today* 17 (1983): pp. 26–31.

27. Bartol and Martin, *Management,* p. 407.

28. Liebler and coauthors, *Management Principles,* pp. 181–83.

29. American Dietetic Association, *Role Delineation for Registered Dietitians and Entry-Level Dietetic Technicians* (Chicago: American Dietetic Association, 1990), pp. 255–90.

30. The discussion of staffing was adapted from Liebler and coauthors, *Management Principles,* pp. 246–66.

31. Bartol and Martin, *Management,* pp. 410–11.

32. F. Rice, Champions of communication, *Fortune* 123 (1991): 111–112, 116, 120.

33. B. R. Nathan and coauthors, Interpersonal relations as a context for the effects of appraisal interviews on performance and satisfaction: A longitudinal study, *Academy of Management Journal* 34 (1991): 352–69.

34. A. A. Chesney and E. A. Locke, Relationships among goal difficulty, business strategies, and performance on a complex management simulation task, *Academy of Management Journal* 34 (1991): 400–24.

35. J. G. Goodale, Seven ways to improve performance appraisals, *HR Magazine* 38 (1993): 77–80.

36. As cited in M. Brown and B. P. McCool, High-performing managers: Leadership attributes for the 1990s, in *Human Resource Management in Health Care*, ed. M. Brown (Gaithersburg, Md.: Aspen Publishers, 1992), p. 22.

37. W. Bennis, Learning some basic truisms about leadership, *National Forum* 71 (1991): 13.

38. J. D. Batten, *Tough-Minded Leadership* (New York: AMACOM, 1989), p. 2.

39. Bartol and Martin, *Management,* p. 480.

40. S. W. Morse, Leadership for an uncertain century, *National Forum* 71 (1991): 2–4.

41. B. Czarniawska-Joerges and R. Wolff, Leaders, managers, entrepreneurs on and off the organizational stage, *Organization Studies* 12 (1991): 529–46.

42. W. Bennis, *On Becoming a Leader* (Reading, Mass.: Addison-Wesley, 1989), pp. 39–41.

43. R. McGarvey, Goal-getters, *Entrepreneur* 21 (1993): 144.

44. P. F. Drucker, *The Practice of Management* (New York: Harper & Row, 1986), pp. 302–11.

45. W. Roberts, *Leadership Secrets of Attila the Hun* (New York: Warner Books, 1987), p. 104.

46. C. M. Falbe and G. Yukl, Consequences for managers of using single influence tactics and combinations of tactics, *Academy of Management Journal* 35 (1992): 638–52.

47. Bartol and Martin, *Management,* p. 520.

48. D. K. Denton, *Recruitment, Retention, and Employee Relations* (Westport, Conn.: Quorum Books, 1992), pp. 155–71.

49. Roberts, *Leadership Secrets,* p. 105.

50. M. S. Corey and G. Corey, *Groups—Process and Practice* (Belmont, Calif.: Wadsworth, 1992), pp. 150-53.

51. Liebler and coauthors, *Management Principles,* pp. 246–66.

52. Bartol and Martin, *Management,* p. 594.

53. American Dietetic Association, *Role Delineation Study,* pp. 273–78.

54. T. D. Lynch, *Public Budgeting in America* (Englewood Cliffs, N.J.: Prentice-Hall, 1985), p. 4.

55. The discussion of top-down, bottom-up, and zero-based budgeting was adapted from Bartol and Martin, *Management,* pp. 644–46.

56. D. D. Roman, *Managing Projects—A Systems Approach* (New York: Elsevier Science Publishing Company, 1986), p. 129.

57. H. H. Schmitz, Decision support: A strategic weapon, in *Healthcare Information Management Systems,* ed. M. J. Ball, et al. (New York: Springer-Verlag, 1991), pp. 42–48.

58. Bartol and Martin, *Management,* pp. 704–5.

59. A. J. Morrison and K. Roth, Developing global subsidiary mandates, *Business Quarterly* 57 (1993): 104–10.

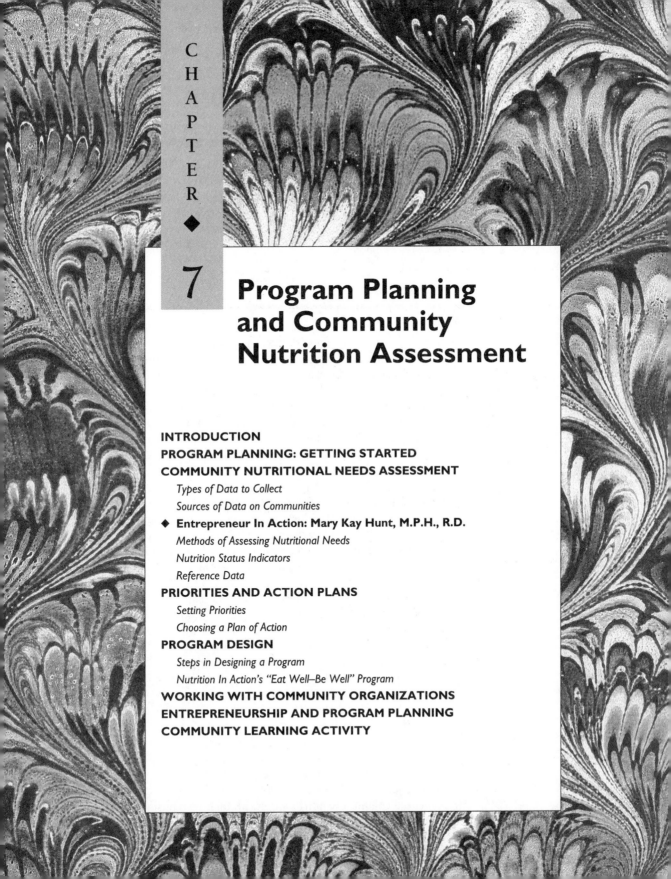

C H A P T E R ◆ 7

Program Planning and Community Nutrition Assessment

I think it could be plausibly argued that changes of diet are more important than changes of dynasty or even of religion.

—George Orwell

Introduction

Malnutrition has been labeled the world's number one health problem. Among children, it affects death rates, physical growth, mental development, and the severity and frequency of illness. Among adults, it contributes to morbidity and mortality and increases disease risk.[1] Although it has many causes, malnutrition is largely an ecological problem. That is, it is a function of the amount of foods and nutrients available to individuals within a community. Food availability depends upon environmental conditions, such as local agricultural practices, soil conditions, and methods of food storage, transport, and marketing. It depends, too, on the political climate of the community, region, and nation and on certain cultural factors, such as traditional cooking practices, religious beliefs, and meal patterns.[2]

Because it is associated with extremes of food intake, from chronic food insecurity among some population groups to chronic overconsumption among others, malnutrition can be widely distributed within a community. Identifying individuals who are malnourished is a major focus of community assessment. In determining the distribution of malnutrition within a community, information is needed about the ecological factors that affect food intake and nutrition status. Since it is not possible or cost-effective to collect data on all of these factors, the community nutritionist must determine which data would be useful to program planners and help convince policymakers that a nutritional need exists.

This chapter describes how community nutritionists collect data on a community's nutritional needs and how programs are designed to meet those needs. As you study this chapter, bear in mind that program planning and community assessment seldom proceed precisely in the manner described here. For example, an organization's decision about where it will spend its time and effort, a process called priority setting, may occur early on instead of toward the end as we show it. Even so, this chapter walks you through the steps that could occur if you were a community nutritionist responsible for program planning in a health department or voluntary health agency. The program planning principles described here apply equally to intrapreneurs in traditional health care settings and to entrepreneurial community nutritionists with their own business.

Program Planning: Getting Started

Recall from Chapter 6 that the program planning process begins with defining the community's nutritional problems and conducting a needs assessment. Although these steps appear to occur in tandem, in reality they often occur simultaneously, as shown in Figure 7-1. Some factor within or outside the organization starts the process. The stimulus might be a perceived need, as when a community nutritionist learns from her talks with social workers that some elderly people are not taking advantage of the community's Meals-on-Wheels program. The stimulus might be a mandate handed down from an organization's national office. For example, when the national office of the American Heart Association (AHA) determines that nutrition and physical activity are the organization's national health promotion initiatives for the coming year, local AHA offices must determine whether their existing programs meet the organization's mandate in these areas.

Research findings sometimes trigger the planning process. The report of the National Cholesterol Education Program on the detection, evaluation, and treatment of high blood cholesterol in adults was published in 1988 and described the major risk factors for coronary heart disease and their relationship to blood cholesterol levels. The report led some hospitals and health departments to review their

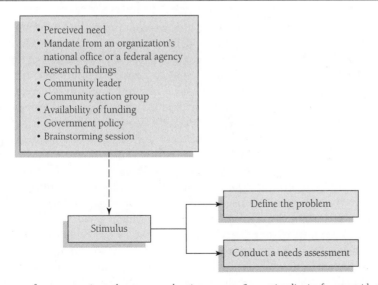

FIGURE

7-1

How the Program Planning Process Gets Started

One or more factors may trigger the program planning process. Some stimuli arise from outside the organization, for example, from the actions of community leaders. Others are internal, as when an agency develops a strategic plan that provides programmatic direction. The activities involved in defining the nutritional problem and conducting a needs assessment often occur simultaneously.

programs for reducing the risk of cardiovascular disease within their communities and, in some cases, to develop new programs to promote cardiovascular health.[3]

Other possible stimuli are listed in Figure 7-1. This list is not meant to be comprehensive but rather to indicate that any number of things can trigger the program planning process. Sometimes several stimuli operate conjointly. In any case, the result is that the organization is activated to determine whether the community has a nutritional need that is not being met. The organization begins by asking employees such as the community nutritionist, epidemiologist, and other personnel to gather information about the perceived problem. In some instances, this research phase helps the organization decide whether it should or should not develop a program, in which case the research is called a **feasibility study**. When the organization has already decided to develop a program, the research is undertaken to help determine what the program should look like. In other words, a **needs assessment** is conducted to help define the nutritional problem, identify discrepancies between the ideal and existing states, and suggest ways in which the program can be structured to address the problem.[4]

Although the focus and use of the information derived from these two types of research differ slightly, they use a similar process and methods to obtain the information. Since we are interested in program design, we will not concern ourselves here with the feasibility study but will proceed to a discussion of needs assessment.

Feasibility study Research activities designed to help an organization determine whether a program should or should not be developed.

Needs assessment Research activities designed to help an organization determine how a program should be developed.

Community Nutritional Needs Assessment

In Chapter 1 we defined a community as a grouping of people who reside in a specific locality and interact through a definite social structure to fulfill a wide range of daily needs. The discipline of community medicine, we pointed out, targets the health care needs of people living in their community and treats that community as a "patient." In much the same fashion, **community needs assessment** views the community as a patient and is concerned with evaluating the health and nutrition status of the community as a whole, determining what the community's nutritional needs are, and identifying places where those needs are not being met.[5]

Organizations approach the community nutritional needs assessment by first *planning* how it will proceed. The amount of time available to conduct the needs assessment, the staff members responsible for conducting it, and the scope of the assessment must all be specified. If the needs assessment is fairly limited in scope, it can be undertaken by one person. In most cases, however, the needs assessment is carried out by a team of people with expertise in nutrition, epidemiology, statistics, management, and survey design and analysis. In this chapter, the community nutritionist is given primary responsibility for conducting the community nutritional needs assessment. She begins by setting the parameters of the assessment and determining the types of data that must be collected to help paint a picture of the community's nutritional problem or need. The steps she might take are diagrammed in Figure 7-2 and described in the discussion that follows.

Community needs assessment Evaluating the community as a whole in terms of its health and nutrition status, its needs, and the resources available to address those needs.

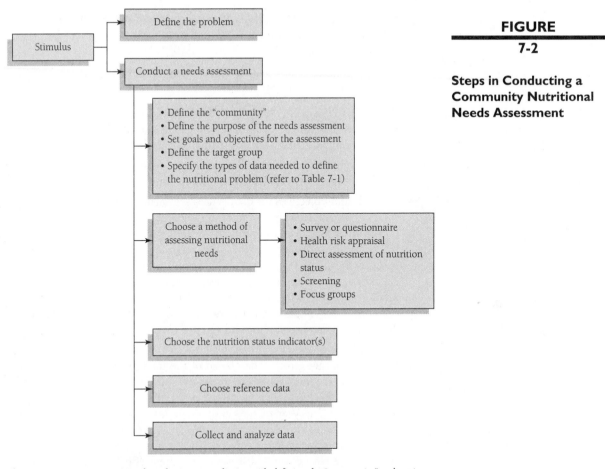

FIGURE

7-2

Steps in Conducting a Community Nutritional Needs Assessment

Planning a community nutritional needs assessment begins with defining the "community" and setting the parameters of the assessment, including the target group and types of data required. The method of obtaining data depends upon the purpose of the assessment and the personnel, money, and time available for it. Before any data are collected, the nutrition status indicators and reference data must be chosen.

◆ Define "community." The scope of the "community" must be specified. The "community" might include the people living within the city limits or the greater metropolitan area bounded by certain suburbs. Sometimes the "community" is a geographical region, state, nation, or several countries. In this chapter, the community is a typical municipal unit such as a city.

◆ Determine the purpose of the nutritional needs assessment. A needs assessment is typically undertaken to gather information about the social, political, economic, and environmental factors that influence the need and the population at risk. Specifying the purpose of the assessment helps the community nutritionist concentrate his efforts on gathering data related to the perceived nutritional problem. The community nutritional needs assessment may have one or more of the purposes shown on page 204.[6]

◆ Identify groups within the community who are at risk nutritionally.

◆ Identify the community's most critical nutritional needs and set priorities among them.

◆ Determine whether existing resources and programs meet the community's nutritional needs.

◆ Tailor a program to a specific population.

◆ Provide baseline information for developing action plans to address nutritional needs and for evaluating the program.

◆ Plan actions to improve nutrition status, using methods that are feasible and focus on established health priorities.

◆ Set goals and objectives for the needs assessment. This is an essential step, as the goals and objectives determine the types of data collected and how they will be used. For example, the overall goal might be to evaluate the intake of dietary calcium among the community's Hispanics and blacks; specific objectives might include determining the major food sources of calcium among these groups and assessing the adequacy of their calcium intake compared with the Recommended Dietary Allowance (RDA) for calcium. Specific data needed in this case would include estimates of the population's food, calcium, and energy intakes. The needs assessment cannot proceed without clearly defined goals and objectives.

◆ Define the target group. The choice of the target group is influenced by the initial perception about the nutritional problem. Sometimes the needs assessment begins with one target population (e.g., all women with infants under one year of age) and concludes with a more refined focus (e.g., teenagers with infants under one year of age). Usually, however, the target group remains constant over the course of the needs assessment (e.g., people with chronic diseases, black men with hypertension, female athletes with amenorrhea).

◆ Define the types of data needed. The types of data required depend on the purpose, goals, and objectives of the assessment. Some data may already be available in the literature or from government sources, while others will need to be collected and analyzed. In general, data are used to identify a high-risk population, define areas where nutritional needs are not being met, identify duplication of nutrition services, or develop directories of services. The types of data collected in a community nutritional needs assessment and their sources are described in the next sections.

Consult Appendix H for a description of Healthy Communities 2000: Model Standards *and how communities can use this guidebook for achieving health and nutrition objectives.*

◆ TYPES OF DATA TO COLLECT

The community nutritionist must assemble many types of data to determine whether a nutritional need exists within the community. Both qualitative and quantitative data are useful in characterizing the community, its values, health problems, and needs. The types of data needed for the community nutritional needs assessment are listed in Table 7-1 and described on the next pages.

Community organizational power and structures

◆ Organization of government (city, county, state, etc.)

◆ Organization of health department (city, state, etc.)

◆ Local, state, and national organizations with a health mandate—e.g., American Heart Association, American Cancer Society, American Dietetic Association, American Public Health Association

◆ Community groups and their leaders

◆ Reporters and other people with the media

◆ Members of the Chamber of Commerce

Community characteristics

◆ Demographic data and trends:

    ◆ Total population by age, sex, race, marital status, etc.

    ◆ Distribution of population subgroups—e.g., % of population that is black, Hispanic, Asian, etc.; % that is foreign born

    ◆ Size and composition of households—e.g., number of family members in households, number of children in households, % of all households consisting of husband-wife families, % of single-parent families

◆ Economic data and trends:

    ◆ Income of families and unrelated persons living in households

    ◆ Median income of families

    ◆ % of families with incomes below the poverty level

    ◆ Number of families receiving Aid to Dependent Children

    ◆ Number of individuals receiving food stamps

    ◆ Number of individuals receiving public assistance

    ◆ Unemployment statistics—e.g., % of households with one or more unemployed members

    ◆ Tangible wealth—e.g., ownership of land and livestock; ownership of items such as personal computers, power boats, and microwave ovens

◆ Sociocultural data and trends:

    ◆ Labor force characteristics—e.g., occupation, industry, class of workers, hours worked

    ◆ Language spoken at home

    ◆ Education—e.g., median school years completed by individuals 25 years of age and older; individuals who completed high school, literacy levels of school-children and adults

Continued

TABLE

7-1

Types of Data to Collect When Conducting a Community Nutritional Needs Assessment

Sources: Adapted from C. Campbell, 1990 Census public use microdata samples (PUMS), *ICPSR Bulletin* 13 (1993): 1–4; D. B. Jelliffe and E. F. P. Jelliffe, *Community Nutritional Assessment* (Oxford: Oxford University Press, 1989), p. 150; A. D. Spiegel and H. H. Hyman, *Strategic Health Planning: Methods and Techniques Applied to Marketing and Management* (Norwood, N.J.: Ablex Publishing, 1991), pp. 90–91; U.S. Department of Health and Human Services, Public Health Service, *Health United States 1991 and Prevention Profile* (Hyattsville, Md.: Public Health Service, 1991); and Report examines nation's only county food council, *Nutrition Week* 23 (1993): 4–5.

◆ **Community organizational power and structures.** Some qualitative data help the community nutritionist understand how the community operates politically and who wields power within the system. The organization charts for government agencies and "city hall" provide information about how the community delivers health services and develops health policy. Knowing the key players in local health organizations and community, business, and media groups helps the community nutritionist identify health and nutrition programs and the concerns of community leaders.

TABLE

7-1

Types of Data to Collect When Conducting a Community Nutritional Needs Assessment— *Continued*

♦ Ecological data and trends:
   ♦ Water supply—e.g., source of water, distance from residence, water quality
   ♦ Type of housing—% of year-round housing that are single dwelling units; housing characteristics, such as units in structure, year structure was built, number of rooms and bedrooms, plumbing, heating, and kitchen facilities
   ♦ Condition of housing—e.g., % of standard housing with an exterior frame made of brick, wood, or concrete block
   ♦ Geography and climate
   ♦ Food systems—e.g., national, regional, and local food distribution networks; extent of emergency and supplemental feeding systems; food wholesale and retail systems; and amount of food grown locally

Community health

♦ Mortality statistics—e.g., death rates according to age, sex, cause, location, etc.
♦ Morbidity statistics—e.g., frequency of symptoms and disabilities, distribution of disease conditions
♦ Fertility and natality statistics—e.g., age and parity of mother, duration of pregnancy, % of mothers who get prenatal care, number of unmarried mothers, infant's birth weight, type of birth (i.e., single, twin), fertility rate, infant mortality
♦ Communicable diseases—e.g., incidence and distribution
♦ Occupational diseases—e.g., incidence and distribution
♦ Leading causes of death
♦ Life expectancy
♦ Determinants and measures of health—e.g., vaccinations, disability days, cigarette smoking, use of selected substances (alcohol, marijuana, cocaine), hypertension, obesity, serum cholesterol levels, exposure to lead, occupational injuries, incidence of foodborne disease
♦ Food and nutrient intake—e.g., food group intake, nutrient and energy intakes, nutritional adequacy of diets compared with the RDA[a]
♦ Use of health resources—e.g., frequency of patient contact with physicians, number of office visits to physicians and dentists
♦ Health care resources—e.g., persons employed in health service, number of active physicians and other health personnel
♦ Inpatient care—e.g., days of care and average length of stay in hospitals, number and types of operations, number of nursing home residents
♦ Facilities—e.g., short-stay and long-term hospitals, community hospital beds

Existing community services and programs

♦ Government-funded food assistance programs—e.g., number of referrals
♦ Nutrition services and programs offered by hospitals, clinics, community health centers, fitness centers, YMCA/YWCAs,[b] the public health department, voluntary health organizations, schools, universities, colleges, civic groups
♦ Primary care services—e.g., location, accessibility
♦ Soup kitchens
♦ Food pantries
♦ Programs and services offered by nutritionists, dietitians, and other health professionals

[a]RDA = Recommended Dietary Allowances.
[b]YMCA/YWCA = Young Men's/Women's Christian Association.

Without this knowledge, it is difficult to use the community's political process effectively to address nutritional problems.

♦ **Community characteristics.** Demographic, economic, sociocultural, and ecologic data help define the community, how and where its people live, and how much money they have to spend on food. Depending upon the purpose of the needs assessment, the community nutritionist may use data on household size, availability of kitchen appliances, family income, education level of heads of household, and the community's food distribution systems to assess food availability and the many factors that influence food consumption.

The factors that influence food consumption are described in Chapter 8.

♦ **Community health.** A variety of health statistics are used to paint a picture of the community's health. Some health data deal with the causes and rates of disease, disability, and death; others focus on key life stages or events. Community health data help the nutritionist identify persons who are malnourished and describe the population's health and nutritional problems.

♦ **Existing community services and programs.** Obtaining data on the community's existing health and nutrition services helps pinpoint gaps where services are needed. Data on both nutrition services and general health services such as primary care are needed. An inventory of the community's nutrition services and programs can be built by (1) identifying the nutrition services and programs available through government agencies, health organizations, and civic groups; (2) cataloging the educational services and materials offered by voluntary health organizations such as the American Red Cross, National Council on Alcoholism, American Heart Association, and American Cancer Society, and in Canada, the Canadian Diabetes Association and Canadian Arthritis and Rheumatism Society, among others; and (3) identifying the programs and services delivered by local nutritionists, dietitians, and other health professionals. In addition, national information centers such as the U.S. National Health Information Clearinghouse (listed together with other clearinghouses and information centers in Appendix B) can be contacted for general information about the availability of educational materials, programs, and referral services.

There are few situations where *all* of the data listed in Table 7-1 need to be collected. As you might imagine, one purpose of planning the needs assessment is to determine with as much precision as possible the specific data required to define the nutritional problem. It is seldom necessary, expedient, or possible to collect and use all data available about the community. Consider the following examples:

♦ Recent data from the second NHANES and the Mexican-American population of the Hispanic HANES (HHANES-MA) revealed that overweight is more prevalent among American Indian children of all ages and both sexes than among other U.S. children.[7] Although your community's schools have a health curriculum, it has only one module on nutrition and fitness. A coalition of community nutritionists, health professionals, educators, and school trustees is concerned that the schools are not giving enough attention to physical activity and nutrition. The coalition conducts a needs assessment to determine the prevalence of overweight among schoolchildren, especially American Indian and Hispanic children (the two largest minority groups in your community), who live within a 50-mile radius of the city. The types of data needed include (1) demographic data (e.g., age, sex) and location and type of school; (2) health data such as height and weight, which can be used to calculate body mass index; and (3) information about the existing curriculum and health and fitness programs available in the schools. Based on the outcome of the needs assessment, the coalition might pursue one of these options: (1) influence school administrators to expand the number of nutrition and fitness modules within the curriculum; (2) alter extracurricular programs in schools to include a greater focus on weight control; or (3) both influence school policy and change the extracurricular programs.

◆ The local health department is aware of the importance of weight control for maintaining good health among black women, who have a high prevalence of obesity in the United States.[8] The department's health and wellness office wants to increase its initiatives to control weight and improve health among the city's black women. Before developing a strategy for achieving this goal, the department needs more information about the factors that contribute to overweight among black women. The department's community nutritionist reviews the spectrum of data that could be collected and decides to focus on the weight-related attitudes and behaviors of black women, especially those dealing with body image, lifestyle patterns, meal patterns, motivations for weight loss, and the kinds of weight-control strategies they have tried in the past. The following data are needed: (1) demographic data (age, household size); (2) economic data (family income, occupation); (3) medical data (current weight, weight at 18 years, general medical history, parity, smoking history, weight-loss history); (4) food-related behaviors (meals skipped, meal and snack patterns, food choices, use of alcohol); (5) attitudes (level of satisfaction about body weight and image, belief in personal ability to lose weight); (6) lifestyle behaviors (activity level, exercise patterns); and (7) the extent to which black women use the community's fitness centers and weight management programs. Using these data, the community nutritionist develops a strategy for increasing black women's awareness of the health implications of overweight, their knowledge about good nutrition and exercise, and their willingness to participate in weight-management programs.

These examples are fairly simple. In contrast, consider the types of data required to evaluate the health and nutrition status of homeless people living in your community. Because homelessness cuts across all age and ethnic groups, a broad spectrum of data on homeless people and the community's resources for dealing with their health and nutritional problems is needed. In the next section, we describe how to locate information about a target population.

◆ SOURCES OF DATA ON COMMUNITIES

Collecting data for the community nutritional needs assessment involves a combination of legwork and networking. Consult Table 7-2 for a summary of sources of data on community structures, characteristics, health, and existing services and programs.

The collection of data typically begins in the library with a search of the medical, nutrition, and public health databases to review the literature on the nutritional problem. Computerized searches make it easier to locate books, journals, and other relevant publications. The government documents section, found in most public and university libraries, contains compilations of vital health statistics and reports on public health issues that relate to the community. Local historical records can also be useful. Information available in newspaper archives, old maps, parish or county records, and other documents can provide a history of a local public health problem and the public attention given to it.

Information about electronic bulletin boards and other electronic resources for community nutritionists is gven in Appendix B.

Many demographic and socioeconomic data can be located in publications of the U.S. Bureau of the Census, Bureau of Labor Statistics, Department of Agriculture, and Department of Health and Human Services. The decennial Census of Population and Housing, for example, which is conducted by the Bureau of the Census, provides data on states, counties, local units of government, school districts, and congressional districts.[9] Census data typically describe age and sex distributions, births and deaths, labor force characteristics (e.g., occupation, industry, hours worked), income, housing characteristics (e.g., year built, number of rooms, plumbing, heating, kitchen facilities), and other demographic variables. Many libraries are repositories for census data.

Additional legwork helps locate health statistics and related health reports from local, county, and state health departments; social welfare agencies; birth, death, marriage, and divorce registries; and courts. The annual reports of local hospitals, clinics, and health centers provide information on the types of health problems within the community, the existence of screening programs for detecting nutritional problems, and the resources available to deal with them.[10]

Background information on the community or region's health status can be secured from federal and state public health agencies and from international agencies such as the Food and Agriculture Organization (FAO) and the World Health Organization (WHO), which may have regional offices that can furnish relevant population health data. Since 1954, for example, the Pan American Health Organization has published a series of quadrennial reports that document the health progress attained by its members. Entitled *Health Conditions in the Americas,* the reports provide general information on the region's social and political climate, primary demographic characteristics, mortality data, and health conditions, focusing on women, children, and the elderly.[11]

If needed health data are not available from local or regional sources, it is sometimes necessary to resort to secondary data sources such as data archives,

TABLE
7-2

Sources of Data for the Community Nutritional Needs Assessment

Community organizational power and structures
- Government manuals (city, county, state, nation)
- Discussions with key informants in:
  - Voluntary health organizations
  - Civic groups
  - Business groups
  - Hospitals, clinics, health centers
  - Health department
  - Professional associations
  - Schools
- Discussions with health or other professionals:
  - Nutritionists, dietitians
  - Physicians
  - Nurses
  - Social Workers
  - Educators
  - Administrators

Community characteristics
- Bureau of the Census
- Bureau of Labor Statistics
- Department of Health and Human Services—e.g., *Health United States and Prevention Profile*
- Department of Agriculture
- Social Security Administration
- State and local health departments
- State labor departments
- Local voter registration lists
- Research findings published in journals, books, reports, etc.
- Secondary sources of data (e.g., ICPSR)[a]

Community health
- Bureau of Vital Statistics
- National Center for Health Statistics[b]
- Department of Health and Human Services and its offices such as the Public Health Service

Continued

which serve as repositories for thousands of surveys conducted over the last two decades. Data archive services have collected and catalogued the surveys of many communities. The services usually charge a fee for data tapes and supporting documentation. The University of Michigan's Institute for Social Research, for example, has become the largest university-based center for interdisciplinary research in the United States. Its major research themes include the Monitoring the Future survey, a continuing survey of the lifestyles and values of young people; studies of occupational stress, social support, and health; studies of aging and its problems; and studies of the social environment surrounding serious medical problems such as AIDS and sudden infant death syndrome. The institute also houses

◆ Within the Public Health Service:
  ◆ National Institutes of Health—data are available from the National Heart, Lung, and Blood Institute; National Cancer Institute; National Institute of Child Health and Human Development; National Institute on Aging, etc.
  ◆ Centers for Disease Control and Prevention
  ◆ Food and Drug Administration
  ◆ Indian Health Service
◆ Department of Agriculture—data are available from:
  ◆ Human Nutrition Information Service
  ◆ Agricultural Research Service
◆ Federal Monitoring and surveillance activities—e.g., National Health and Nutrition Examination Survey, National Health Interview Survey, National Maternal and Infant Health Survey, etc.[c]
◆ State and local health departments
◆ Local hospitals, clinics, and health centers
◆ Research findings published in journals, reports, etc.
◆ Health statistics published directly by government agencies or summarized in widely distributed journals—e.g., *Morbidity and Mortality Weekly Report* published by the Centers for Disease Control and Prevention and summarized in the *Journal of the American Medical Association; Vital and Health Statistics,* prepared by the National Center for Health Statistics; and the *Health United States and Prevention Profile,* published by the Public Health Service

Existing community services and programs

◆ Government agencies
◆ Hospitals, clinics, health centers, and fitness centers
◆ Voluntary health organizations
◆ Civic and business groups
◆ Schools, colleges, universities
◆ Key informants, government officials, and community leaders
◆ Nutritionists, dietitians, and other health professionals

[a]ICPSR = Inter-university Consortium for Political and Social Research.
[b]The National Center for Health Statistics is part of the Centers for Disease Control and Prevention.
[c]Some health statistics and food intake data collected by various government agencies such as the Department of Agriculture and the National Institutes of Health are available from the National Technical Information Service, U.S. Department of Commerce, Springfield, VA 22161. Appendix C contains a complete list of the surveys that comprise the national nutrition monitoring and surveillance system.

TABLE
_____

7-2

Sources of Data for the Community Nutritional Needs Assessment— *Continued*

the Inter-university Consortium for Political and Social Research (ICPSR), a social science data archive and distribution facility for computer-readable survey data. Data from the National Health Interview Survey, for example, are free to consortium members; nonmembers must pay an access fee to use the data. The ICPSR's databases include the Census of Population and Housing and the General Social Survey (a survey of social indicators such as socioeconomic status, social mobility, social control, and the family), among many others. The ICPSR also oversees the National Archive of Computerized Data on Aging, a database that covers such areas as the demographic, social, and economic characteristics of

◆ ENTREPRENEUR IN ACTION

Introducing Mary Kay Hunt, M.P.H., R.D.

◆ HER BACKGROUND . . .

Mary Kay Hunt has been directly involved in several of the most significant community-based nutrition intervention studies of the last decade: the Minnesota Heart Health Program, the Pawtucket Heart Health Program, the Centers for Disease Control/South Carolina Heart to Heart Project, the Treatwell Program, and WellWorks, a national work-site health promotion study. She is currently Associate Director of Community-based Research at the Dana-Farber Cancer Institute in Boston. In this capacity, she is involved in the design, implementation, and measurement of individual and organizational change in risk factors associated with nutrition, smoking, occupational health, and breast cancer. Hunt is an intrapreneur—a creative and innovative thinker who works to improve the public's health from within a large organization.

◆ SHE HAS THIS TO SAY ABOUT ENTREPRENEURSHIP . . .

"Entrepreneurship requires systematic, purposeful activity. To me this means careful, planned, and scientifically based activity—not impulsive and risky strategies for the sake of taking risks. I believe that risk taking and creative thinking and action are *essential* to moving healthy eating habits to the status of social norms in society. Community nutritionists need to look to models for reaching large numbers of people with understandable food messages using the tools of mass communication and collaboration across agencies and sectors."

Hunt is familiar with the challenge of forging new ground. "In launching some of these innovative community projects," she says, "there was no template to follow. We had to create a model based upon the principles of nutrition science and human behavior. Because we were creating the model, we learned many things by trial and error! We took risks—some of which were successful and moved us ahead and some of which weren't and caused us to go back to the drawing board. The surprising thing was that these innovations tended to take us places we could not foresee. For example, on the WellWorks project, our concern about hazardous materials in work processes enabled us to gain access to production workers to deliver nutrition programs. Without a doubt, the most innovative aspects of these projects came as a result of really listening to what people told us, adapting it to nutrition, and putting the intervention into operation."

Another facet of entrepreneurship that concerns Hunt is ethical decision making. "Ethical decisions are frequently encountered in the practice of community nutrition today. For example, questions of scientific precision arise continually in creating eating pattern messages that are meaningful to the general public, and ethical issues are always a consideration when forming collaborative partnerships with private industry and other sectors."

What message would she want students to take with them into the field? "Learn to live with ambiguity. By this I mean: be willing to act after prudent planning but before 100 percent of the facts are in or when you do not share 100 percent of the objectives of your collaborators or when it hasn't been done before or when you might not please 100 percent of your colleagues or when you are not 100 percent sure of the outcome. Learn to live with ambiguity, but don't be afraid to take risks."

older adults, their mental and physical health and well-being, and their health care needs.[12]

Another archival facility is the Institute for Research in Social Science at the University of North Carolina (UNC). The institute serves primarily the UNC social science faculty, but some services are available to non-UNC faculty on a cost-recovery basis. The institute is a source for nonproprietary opinion data, such as the Louis Harris public opinion data; national census data; and data from the World Fertility Surveys and the Demographic and Health Surveys.[13] Information about these archives, including how data tapes can be ordered, is given in Appendix B.

Networking also helps locate data for the needs assessment. By contacting other nutritionists, health professionals, and leaders within your community or state or national organizations, you may learn of newly published documents or unpublished data that can be made available to you in preliminary form. Networking keeps you informed about the programs and projects of other health agencies and community groups.

◆ METHODS OF ASSESSING NUTRITIONAL NEEDS

Assessing a community's nutritional needs generally involves a combination of preparing an inventory of existing health services and collecting specific data on the health and nutrition status of individuals living in the community. The methods for assessing nutritional needs must be simple, cost-effective, and doable within a reasonable time frame. Although the ultimate goal is to get a picture of the nutritional needs of the *community*, the assessment must begin by collecting data about *individuals* within the community. In this section, we will examine some of the methods used in community nutritional needs assessment. Refer to Figure 7-2 on page 203 to refresh your memory about where we are in the process of conducting a needs assessment.

Nutrition Surveys and Questionnaires   In gathering health and nutrition data, community nutritionists are usually faced with two choices: (1) use data already collected about the target population, or (2) design and conduct a survey because data on the target group are not available. Both options are examined in the next paragraphs.

◆ Using available survey data. Depending upon the questions you ask about your community's health and nutrition status, the most expedient and cost-effective course may be to use data already available on your target population to help you determine your community's nutritional needs. Data about your target population can be gathered from large-scale population surveys, such as those conducted by the National Nutrition Monitoring System (NNMS), or from small surveys of special populations conducted in your community or region. It is usually desirable to have both types of data on hand.

NNMS survey data provide a national perspective on your target population and the factors that contribute to its nutritional needs in other regions of the country. The NNMS surveys collect many types of data on the U.S. population and certain subgroups such as infants and children, the elderly, and individuals who are trying to lose weight. Common measurements made in NNMS surveys include those related to health and nutrition status, food and nutrient intake, dietary knowledge and attitudes, and/or sociodemographic and economic factors. Refer to Table 7-3 for a description of data collected for three NNMS surveys.

In most cases, NNMS survey data can be obtained from the National Technical Information Service either as a printed publication or on tape. Some data tapes and publications are available from the sponsoring

TABLE 7-3	Data Collected in Three Surveys of the National Nutrition Monitoring System and How to Obtain Them		
SURVEY	**TARGET POPULATION**	**TYPES OF DATA COLLECTED**	**HOW TO OBTAIN DATA**
National Health and Nutrition Examination Surveys (NHANES I, II, and III)*	Civilian noninstitutionalized persons, aged 1 through 74 years	◆ Dietary intake ◆ Body measurements ◆ Biochemical analyses of whole blood and serum ◆ Blood pressure ◆ Electrocardiogram ◆ Urine tests ◆ X rays of hand, wrist, cervical and lumbar spine, chest ◆ Dental examinations	Public-use data tapes are available from the National Technical Information Service.
National Health Interview Survey— Supplement on Aging	Civilian noninstitutionalized persons, aged 55 years and over	◆ Family structure ◆ Community services ◆ Occupation ◆ Health conditions ◆ Activities of daily living ◆ Health opinions ◆ Living arrangements ◆ Social support ◆ Retirement ◆ Home care, hospice ◆ Meal services ◆ Difficulty preparing meals ◆ Difficulty eating	Public-use data tapes from the 1984 Supplement on Aging Data Set are available from the National Center for Health Statistics of the Centers for Disease Control and Prevention.
Pediatric Nutrition Surveillance System (PedNSS)	Low-income, high-risk children 0 to 17 years, especially those 0 to 5 years of age	◆ Anthropometry (height and weight) ◆ Birth weight (< 2500 grams) ◆ Hematology (hemoglobin, hematocrit)	PedNSS data are returned to individual participating states. Some states produce tabulations of PedNSS data and reports using CDC PedNSS software.

*The types of data collected for the NHANES I differ slightly from those collected for the NHANES II and III.

Source: U.S. Department of Health and Human Services, U.S. Department of Agriculture, *Nutrition Monitoring in the United States: The Directory of Federal Nutrition Monitoring Activities* (Hyattsville, Md.: U.S. Government Printing Office, DHHS Pub. No. 89–1255–1, 1989), pp. 1–2, 4, 6, and 19.

agency (e.g., U.S. Department of Agriculture, National Institute of Child Health and Human Development), secondary data sources such as ICPSR, or the U.S. Government Printing Office. In addition, many health and nutrition data are published in periodicals such as the *Journal of the American Dietetic Association, Public Health Reports,* and the *New England Journal of Medicine.* Consult the Public Health Service's publication, *Nutrition Monitoring in the United States: The Directory of Federal Nutrition Monitoring Activities,* for a list of NNMS surveys and pertinent journal publications of survey findings and a description of where NNMS survey data can be obtained.[14]

A list of the National Nutrition Monitoring System surveys appears in Appendix C.

Your decision to use NNMS survey data will be influenced by the level of detail you need about the target population, the personnel and facilities available for sorting and analyzing the data, and budget constraints. The cost of purchasing data ranges from $100 to $1,500.

National survey data do not always reflect the nutrition status or food intake of the target population in a particular community. Consider this scenario: national CSFII survey data indicated that black women aged 19 to 50 years consumed on average about 54 percent of the RDA for calcium in 1986; however, a 1993 survey of black women living in your community's inner-city district found that their mean intake of calcium was only 48 percent of the RDA.[15] In this situation, the national data may not reflect your community particularly well, but they may be a good benchmark against which to compare your target population. The question for you as a community nutritionist is why some black women in your community have a calcium intake lower than the national average. Thus, small surveys carried out locally provide insights into *your* community's needs and values. They tend to be more relevant to defining your community's nutritional problems and needs than large, national surveys.

◆ **Designing and conducting a survey.** In some situations, data on your target population are not readily available, in which case you may have to design and conduct a survey to obtain the needed data. Conducting a **nutrition survey** involves more than heading out with a clipboard and a list of questions to interview people as they come into your clinic. Survey design and analysis is a discipline in itself, and the process of conducting a community survey usually requires a team of experts with knowledge of survey research, statistics, epidemiology, public health, and nutrition. Although a detailed discussion of survey methodology is beyond the scope of this book, a few comments are in order about the issues to consider when designing a nutrition survey or adapting an existing survey for your own purposes.

Nutrition survey An instrument designed to collect data on the nutrition status and dietary intake of a population group.

"Planning a survey consists of making a series of scientific and practical decisions."[16] The first step is to determine the purpose of the survey. Most nutrition surveys are carried out to assess the food consumption of households or individuals, evaluate eating patterns, estimate the adequacy of the food supply, assess the nutritional quality of the food supply, measure the nutrient intake of a certain population group, study the relationship of diet and nutrition status to health, or determine the effectiveness of an education program.[17] A nutrition survey does not have to be complex and gargantuan to be meaningful, but it must have a well-defined purpose.

Next, decisions must be made about who will design the survey, who will conduct it, and how it will be carried out. The target population must be specified, the survey instrument designed and pretested, and the method of assessing nutrition status or dietary intake chosen. The personnel responsible for conducting the survey and analyzing data must be trained. Numerous other decisions must be made about the feasibility of the survey, the reliability and validity of the instrument, the costs of carrying it out, and the way the data will be analyzed and used. At every step in the planning process, there are practical constraints related to time and money.[18]

Whether the survey consists of a telephone interview or a questionnaire mailed to respondents, one of the most important aspects of survey design is preventing bias and ambiguous language from creeping into the survey questions.[19] Writing a survey question that is easy for respondents to understand *and* gives you the nutrition information you want is no simple task. Examine the questions in Table 7-4. The first question is fairly straightforward. Most consumers know what fruits are, and they can estimate their fruit intake with a reasonable degree of accuracy. The second question is more difficult to answer. Respondents must know what a fat is and recognize butter, stick margarine, tub margarine, lard, fatback, bacon fat, and vegetable shortening as fats that are used in cooking. They must then estimate how frequently they use one or more of these fats (plus vegetable oils) in cooking, a complex calculation for most consumers. The third question likewise presents a problem. Respondents must decide what the survey question means by "mayonnaise" and "salad

TABLE

7-4

Examples of Survey Questions Designed to Obtain Information about Fiber and Fat Intake

SURVEY QUESTION	RESPONSE
◆ Not counting juices, how many fruits do you usually eat per day or week?	_____ fruits per _____ day, week
◆ How often do you use fat or oil in cooking?	_____ times per _____ day, week, month
◆ How many servings, on average, do you eat of mayonnaise or salad dressing (serving size = 2 tablespoons)?	_____ never or <1 per month _____ 1–3 per month _____ 1–4 per week _____ 5–7 per week _____ 2 or more per day

Sources: The first two questions were taken from the National Cancer Institute's Health Habits and History questionnaire (Bethesda, Md.: National Cancer Institute, 1987), p. 4. The third question was adapted from the University of Minnesota Healthy Worker Project questionnaire (Minneapolis, Minn.: University of Minnesota, 1987), p. 3.

dressing." Is the question asking about all such products, regardless of their fat content, or only regular, full-fat mayonnaise and salad dressings? These examples demonstrate how difficult it can be to obtain accurate information about food intake and dietary practices.

Surveys are important tools in assessing the health and nutrition status of individuals, but they must be carefully designed and carried out to provide valid and reliable information. Consult Table 7-5 for a list of questions to ask when designing a survey for your nutritional needs assessment.

Health Risk Appraisals The health risk appraisal (HRA) is a type of survey instrument used to characterize a population's general health status. We mention it here in a separate category because it is widely used in worksites, government agencies, universities, and other organizations as a health education or screening tool.[20]

The HRA is a kind of "health hazard chart" that asks questions about the lifestyle factors that influence disease risk.[21] A typical HRA asks questions about

---

◆ **Is the survey valid and reliable?** Will it measure what it is intended to measure, and, assuming that nothing changed in the interim, will it produce the same estimate of this measurement on separate occasions?

◆ **Are norms available?** That is, are reference data or population standards available against which the data from your target group can be compared?

◆ **Is the survey suitable for the target population?** A survey designed to obtain health and nutrition data on free-living elderly people may not be appropriate for the institutionalized elderly.

◆ **Are the survey questions easy to read and understand?** Survey questions must be geared to the target population and its level of literacy, reading comprehension, and fluency in the primary language. Having a readable survey is especially important if it is to be self-administered.

◆ **Is the format of the questionnaire clear?** If the questionnaire is not laid out carefully, respondents may become confused and inadvertently skip questions or sections.

◆ **Are the responses clear?** A variety of scales and responses may be used in designing a survey. Some questions may require filling in blanks or providing simple yes/no or true/false answers. Others may ask respondents to rank-order their responses from "seldom/never use" to "use often/always." The trick when selecting such scales is to choose one that allows you to discriminate between responses but doesn't provide so many categories that respondents are overwhelmed.

◆ **Is the survey comprehensive but brief?** Often the length of the survey must be limited to ensure that respondents complete it within a reasonable time frame. With long questionnaires, respondents are likely to answer questions hurriedly and mark the same answer to most questions.

◆ **Does the survey ask "socially loaded" questions?** Each survey question should be evaluated for how it is likely to be interpreted. Questions that imply certain value judgments or socially desirable responses should be rewritten. This is especially important when dealing with respondents from cultures other than your own.

TABLE

7-5

Questions to Ask When Designing a Survey
Source: Adapted from L. Fallowfield, *The Quality of Life* (London: Souvenir Press, 1990), pp. 40–45.

age, sex, height, weight, marital status, body frame size, exercise habits, consumption of certain foods (e.g., fruits and vegetables) and ingredients (e.g., sodium), intake of alcohol, job satisfaction, hours of sleep, smoking habits, and medical checkups or hospitalizations. A portion of the U.S. Army's HRA questionnaire is shown in Figure 7-3.

HRAs are used to alert individuals about their risky health behaviors and how such behaviors might be modified, usually through a lifestyle modification program.[22] For example, a health risk questionnaire was used at a trucker trade

---

FIGURE 7-3   **A Portion of a Health Risk Appraisal Form**

Source: Used with permission from The Office of the Surgeon General, U.S. Army, Personal Readiness Division.

show to assess the health status of truck drivers. Truckers who stopped at the trade show enjoyed free food, music, raffles, and other events. At one booth, truckers received free blood pressure measurements and health education materials and were asked to complete a survey of their health risk factors, health status, and driving patterns. An analysis of the survey results showed that truck drivers tend to smoke cigarettes, be sedentary and overweight, and be unaware that they had high blood pressure. Thus, health promotion programs are needed for truck drivers who have no "fixed" worksite base and could benefit from lifestyle changes.[23]

Direct Assessment of Nutrition Status   Another method of determining nutritional needs is to conduct a direct assessment of individuals. Direct assessment methods use dietary, laboratory, anthropometric, and clinical measurements of individuals to identify those with malnutrition or a nutritional deficiency state. These methods may be used alone or in combination. Each direct nutrition assessment method is described briefly here. A detailed description of how these methods are used with population groups such as pregnant women, infants, children, and adults is given in Chapters 12–14.

◆ **Dietary assessment.** Dietary methods are used to determine an individual or population's usual dietary intake and to identify potential dietary inadequacies. Dietary inadequacies represent stage 1 of the nutrient depletion scheme shown in Table 7-6. The primary methods of measuring the food consumption of individuals include the 24-hour recall method, food records, diet histories, and the food frequency questionnaire. At the household level, food records and inventory methods are used to estimate food consumption; population dietary intakes are estimated using food balance sheets and market databases.[24]

◆ **Laboratory methods.** Laboratory methods can be used to identify individuals at risk of a nutrient deficiency (stages 2–5 in Table 7-6), since tissue stores of nutrients gradually become depleted over time. The depletion may result in alterations in the level or activity of some nutrient-dependent

STAGE	DEPLETION STAGE	METHOD(S) USED TO IDENTIFY
1	Dietary inadequacy	Dietary
2	Decreased level in reserve tissue store	Biochemical
3	Decreased level in body fluids	Biochemical
4	Decreased functional level in tissues	Anthropometric/biochemcial
5	Decreased activity in nutrient-dependent enzyme	Biochemical
6	Functional change	Behavioral/psychological
7	Clinical symptoms	Clinical
8	Anatomical sign	Clinical

TABLE

7-6

General Scheme for the Development of a Nutritional Deficiency

Source: With permission from: Sahn DE, Lockwood R, Scrimshaw NS. *Methods for the Evaluation of the Impact of Food and Nutrition Programmes.* Tokyo; United Nations University, 1984.

enzymes or the levels of metabolic products. Thus, laboratory methods are used to detect subclinical nutrient deficiencies. Static biochemical tests measure a nutrient in biological tissues or fluids or the urinary excretion rate of the nutrient. Examples of static tests include the platelet concentration of α-tocopherol and urinary 3-hydroxyproline excretion. Functional biochemical tests measure the biological importance of a nutrient and the consequences of the nutritional deficiency. Functional biochemical tests include taste acuity, a measure of zinc status; dark adaptation, a measure of vitamin A status; and capillary fragility, a measure of vitamin C deficiency. Functional tests are generally too invasive and expensive to employ in most field surveys of nutrition status.

◆ **Anthropometric methods.** Measurements of the body's physical dimensions and composition are used to detect moderate and severe degrees of malnutrition and chronic imbalances in energy and protein intakes. The most common growth indices include measurements of stature (height or length), weight, and circumference of the head. Measurements of skinfolds, mid-upper-arm circumference, and the waist-hip circumference ratio are used to derive equations that predict muscle and fat mass. Anthropometric measurements are useful in large-scale community assessment programs, because they involve simple, safe, noninvasive procedures, require only inexpensive and portable equipment, and produce accurate and precise data when obtained by trained personnel. Such measurements are used to estimate an individual's long-term nutritional histo-

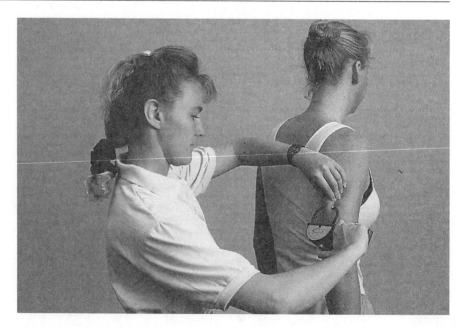

Skinfold and other anthropometric measurements are commonly used in nutrition assessment as early warning signs of changes in nutrition status.

ry. They do not provide data on short-term nutrition status, nor can they provide information about specific nutritional deficiencies.[25]

◆ **Clinical methods.** Clinical assessment of health status consists of a medical history and a physical examination to detect **physical signs** and **symptoms** associated with malnutrition. The medical history includes a description of the individual (patient) and his living situation (for example, married or single, children, employment). It typically obtains information about existing clinical conditions, previous bouts of illness, hospitalizations and surgical procedures, use of medications, presence of congenital conditions, smoking status, existence of food allergies and intolerances, and usual levels of physical activity. In the physical examination, the clinician evaluates the major organ systems: skin, muscular and skeletal, cardiovascular, gastrointestinal, and nervous. The hair, face, eyes, lips, tongue, teeth and gums, and nails are also examined for signs associated with malnutrition. Consult Appendix E for a description of the physical signs that may indicate or suggest malnutrition and a summary of the most important risk factors that contribute to malnutrition.[26]

Physical signs The observations made by a qualified examiner during a physical examination.

Symptoms The manifestations reported by the patient during a physical examination.

Screening   Screening is an important preventive health activity designed to reverse, retard, or halt the progress of a disease by detecting it as soon as possible. Screening occurs in both clinical practice and community settings, using procedures that are safe, simple, and cheap. Table 7-7 lists some common screening procedures. In community screening programs, people from the community are invited to have an assessment made of a health risk or behavior (e.g., blood cholesterol). Their screening value is then compared with a predetermined cutpoint or risk level (e.g., the classification of high, borderline-high, and desirable blood cholesterol levels published by the National Cholesterol Education Program).

TABLE

7-7

Common Screening Procedures in Clinical Practice and Community Settings

SCREENING PROCEDURE	TARGET POPULATION
◆ Clinical practice	
Taking a medical history	All ages, both sexes
Height and weight	All ages, both sexes
Phenylketonuria (PKU)	Newborn infants
Posture (for detection of scoliosis)	Children over 3 years of age
Vision	Children over 3 years of age
Hearing	Children over 3 years of age
Tuberculin test	Children over 1 year of age
◆ Community settings	
Health risk appraisal	Primarily adults over 18 years of age
Blood pressure	Adults over 18 years of age
Blood cholesterol level	Adults over 18 years of age

Sources: Adapted from J. M. Last, *Public Health and Human Ecology* (East Norwalk, Conn.: Appleton & Lange, 1987), p. 13, and *The Merck Manual,* ed. R. Berkow, 15th ed. (Rahway, N.J.: Merck Sharp & Dohme Research Laboratorie   ,7), pp. 1814–20.

Individuals whose screening value suggests an elevated risk are referred to a nutritionist, doctor, or other health professional for follow-up and treatment. Screening programs are not meant to substitute for a health care visit or routine medical monitoring for people already receiving treatment, but they do have educational value and serve to identify high-risk persons.[27]

Examples of screening programs abound. The Screening Plus program was a worksite blood pressure management program developed by the Pawtucket Heart Health Program in cooperation with the Rhode Island Department of Health and the Rhode Island affiliate chapter of the American Heart Association. The program provided blood pressure measurements and long-term follow-up for people with elevated blood pressure in all Rhode Island worksites, regardless of size.[28] Another example is the Nutrition Screening Initiative, a project designed to promote nutrition screening and improved nutritional care in the United States, especially among older adults.[29]

More information about the Nutrition Screening Initiative is provided in Chapter 14.

Focus Groups   One method of obtaining information about the community's values and concerns is to hold focus group interviews. **Focus groups** usually consist of 5 to 12 people who meet in sessions lasting about one to three hours. The group members are brought together to talk about their concerns, experiences, beliefs, or problems. Focus group participants are sometimes asked to provide opinions about products or creative concepts such as advertising campaigns or program logos. The sessions are led by a trained moderator who is skilled at putting people at ease, asking questions in a nonthreatening manner, and promoting group interaction. The information obtained from focus group interviews is then used to change a marketing strategy, product, or program.

Focus group An informal group of about 5 to 12 people who are asked to share their concerns, experiences, beliefs, opinions, or problems.

Focus group interviews provide qualitative information that helps managers develop a plan of action. They are less expensive to conduct than face-to-face interviews, and they help managers obtain information of a sensitive nature or that might otherwise be difficult or costly to get.[30] The Johns Hopkins Hospital staff, for example, used focus groups to help them understand why some clients were not complying with cardiovascular health promotion programs to control hypercholesterolemia. Participants were asked questions about health, high blood cholesterol, current diet, food preferences, grocery shopping, and the types of education programs and materials they usually used. The staff learned that clients preferred to be taught by professionals in small groups and liked to hear from individuals who had successfully lowered their blood cholesterol. Changes were made in the delivery of the health promotion program based on the focus group interviews.[31]

◆ NUTRITION STATUS INDICATORS

Nutrition status indicator A quantitative measure used as a guide to screen, diagnose, and evaluate interventions in individuals.

Some measures of health or nutrition status are required when conducting the nutritional needs assessment (refer to Figure 7-2). These measures, called **nutrition status indicators**, are quantitative measures that serve as guides "to screen, diagnose, and evaluate interventions in individuals."[32] Nutrition status indicators are often used to estimate the magnitude of a nutrition problem, its distribution within the population, its cause, and the effects of programs and policies designed to alleviate the problem. They are used by researchers, program planners, health professionals, and policymakers for analyzing health and nutritional problems.

Because there is no single "best" indicator, several may be used in the nutritional needs assessment. For example, major indicators of poor nutrition status in older U.S. adults include a weight loss of 10 pounds or more, being underweight or overweight, or having a serum albumin below 3.5 grams per deciliter, an inappropriate food intake, a mid-arm muscle circumference < 10th percentile, and folate deficiency, among others.[33] Nutrition status indicators exist for vitamin, mineral, and protein status and energy intake. Efforts are underway to develop accurate and reliable indicators of hunger and overall nutrition status. Table 7-8 lists the core nutrition status indicators recommended for the assessment of populations that are difficult to survey, such as homeless people, migrants, and institutionalized persons.[34]

◆ REFERENCE DATA

In addition to specifying the nutrition status indicators, the community nutritionist must choose the reference data against which the outcomes will be compared. For example, if she is evaluating the nutrition status of children whose mothers

NUTRITION CONCERN	INDICATOR
Obesity	Weight for length
	Weight for height
Hypercholesterolemia	Serum total cholesterol
Hypertension	Brachial artery pressure
Iron status	Complete blood count
Food insecurity	Food consumption:
	◆ Patterns over time
	◆ Types of foods
	◆ Frequency of consumption
	◆ Variety of foods
	Self-reports of:
	◆ Food sufficiency
	◆ Constraints to obtaining food
	Sources of food
Drug-nutrient interactions	Assessment of specific nutrient(s) affected by drugs and alcohol
Protein-energy malnutrition	Height
	Weight for height
	Weight change
	Skinfolds
	Body circumference
	Edema
Folate status as a marker for quality of diets limited in variety and quantity of foods	Serum and red blood cell folate concentrations
Vitamin A status	Serum retinol

TABLE

7-8

Indicators for the Assessment of Nutrition Status among Migrant Workers, the Homeless, and Other Difficult-to-Sample Populations
Source: S. A. Anderson, Core indicators of nutritional state for difficult-to-sample populations. © J. Nutr.: Vol. 120, p. 1585, American Institute of Nutrition.

are participating in the Special Supplemental Food Program for Women, Infants, and Children (WIC), she might choose height, weight, and hemoglobin as the nutrition status indicators. To evaluate the children's growth and development, she might choose the reference growth data for children published by the U.S. National Center for Health Statistics (NCHS). The NCHS curves for evaluating the physical growth of children are based on a large, nationally representative sample of U.S. children. The nomograms showing the reference data for stature and weight for age for U.S. girls and boys aged 2 to 18 years are given in Appendix E. For evaluating the iron status of WIC children, the community nutritionist might use reference data for hemoglobin from the NHANES II survey for children of the same age and sex.[35]

Nutrient intake data are usually compared with the RDA or, in Canada, the Recommended Nutrient Intakes. Reference data for comparison purposes can also be obtained from countries where national surveys of dietary intakes have been carried out. In situations where no reference data for a country exist, the FAO and/or WHO requirements for nutritional intake can be used.[36]

The activities associated with community assessment are basically the same whether the community is global or local; the difference in effort is generally one of scale. On the global level, the WHO and its regional offices spearhead the effort to collect data, evaluate existing programs, and review the political and social climates of countries around the world with an eye to developing international policies and activities to relieve malnutrition worldwide. Global data collection, in particular, requires a significant commitment of resources and personnel. These assessment efforts are usually undertaken in cooperation with such groups as the Administrative Committee on Coordination/Subcommittee on Nutrition of the United Nations (UN), which harmonizes the nutrition polices and activities within the UN system.[37] On the national level, the federal government coordinates population-wide nutrition research and survey activities. Locally, community assessment is usually undertaken by the city's department of public health or some other municipal health agency. As an entrepreneurial community nutritionist, however, you may need to conduct your own community assessment as part of your program planning.

Priorities and Action Plans

When the relevant data have been collected and the nutrition problem properly defined, a decision must be made about what action should be taken to address the problem. As Figure 7-4 indicates, the decision is influenced by the health priorities of the organization and the community.

◆ SETTING PRIORITIES

Setting priorities involves deciding *who* is to get *what* at *whose expense.*[38] Setting priorities among competing health and nutritional needs is difficult, as communi-

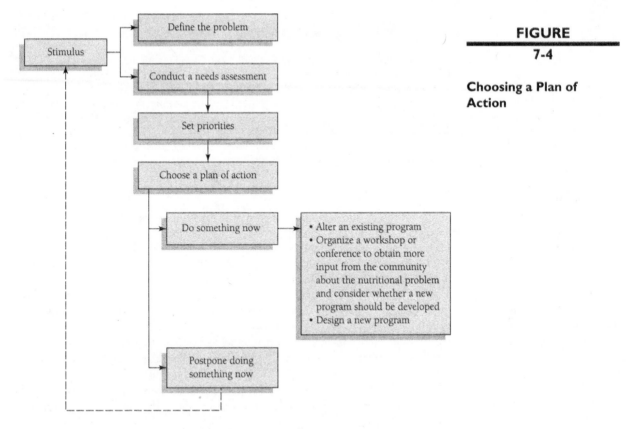

FIGURE

7-4

Choosing a Plan of Action

Once the needs assessment is completed, the importance of the nutritional problem relative to other community health and nutritional problems must be evaluated. If the problem receives a high priority rating, a decision must be made about how to proceed. In some cases, no action is taken at the present time, but the problem is monitored for future action. In other cases, a decision is made to do something to address the nutritional problem. The nature of the plan of action depends upon the organization's mandate, the resources and personnel available, and other factors.

ties have many public health problems that deserve to be addressed. Considering the fierce competition for scarce resources, how do community and organization leaders decide where to put their efforts and money?

No one method exists for ranking problems, although various scoring systems that rank risk factors by relative importance have been proposed. A few principles that provide guidance in identifying problems of the highest priority are listed in Table 7-9. In general, an organization begins the priority setting process by evaluating the outcome of the needs assessment, which provides information about the dimensions of the nutritional need within the community, including its severity, extent, and frequency; its distribution across the urban, rural, or regional setting and across age groups; its causes; and the mortality and morbidity associated with the nutritional problem. The needs assessment may

TABLE
7-9

Principles Involved in Setting Priorities

- ◆ Community priorities, preferences, and concerns should be given priority.
- ◆ Higher priority should be given to common problems than to rare ones.
- ◆ Higher priority should be given to serious problems than to less serious ones.
- ◆ The health problems of mothers and children that can easily be prevented should have a higher priority than those that are more difficult to prevent.
- ◆ Higher priority should be given to health problems whose frequencies are increasing over time than to those whose frequencies are declining or remaining static.

Source: Adapted from D. B. Jelliffe and E. F. P. Jelliffe, *Community Nutritional Assessment* (Oxford: Oxford University Press, 1989), p. 452. By permission of Oxford University Press.

Cluster analysis A statistical method for studying the interrelationships among two or more variables.

also provide information about the cost of treating versus preventing the condition and the social consequences of not intervening.[39]

The organization then considers the seriousness of the problem relative to other nutrition and health problems within the community and other priorities within the organization. It may prioritize problems by using a statistical method such as **cluster analysis** to help describe the distribution of various problems in the community. The outcome of one cluster analysis is shown in Figure 7-5, which graphically depicts the stroke mortality in Florida. The organization may also ask its managers and health personnel to rank existing health and nutritional problems and make recommendations about where the organization should direct its efforts. Using these and other approaches, a list of the community's problems is compiled. Note in Table 7-10 that one community's health problems cut across several of the organization's departments: nutrition, infectious diseases, and chronic diseases.

In a perfect world, the organization would have ample personnel, money, and other resources to spend on each of the community's problems. There would be no need for priority setting. In reality, no organization ever has enough resources to address all public health problems, and the decisions about which problems receive attention are not always rational, right, or fair. The process of setting priorities is influenced by the community's political power base, federal and state public health priorities, public opinion, and the beliefs of the organization's senior management and board of directors. In most organizations, the chief executive officer and the board of directors help senior managers set major priority areas by developing organizational goals. Senior managers, in turn, relay the organization's mandate to their employees. Lower-level managers are often given some leeway in setting program goals in their areas. The organization's final priority areas generally reflect its ranking of the importance of public health problems and its assessment of the feasibility of implementing solutions.

◆ CHOOSING A PLAN OF ACTION

The community nutritionist is now ready to make a decision. He has on hand a definition of the community's nutritional problem, the results of the needs assessment, and the organization's priorities for action. Now what? As shown in Figure 7-4, the community nutritionist has two choices: do something now or postpone

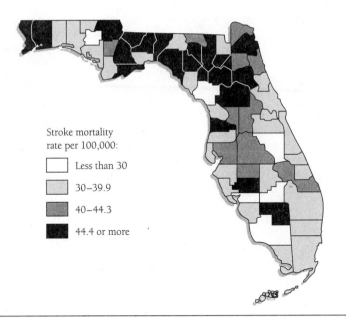

Stroke mortality
rate per 100,000:

☐ Less than 30

▨ 30–39.9

▨ 40–44.3

■ 44.4 or more

FIGURE

7-5

Data on the Number of Stroke Deaths in Florida Counties, 1979–81

Source: P. Z. Siegel and coauthors, North Florida is part of the stroke belt, *Public Health Reports* 107 (1992): 542.

doing something about the nutritional problem until a later date. Deciding to do nothing at the moment is sometimes the only choice. The organization may not have enough money to fund an intervention or the personnel to carry it out, or the political climate may not favor an intervention. When this situation occurs, the problem is not forgotten, but it is moved to the back burner for further monitoring. There it becomes a "stimulus" that can trigger the program planning process at some future date.

When a decision is made to do something now, the question becomes: What should we do? Deciding to take action does not necessarily mean that a new program to address the problem will be developed. Other options exist, as shown in Figure 7-4. The community nutritionist might elect to organize a workshop or conference to obtain additional data on the problem or pull together community leaders—sometimes called stakeholders—to explore future actions. Or he might decide to alter an existing program by developing new educational materials, enlarging a marketing campaign, or changing the mechanism for delivering the program. Finally, he might decide to develop a new program to address the community's nutritional problem, in which case he may choose to write a grant proposal to apply for money to pilot test his idea. In the next section, we consider how to plan a new program.

Information about grant writing is given in Appendix F.

Program Design

New programs are usually developed when the community nutritional needs assessment reveals a gap in services. For example, the Heart & Stroke Foundation

TABLE

7-10

Ranking of Health and Nutritional Problems by a State Health Department

Sources: Adapted from W. Carr, *Measuring Avoidable Deaths and Diseases in New York State,* Paper Series 8 (New York: United Hospital Fund, 1988), p. 48, and U.S. Department of Health and Human Services, Public Health Service, *Health United States and Prevention Profile, 1991* (Hyattsville, Md.: Public Health Service, 1991), pp. 158–60.

DISEASE OR CONDITION	PRIORITY CLUSTER
Lung cancer among blacks	First priority
Tuberculosis among blacks	
AIDS	
Iron deficiency among blacks	
Tuberculosis among Hispanics	
Lung cancer among adults (18–75+ years)	
Prostate cancer among Caucasian males	
Stroke	
Lung cancer among Caucasians	Second Priority
Anemia among Caucasians	
Anemia among blacks	
Iron deficiency among Hispanics	
Diabetes mellitus	
Emphysema	
Breast cancer among women	
Pneumonia among blacks and American Indians	Third Priority
Cirrhosis	
Accidents among young males	
Bladder cancer among blacks	

of Manitoba decided to develop, evaluate, and implement a school-based cafeteria nutrition program. Its decision was based on the outcome of a community assessment indicating that no such program existed and that local school trustees, educators, administrators, and nutritionists perceived a need to provide nutrition guidance to school foodservice managers.[40]

It is one thing to recognize that a need exists, however, and another to design a program that effectively meets that need. Designing a program that puts together the services and materials with the best chance of achieving the program's objectives requires work and planning. Many factors must be considered: personnel; money for equipment, travel, education materials, and marketing campaigns; facilities for offering the program; and the location of the target population.[41] In the next section, we consider how a community nutritionist might design a program to meet a community's nutritional need.

◆ STEPS IN DESIGNING A PROGRAM

The steps involved in designing a program are outlined in Figure 7-6. This figure is not meant to be taken literally, as some steps may occur concurrently. Decisions about the program format, for example, may be made at the same time that the intervention strategies and educational messages are chosen.

Even though Figure 7-6 is not carved in stone, the first step in program design always involves setting goals and objectives—that is, determining what the program is designed to accomplish and who it is for. Both outcome and process objectives are important. Next, an **intervention strategy** is chosen. The intervention strategy is the approach for achieving the program's goals and objectives and

Intervention strategy An approach for achieving the program's goals and objectives.

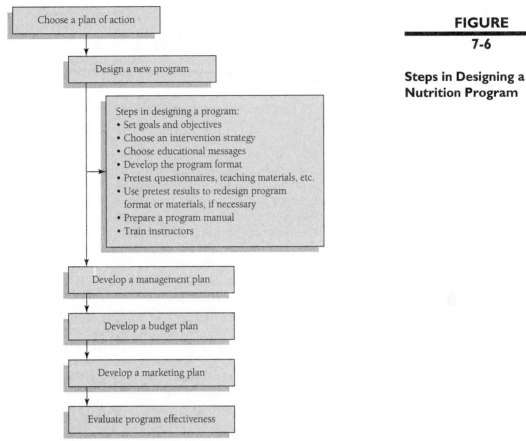

FIGURE

7-6

Steps in Designing a Nutrition Program

A program's format is dictated partly by the program's goals and objectives, the nature of the nutritional problem being addressed, and the target population. Learner objectives should be developed for each session, and teaching materials that best convey the nutrition message should be chosen. Once the program elements have been developed and tested, the management, budget, and marketing plans must be finalized. Refer to Chapter 6 for a discussion of management and budgeting and Chapter 9 for marketing. The process of program evaluation is described in Chapter 10.

addresses the question of *how* the program will be implemented to meet the nutritional need. Potential intervention strategies include the following:

◆ Classes on nutrition for small groups of people. An example of this type of program is the Growing as a Single Parent (GASP) program designed to teach young single mothers about the importance of good nutrition during and after pregnancy, the basic principles of infant and child nutrition, and stress management.[42]

◆ Programs in organizations such as worksites, schools, and grocery stores that target both individuals within the organization and the organization as a whole. Examples of these programs include the worksite-based

Treatwell Program, described in Chapter 8, and point-of-purchase food labeling programs in university residence halls or other locations.[43]

◆ Mass education campaigns that target the general public, such as the National Cancer Institute's 5 A Day program and the ADA's Project LEAN (*Lowfat Eating for America Now*).[44]

When choosing an intervention strategy, the community nutritionist considers how best to motivate people to make dietary or other behavior changes. In some situations, she might help people change their perceptions about a risky health behavior, learn new skills in preparing low-fat foods, change their eating habits, or identify barriers to making dietary changes. In other situations, she might use mass marketing techniques to motivate and educate the general public. Behavior change strategies are described in more detail in Chapter 8.

The next step in the program planning process is to choose the dietary messages that will educate people about healthy eating patterns and food choices. There are several reasons for promoting dietary messages as part of the nutrition education component of the program: (1) dietary messages help consumers make judicious food choices for good health and well-being; (2) through nutrition education, consumers are able to evaluate the nutrition information they receive; and (3) dietary messages and other nutrition education efforts reinforce consumer knowledge about diet and nutrition and correct faulty knowledge. The purpose of nutrition education in general, and the dietary messages in particular, is to help consumers deal with their confusion about foods and diets and to help them make the kinds of food choices that will promote good eating habits and good health.[45]

In most cases, dietary messages for the general public are based on the dietary guidelines or the RDAs. Dietary messages may focus on nutrients, such as fat, sodium, or calcium, or eating patterns, such as the advice in "The Food Guide Pyramid" brochure to "eat a variety of foods." Dietary messages should be based on sound scientific evidence and presented consistently in all educational materials. They should also be simple and easy for consumers to understand. Refer to Figure 5-3 for a description of the dietary messages that accompany the Food Guide Pyramid and Figure 5-4 for the U.S. dietary guidelines.

The program format must also be designed. This is a challenging task, for there are probably as many types of formats as there are nutrition programs in existence today! Some programs consist primarily of individual sessions designed to teach basic nutrition principles. Others such as WIC combine individual and group educational sessions. Still others use group sessions and mass marketing techniques. The possible combinations of educational strategies are endless. Regardless of the final format, an outline of the program activities and a list of **learner objectives** must be prepared. The learner objectives help the community nutritionist describe what program participants should learn by the end of the session, course, or other activity.

Learner objectives A set of goal statements designed to show what program participants can expect to have learned on completing the program.

If the program is going to be delivered through a series of classes, for example, a class outline describing the topics to be covered at each session is developed. Learner objectives and activities are formulated for each class. Teaching materials, such as slides, overhead transparencies, fact sheets, handouts for class participants, and food models, are selected. If appropriate teaching materials do not exist, they must be designed. It is usually helpful to prepare a list of the items needed for each class period.

Questionnaires and teaching materials developed for the class are tested for readability and effectiveness. Sometimes it helps to teach the classes to small groups of people who are similar to the target population as a means of evaluating the topics and flow of ideas. Then, the order of lessons or types of teaching materials are adjusted as required. Once the program of instruction is set, a teaching manual can be assembled. Finally, the instructors responsible for delivering the program are trained in how to present the material and answer questions that participants may have.

◆ NUTRITION IN ACTION'S "EAT WELL–BE WELL" PROGRAM

Let's consider how Nutrition in Action designed its ABC Fitness Program. Recall from Chapter 6 that our hypothetical fitness program was developed for worksites. Its goal is to improve the fitness levels and eating habits of employees. Its nutrition objective is to reduce employees' fat intake to less than 30 percent of total calories. (Refer to Table 6-4 for a list of the program's outcome and process objectives.)

Nutrition in Action staff considered several factors in designing the nutrition component of the program: amount of staff time available to implement the program in local worksites, cost of materials, and the best format for worksites based on their reading of the literature, discussions with other nutritionists, and personal experience. For the nutrition component, they chose a format consisting of eight sessions, each 30 minutes long, and named the program "Eat Well–Be Well." They decided on the following general topics to be covered in the sessions:[46]

- ◆ The ABC's of good nutrition
- ◆ Focus on fats—cooking fats and oils
- ◆ Focus on fats—meats
- ◆ Focus on fats—dairy products
- ◆ Fiber
- ◆ Cooking for good health
- ◆ Making sense of the supermarket
- ◆ Dealing with dining out

After choosing the topics to be covered, the staff "fleshed out" each session by defining its purpose, the learner objectives for the class, an in-class activity (designed to make the class lively and entertaining), a take-home activity (designed to keep participants involved in the learning process), and a list of handouts for the class. Table 7-11 describes these items for the first three sessions.

Once the sessions have been fleshed out, a manual is prepared to help instructors teach the classes and maintain consistency from one worksite to another. The manual would include the items shown in Table 7-11, together with a list of materials needed to teach each session. For recipe demonstrations, all cooking utensils, storage containers, and food supplies needed are listed.

TABLE 7-11   **Session Plans for Nutrition in Action's "Eat Well–Be Well" Program**

SESSION	PURPOSE	LEARNER OBJECTIVES	CLASS ACTIVITY	TAKE-HOME ACTIVITY	HANDOUTS
1	Introduce participants to the principles of good nutrition: variety, balance, and moderation	At the end of the 30-minute class, participants will be able to: ◆ Identify foods from the basic food groups ◆ Describe 3 reasons why eating well is important ◆ Define "fat" and "fiber"	Participants complete "Rate Your Plate."	Participants keep a 3-day food diary of all foods and beverages consumed.	◆ USDA brochure— The Food Guide Pyramid ◆ "Rate Your Plate" ◆ 3-day food diary with instruction sheet
2	Describe major food sources of fat, with a focus on cooking fats and oils	At the end of the 30-minute class, participants will be able to: ◆ Describe the energy value of fats and oils ◆ Describe in general terms the differences between saturated, monounsaturated, and polyunsaturated fats and their effects on blood lipids ◆ Identify hidden sources of fat ◆ Reduce use of fats and oils in cooking	Participants play a "Find the Fat" game.	Participants try one new fat-reduced product and rate its acceptability in terms of taste and convenience *or* reduce the amount of fat in one of their favorite family recipes and rate its acceptability.	◆ "Find the Fat" game ◆ Fact sheet on fats ◆ Comparison chart of composition of dietary fats
3	Describe meats and how lean meats can fit into a low-fat eating plan	At the end of the 30-minute class, participants will be able to: ◆ Identify lean cuts of meat ◆ Describe marbling and visible fat ◆ Describe ways to reduce the amount of meat fat in their eating patterns ◆ Describe the recommended daily intake of meat/meat products ◆ Describe the recommended portion size of meat	◆ Participants rank meats and meat-containing products from lean to high fat using food models. *or* ◆ Participants try vegetable/beef stir-fry prepared during class.	Participants take a recipe to prepare at home.	◆ Fact sheet showing recommended serving sizes for meats ◆ Brochure describing the "skinniest six" cuts of meat

Of course, program design does not end with the preparation of the manual. Other program elements must be considered before the program is finalized. As Figure 7-6 indicates, management, budget, and marketing plans must be developed to ensure that the organization's personnel and resources are used efficiently in delivering the program. Once the program is underway, a formal evaluation of its effectiveness is conducted. (Program evaluation is described in Chapter 10.)

Working with Community Organizations

Addressing a community's particular nutritional need may require the formation of a task force or committee to build a consensus on the issue and ensure that the people with the most knowledge about the problem are involved in developing a solution. Recall that earlier we described a cafeteria-based nutrition program for schools in Manitoba, Canada. Consider how this program came about. Nutritionists in Winnipeg were concerned about the eating habits of high school students. Although improving students' eating patterns was considered a priority and the idea of developing a program to address this issue had support among the city's nutritionists, the concept languished until the director of education at the Heart and Stroke Foundation of Manitoba organized a committee to design, implement, and evaluate a school foodservice program. Volunteer committee members were drawn from a variety of Winnipeg organizations—Manitoba Education and Training, Manitoba Health, the Manitoba Milk Producers' Marketing Board, and the Beef Information Centre, among others. These diverse professionals, with expertise in nutrition, home economics, education, nursing, school administration, and foodservice, designed an environmental program—called the FitzIn Program—to help school foodservice managers purchase, prepare, serve, and market low-fat and reduced-fat foods. The program goal was to build a coalition of administrators, teachers, foodservice employees, parents, school board members, and students to promote healthful food choices in school cafeterias or canteens. The program was developed in stages over a two-year period and made available to all provincial high schools in 1993.

This type of community organization can be a powerful method of addressing a community problem. Its strength lies in the makeup of the interagency committee; the members represent a broad cross section of interested groups and agencies, each bringing his or her own unique perspective about the community problem to the drawing board. The project's success is due to the members' ability to put aside the hidden agendas of participating agencies and individuals, commit themselves to a common community goal, and forge a new program. Increasingly, such community planning units are forming partnerships with local government and business sectors to carry out developmental projects. Such partnerships can include administrative and programmatic linkages. Agencies can be linked administratively through joint budgeting or by combining funds (joint funding) to realize a shared goal. They may also share services to obtain and process information, keep records, manage grants, evaluate projects, or develop standards and guidelines. Programmatic linkages occur when agencies share staff on a particular project or agree to centralize staff development programs.[47] Interagency linkages are increasingly viewed as an effective means of applying resources and personnel to a community need.

Entrepreneurship and Program Planning

In her book, *The Popcorn Report,* Faith Popcorn discusses the leading consumer trends of the decade and describes the importance of developing a vision of the future. One of her book's chapters bears the title, "You have to see the future to deal with the present."[48] These are apt words for community nutritionists with responsibility for identifying a community's nutritional needs and developing programs to meet those needs. A good, effective nutrition program is not achieved by accident, but by planning today to meet the needs of tomorrow.

Although the concept of "program planning" sounds deadly dull, in truth, it is one of the most exciting aspects of the community nutritionist's job, because it lends itself well to the creative process. Go back to Chapter 1 and review Table 1-2. Three-quarters of the entrepreneurial activities listed there are essential aspects of the planning process. The excitement of planning stems from the constantly changing environment. As Faith Popcorn put it, "Remember, trends never end. And the future is never here."[49] As a community nutritionist, you can promote entrepreneurship in the program planning process by seeking innovative ideas related to goal setting, the use and development of resources, and program design.

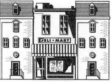 **COMMUNITY LEARNING ACTIVITY**

Continue using the target population and scenario you selected in Chapter 6 and complete the following activities:

1. Design the program. Develop a class outline, list of topics to be covered in each session, and learner objectives. Choose the teaching materials and handouts you would use in conveying important nutrition messages.

2. If you were to pull together a task force to assist you in planning the program, who would you invite to participate? List their organizations and backgrounds. Why would these particular people be useful?

3. Examine the following list of common nutritional disorders. How would you prioritize these nutritional problems in your community?

   ◆ AIDS

   ◆ Cardiovascular disease

- Diabetes
- Iron-deficiency anemia
- Hypercholesterolemia
- Hypertension
- Overweight
- Macrocytic anemias (e.g., folate deficiency)
- Nutrient deficiencies (e.g., protein deficiency, avitaminoses)
- Osteoporosis
- Stroke
- Underweight

NOTES

1. A. Berg, *The Nutrition Factor* (Washington, D.C.: The Brookings Institution, 1973), pp. 1–8.
2. D. B. Jelliffe and E. F. P. Jelliffe, *Community Nutritional Assessment* (Oxford: Oxford University Press, 1989), pp. 142–55.
3. Expert Panel, Report of the National Cholesterol Education Program Expert Panel on detection, evaluation, and treatment of high blood cholesterol in adults, *Archives of Internal Medicine* 148 (1988): 36–69.
4. M. P. O'Donnell, *Design of Workplace Health Promotion Programs* (Rochester Hills, Mich.: American Journal of Health Promotion, 1986), pp. 17–20.
5. G. Christakis, Community assessment of nutritional status, in H. S. Wright and L. S. Sims, *Community Nutrition—People, Policies, and Programs* (Belmont, Calif.: Wadsworth, 1981), pp. 83–97.
6. The description of the purposes of community nutritional needs assessment was adapted from Wright and Sims, *Community Nutrition—People, Policies, and Programs*, pp. 83–97; Jelliffe and Jelliffe, *Community Nutritional Assessment*, p. 12; and Office of Disease Prevention and Health Promotion, Public Health Service and American Dietetic Association, *Worksite Nutrition—A Guide to Planning, Implementation, and Evaluation* (Chicago: American Dietetic Association, 1993), pp. 14–15.
7. M. Y. Jackson, Height, weight, and body mass index of American Indian schoolchildren, 1990–1991, *Journal of the American Dietetic Association* 93 (1993): 1136–40.
8. S. Kumanyika and coauthors, Weight-related attitudes and behaviors of black women, *Journal of the American Dietetic Association* 93 (1993): 416–22.
9. P. R. Voss and coauthors, Role of secondary data, in *Needs Assessment: Theory and Methods*, ed. D. E. Johnson et al. (Ames, Iowa: Iowa State University Press, 1987), pp. 156–70.
10. Jelliffe and Jelliffe, *Community Nutritional Assessment*, pp. 355–83.
11. Pan American Health Organization, *Health Conditions in the Americas*, vol. 1 (Washington, D.C.: Pan American Health Organization, 1990).
12. Information about the University of Michigan data archive services was obtained from a booklet published by the Institute for Social Research, University of Michigan (Ann Arbor, Mich.); Catalog of Data Collections (Ann Arbor, Mich.: Inter-university Consortium for Political and Social Research, 1992); and C. Campbell, 1990 Census public use microdata samples (PUMS), *ICPSR Bulletin* 13 (1993): 1–7.
13. Information about the Institute for Research in Social Science was obtained from a booklet published by the institute at the University of North Carolina (Chapel Hill, N.C., 1991).
14. Department of Health and Human Services and Department of Agriculture, *Nutrition Monitoring in the United States: The Directory of Federal Nutrition Monitoring Activities* (Hyattsville, Md.: U.S. Government Printing Office, DHHS Pub. No. 89–1255–1, 1989).
15. U.S. Department of Agriculture, Human Nutrition Information Service, Nutrition Monitoring Division, *Nationwide Food Consumption Survey—Continuing Survey of Food Intakes by Individuals*, Women 19–50 years and their children 1–5 years, 1 day (Washington, D.C.: U.S. Department of Agriculture, 1987), p. 5.
16. C. E. Woteki and coauthors, Selection of nutrition status indicators for field surveys: The NHANES III design, *Journal of Nutrition* 120 (1990): 1440–45.
17. J. H. Sabry, Purposes of food consumption studies, in

M. E. Cameron and W. A. Van Staveren, *Manual on Methodology for Food Consumption Studies* (Oxford: Oxford University Press, 1988), pp. 25–31.

18. I. H. E. Rutishauser, Practical implementation, in Cameron and Van Staveren, *Manual on Methodology for Food Consumption Studies,* pp. 223–45.

19. C. A. Woodward and L. W. Chambers, *Guide to Questionnaire Construction and Question Writing* (Ontario: Canadian Public Health Association, 1983), pp. 1–33.

20. R. A. Spasoff and I. W. McDowell, On the efficacy of health hazard/health risk appraisal, *Health Services Research* 22 (1987): 467–97.

21. V. J. Schoenbach, Appraising health risk appraisal (editorial), *American Journal of Public Health* 77 (1987): 409–11.

22. K. W. Smith and coauthors, The validity of health risk appraisal instruments for assessing coronary heart disease risk, *American Journal of Public Health* 77 (1987): 419–24.

23. J. J. Korelitz and coauthors, Health habits and risk factors among truck drivers visiting a health booth during a trucker trade show, *American Journal of Health Promotion* 8 (1993): 117–23.

24. R. S. Gibson, *Principles of Nutritional Assessment* (New York: Oxford University Press, 1990), pp. 3–20.

25. Ibid., pp. 155–62.

26. M. Nestle, *Nutrition in Clinical Practice* (Greenbrae, Calif.: Jones Medical Publications, 1985), pp. 64–65.

27. Information about screening was adapted from J. M. Last, *Public Health and Human Ecology* (East Norwalk, Conn.: Appleton & Lange, 1987), pp. 12–15, and U.S. Department of Health and Human Services, National Institutes of Health, *Report of the Expert Panel on Population Strategies for Blood Cholesterol Reduction* (Bethesda, Md.: National Institutes of Health, NIH Pub. No. 90–3046, 1990), pp. 101–2.

28. R. C. Lefebvre and coauthors, Theory and delivery of health programming in the community: The Pawtucket Heart Health Program, *Preventive Medicine* 16 (1987): 80–95.

29. Nutrition Screening Initiative, *Implementing Nutrition Screening and Intervention Strategies* (Washington, D.C.: Nutrition Screening Initiative, 1993).

30. C. E. Basch, Focus group interview: An underutilized research technique for improving theory and practice in health education, *Health Education Quarterly* 14 (1987): 411–48.

31. R. B. Masters and coauthors, The use of focus groups in the design of cholesterol education intervention programs, *American Journal of Health Promotion* 8 (1993): 95–97.

32. J-P. Habicht and D. L. Pelletier, The importance of context in choosing nutritional indicators, *Journal of Nutrition* 120 (1990): 1519–24.

33. Nutrition Screening Initiative, *Implementing Nutrition Screening and Intervention Strategies,* p. 3.

34. S. A. Anderson, Core indicators of nutritional state for difficult-to-sample populations, *Journal of Nutrition* 120 (1990): 1559–1600.

35. The discussion of reference data was adapted from Gibson, *Principles of Nutritional Assessment,* pp. 209–46 and 349–76, and F. E. Johnston and Z. Ouyang, Choosing appropriate reference data for the anthropometric assessment of nutritional status, in *Anthropometric Assessment of Nutritional Status,* ed. J. H. Himes (New York: John Wiley & Sons, 1991), pp. 337–46.

36. Gibson, *Principles of Nutritional Assessment,* pp. 137–53.

37. Administrative Committee on Coordination— Subcommittee on Nutrition, United Nations, *Update on the Nutrition Situation* (Geneva: World Health Organization, 1989).

38. A. D. Spiegel and H. H. Hyman, *Strategic Health Planning: Methods and Techniques Applied to Marketing and Management* (Norwood, N.J.: Ablex Publishing, 1991), p. 203.

39. Jelliffe and Jelliffe, *Community Nutritional Assessment,* pp. 452–64.

40. The reports on the evaluation of the FitzIn Program are available from the Heart & Stroke Foundation of Manitoba, Winnipeg, Manitoba, Canada R3B 2H8.

41. P. M. Kettner, R. M. Moroney, and L. L. Martin, *Designing and Managing Programs* (Newbury Park, Calif.: Sage Publications, 1990), pp. 21–23.

42. B. B. Morlang and J. C. Robbins, Education program for pregnant teenagers, *Journal of Nutrition Education* 24 (1992): 50D.

43. M. K. Hunt and coauthors, Impact of a worksite cancer prevention program on eating patterns of workers, *Journal of Nutrition Education* 25 (1993): 236–44; L. B. Larson-Brown, Point-of-choice nutrition education in a university residence hall cafeteria, *Journal of Nutrition Education* 25 (1993): 350–51; and K. Glanz, Nutrition education for risk factor reduction and patient education: A review, *Preventive Medicine* 14 (1985): 721–52.

44. Information on the 5 A Day program can be obtained from the National Institutes of Health, Bethesda, Md. (Press office phone: 301-496-6641). Information on Project LEAN can be obtained from the National Center

for Nutrition and Dietetics, American Dietetic Association, Chicago, Ill. (Phone: 312–899–4853).

45. F. J. Stare and coauthors, Nutrition education in America: From day one, *World Review of Nutrition and Dietetics* 47 (1986): 1–29, and *Teaching Nutrition: A Review of Programs and Research,* ed. J. P. Nestor and J. A. Glotzer (Cambridge, Mass.: Abt Books, 1981), pp. ix–xvii.

46. The outline for the "Eat Well–Be Well" nutrition program was adapted from the Treatwell Program.

Information about the Treatwell Program's "Eatwell" series is available from the Dana Farber Cancer Institute, Community-based Programs, Department of Epidemiology and Cancer Control, Boston, MA. 02115.

47. A. Lauffer, *Social Planning at the Community Level* (Englewood Cliffs, N.J.: Prentice-Hall, 1978), pp. 187–207.

48. F. Popcorn, *The Popcorn Report* (New York: HarperCollins, 1991), p. 12.

49. Popcorn, *The Popcorn Report,* p. 200.

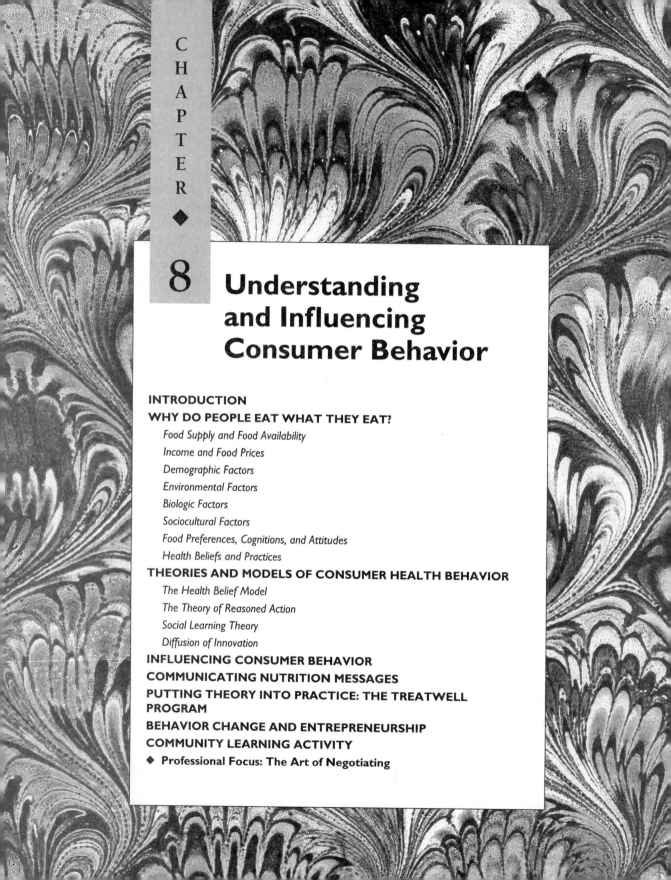

Understanding and Influencing Consumer Behavior

Something to Think About . . .

Everyone and no one can define "innovation." This is because what is innovative is in the eye of the beholder. If a person has seen, heard, or tried something, it is no longer new to him. An innovation, then, is something that is perceived as new by an individual at any given time in any community. This may be a shaky base for science, but it is an insight that must be dealt with when attempting to design change strategies.

—N. E. Hearn, *Phi Delta Kappan* (1972)

Introduction

In 1937 an inventor introduced a new product to the grocery store: the shopping cart. Until that time, people had shopped for their groceries using a small bag or basket. The inventor perceived the convenience and ease of using a cart on wheels for this activity and advertised his product with the question, "Can you imagine winding your way through a spacious food market without having to carry a cumbersome shopping basket on your arm?"[1] Unfortunately, most people refused to accept the innovation. When queried about their behavior, customers claimed that the shopping cart looked like a baby carriage and said they felt that it called into question their strength and independence. To get around this perception, the inventor hired women and men of various ages to come into his supermarkets and use the shopping carts to buy their groceries. This simple approach had the desired effect. Other customers saw the carts being used and elected to use them, too.[2]

This story illustrates two concepts about consumer behavior. First, consumer behavior is complex. By **consumer behavior**, we are referring to the "process by which consumers make decisions . . . [and specifically] with how consumers acquire, organize, and use information to make consumption choices."[3] If the decision to use a shopping cart for the first time is difficult for some consumers, imagine how complicated the process is by which consumers decide what goes *into* their shopping carts.

Consumer behavior The process by which consumers acquire, organize, and use information to make purchasing decisions.

Secondly, understanding consumer behavior is the first step toward developing strategies for influencing—and eventually changing—consumer behavior. In the shopping cart example, the inventor sought to change consumers' perception of his invention. The fact that today most consumers take the convenience of shopping carts for granted indicates that the social norm related to shopping carts has changed. Changing consumers' perceptions and changing social norms are two behavior change strategies. Many other behavior change strategies exist and are used by marketers and community nutritionists alike to influence consumer food consumption and eating patterns.

This chapter describes some of the factors that influence consumer food-related behavior, examines a few of the major theories of consumer behavior, and outlines some strategies that community nutritionists can use to help consumers change their eating behavior.

Why Do People Eat What They Eat?

Like other organisms, humans must eat to live. One of our prime motivations is securing nourishing food. In Abraham Maslow's hierarchy of needs, shown in Figure 8-1, physiological needs are basic requirements such as obtaining food, water, and shelter. Safety needs pertain to things that make us feel secure and safe. Storing food for future use, for example, gives us a sense of security. Once we feel safe and secure, we begin fulfilling needs through our relationships with other people (belongingness). Sharing foods with family members and friends expresses hospitality and friendliness and makes us feel a part of the group. At the level of esteem needs, we focus on developing a positive self-image and having our contributions and ideas valued by other people. Sometimes we buy certain foods like champagne and caviar to send a signal about our social status or to celebrate achievements. Finally, self-actualization needs refer to those involved in developing our full potential. Maslow believed that once a need is fulfilled, the need ceases to be a motivator and we begin to focus on fulfilling needs at higher levels. In other words, once we ensure ready access to nourishing food (physio-

FIGURE

8-1

Maslow's Hierarchy of Needs

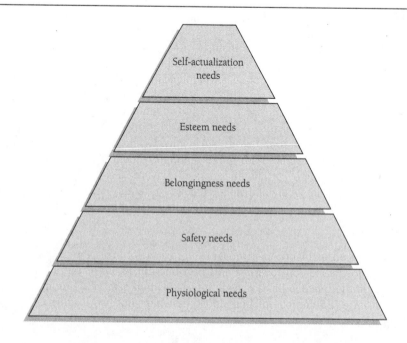

logical and safety needs), we use foods to fulfill needs relating to belonging, self-esteem, and self-actualization.[4]

For humans, then, foods are more than simply a source of nutrients and nourishment. They are also used to express friendliness and hospitality, maintain and strengthen personal relationships, enhance social status, relieve stress, and express religious and cultural beliefs.[5] Foods have symbolic meanings for humans, and the symbolic values we give to foods, together with other factors, influence the decisions we make about them.

In this section, we examine some of the factors that influence food consumption using the model shown in Figure 8-2. The model was adapted from one developed by the Expert Panel on Nutrition Monitoring of the Federation of American Societies for Experimental Biology (FASEB).[6] Other models of dietary behavior also exist, such as the lifestyle model developed by G. H. Pelto.[7] The model in Figure 8-2, like other models, is imperfect in that it does not define the determinants of food consumption precisely and does not specify which determinants are the best predictors of food-related behavior. Even so, it serves as a framework for understanding the many factors that influence our food choices.

◆ FOOD SUPPLY AND FOOD AVAILABILITY

Food choices are influenced by the types and amounts of foods available to consumers through the food supply, which is itself shaped by many forces. The food

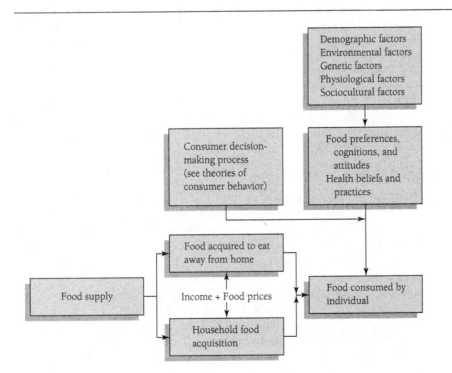

FIGURE

8-2

A Conceptual Model of the Factors Affecting Food Consumption
Source: Adapted from C. E. Woteki and M. T. Fanelli-Kuczmarski, The national nutrition monitoring system, in *Present Knowledge in Nutrition*, p. 416. Reprinted with permission from *Present Knowledge in Nutrition*, 6th ed., International Life Sciences Institute. Note: The complete model showing the relationships of food to health is shown in Figure 5-1 on page 127.

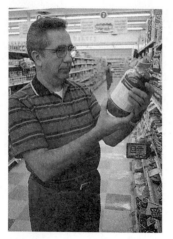

Even when consumers are knowledgeable about foods and nutrition, they do not always use their knowledge to make wise food choices.

supply is a product of the geographical area, climate, soil conditions, labor, and capital available for building the agricultural base. These factors determine the types of foods that can be grown locally. Foods imported from other countries and the extent of the food distribution system affect food availability, as do the resources and facilities that exist for food processing and production. The regulatory environment influences consumer food-related behavior through the policies and regulations that govern food production, processing, distribution, and advertising. Public policy, for example, affects consumers' food-purchasing behavior through food-labeling regulations.

Individual food intake is affected by the foods purchased for consumption at home or away from home, although not all foods purchased for consumption are actually consumed. Some foods brought into a household for consumption are eaten by family pets or discarded due to spoilage.[8]

◆ INCOME AND FOOD PRICES

Income and food prices are two economic factors that affect food consumption. The relationship between income and food consumption is expressed by the Engel function, which is named for Ernst Engel, a Prussian mining engineer who was interested in sociologic issues. Engel published a study in 1857 showing that the poorer a family is, the greater the proportion of income it must spend on food purchases. The modern equivalent of this function states that as a consumer's income increases, the proportion of income spent on food decreases. Data from 1988 reveal that households with incomes over $50,000 spent just 8.5 percent of their income on food, whereas the poorest households with incomes less than $5,000 spent 82.1 percent of their income on food purchases.[9]

Food prices affect consumption patterns. Some of the trends in meat consumption over the last two decades may be due to changes in relative prices: consumption of poultry increased because its price rose slightly relative to the price of beef, which increased considerably.[10] Generally, households with higher incomes have more money to spend on food and choose whatever foods they want, regardless of price. Low-income households are more likely to have limited food budgets and to be concerned with price and value.[11]

◆ DEMOGRAPHIC FACTORS

Many demographic factors such as age, sex, race, and education influence food choices. Age affects food consumption because nutrient and caloric needs, as well as food preferences, change as people age. Older people tend to choose traditional foods and meal patterns, eat fewer fried foods, use less table salt, and eat away from home less often than younger groups.[12] Men and women exhibit modest differences in food choices, with women consuming slightly more citrus fruits, yogurt, coffee, tea, and low-calorie carbonated beverages than men, who report eating more luncheon meats, whole milk, meat sandwiches, and desserts than women. Ethnicity influences food consumption. Nonwhites are more likely to eat rice, pork, fish, poultry, eggs, and legumes and less likely to drink milk or consume milk products, butter, margarine, beef, or desserts than whites.[13] Finally, educated people, especially those with college degrees, tend to be better informed about diet and nutrition, eat away from home more often, and try new foods more readily than people with less education.[14]

◆ ENVIRONMENTAL FACTORS

Environmental factors such as advertising, packaging, label information, convenience, availability of stoves and refrigerators, and location of food stores affect food choices. Advertising is especially influential. A survey of four widely circulated women's magazines found that the number of food and beverage advertisements making health and nutrition claims increased significantly between 1975 and 1990.[15] The impact of advertising is reinforced by data from a survey conducted by the American Dietetic Association (ADA), which found that 51 percent of consumers looked first to magazines as a source of information about diet and nutrition, followed by television/radio (34 percent) and the food/lifestyle sections of newspapers (26 percent).[16]

◆ BIOLOGIC FACTORS

From a biologic standpoint, the consumer's genetic endowment affects food utilization, individual health status, and nutritional needs, all of which can influence eating patterns. Examples of conditions with a genetic component that affect food consumption include lactose intolerance and celiac disease.[17] An individual's physiological status also affects food choices and nutrient needs. The physiological changes that occur during pregnancy affect nutrient needs and nutrient utilization. Pregnant women are advised to eat a balanced diet and to gain weight steadily over the course of their pregnancy. Some women, however, develop food cravings and aversions that disrupt their normal eating patterns. A survey of pregnant adolescents found that most (86 percent) had cravings during pregnancy for sweets, especially chocolate; fruits and fruit juices; pizza; pickles; and ice cream. Some had food aversions to meats, eggs, and, paradoxically, pizza.[18] Space flight likewise results in physiological changes that can produce motion sickness, nausea, anorexia, and other symptoms affecting eating patterns.[19]

◆ SOCIOCULTURAL FACTORS

Social and cultural factors influence food consumption. Food choices, for example, are strongly influenced by social groups. Primary **social groups** like families, friends, and work groups are more likely to affect behavior directly, and within this category, the family exerts the most influence.[20] This is not surprising, as the family is the first social group to which an individual belongs, and under most circumstances, it is the group to which an individual belongs for the longest period of time. The family is a paramount source of values for its members, and its values, attitudes, and traditions can have lasting effects on their food choices.

    Friendships, work groups, and other social networks also influence consumer behavior. Consider a primary maxim of reputable weight-loss programs: build social support. A recognized key to successfully losing weight is securing

Social group A group of people who are interdependent and share a set of norms, beliefs, values, or behaviors.

Culture The knowledge, beliefs, customs, laws, morals, art, and any other habits and skills acquired by humans as members of society.

the support of a spouse, significant others, friends, and even coworkers, all of whom are in a position to support weight-loss efforts.[21]

Our cultural environment also affects our food behavior. By **culture**, we are referring to "the integrated pattern of human knowledge, belief, and behavior that depends upon man's capacity for learning and transmitting knowledge to succeeding generations."[22] Many of our food habits arise from the traditions, customs, belief systems, technologies, values, and norms of the culture in which we live. Every culture has particular foodways or activities related to food. These include the activities surrounding procuring, distributing, manipulating, storing, consuming, and disposing of foods and even which foods are considered edible. North of the U.S.-Mexican border, for example, insects are seldom eaten, but in Mexico, the appetizer *los gusanos fritos* (fried caterpillars) may grace the menu in the finest restaurants.

Religious beliefs also affect the food choices of millions of people worldwide. Many religions, including Islam, Hinduism, Buddhism, Judaism, and Seventh-Day Adventism, specify the foods that may be eaten and how they should be prepared. Hinduism, for example, is the principal religion of India, and its food laws are steeped in ritual and meaning. Because the caste system is an integral part of Indian society, there are strict guidelines on how and with whom foods should be consumed. Among Brahmins, the highest caste, the eater must be pure, meaning among other things that he has not come into contact with a lower-caste individual or animal. This rule dictates that a host generally does not eat with his guests. Thus, meals are not the noisy, busy, conversation-filled activities typical of North American families; for Hindus, the focus of mealtime is eating, not conversation or socializing.[23] While the daily food choices of Christians in the Western world are not generally dictated by the basic doctrines of the Roman Catholic and Protestant churches, some Christian church sacraments such as Holy Communion use food (bread and wine) symbolically. The principal dietary practices of several major religions are summarized in Table 8-1.

◆ FOOD PREFERENCES, COGNITIONS, AND ATTITUDES

The demographic, environmental, and other factors just described shape many of our personal attributes such as food preferences, cognitions, and attitudes. These attributes in turn affect our food choices.

Humans enjoy a wide range of tastes that add to the pleasure of eating. Preferences or likings for certain tastes and foods appear to develop quite early in humans. Not surprisingly, parents and their children tend to have similar food preferences. The early experiences children have with salty and sweet foods, for example, tend to shape their later preferences for these foods.[24] Food preferences are shaped not only by family eating patterns but also by regional tastes. Mexican food is popular in western regions of the United States, whereas the Northeast prefers Italian foods.[25]

Cognitions The knowledge and awareness we have of our environment and the judgments we make related to it.

Food choices are affected by our **cognitions** or what we think. It seems logical that consumers who have learned about food composition and healthful eating practices have the knowledge base needed to select foods for good health, but consumers do not always practice what they have learned. The ADA's 1993 sur-

RELIGION	FOOD LAWS AND DIETARY PRACTICES
Buddhism	The central tenet of Buddhism is vegetarianism, which stems from the dual concepts of Karuna (compassion) and Karma (action, conduct). In the eyes of a Buddhist, to eat meat is to destroy the seeds of compassion. Foods of plant origin are considered appropriate for consumption except for the "five pungent foods": garlic, leek, scallion, chives, and onion. These foods are considered unclean and are believed to generate lust when eaten cooked and rage when eaten raw.
Hinduism	The Hindus believe that food was created by the Supreme Being for the benefit of humans. Many Hindus are vegetarians, but some, particularly in cold, northern areas of India, eat meat except for beef, which is prohibited.
Islam	Islamic food laws are derived from the Koran, the divine book given by Allah (the Creator) to Muhammad (the Prophet). Islamic food laws prohibit the consumption of unclean foods, such as carrion or dead animals, flowing or congealed blood, swine, animals slaughtered without pronouncing the name of Allah on them, animals killed in a manner that prevents their blood from being fully drained from their bodies, intoxicants of all types, carnivorous animals with fangs (e.g., lions, dogs, wolves, and tigers), birds with sharp claws (birds of prey, such as falcons, eagles, owls, and vultures), and land animals without ears (e.g., frogs and snakes).
Judaism	The traditional dietary laws of Judaism prohibit the consumption of swine, carrion eaters, and shellfish and specify other dietary practices, such as the ritual slaughtering of animals and the ritual breaking of bread at each Sabbath meal. The term *kosher* indicates that the food so labeled was not derived from any prohibited animal, bird, or fish; the animal or bird was slaughtered by the appropriate ritual method; the meat was salted to remove the blood; and milk and meat were prepared in separate utensils and containers and not cooked together.
Seventh-Day Adventism	Seventh-Day Adventists believe the body is the temple of the Holy Spirit. Thus, their dietary practices focus on health. Vegetarianism is the foundation of their dietary standard, although not all adherents are strict vegans. Other dietary standards call for abstaining totally from alcoholic beverages and avoiding certain "hot" spices and condiments such as pepper and chili, aged cheeses, and caffeine-containing beverages. The church recommends that its members eat a wholesome diet, consisting of whole grains, fruits, nuts, vegetables, a little milk, and occasional eggs.

TABLE 8-1

Food Laws and Dietary Practices of Several Major Religions

Sources: For Buddhism, Y. Huang and C. Y. W. Ang, Vegetarian foods for Chinese Buddhists, *Food Technology* 46 (1992): 105–8. For Hinduism, A. Kilara and K. K. Iya, Food and dietary habits of the Hindu, *Food Technology* 46 (1992): 94–104. For Islam, M. M. Chaudry, Islamic food laws: Philosophical basis and practical implications, *Food Technology* 46 (1992): 92–93, 104. For Judaism, *The New Encyclopaedia Britannica* (Chicago: Encyclopaedia Britannica, 1985), pp. 444–451 and the Macropaedia, pp. 968–69. For Seventh-Day Adventism, G. C. Bosley and M. G. Hardinge, Seventh-Day Adventists: Dietary standards and concerns, *Food Technology* 46 (1992): 112–13.

vey of consumer dietary habits found that about one in four Americans rated themselves as very knowledgeable about the recommended dietary guidelines. Yet, when asked to state the specific guidelines for cholesterol and fat intake, few participants could do so.[26] So, although nutrition knowledge can influence food-related behavior, the effect does not appear to be large. Having access to information about food and nutrition does not ensure that consumers will adopt healthful eating practices.[27]

One of the most complex areas of consumer behavior is the relationship of **attitude** to behavior. Early attitude research, conducted at the turn of the century, suggested that an individual's behavior was determined to a great extent by his

Attitude The positive or negative evaluation of performing a behavior.

attitude toward that behavior. Beginning in the 1930s, however, some researchers began to suspect that there was no predictable relationship between attitude and any given behavior. By the 1970s, some investigators concluded that attitudes could not be used to predict behavior; they maintained that the inconsistencies between attitude and behavior could be explained by any number of other variables, such as competing motives, conflicting attitudes, and individual differences.[28] Today, attitudes are believed to influence behavior indirectly.

◆ HEALTH BELIEFS AND PRACTICES

Beliefs about foods, diet, and health influence our food choices. Two examples of the power of health beliefs can be drawn from different cultures. In Senegal, pregnant women avoid spicy condiments and foods, but they indulge their cravings for curdled milk, palm oil, meat, butter, and the traditional millet porridge. The Senegalese believe that if pregnant women are not allowed to satisfy their food cravings, their babies may be born with birthmarks.[29]

According to traditional Chinese beliefs, illnesses are caused by an excess of either yin (the dark, cold, feminine aspect) or yang (the bright, hot, masculine aspect) energy. Foods and herbs, which themselves may be either yin or yang, are prescribed to treat certain symptoms of disease. Yang foods such as hot soups made from chicken, pork liver, or oxtail are prescribed to treat the clinical manifestations of excess yin such as dry cough, muscle cramps, and dizziness. Yin foods include fish, most vegetables, and some fruits like bananas; they are used to treat the symptoms of hives and dry throat, which are believed to be caused by excess yang energy.[30] Thus, health beliefs influence many consumer health practices, including leisure-time activities, eating certain comfort foods during illness, using vitamin supplements, and choosing snack foods.

Theories and Models of Consumer Health Behavior

Simply knowing the factors that affect consumers' food choices does not tell us *how* consumers make their decisions. Many theories have been proposed to explain the decision-making process as it relates to health. Such theories are important because they suggest the questions that scientists or managers should ask to understand consumer behavior. They also help in interpreting study outcomes and choosing strategies to influence behavior. Theories are sometimes presented in the form of *models,* which are simple images of the decision-making process. It is not possible to describe every health behavior theory in this chapter, but four deserve mention: the Health Belief Model, Theory of Reasoned Action, Social Learning Theory, and Diffusion of Innovation. In this section, we will briefly examine each theory and then consider how it can be applied in practice.

◆ THE HEALTH BELIEF MODEL

The Theory   The Health Belief Model was developed in the 1950s by social psychologists with the U.S. Public Health Service as a means of explaining why people, especially people in high-risk groups, failed to participate in programs designed to detect or prevent disease. The study of a tuberculosis screening program led G. M. Hochbaum to propose that participation in the program stemmed from an individual's perception of both her susceptibility to tuberculosis and the benefits of screening. Furthermore, an individual's "readiness" to participate in the program could be triggered by any number of environmental events, such as media advertising.[31] Since Hochbaum's analysis, the Health Belief Model has been expanded to include all preventive and health behaviors, from smoking cessation to complying with diet and drug regimens.

The key components of the Health Belief Model are shown in Table 8-2. The first component is the perception of a threat to health, which has two dimensions. An individual perceives that she is at risk of contracting a disease and is concerned that having the disease carries serious consequences, some of which may be physical or clinical (for example, death or pain), while others may be social (such as infecting family members or missing time at work). The second component is the expectation of certain outcomes related to a behavior. In other words, the individual perceives that a certain behavior (for example, choosing low-fat foods to facilitate weight loss) will have benefits. Bound up in the perception of benefits is the recognition of the barriers to successfully adopting the behavior (choosing low-fat foods requires skill in label reading and knowledge of food composition). The third component is **self-efficacy** or "the conviction that one can successfully execute the behavior required to produce the outcomes."[32] A key tenet of losing weight, for example, is the belief that one *can* lose weight. Other variables, such as education and income level, age, sex, and ethnic background, influence health behaviors in this model, but they are believed to act indirectly.

Self-efficacy The belief that one *can* make a behavior change.

◆ Threat:
  ◆ Perceived susceptibility to an ill-health condition (or the acceptance of a diagnosis)
  ◆ Perceived seriousness of the condition
◆ Outcome expectations:
  ◆ Perceived benefits of a specified action
  ◆ Perceived barriers to taking that action
◆ Efficacy expectations: The belief in one's ability to carry out the recommended action (self-efficacy)

Note: Sociodemographic factors such as education, age, sex, race, ethnicity, and income are believed to influence behavior indirectly by affecting perceived threat, outcome expectations, and efficacy expectations.

TABLE

8-2

Major Components of the Health Belief Model

Source: I. M. Rosenstock, The Health Belief Model: Explaining health behavior through expectancies, in *Health Behavior and Health Education—Theory, Research, and Practice,* ed. K. Glanz, F. M. Lewis, and B. K. Rimer (San Francisco: Jossey-Bass, 1990), p. 46. Copyright 1990 by Jossey-Bass, Inc., Publishers. Used with permission.

The Application Food safety is an important issue for consumers, but there is little information about how consumers respond to the danger of unsafe foods or what actions they take to avoid contaminated foods. To explore these issues, R. B. Schafer and his coworkers at Iowa State University used the Health Belief Model as the basis for understanding consumer food safety behavior.[33] Food safety behavior was defined in terms of nine behaviors related to selecting and preparing food and seeking information. Specific behaviors included buying organically grown food, washing or peeling fresh produce, and reading articles about food safety. The researchers surveyed 630 adult Iowa residents about their belief that unsafe food poses a personal health hazard (i.e., a perceived threat), the extent to which they engaged in health behaviors (outcome expectations), how strongly they believed food safety could be controlled (self-efficacy), and which food safety behaviors they practiced. Sociodemographic data such as age, sex, marital status, education, and income were also obtained.

An analysis of the survey results showed that the most frequently reported food safety actions involved food preparation practices such as washing foods before use. Respondents who perceived food safety as a personal threat and who engaged in healthy behaviors such as eating breakfast and not smoking were more likely to take steps to control food safety than those with low scores on these measures. Respondents with high levels of self-efficacy responded to the danger of contaminated foods by washing and handling foods carefully. There were differences in food safety behavior based on age and sex, with younger respondents being less aware of and concerned about food safety risks than older people. Women undertook more safe food-handling practices than men.

Community nutritionists can use the principles of this theory to design effective educational materials and programs. In this example, food safety education programs can be designed to include skill-building tasks as a way to increase clients' self-efficacy. Specific skills related to handling meat, keeping cutting boards clean, and storing perishable foods can be taught to clients. Secondly, community nutritionists can be alert to times when consumers are likely to perceive a health threat and change their behavior significantly. For example, some consumers may eliminate foods or entire food groups from their diet because of concerns about pesticides. Teaching consumers about pesticide risk and how to reduce their exposure to pesticides will temper their concern. Finally, community nutritionists can identify barriers to taking action to improve health and develop strategies for helping clients overcome these barriers. Handouts that present food safety practices in a simple, graphic format can be designed for consumers whose knowledge about such practices is limited. These concepts can be applied to many other food and nutrition issues.

◆ THE THEORY OF REASONED ACTION

The Theory The Theory of Reasoned Action was developed by I. Ajzen and M. Fishbein. It "predicts a person's intention to perform a behavior in a well-defined setting."[34] The theory is a fundamental model for explaining social action and can be used to explain virtually any health behavior over which the individual has control. According to the model, behavior is directly determined by a person's intention to perform the behavior. **Intentions** are defined as the "instructions people give to themselves to behave in certain ways."[35] Intentions are the scripts that people use for their future behavior. In forming intentions, people tend to consider the outcome of their behavior and the opinion of significant others before committing themselves to a particular action. In other words, intentions are influenced by attitudes and **subjective norms**. Attitudes are determined by the individual's belief that a certain behavior will have a given outcome and by an evaluation of the actual outcome of the behavior. Subjective norms are determined by the individual's normative beliefs. In forming a subjective norm, the individual considers the expectations of various other people.

A modification of the theory was proposed by R. P. Bagozzi, who argued that "attitudes and subjective norms are not sufficient determinants of intentions and that intentions are not a sufficient impetus for action."[36] Bagozzi and his colleagues developed a new model, the Theory of Trying, shown in Figure 8-3, to explain the relationship of attitudes and intentions to behavior. In the new model, such factors as past experience (success or failure) with the behavior, the existence of mechanisms for coping with the behavior outcome (e.g., having a strategy for not meeting a weight-loss goal), and emotional responses to the process all influence the intention to try a behavior. Bagozzi and his colleagues hypothesized that when intentions are well formed, they are strong mediators of behavior; when intentions are poorly formed, however, their influence on behavior is diminished, while that of attitudes grows stronger.[37]

The Application One challenge for nutritionists working with overweight individuals is reducing attrition from weight-reduction programs. Why do people

Intention A determination to act in a certain way.

Subjective norm The perceived social pressure to perform or not perform a behavior.

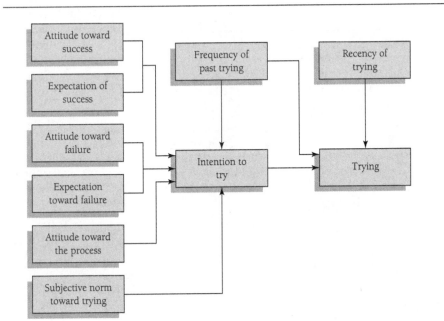

FIGURE

8-3

The Theory of Trying
Source: R. P. Bagozzi, The self-regulation of attitudes, intentions, and behavior, *Social Psychology Quarterly* 55 (1992): 179. Used with permission of R. P. Bagozzi and the American Sociological Association.

drop out of such programs and what can be done to prevent dropout? To help understand the factors contributing to attrition, C. A. Pratt and her colleagues at Virginia Polytechnic Institute and State University surveyed 309 adults enrolled in a 10-week weight-reduction program.[38] The model they developed for studying attrition was based on the Theory of Reasoned Action. Thus, intention to drop out was assumed to be the immediate determinant of dropout. The model also included other factors believed to affect attrition, such as attitudes, level of support from family and friends, the participants' expectations of success, and their perception of their ability to control eating and lose weight.

The survey results indicated significant differences between people who completed the program and those who dropped out. Because the data did not support the original model, however, Pratt and her coworkers formulated a new model, shown in Figure 8-4. The factor with the greatest effect on program completion was the extent to which participants believed they could control their eating and exercise habits and their level of motivation and commitment to the program (self-assurance). Demographic characteristics, level of social support, and comfort level in class (social ease) had little effect on program completion.

For community nutritionists working in a variety of settings, this model suggests ways of influencing consumer behavior to produce a positive outcome. In our example, knowing that self-assurance is linked with program completion signals a need to enhance self-esteem and self-efficacy among program participants. (The attribute "self-assurance" used in this model resembles "self-efficacy" in the Health Belief Model.) For example, a screening tool can be used to determine whether clients entering the program are ready to try to lose weight, how successful they have been at losing weight in the past, their confidence level in reaching weight-loss goals, and their level of commitment to the program. Additional

---

FIGURE
8-4

A Model of the Factors Influencing the Completion of a Weight-Reduction Program

Source: Adapted from C. A. Pratt, C. Gaylord, and G. W. McLaughlin, A multivariate analysis of the attitudinal and perceptual determinants of completion of a weight-reduction program, *Journal of Nutrition Education* 24 (1992): 18. Used with permission from Society for Nutrition Education.

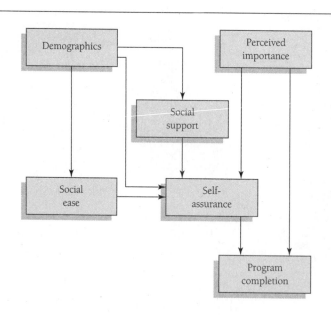

checkpoints for readiness and self-assurance can be built into the program as a means of keeping clients on track toward their goal. This model can be used to help understand and influence other food-related behaviors, such as trying low-fat products and eating five or more fruits and vegetables daily.

◆ SOCIAL LEARNING THEORY

The Theory   Social Learning Theory (SLT) explains behavior in terms of a model in which behavior, personal factors such as cognitions, and the environment interact constantly, such that a change in any one area has implications for the others. For example, a change in the environment (the loss of a spouse's support for a weight-loss effort) produces a change in the individual (a decrease in the incentive to lose weight) and consequently a change in the behavior (a low-fat eating pattern is abandoned). The theory was developed to explain how people acquire and maintain certain behaviors, and it serves as a basis for intervention strategies.

The major concepts in SLT, many of which were formulated by A. Bandura, and their implications for interventions are given in Table 8-3. In this context, the environment includes both the social realm (family, friends, peers, coworkers) and the physical realm (the workplace, the layout of a kitchen), and it provides cues for reinforcing or diminishing behavior. A strength of SLT is that it focuses on certain target behaviors rather than on knowledge and attitudes.[39]

TABLE 8-3	Key Concepts in Social Learning Theory and Their Implications for Behavioral Intervention	
CONCEPT	DEFINITION	IMPLICATIONS
Environment	Factors that are physically external to the person	Provide opportunities and social support
Situation	Person's perception of the environment	Correct misperceptions and promote healthful norms
Behavioral capability	Knowledge and skill to perform a given behavior	Promote mastery learning through skills training
Expectations	Anticipatory outcomes of a behavior	Model positive outcomes of health behavior
Expectancies	The values that the person places on a given outcome and incentives	Present outcomes of change that have a functional meaning
Self-control	Personal regulation of goal-directed behavior or performance	Provide opportunities for self-monitoring and contracting
Observational	Behavioral acquisition that occurs by watching the actions and outcomes of others' behavior	Include credible role models of the targeted behavior
Reinforcements	Responses to a person's behavior that increase or decrease the likelihood of recurrence	Promote self-initiated rewards and incentives
Self-efficacy	The person's confidence in performing a particular behavior	Approach behavior change in small steps; seek specificity about the change sought
Emotional coping responses	Strategies or tactics that are used by a person to deal with emotional stimuli	Provide training in problem solving and stress management

Source: C. L. Perry, T. Baranowski, and G. S. Parcel, How individuals, environments, and health behavior interact: Social Learning Theory, in *Health Behavior and Health Education—Theory, Research, and Practice*, ed. K. Glanz, F. M. Lewis, and B. K. Rimer (San Francisco: Jossey-Bass, 1990), p. 166. Copyright 1990 by Jossey-Bass, Inc., Publishers. Used with permission.

The Application Using the health objective for the year 2000 that calls for increasing fruit and vegetable intake to five or more servings per day, a group of behavioral scientists and nutritionists conducted focus group interviews with fourth- and fifth-grade students in the public schools of one Georgia county. The children were asked to grade posters depicting dietary information about fruits and vegetables and to describe their own suggestions for making dietary changes.[40]

SLT was selected as the model, because it was perceived as being valuable in designing school nutrition education programs. The important components of SLT for this application were the *environment* (if fruits and vegetables are not available within the environment, children cannot consume them), *expectancies* (children who like and enjoy fruits and vegetables will consume them), and *behavioral capability* (children with the ability and confidence to control their environment are likely to eat fruits and vegetables).

A number of behavior change strategies grew out of the focus group interviews. First, increasing access to fruits and vegetables enhances their intake. Children who are exposed to fruits and vegetables in their home, school, and play environments have a greater preference for them. In addition, children's food preferences can be shaped by *modeling* (the "observational" concept in Table 8-3). The children reported being influenced by athletes and pictures of children their own age (but not celebrity children). They believed they could be influenced by older adults such as grandparents but not by adults their parents' ages. Although they mentioned Bart Simpson as a popular cartoon character, he was not thought to be a good role model because he probably would not eat fruits and vegetables!

The children reported liking most fruits, but there were many vegetables they did not like. They had definite preferences for the sensory qualities of these foods. For example, they did not like ugly, wrinkled, purple, or yellow fruits and vegetables, and they preferred crunchy and raw fruits and vegetables over soft or "smooshie" ones. They would not give up a dessert for a piece of fruit, and they believed the dietary goal of eating five or more fruits and vegetables per day was unreasonably high. These results suggest that simple activities like taste tests at home or school can increase children's enjoyment of fruits and vegetables.

The focus group interviews revealed that children need skills to handle certain critical situations, which usually arise when they must make a decision about whether to eat a food. These critical situations may occur in any of the several environments listed in Table 8-4. Children with strong decision-making skills are able to handle difficult food choices, such as whether to eat fruit or a candy bar.

Community nutritionists can use the SLT model in other settings. The following SLT concepts can be used in classes designed to teach the principles of a low-fat, low-cholesterol diet plan:

- ◆ Environment—Invite spouses or significant others to attend classes.
- ◆ Behavioral capability—Provide simple recipes for program participants to try at home.
- ◆ Expectations—Provide a checklist of benefits of eating a low-fat, low-cholesterol diet.

TABLE 8-4	Critical Situations for Children for Purchasing, Selecting, or Consuming More Fruits and Vegetables	
ENVIRONMENTS	**AVAILABILITY ASPECT**	**CRITICAL SITUATIONS**
Grocery stores	Purchase	What fruits and vegetables to put on shopping list
		What fruits and vegetables to buy and/or ask parent to buy
		What fruits and vegetables to place in shopping cart
Home	Selection	Whether to eat cookies or fruit for a snack
	Preparation	What sauces or seasonings to ask for
	Consumption	Whether or not to eat the fruit for dessert
Convenience stores	Purchase	Whether to buy candy or fruit
Fast-food places	Selection	To select a salad or a sandwich
		To select ice cream or fruit salad
		To select the tacos (with vegetables) or the enchiladas
	Consumption	To eat the salad or not

Source: T. Baranowski and coauthors, Increasing fruit and vegetable consumption among 4th and 5th grade students: Results from focus groups using reciprocal determinism, *Journal of Nutrition Education* 25 (1993): 118. Used with permission from Society for Nutrition Education.

- ◆ Observational—Invite a previous program participant to speak to the class about his success in following a low-fat eating pattern.
- ◆ Self-efficacy—Ask participants to keep a log of all new low-fat foods they try or prepare during the week.

◆ DIFFUSION OF INNOVATION

The Theory People often cannot or will not change their behavior, and many do not adopt innovations easily (recall the story about shopping carts at the beginning of this chapter). Even so, some people are more daring than others. Such people are the vanguard in the **diffusion of innovation**, the process by which an innovation spreads and involves an ever-increasing number of individuals within a population.[41] The Diffusion of Innovation model was developed by E. M. Rogers and F. F. Shoemaker in the 1970s to explain how a product or idea becomes accepted by a majority of consumers. The model consists of four stages:[42]

- ◆ **Knowledge.** The individual is aware of the innovation and has acquired some information about it.
- ◆ **Persuasion.** The individual forms an attitude either in favor of the innovation or against it.
- ◆ **Decision.** The individual performs activities that lead to either adopting or rejecting the innovation.
- ◆ **Confirmation.** The individual looks for reinforcement for his decision and may change it if he is exposed to counter-reinforcing messages.

Innovations spread throughout a population largely by word of mouth. The speed of diffusion is a function, in part, of the number of people who adopt the

Diffusion of innovation The process by which a new idea, product, or service spreads throughout a population.

innovation. Consumers can be classified according to how readily they adopt new ideas or products. *Innovators* are those people who adopt the innovation quite readily, usually without input from significant others. Innovators tend to be integrated socially within their communities, perceive themselves as popular, and be financially privileged. This group is small. *Early adopters* are also integrated into the social fabric of their communities and are well respected by their families and peers. Opinion leaders are found most frequently within this group. Members of the *early majority* tend to be cautious in adopting a new idea or product, but they have considerable contact with early adopters and hence display some opinion leadership. Persons in the *late majority* are characterized by skepticism. They are moved to adopt an innovation only through constant peer pressure. Most members of this group have a lower income, social status, and educational level than early adopters. Finally, the *laggards* represent the last to adopt an idea, service, or product, although they will adopt it eventually. Members of this group tend to come from small families, to be single and older, and to have lower incomes than other groups. They also are bound tightly to tradition. Figure 8-5 shows the S-shaped diffusion curve representing the percentage of people who adopt an innovation over time.[43]

The Application Health educators at the University of North Carolina at Chapel Hill were interested in measuring the diffusion of tobacco prevention curricula (the "innovation") across junior high schools in North Carolina over a four-year period.[44] The tobacco prevention programs being disseminated were

---

FIGURE

8-5

The S-Shaped Diffusion Curve

Source: G. Macdonald, Communication theory and health promotion, in *Health Promotion*, ed. R. Bunton and G. Macdonald (New York: Routledge, 1992), p. 186. Used with permission.

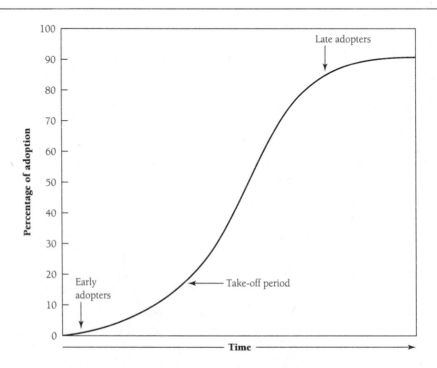

(1) *Growing Healthy,* (2) *Teenage Health Teaching Modules,* and (3) *Project SMART.* The educators developed and tested several instruments to evaluate awareness of the curricula, extent of adoption, level of implementation, level of success with the curricula, and the degree to which the curricula became integrated within school districts.

The mid-study assessment of diffusion indicated that 16 of 21 districts had adopted at least one of the programs. Drawing on the Diffusion of Innovation model, the educators noted that the greater the levels of awareness, concern, and interest, the greater the likelihood of adopting the curricula. School districts with an organizational climate that favored innovation were more likely to adopt the programs. The curricula were implemented most successfully in districts where teachers used the programs extensively and school administrators believed that the curricula met their goals and provided important benefits.

The concept of diffusion is important for community nutritionists. Consider the USDA's Food Pyramid. It first received a cursory explanation in newspapers and popular news magazines and on television. Then, a brochure describing the pyramid was released to nutritionists and other health professionals. Within a year after the Food Pyramid was introduced, it appeared on refrigerator magnets, posters, and T-shirts and in educational brochures developed by food companies. Consumers are gradually becoming aware of the new dietary guidance system. The diffusion process was facilitated by the actions of the federal government, nutritionists, food companies, and the media.

Consumers sometimes resist innovative ideas, products, and services. Why? Consumers may resist an innovation because it changes the status quo and disrupts established routines. The greater the perturbation in the status quo, the greater the resistance to the innovation. When tofu was introduced into the U.S. market, consumers did not accept it readily because different cooking skills and new recipes were required to incorporate it into meals. Consumers may also resist an innovation because it conflicts with their beliefs. Consumers who believe that honey is the best natural sweetener refrain from using high-intensity sweeteners because they believe artificial sweeteners are less "pure" and wholesome.[45] In general, innovations that are complex and difficult to understand, use, and communicate to others are more likely to be resisted than simple innovations.[46]

Influencing Consumer Behavior

Community nutritionists often design their programs and messages to target groups of people in different settings. Such "macro" level interventions may influence small groups such as families and peer groups; organizations such as schools, churches, worksites, fitness centers, and grocery stores; and entire communities.

Working toward behavior change at the macro level is challenging. Every group differs in terms of its purpose and format and the composition and number of its members. Consequently, behavior change strategies are dictated partly by

In taste tests conducted nationwide, chocolate lovers were blindfolded and asked to compare five leading brands of chocolate. The result?

3 OUT OF 4 INDIVIDUALS ACTUALLY RESENTED HAVING BEEN BLINDFOLDED

the nature of the group. A community nutritionist has less influence with participants in a single, two-hour group workshop than with participants in a 12-week group program, simply because there is less time in the workshop for building trust and rapport and helping participants develop specific behavioral goals.

The macro approach to behavior change is attractive, because it makes it possible to reach large numbers of people at a relatively low cost. Support for early adopters of positive health and nutrition behaviors can be sustained over time, thus exposing other members of the group, organization, or community to the positive behaviors of the early adopters, who serve as role models. The macro approach to behavior change has disadvantages, however. The main criticism is that because the intervention occurs at the group level, helping individuals within the group maintain lifestyle changes is difficult. Skills training and goal setting are more difficult in a group than with one-on-one interventions. Because groups of people are the primary targets of macro interventions, it is not possible to evaluate an individual participant's eating habits and readiness for change. In addition, some individuals become more resistant to behavior change during large-scale interventions, such as community antismoking campaigns.[47]

Despite its limitations, the macro approach has been used successfully in the areas of smoking cessation, weight loss, and reduction of cardiovascular disease risk. Table 8-5 gives examples of macro-level interventions and the behavior change strategies used to help people improve their eating habits.

Communicating Nutrition Messages

One of the most challenging tasks facing community nutritionists is translating official dietary guidelines into practical eating patterns that consumers can understand and implement. Consider the oft-quoted recommendation of the U.S. feder-

TABLE 8-5	Examples of Macro-Level Interventions and Behavior Change Strategies	

LEVEL OF INTERVENTION	EXAMPLE	BEHAVIOR CHANGE STRATEGIES
Group	New Haven Summer Youth Nutrition Education Program—a 5-year curriculum designed for teenagers to use in teaching younger children. (This approach is sometimes called "train the trainer.")	◆ Increase the nutrition knowledge of teenagers by teaching them how to teach the curriculum. ◆ Develop nutrition skills through activities (e.g., preparing snack recipes, completing crossword puzzles and dot-to-dot pictures). ◆ Enhance modeling of good eating behaviors through the teenagers. ◆ Reinforce nutrition concepts being taught to teenagers and children by coupling program messages with foods offered through the Summer Food Service Program. ◆ Build self-efficacy by encouraging teenagers to develop their own ideas for teaching children good eating habits.
Organization	Heart Smart school-based cardiovascular program—designed to help schoolchildren adopt healthy lifestyles through increased self-esteem and self-confidence.	◆ Build mastery of new behaviors by having children prepare snacks and heart-healthy lunches and practice jogging techniques and stretching exercises. ◆ Use modeling to influence children and reinforce good eating behaviors—e.g., parents exercise with their children. ◆ Increase knowledge about healthy behaviors through program activities. ◆ Provide feedback to children and their parents through taste testing, pulse counting during exercise, and relaxation techniques.
Community	Project LEAN (Low-fat Eating for America Now)—a national campaign to reduce dietary fat consumption.	◆ Use fact sheets, feature stories and other educational materials to increase consumers' skills in buying and preparing low-fat foods and choosing low-fat foods when they dine out. ◆ Use Project LEAN public service announcements to communicate the dietary messages. ◆ Use appropriate communication channels for the campaign—e.g., mass media (newspapers, radio and TV, magazines, billboards, transit cards, etc.), food delivery sites (e.g., worksites, schools, cafeterias, grocery stores, and restaurants), peer groups (e.g., community groups, professional groups, etc.), and face-to-face situations (e.g., counseling programs). ◆ Use one or more tactics to reach the target population—e.g., build a community coalition; generate local or statewide publicity; work with grocery stores, restaurants, worksites, and schools; and hold special events.

Sources: For the New Haven program, J. A. Anliker and coauthors, Impacts of a multi-layered nutrition education program: Teenagers teaching children, *Journal of Nutrition Education* 25 (1993): 140–43. For Heart Smart, S. M. Hunter and coauthors, Heart Smart: A multifaceted cardiovascular risk reduction program for grade school students, *American Journal of Health Promotion* 4 (1990): 352–60. For Project LEAN, National Center for Nutrition and Dietetics, *Idea Kit for State and Community Programs to Reduce Dietary Fat* (Chicago: American Dietetic Association, 1989).

al government regarding total fat intake, cited directly from the USDA's brochure, *Eating Right with the Dietary Guidelines:*

> **Total Fat.** Your goal for fat depends on your calorie needs. An amount that provides 30 percent or less of calories is suggested.[48]

When presented with this recommendation, consumers often ask, "What kinds of foods should I eat to ensure that my total fat intake is less than 30 percent of total calories?" "Is it okay to eat a food that provides 50 percent of its calories from fat?" "Should I avoid eating fat altogether?" Consumers often find this concept difficult to grasp—and rightly so. No one, not even a nutritionist, knows whether his diet provides the recommended intake of fat unless detailed records of all foods and beverages consumed daily are kept and analyzed.

The task for community nutritionists is to translate such recommendations into a more useful format for consumers. For example, helping consumers understand a dietary pattern that provides 30 percent or less of calories as fat means showing them what such a pattern looks like in terms of the foods that can be eaten at meals and for snacks. It also means providing them with information about the fat content of foods and listing foods that are high in fat as well as those that are low in fat. It means teaching them how to read and use food labels. Plus, it requires helping consumers appreciate the concerns of federal agencies and public health officials about fat intake and why they are being advised to lower their intake of this nutrient.

Keep these points in mind as you work to translate dietary guidelines and other nutrition concepts for consumers:[49]

◆ **Keep it simple.** Ask yourself what consumers *need* to know in order to implement a specific guideline and build your advice on that. You will find that because *you* know much more than *consumers* need to know, you may have difficulty developing general, easy-to-understand statements about foods and eating patterns. The challenge is to explain or interpret a nutrition message so that the client understands and can act on it.

◆ **Use "consumer" language.** Terms such as "low-density lipoprotein," "monounsaturated fatty acid" and " complex carbohydrate" are all part of your nutrition vocabulary. While you know the technical definition of dietary fiber, consumers understand dietary fiber as "that part of whole grains, fruits, vegetables, beans, nuts and seeds that humans cannot digest."[50] Whenever possible, strive to translate complex scientific terms into simple, conversational language consumers use in their everyday lives. Consider using the SMOG Readability Formula (given in Appendix G) to simplify and improve the readability of your educational materials. Proceed from simple ideas to more complex ones.

◆ **Use illustrations.** To increase the readability of your materials, use illustrations to demonstrate basic concepts. Some basic cooking skills and recipes, for example, can be taught exclusively through the use of graphics.

◆ **Recommend specific behaviors.** People are better able to make behavior changes when they are given or are allowed to formulate specific behavior goals. The recommendation to "drink alcohol in moderation" is less specific and less likely to have a behavioral impact than the recommendation to "limit your alcohol intake to 1 drink a day if you are a woman, and 2 drinks a day if you are a man."

◆ **Use examples.** Examples demonstrate how a consumer can apply a dietary guideline to her eating patterns. For example, one of the USDA's dietary guidelines calls for the use of salt and sodium in moderation. A food tip to help consumers apply this advice states: Use salt sparingly, if at all, in cooking and at the table.

◆ **Use positive rather than negative messages.** One hurdle for many consumers, especially dieters, is overcoming the belief that dietary changes require that they totally give up their favorite foods. Rather than say "Eliminate all high-fat dairy foods from your diet," say "Substitute nonfat yogurt, skim or 1 percent milk, and other low-fat dairy products for higher-fat dairy products."

◆ **Use humor, if appropriate.** Most people enjoy a good chuckle about the challenges of learning new eating habits, but be sure to pretest your cartoons or other humorous elements to make sure that they don't offend.

◆ **Make your message relevant to your target audience.** Consumers are more likely to remember and act on a dietary message that is realistic, interesting, informative, and relevant to them personally.

Putting Theory into Practice: The Treatwell Program

How do community nutritionists use the theories and models of consumer health behavior to fashion nutrition programs? One example of how theory is put into practice is the Treatwell Program, a worksite-based health promotion program designed to promote dietary changes to reduce cancer risk.[51] The Treatwell Program was developed as part of a study funded by the National Cancer Institute (NCI). Sixteen worksites in Massachusetts and Rhode Island were recruited to participate in the development, testing, and evaluation of the 15-month program. Eight worksites received the nutrition intervention; the other eight worksites served as a comparison group.

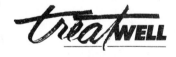

Educational Messages The educational messages used in the Treatwell Program were based on the NCI's dietary goals, which call for reducing total dietary fat consumed to 30 percent of total calories and increasing dietary fiber consumed to 20–30 grams per day.[52] A set of eating pattern guidelines, shown in Figure 8-6, was developed to translate the NCI dietary recommendations into a practical eating guide for employees in the intervention worksites. One or more of these dietary messages was emphasized in all program activities, including taste tests, brown-bag lunches, nutrition classes, and point-of-purchase labeling in the worksite cafeteria.[53]

FIGURE

8-6

Treatwell Eating Pattern Guidelines

Source: G. Sorensen and coauthors, Work-site nutrition intervention and employees' dietary habits: The Treatwell Program, *American Journal of Public Health* 82 (1992): 880. Copyright 1992 American Public Health Association.

Trim fat:

◆ Choose fish, skinned turkey and chicken, and trimmed lean red meat. Keep the amount at 6 oz or less, cooked, a day.

◆ Choose low-fat dairy products: skim, 1%, or 2% milk; low-fat yogurt; ice milk; and low-fat cheeses.

◆ Use half the amount of fat or oil you normally use in cooking and baking, and at the table.

Add fiber:

◆ Eat at least one serving of high-fiber cereal every day.

◆ Eat one or more servings of fruit at each meal and for snacks.

◆ Eat one or more servings of vegetables at lunch and dinner.

◆ Eat at least one of these foods at each meal: whole-grain bread, rice and/or pasta; potato; or dried beans, peas, or lentils.

The Intervention Model   The Treatwell Program intervention model drew from Social Learning Theory, Diffusion of Innovation, and the principles of community organization. The theoretical model for the intervention, shown in Figure 8-7, was based on the model used in the Pawtucket Heart Health Program.[54]

Worksite Organization and Mobilization   A key element of the Treatwell Program was recognizing that a program is most likely to be adopted when it fits within the organization's value system and "culture." To achieve this fit, the program secured the support of top management. Supportive managers endorsed Treatwell activities, attended company-wide events, helped solve logistical problems, and approved employee involvement in Treatwell activities. The program also assessed the worksite norms and culture through a series of interviews with employees and key informants and organized an employee advisory board within each intervention worksite to plan, promote (market), and implement the intervention activities. The employee advisory board helped tailor the program to meet the needs and interests of the individual worksite.

Program Focus   The Treatwell Program interventions targeted both individual employees and the worksite environment. At the individual level, a "core" group of classes was offered at all intervention sites. These included a 7-session "Eat Well" class designed to help participants develop the skills needed to purchase and prepare low-fat, high-fiber foods; a 10-session "Wise Weighs" weight-management program; and a one-hour slide-tape presentation ("Taking Control") of the American Cancer Society. Interested employees signed up for these classes, most of which were held on-site over the lunch hour. At the environmental level, the program worked with the foodservice manager and his or her employees to increase the number of low-fat, high-fiber foods offered in the worksite cafeteria and to reduce barriers to selecting healthful foods. The Treatwell logo on point-of-purchase labeling helped employees identify low-fat, high-fiber foods for sale in the cafeteria. Activities targeting the environmental level reached more employees than those targeting individual employees.

Behavior Change Strategies   Individual behavior change and environmental change strategies were planned as part of the Treatwell Program and are shown in

FIGURE

8-7

The Treatwell Intervention Model

Source: G. Sorensen and coauthors, Promoting healthy eating patterns in the worksite: The Treatwell intervention model, *Health Education Research* 5 (1990): 508, by permission of Oxford University Press.

Table 8-6. Promotional and motivational strategies were designed to interest employees in changing their eating behaviors, create a climate for change, and provide information about the relationship of eating patterns to cancer risk. In one worksite, for example, a cholesterol screening was held to interest employees in the program. This worksite-wide event presented the Treatwell eating pattern guidelines and provided a taste test of a low-fat food. The event reached 26 percent of the workforce in one day.

Strategies for skills training included active participation in Treatwell events and role modeling. All Treatwell activities focused on one or more of the dietary messages as a means of enhancing employees' skill level and confidence in choosing and preparing low-fat, high-fiber foods. Another strategy focused on building social support for dietary change, mainly through the employee advisory boards and group activities. Finally, employee advisory board members, foodservice managers, and other opinion leaders within the intervention worksites were trained to provide peer education as a means of spreading the Treatwell messages.

The Outcome   A food frequency questionnaire was used to measure dietary intake among a cohort of employees from both intervention and comparison worksites. Dietary fat intake decreased to a greater extent among employees in the intervention sites compared with the control sites; dietary fiber intake did not differ between the intervention and control worksites. Greater differences in dietary fat and fiber intake might have occurred with a longer programming period. This study provided evidence that a worksite-based nutrition intervention program can influence employees' dietary habits.[55]

Behavior Change and Entrepreneurship

No single theory or strategy is sufficient for changing eating habits, because food choices result from the complex interactions of individual, environmental, socio-

TABLE 8-6	**Summary of the Treatwell Program's Behavior Change Strategies**

PROGRAM FOCUS	BEHAVIOR CHANGE STRATEGIES			
	Promotion/ Motivation	Skills Training	Social Support	Maintenance/ Generalization
Individual	◆ Use members of employee advisory board as opinion leaders and role models. ◆ Organize a "kickoff" to introduce the program. ◆ Organize other worksite-wide programs such as a cholesterol screening, barbecue, holiday party, and taste tests. ◆ Offer incentives for behavior change (e.g., sponsor weight-loss competitions between departments, award prizes like T-shirts for meeting short-term goals).	◆ Distribute educational materials showing one or more Treatwell eating pattern messages. ◆ Implement "core" programs to build skills needed to purchase and prepare low-fat, high-fiber foods, read labels, and modify recipes.	◆ Build support for food behavior changes through brown-bag lunches, classes, and other program activities. ◆ Develop educational materials that employees can take home as a way to reinforce behavior changes in other environments. ◆ Have respected company leaders give testimonials about the program. ◆ Invite employees' families to participate in some events.	◆ Train members of the employee advisory board to teach other employees about the eating pattern messages. ◆ Encourage employees to use their new skills in other settings (e.g., grocery stores, restaurants, at home). ◆ Use point-of-purchase labeling and changes in menu selections to support program goals long term.
Environment	◆ Obtain support from top management. ◆ Develop a program logo and nutrition messages that can be used in worksite areas such as the cafeteria. ◆ Use posters, table tents, and other promotional items to disseminate nutrition messages.	◆ Teach low-fat, food purchasing, and serving practices to worksite foodservice managers. ◆ Label low-fat, high-fiber foods with the Treatwell logo in the cafeteria and vending machines.	◆ Use employee advisory board to encourage and support food behavior changes. ◆ Use the cafeteria as a focus for enhancing behavior change.	◆ Identify a corporate sponsor to serve as an advocate for the program within the organization. ◆ Build "ownership" through employee involvement in planning and implementing activities. ◆ Ensure visibility of the program. ◆ Develop an implementation manual. ◆ Tailor activities to worksite culture.

Source: G. Sorensen and coauthors, Promoting healthy eating patterns in the worksite: The Treatwell intervention model, *Health Education Research* 5 (1990): 505–15.

cultural, and biological factors. By using a variety of theories of human behavior to identify, explain, and predict the determinants of food consumption, you will be more effective in helping consumers adopt healthful eating habits.[56] A well-designed and well-executed effort to change eating patterns can make a difference. In Brazil, breastfeeding promotion programs resulted in a 12 percent reduction in infant mortality.[57] In addition to behavior change theories, you can draw on the two basic principles of entrepreneurship—creativity and innovation—to fashion a catchy jingle or slogan, create new action figures for young audiences, or use new educational media such as laser disk technology to help consumers acquire and maintain positive food-related behaviors. Entrepreneurial community nutritionists think of new ways to craft their nutrition messages, educational materials, and programs to reach their client base, especially high-risk groups and the underserved.

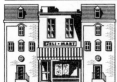

COMMUNITY LEARNING ACTIVITY

In this Community Learning Activity, you will choose behavior change strategies and dietary messages for your program's target population.

1. Describe some of the cultural, social, environmental, and individual factors that may affect their food consumption patterns. Base your conclusions on what you know about your population and the community in which you live now.

2. Develop three dietary messages for your target group. These should be explicit statements that will help your target audience make healthful dietary decisions and around which some of your marketing efforts can be built. (Consult the Treatwell eating pattern guidelines on page 260.)

3. For each dietary message, identify one strategy for achieving behavior change. Use any or all of the consumer behavior theories described in this chapter. Then, for each behavior change strategy, outline the primary intervention activities you plan to use. For example, your overall plan might look like this:

Dietary Message:	Choose low-fat dairy products.
Change Strategy:	Increase self-efficacy.
Behavior Theory:	Health Belief Model, Theory of Trying
Intervention Activities:	**1.** Develop education materials such as posters and table tents that show the fat content of dairy products.
	2. Identify barriers to choosing low-fat dairy products: e.g., consumers have never tasted low-fat dairy products such as yogurt.
	3. Develop strategies for removing barriers: e.g., conduct a taste test of low-fat yogurt and provide a recipe using the product.

4. Outline the factors that may prevent your dietary messages from being adopted by your target population (i.e., the barriers to diffusion of innovation).

5. Describe the factors you would need to consider in developing your intervention activities if your target population consisted of a particular ethnic group (for example, Latinos, Pakistanis, Asians).

The Art of Negotiating

Whether we like it or not, we are all negotiators. Every day of our lives, we negotiate with family, friends, and coworkers to get something we want. Although each of us negotiates something every day, most of us don't negotiate particularly well. We tend to find ourselves in situations where the negotiations leave us feeling frustrated, taken advantage of, dissatisfied, or just plain worn out. This is unfortunate, because negotiation is the heart of all business deals.

The reason why people sometimes emerge from negotiations feeling this way is that they tend to see only two ways to negotiate: hard or soft.[1] Hard negotiators view the other participants as adversaries. Their goal is victory—their side wins, while the other side loses. Hard negotiators tend to distrust the other party and make threats. They perceive the negotiation process as a contest of wills. Soft negotiators, by comparison, think of the participants as friends. Their goal is agreement among the parties. They tend to be trusting, avoid a battle of wills, change positions easily, and make concessions to maintain the relationship. Many of us use soft negotiation tactics in our dealings with our parents, siblings, friends, or other persons who are important to us.

Are these the only ways to negotiate? There is a better way to negotiate than either the soft or the hard approach, according to Roger Fisher and William Ury of the Harvard Negotiation Project. The method they developed is called *principled negotiation*. Its main precept is that a decision about an issue should be based on its merits, not on what each side says it will or will not do. The method can be boiled down to four basic elements:

◆ People—Separate the people from the problem.

◆ Interests—Focus on interests, not positions.

◆ Options—Generate a variety of possibilities before deciding what to do.

◆ Criteria—Insist that the result be based on some objective standard.

◆ SEPARATE THE PEOPLE FROM THE PROBLEM

When people sit down at the bargaining table, they bring with them certain perceptions about the relationships among the participants and about the problem itself. Whether these perceptions are accurate or false, they pervade the proceedings. There is a tendency to confuse the participants' relationships with the "issue" or "problem." One of the first steps to take in negotiating is to separate the problem from the people and deal with relationship and problem goals separately. This means thinking about how to get good results from the negotiation and what kind of relationship is likely to produce those results.

Another challenge to negotiating is having to deal with a problem when emotions are running high. People sometimes come to the bargaining table with strong feelings. They may be angry or frightened, feel threatened or misunderstood, or be worried about the outcome. A good way to handle the emotional aspect of the negotiation process is to recognize the emotions and give them legitimacy. The bottom line, write Fisher and Brown, is to "do only those things that are both good for the relationship and good for us."[2]

Continued

◆ PROFESSIONAL FOCUS—*Continued*

◆ FOCUS ON INTERESTS, NOT POSITIONS

The purpose of negotiating is to serve our interests. Interests motivate people to reach certain decisions. The primary problem in most negotiations is not the difference in positions, but the conflicts between the two sides' needs, fears, desires, and concerns—in other words, interests. In addition, most of us tend to think that the other party's interests are similar to our own. This is almost never the case. When negotiating, begin by defining, as precisely as possible, your own interests and allow the other participants to define theirs. Work through the discussion until mutual interests are identified.[3]

◆ CONSIDER A VARIETY OF OPTIONS

We sometimes approach a negotiating session with only one outcome in mind. We operate with blinders on and fail to see other dimensions to the problem that may be a source for possible solutions. To get around this barrier, bring the participants together to brainstorm about potential solutions and options. In a good brainstorming session, judgments about possible solutions are suspended, and everyone involved in the negotiation is allowed to contribute ideas. At the end of the session, the parties discuss the various options, picking several that offer the most promise. The parties then allow themselves time to evaluate each of these "best and brightest" ideas and consider which of them, if any, would best suit their purpose. Once again, when exploring options, consider the interests of both parties.

◆ USE OBJECTIVE CRITERIA

Suppose your roommate wants to buy your car, but you cannot agree on a price. She thinks your asking price is too high; you think her offer is too low. Where do you go from here? One option is to consult the Blue Book price for your car's make and model. Another is to examine the newspaper listings of used cars for sale to determine the asking price for cars like yours. These options are the criteria or standards that help you reach an agreement. The type of criteria you use will depend upon the nature of the issue being negotiated. In this case, the criterion was the fair market value of your car. In other situations, a court decision, tradition, precedent, scientific judgment, cost, or moral standard might serve as well. The important thing is to choose an objective standard that all parties are comfortable with.

◆ BUILD GOOD RELATIONSHIPS

The negotiating process is much like a tango—a little give and take on both sides. Regardless of the issue, a "good" negotiation is fueled by a good relationship. When next you enter into a negotiation, take a few minutes to evaluate your relationship with the other person or party. The questions in the boxed insert will help you determine how good your working relationship is and where improvements can be made. With practice you can help build good working relationships.

Continued

Does Our Relationship Work?

Do we want to work together?

In a good relationship, people want to work together. They respect each other and actively pursue strategies for sorting out differences. They work to keep problems to a minimum.

Are we reliable?

Good relationships are built on trust and constancy. All parties have confidence that verbal and written commitments will be kept. The parties work to allay any concerns about trustworthiness.

Do we understand each other?

Even in the best of working relationships, there will be differences of opinion, values, perceptions, and motives. In good relationships, the parties strive to accept each other and work toward understanding their differences.

Do we use our powers of persuasion effectively?

In good relationships, persuasion is used to influence and inform the other party about an issue or proposed action. The parties refrain from using coercive tactics and rely instead on rational, logical discussions of the merits of a particular position or action.

Do we communicate well?

Good communication is based on sound and compassionate reasoning. In good relationships, sensitive issues can be discussed in a supportive environment, one where candor is valued. The parties in a good relationship communicate often, consult each other before making decisions, and practice "active listening," where the parties work to hear each other with an open, flexible mind.

Sources: J. D. Batten, *Tough-Minded Leadership* (New York: AMACOM, 1989), pp. 122–32; M. DePree, *Leadership is an Art* (New York: Doubleday, 1989), pp. 89–96; and R. Fisher and S. Brown, *Getting Together—Building a Relationship That Gets to Yes* (Boston: Houghton Mifflin, 1988), pp. 178–79.

◆ WORK TOWARD SUCCESS

Good negotiating means that all parties leave the bargaining table feeling they have won. The successful negotiation is one in which the outcome meets both parties' interests. It is seen to be fair. The solution was arrived at with an efficient use of everyone's time. Neither party feels that they are at a disadvantage. And the solution will be implemented according

Continued

◆ PROFESSIONAL FOCUS—*Continued*

to plan. A successful negotiation leaves the parties feeling respect for their counterparts and a desire to work together again.[4]

1. The discussion of hard and soft negotiators was adapted from R. Fisher and W. Ury, *Getting to Yes—Negotiating Agreement without Giving In* (New York: Penguin Books, 1981), pp. 8–9.
2. The quotation was taken from R. Fisher and S. Brown, *Getting Together—Building a Relationship That Gets to Yes* (Boston: Houghton Mifflin, 1988), p. 38.
3. K. Albrecht and S. Albrecht, Added value negotiating, *Training* 30 (1993): 26–29.
4. J. Allan, Talking your way to success, *Accountancy* 111 (1993): 62–63.

NOTES

1. The man who put your groceries on wheels, *New York Post,* April 28, 1977, p. 37.
2. D. Cohen, *Consumer Behavior* (New York: Random House, 1981), p. 427.
3. As cited in B. Sternthal and C. S. Craig, *Consumer Behavior: An Information Processing Perspective* (Englewood Cliffs, N.J.: Prentice-Hall, 1982), pp. 6–7.
4. K. M. Bartol and D. C. Martin, *Management* (New York: McGraw-Hill, 1991), pp. 448–49.
5. M. L. Axelson, The impact of culture on food-related behavior, *Annual Review of Nutrition* 6 (1986): 345–63.
6. Life Sciences Research Office, Federation of American Societies for Experimental Biology, *Nutrition Monitoring in the United States: An Update Report on Nutrition Monitoring* (Washington, D.C.: U.S. Government Printing Office, DHHS Pub. No. 89–1255, 1989), p. 9.
7. G. H. Pelto, Anthropological contributions to nutrition education research, *Journal of Nutrition Education* 13 (1981): S2–S8.
8. W. L. Rathje and E. E. Ho, Meat fat madness: Conflicting patterns of meat fat consumption and their public health implications, *Journal of the American Dietetic Association* 87 (1987): 1357–62.
9. B. Senauer, E. Asp, and J. Kinsey, *Food Trends and the Changing Consumer* (St. Paul, Minn.: Eagan Press, 1991), pp. 133–53.
10. B. Senauer, Economics and nutrition, in *What Is America Eating?* (Washington, D.C.: National Academy Press, 1986), pp. 46–57.
11. M. Krondl and D. Lau, Social determinants in human food selection, in *The Psychobiology of Human Food Selection* (Westport, Conn.: AVI Publishing Company, 1982), pp. 139–51.
12. L. C. Medeiros and coauthors, Dietary practices and nutrition beliefs through the adult life cycle, *Journal of Nutrition Education* 25 (1993): 201–4.
13. F. J. Cronin and coauthors, Characterizing food usage by demographic variables, *Journal of the American Dietetic Association* 81 (1982): 661–73.
14. Senauer and coauthors, *Food Trends and the Changing Consumer,* pp. 92–94.
15. B. W. Hickman and coauthors, Nutrition claims in advertising: A study of four women's magazines, *Journal of Nutrition Education* 25 (1993): 227–35.
16. American Dietetic Association, *Survey of American Dietary Habits* (Chicago: American Dietetic Association, 1993).
17. F. J. Simoons, Geography and genetics as factors in the psychobiology of human food selection, in *The Psychobiology of Human Food Selection* (Westport, Conn.: AVI Publishing Company, 1982), pp. 205–24.
18. J. F. Pope and coauthors, Cravings and aversions of pregnant adolescents, *Journal of the American Dietetic Association* 92 (1992): 1479–82.
19. H. W. Lane and L. O. Schulz, Nutritional questions relevant to space flight, *Annual Review of Nutrition* 12 (1992): 257–78.
20. Cohen, *Consumer Behavior,* pp. 76–127.
21. K. D. Brownell, *The LEARN Program for Weight Control* (Dallas: American Health Publishing Company, 1991), pp. 76–77, 117–21.
22. The definition of culture was taken from *Webster's Ninth New Collegiate Dictionary* (Springfield, Mass.: Merriam-

Webster, 1988), p. 314.

23. A. Kilara and K. K. Iya, Food and dietary habits of the Hindu, *Food Technology* 46 (1992): 94–104.

24. J. Borah-Giddens and G. A. Falciglia, A meta-analysis of the relationship in food preferences between parents and children, *Journal of Nutrition Education* 25 (1993): 102–7.

25. Regional food preferences outlined in study of consumer eating trends, *Journal of the American Dietetic Association* 90 (1990): 1727.

26. American Dietetic Association, *Survey of American Dietary Habits,* p. 8.

27. I. M. Parraga, Determinants of food consumption, *Journal of the American Dietetic Association* 90 (1990): 661–63.

28. I. Ajzen and M. Fishbein, *Understanding Attitudes and Predicting Social Behavior* (Englewood Cliffs, N.J.: Prentice-Hall, 1980), pp. 13–27.

29. C. S. Wilson, Nutritionally beneficial cultural practices, *World Review of Nutrition and Dietetics* 45 (1985): 68–96.

30. American Dietetic Association and American Diabetes Association, *Ethnic and Regional Food Practices: Chinese American Food Practices, Customs, and Holidays* (Chicago: American Dietetic Association, 1990), pp. 2–3.

31. I. M. Rosenstock, The Health Belief Model: Explaining health behavior through expectancies, in *Health Behavior and Health Education—Theory, Research and Practice,* ed. K. Glanz, F. M. Lewis, and B. K. Rimer (San Francisco: Jossey-Bass, 1991), pp. 39–62.

32. A. Bandura, *Social Learning Theory* (Englewood Cliffs, N.J.: Prentice-Hall, 1977), p. 79.

33. R. B. Schafer and coauthors, Food safety: An application of the Health Belief Model, *Journal of Nutrition Education* 25 (1993): 17–24.

34. W. B. Carter, Health behavior as a rational process: Theory of Reasoned Action and Multiattribute Utility Theory, in *Health Behavior and Health Education,* pp. 63–91.

35. R. P. Bagozzi and Y. Yi, The degree of intention formation as a moderator of the attitude-behavior relationship, *Social Psychology Quarterly* 52 (1989): 266–79.

36. R. P. Bagozzi, The self-regulation of attitudes, intentions, and behavior, *Social Psychology Quarterly* 55 (1992): 178.

37. Ibid., pp. 178–204.

38. C. A. Pratt and coauthors, A multivariate analysis of the attitudinal and perceptual determinants of completion of a weight-reduction program, *Journal of Nutrition*

Education 24 (1992): 14–20.

39. D. B. Abrams and coauthors, Social learning principles for organizational health promotion: An integrated approach, in *Health and Industry—A Behavioral Medicine Perspective,* ed. M. F. Cataldo and T. J. Coates (New York: John Wiley & Sons, 1986), pp. 28–51.

40. T. Baranowski and coauthors, Increasing fruit and vegetable consumption among 4th and 5th grade students: Results from focus groups using reciprocal determinism, *Journal of Nutrition Education* 25 (1993): 114–20.

41. E. M. Rogers and F. F. Shoemaker, *Communication of Innovations—A Cross-Cultural Approach* (New York: Free Press, 1971).

42. As cited in Cohen, *Consumer Behavior,* pp. 429–30.

43. G. Macdonald, Communication theory and health promotion, in *Health Promotion,* ed. R. Bunton and G. Macdonald (New York: Routledge, 1992), p. 186.

44. A. Steckler and coauthors, Measuring the diffusion of innovative health promotion programs, *American Journal of Health Promotion* 6 (1992): 214–24.

45. S. Ram and J. N. Sheth, Consumer resistance to innovations: The marketing problem and its solutions, *Journal of Consumer Marketing* 6 (1989): 5–14.

46. C. E. Basch and E. M. Sliepcevich, Innovators, innovations and implementation: A framework for curricular research in school health education, *Health Education* 14 (1983): 20–24.

47. Abrams and coauthors, Social learning principles for organizational health promotion, pp. 29–31.

48. *Eating Right with the Dietary Guidelines* (Washington, D.C.: U.S. Department of Agriculture, 1991).

49. Department of Health and Human Services, Public Health Service, *Pretesting in Health Communications* (Bethesda, Md.: National Cancer Institute, NIH Pub. No. 84–1493, 1984), and J. Ruud and coauthors, Developing written nutrition information for adults with low literacy skills, *Journal of Nutrition Education* 25 (1993): 11–16.

50. Dietary fiber—What is it? (brochure), Kellogg Company, 1992.

51. G. Sorensen and coauthors, Promoting healthy eating patterns in the worksite: The Treatwell intervention model, *Health Education Research* 5 (1990): 505–15.

52. R. R. Butrum and coauthors, NCI dietary guidelines: Rationale, *American Journal of Clinical Nutrition* 48 (1988): 888–95.

53. G. Sorensen and coauthors, Work-site nutrition intervention and employees' dietary habits: The Treatwell Program, *American Journal of Public Health* 82 (1992): 877–80.

54. R. C. Lefebvre and coauthors, Theory and delivery of health programming in the community: The Pawtucket Heart Health Program, *Preventive Medicine* 16 (1987): 80–95.

55. M. K. Hunt and coauthors, Impact of a worksite cancer prevention program on eating patterns of workers, *Journal of Nutrition Education* 25 (1993): 236–44.

56. K. Glanz and J. Rudd, Views of theory, research, and practice: A survey of nutrition education and consumer behavior professionals, *Journal of Nutrition Education* 25 (1993): 269–73.

57. A. Berg, More resources for nutrition education: Strengthening the case, *Journal of Nutrition Education* 25 (1993): 278–82.

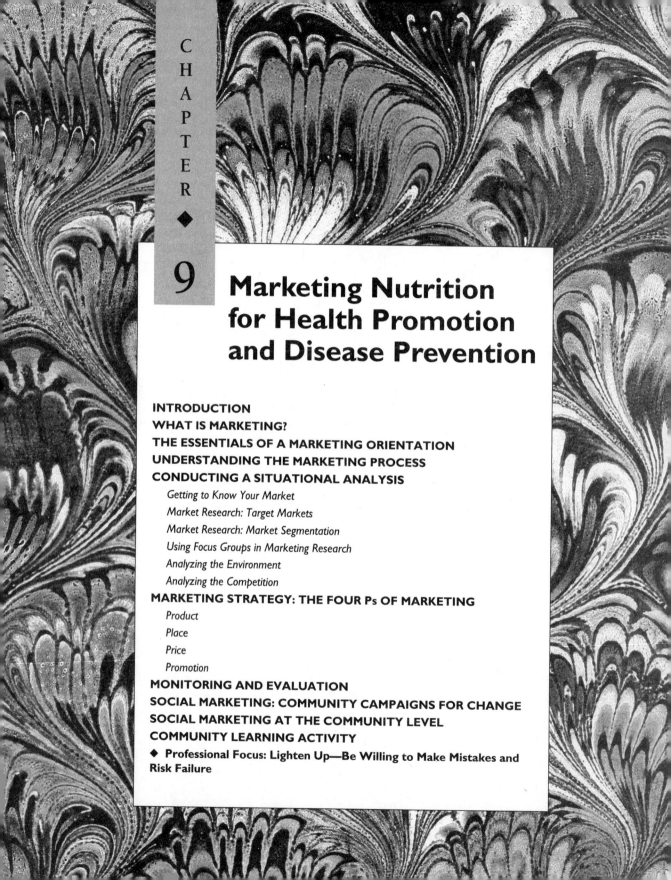

CHAPTER ◆ 9

Marketing Nutrition for Health Promotion and Disease Prevention

Something to Think About . . .

It is clear that social marketing and health education each has something to contribute to the promotion of more desirable health behavior. But what, where, and how much each has to contribute depends on the kind of health behavior being considered. . . . human health behavior is of such vast complexity and variability, is still so little understood, and so difficult to influence, that neither health education nor marketing has all the answers. Neither is fully effective with all kinds of health behavior, in all situations, with all populations, with all program objectives.

The two fields are not rivals but complementary, each contributing its own peculiar set of conceptual and operational skills and tools to the pursuit of the shared goal: improving the health of the public. The key to its achievement is pooling of skills and tools, learning from one another, and—collaboration.

—Godfrey Hochbaum

Introduction

On her way home from work, a New York woman hears a familiar jingle on the car radio reminding her which soap to use for beautiful skin. Halfway around the world, in a remote Sri Lankan village, another woman hears a message on the community radio that teaches her about oral rehydration therapy for her child's diarrhea. Both of these women are part of a target audience for a well-planned marketing campaign. But while the New York woman is listening to traditional Madison Avenue marketing, the woman in Sri Lanka is a "consumer" receiving a relatively new kind of message, grounded in social marketing.[1] The same basic principles lie behind both the commercial and the social approaches to marketing. The aim of both approaches is to strengthen the fit between the nutrition services and programs offered and the needs of the population. As you will see, marketing is for everyone, regardless of their job description. Whether you are a dietitian in private practice attempting to get physicians to refer clients to you, a public health nutritionist developing nutrition education materials for pregnant teens, or a wellness center dietitian trying to develop services for weight loss, you can use marketing strategies. In both business and public health, revenues and profits depend squarely on how well managers identify and meet consumer needs and problems. This chapter provides an overview of the basic marketing principles and strategies and shows how the effective use of marketing can lead to optimal nutrition programs and services for health promotion and disease prevention.

What Is Marketing?

Marketing The analysis, planning, implementation, and control of carefully formulated programs designed to bring about voluntary exchanges of value with target markets for the purpose of achieving organizational objectives. It relies heavily on designing the organization's offering in terms of the target market's needs and desires and on using effective pricing, communication, and distribution to inform, motivate, and service the market.

Buying and selling have a long history, but comprehensive and systematic marketing research developed only in recent decades.[2] Peter Drucker is credited with demonstrating the benefits of marketing to business. In the 1950s, he suggested that the primary focus of any business should be the consumer, not the product.[3]

Commercial **marketing** employs powerful techniques for selecting, producing, distributing, promoting, and selling an enormous array of goods and services to a wide variety of people in every possible political, social, and economic context.[4] Most people would agree that marketing works. Marketing creates products, positions them in the marketplace to meet consumer demand, makes the products available and affordable to particular segments, and motivates consumers to buy and use products by illuminating their benefits.[5] Simply stated, marketing is the process of identifying a need, assisting potential consumers or decision makers in recognizing that need, producing the product or service, and then letting people know that it is available.[6]

Marketing theory is based on a set of methods designed to reconcile an organization's resources with the needs and preferences of consumers. The relationship between the organization and consumer can be viewed as an exchange in which something of value, such as a product or service, is offered to someone who is willing to give something else of value, such as money or time, for it.[7] For example, a community health agency trades services for improved health status in the community. Five familiar examples of exchange relationships are illustrated in Figure 9-1. Many health care organizations engage in exchange relationships much more complex than those depicted in Figure 9-1. Figure 9-2 provides an example. Marketing provides a framework for analyzing, predicting, and managing these exchanges for the benefit of all concerned.[8]

The Essentials of a Marketing Orientation

Marketing is more than just advertising or "selling" oneself or one's program and services as a professional. Too often, people mistakenly believe that an organization that includes a marketing department or hires a market research consultant or advertising agency has become market-oriented. In reality, the organization may have any of three other orientations instead.

A **production orientation** holds that the major task of an organization is to pursue efficiency in production and distribution.

A **product orientation** holds that the major task of an organization is to deliver products, programs, and services it thinks would be good for the market.

Some organizations and businesses have a **production orientation**—they emphasize a smoothly run and efficient production process. Consider the billing offices of third-party insurance companies where customers often report being identified and treated as a number, or the busy primary care clinic where patients wait for long periods so that physicians may maximize their efficiency by seeing a large number of patients.[9]

Other organizations take a more paternalistic approach and focus on their product. The health care field in general has been criticized for having a **product**

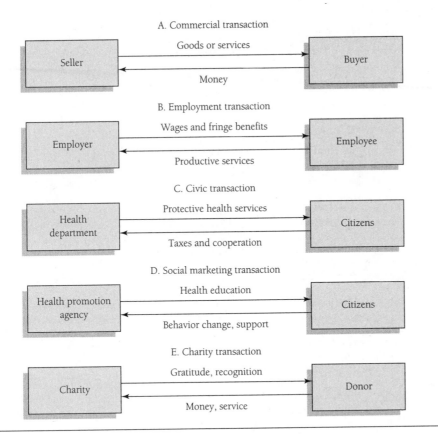

A. Commercial transaction

Seller → Goods or services → Buyer

Buyer → Money → Seller

B. Employment transaction

Employer → Wages and fringe benefits → Employee

Employee → Productive services → Employer

C. Civic transaction

Health department → Protective health services → Citizens

Citizens → Taxes and cooperation → Health department

D. Social marketing transaction

Health promotion agency → Health education → Citizens

Citizens → Behavior change, support → Health promotion agency

E. Charity transaction

Charity → Gratitude, recognition → Donor

Donor → Money, service → Charity

FIGURE 9-1

Examples of Exchange Relationships

Source: Reprinted with permission from P. Kotler and R. N. Clarke, *Marketing for Health Care Organizations* (Englewood Cliffs, N.J.: Prentice-Hall, 1987), p. 48.

orientation. ("We know better than you what is good for you.") Health providers often begin with a program like weight reduction in mind and suspend analysis of the consumer until later.[10] A successful marketing model first researches the wants and needs of the consumer and only then formulates a program, as illustrated in Figure 9-3 on page 275. Still other organizations take a **sales orientation** and attempt to increase the size of their **market** by focusing on promotional techniques. These orientations are referred to as "push" marketing because an agency "pushes" its ideas, services, or products onto consumers.[11]

Organizations with a production, product, or sales orientation are likely to fail because they are trying to sell a product (service, program, or idea) that is not matched to consumers' needs and preferences.[12] Market theory holds that the only effective form of marketing involves a consumer or **marketing orientation.** This approach focuses on satisfying consumers' changing needs and wants. Marketing's concentration on the consumer is its greatest asset and the largest contribution that the marketing discipline can bring to any public health or community program.[13] This type of orientation is sometimes referred to as "pull" marketing because consumers "pull" certain ideas, products, or services out of agencies.[14]

A **sales orientation** holds that the main task of an organization is to stimulate the interest of potential consumers in products and services.

Market Potential customers for a product or service.

A **marketing orientation** holds that the main task of the organization is to determine the needs and wants of target markets and to satisfy them through the design, communication, pricing, and delivery of appropriate and competitively viable products and services.

FIGURE

9-2

An Example of a Complex Exchange Transaction

Source: Adapted from P. Kotler and R. N. Clarke, *Marketing for Health Care Organizations* (Englewood Cliffs, N.J.: Prentice-Hall, 1987), p. 49.

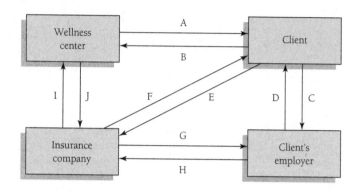

A. The wellness center provides nutrition services to the client.
B. The client provides direct payment and/or guarantee of payment from a third party to the wellness center. In addition, the client utilizes other components of the wellness center (aerobics class, stress management workshop), which the wellness center encourages.
C. The client, as an employee, provides productive work services to the employer.
D. The employer provides monetary compensation for work services, plus partial coverage for the employee's health benefits and insurance.
E. The client makes monthly payments for health insurance beyond that paid by her employer.
F. The insurance company guarantees partial coverage for the client's preventive health services at the wellness center.
G. The insurance company provides a mechanism by which the employer can offer health insurance to the employee's group.
H. The employer makes monthly payments to the insurance company.
I. The insurance company reimburses the wellness center for services rendered.
J. The wellness center guarantees that services will be provided in a cost-efficient manner so that the insurance company will not end up paying out more in reimbursements than it has attracted in payments.

Understanding the Marketing Process

Strategic marketing The process of developing, implementing, and evaluating the strategic fit between the goals and resources of an organization and the needs and wants of a target audience.

Target market One particular market segment pinpointed as a primary customer group.

Strategic **marketing**, which is consumer-oriented as opposed to product-oriented, involves three fundamental steps:[15]

1. A research and analysis component in which the potential markets, environment, and competition are identified and analyzed and **target markets** are selected

2. An implementation or operational component in which programs are elaborated and the **marketing mix** is developed

3. An evaluation and control component in which the exchange relationship is monitored and appropriate corrective actions are taken as needed

These steps are analyzed in detail in the next sections and summarized in Figure 9-4 on page 276.

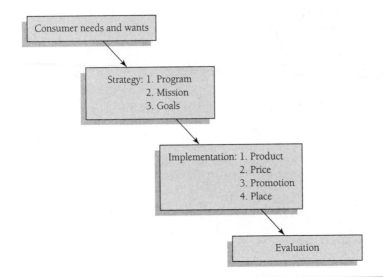

FIGURE

9-3

A Marketing Planning Model for Health Promotion with a Consumer Orientation
Source: Adapted from S. C. Parks and D. L. Moody, A marketing model: Applications for dietetic professionals. © The American Dietetic Association. Reprinted with permission from *Journal of the American Dietetic Association* 86 (1986): 40.

Conducting a Situational Analysis

A situational analysis is a detailed assessment of the environment including an evaluation of the consumer, the competition, and any other factors that may affect the program or business.[16] This step, which is critical to the ultimate success of the entire marketing plan, is sometimes referred to as a SWOT analysis. SWOT, an acronym for strengths, weaknesses, opportunities, and threats, requires a description of the present state of the business or agency, including its strengths and weaknesses, programs, and services, as well as the threats and opportunities present in the external environment (competition, pending legislation, and the like).[17]

◆ GETTING TO KNOW YOUR MARKET

The first step in the marketing process is the identification and analysis of all consumers—one's current and potential markets. Consumers can be categorized as one of three types: users of services, referral sources, or other decision makers.[18] The users of services are the clients themselves or potential consumers. For example, the WIC program identifies its users as low-income pregnant or breast-feeding women and mothers of children under five years of age. The National Dairy Council targets a different market—"leader groups," such as educators, dietitians, health teachers, and dental hygienists.[19]

Referral sources include anyone who refers clients or customers to you. They may include physicians, social workers, teachers, former clients, and others. Other decision makers are those who influence the client's decision to use a ser-

Marketing mix Four universal elements of marketing that are often called the "four Ps"—product, price, place, and promotion. Product encompasses the range of services offered; price encompasses the monetary and intangible value of the product; place refers to where the product is available; promotion is persuasive communication aimed at targeted users.

SWOT An acronym that stands for strengths, weaknesses, opportunities, and threats. A situational analysis technique often used in market research.

FIGURE

9-4

The Strategic Marketing Process

Market research: Conduct a situational analysis
- Identify program mission and goals
- Identify nutrition or health problem
- Identify market segments
- Select and analyze target market
- Analyze competition
- SWOT: Identify strengths, weaknesses, opportunities, and threats
- Describe market niche

Market strategy: Design and implement the appropriate marketing mix to the target market
- Set objectives and goals
- Develop strategies for each element of marketing mix:
  - Product
  - Price
  - Place
  - Promotion
- Develop a timetable for achieving objectives
- Specify the resources required
- Determine the activities needed

Marketing control: Monitor and evaluate results
- Measure results
- Evaluate cost-effectiveness
- Take corrective action
- Reevaluate objectives and marketing strategy
- Make changes as needed

vice or join a program. Such people would include family members (spouses, parents) and third-party payers, among others. It is important to identify these three types of users for your particular setting.

The next step in your analysis is to identify what your consumers want and need. Table 9-1 provides an example of this type of analysis. What are your clients' characteristics, problems, and special needs? What benefits do they desire? Written questionnaires, telephone surveys, direct interviews, and focus groups can be used to gather information about your consumers. A later section of the chapter discusses these market research tools in more detail.

◆ MARKET RESEARCH: TARGET MARKETS

An inherent part of the situational analysis is to determine and target your clients or audiences. Each target market should be viewed as a separate and different audience. For example, one survey of dietitians in private practice found they listed the following as their target populations.[20]

TYPE	CONSUMERS	CHARACTERISTICS	BENEFITS
Users	Men at risk for coronary heart disease (CHD)	Age 40+ with history of CHD and/or known risk factor	Improved quality of life; decreased risk of CHD
Referral sources	Cardiologists Other physicians Social workers Former clients	Health care providers	Improved care of patient; delayed CHD development
Decision makers	Spouse/significant other	Age 40+	Want spouse to be "healthy"

TABLE

9-1

Worksheet to Identify Your Consumers

Source: Adapted from C. B. Matthews, Marketing your services: Strategies that work, *ASHA Magazine* 30 (1988): 23.

◆ Overweight women between 20 and 40 years

◆ Athletic men

◆ Middle-class women for weight reduction

◆ People interested in sports nutrition

◆ People in need of modification of diet and lifestyle

◆ Individuals wanting basic nutrition information and modified diets

◆ Physicians for referrals

◆ Corporations to provide employee workshops

Ideally, if resources are available, you would want to develop a specific marketing mix for each target audience. Once a population group has been identified for targeting, it is important to determine its prevailing patterns of lifestyle, eating, drinking, working conditions, attitudes toward nutrition and health, and current and past state of health.[21]

Most programs or organizations find it unrealistic to service the total target market effectively. For this reason, actual and potential markets should be divided further into distinct and homogeneous subgroups, a process called **market segmentation**. Market segmentation offers the following benefits:[22]

◆ A more precise definition of consumer needs and behavior patterns

◆ Improved identification of ways to provide services to population groups

◆ More efficient utilization of nutrition and health education resources through a better fit between products, programs, and services and consumers

Market segmentation The separation of large groups of potential clients into smaller groups with similar characteristics. Advantages include simpler, more accurate analysis of each group's needs and more customized delivery of service.

As an example of market segmentation, consider as your potential market, the population of adults 45 years or older—sometimes referred to as 45+ consumers. This total market can be divided into several more homogeneous parts, some of which are shown in Figure 9-5. Each of these segments can then be reached with a distinct marketing strategy (to be discussed shortly).

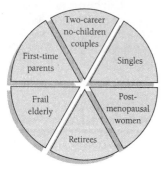

◆ MARKET RESEARCH: MARKET SEGMENTATION

Market research enables community nutritionists to target specific groups for health promotion and disease prevention in terms of their geography, demography, and psychography. This type of analysis is helpful in many ways: (1) targeting those at risk, (2) carrying out strategic marketing planning, (3) developing marketing media strategies, (4) examining the feasibility of various promotional tools (e.g., direct mailing of nutrition education materials), or (5) determining the appropriate mix of nutrition programs and services to offer based on demographics (e.g., concentration of women, infants, children, and the elderly).

Three classes of variables are typically used for market segmentation:[23]

1. Geographical segmentation refers to the grouping of people according to the location of their residence or work (region, county, census tract). This can be done on a simple geographical basis or according to other variables, such as population density or climate.

2. Demographic segmentation is the grouping of individuals on the basis of such variables as age, sex, income, occupation, education, family size, religion, or race.

3. Psychographic segmentation is based on such criteria as personal values, attitudes, opinions, personality, behavior, lifestyle, level of readiness for change, and benefits sought.

An understanding of demographics is essential to the development and targeting of nutrition and public health programs. Consider the public health agency or wellness center with programs attempting to promote such products as smoking cessation, low-fat diets, fitness programs, maternal-infant care, cancer prevention, hypertension screening, diabetes education, infant mortality reduction, and prevention of AIDS.[24] The community agency or wellness center must first analyze the demographics of the areas served by these programs in order to identify its clients. The information to categorize and examine includes the following:

◆ Total population of the area that the program is intended to serve
◆ Rate of change of the population
◆ Age and sex distribution
◆ Racial, ethnic, and religious composition
◆ Socioeconomic status
◆ Housing information
◆ Fertility patterns

Of these, age distribution of the population, trends over time, and fertility rates are particularly important to public health nutrition programs. Major segmentation variables for consumer markets are given in Table 9-2. Figure 9-6 summarizes the steps required for market segmentation and target marketing.

Obviously, the first step in the marketing plan—the situational analysis—demands a significant amount of market research. This research includes the use

VARIABLE	TYPICAL BREAKDOWNS
Geographical	
Region	Pacific, Mountain, West North Central, West South Central, East North Central, East South Central, South Atlantic, Middle Atlantic, New England
County size	A, B, C, D
City size	Under 5,000, 5,000–20,000, 20,000–50,000, 50,000–100,000, 100,000–250,000, 250,000–500,000, 500,000–1,000,000, 1,000,000–4,000,000, over 4,000,000
Density	Urban, suburban, rural
Climate	Northern, southern
Demographic	
Age	Under 6, 6–11, 12–19, 20–34, 35–49, 50–64, 65+
Sex	Male, female
Family size	1–2, 3–4, 5+
Family life cycle	Young, single; young, married, no children; young, married, youngest child under 6; young, married, youngest child 6 or over; older, married, with children; older, married, no children under 18; older, single; other
Income	Under $2,500, $2,500–$5,000, $5,000–$7,500, $7,500–$10,000, $10,000–$15,000, $15,000–$20,000, $20,000–$30,000, $30,000–$50,000, over $50,000
Occupation	Professional and technical; managers, officials, and proprietors; clerical, sales; artisans, forepersons; operatives; farmers; retired; students; homemakers; unemployed
Education	Grade school or less, some high school, graduated high school, some college, graduated college
Religion	Catholic, Protestant, Jewish, other
Race	Asian, Black, Hispanic, Native American, White
Nationality	American, British, French, German, Italian, Japanese, Latin American, Middle Eastern, Scandinavian
Social class	Lower lower, upper lower, lower middle, upper middle, lower upper, upper upper
Psychographic	
Lifestyle	Straight, swinger, longhair, yuppie, conservative, liberal
Personality	Compulsive, gregarious, authoritarian, ambitious, leader, follower, independent, dependent
Behavioristic	
Purchase occasion	Regular occasion, special occasion
Benefits sought	Quality, service, economy, convenience, health
User status	Nonuser, ex-user, potential user, first-time user, regular user
Usage rate	Light user, medium user, heavy user
Loyalty status	None, medium, strong, absolute
Readiness stage	Unaware, aware, informed, interested, desirous, intending to buy
Attitude toward product	Enthusiastic, positive, indifferent, negative, hostile

TABLE 9-2

Major Segmentation Variables for Consumer Markets

Source: Adapted from P. Kotler and R. N. Clarke, *Marketing for Health Care Organizations* (Englewood Cliffs, N.J.: Prentice-Hall, 1987), p. 237.

of both primary (direct) and secondary (indirect) data. Primary data are new data collected for the first time through random sampling surveys, questionnaires and qualitative methods such as personal interviews and focus groups. Table 9-3 describes five methods frequently used to collect primary data about a market.

**FIGURE
9-6**

**Steps in Market
Segmentation and
Target Marketing**
Source: Reprinted with permission
from P. Kotler and R. N. Clarke,
*Marketing for Health Care
Organizations* (Englewood Cliffs, N.J.:
Prentice-Hall, 1987), p. 234.

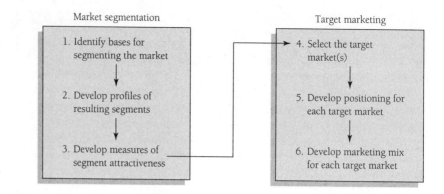

Secondary data are data gathered by somebody else (census data, food consumption surveys, marketing surveys, national polls). Fortunately, some of the data and information that you require for a thorough situational analysis already exist and can be obtained from a number of sources (see Table 9-4). For example, the U.S. Bureau of the Census makes census data available for any given zip code or geographic region. The information contains age, sex, household size, household income, and population growth data.

A number of vendors also provide information about various segments of a population based on demographics, geography, and psychographics. Each vendor has a clustering system that groups individuals on the basis of like characteristics.

◆ USING FOCUS GROUPS IN MARKETING RESEARCH

Qualitative research is frequently used to generate information needed for program design. Focus groups, used in conjunction with formal quantitative surveys, are a popular way to conduct informal qualitative research. Focus groups are useful for probing for the underlying reasons for consumer beliefs or attitudes toward a program or the competition and for pretesting the effectiveness of advertising copy or other promotional tools for a new program or service.

In a focus group interview, a trained moderator guides a small group discussion to gain insights into participants' attitudes, perceptions, and opinions on a designated topic. The group's composition and the discussion are carefully planned to create a permissive, nonthreatening environment conducive to revelation and disclosure. Participants are encouraged to express differing perceptions, ask questions, and respond to comments of other participants, as well as to those presented by the moderator. After several discussions are conducted with groups comprised of similar types of participants, patterns can be identified in participants' attitudes and other factors that influence their opinions of the research topic.[25]

Focus groups can help marketers identify lifestyle variables that will be most appealing in promoting an idea, program, or product or uncover the real reasons why people will not try a product or adopt a practice.[26] The loosely structured interview format encourages this process. In contrast to more structured survey

METHOD	DESCRIPTION
Mail survey	The most frequently used technique in market research; often misused. Tips to improve reliability: Use homogeneous sample, keep length reasonable, pretest and rewrite as necessary.
Telephone survey	Can involve errors as in mail surveys. Helpful to ask: Is the true meaning of the question being reflected by the interviewer, or is it distorted? Is the wording of the question likely to elicit a biased response?
Personal interview	A recommended supplement to mail or telephone surveys; helpful in observing subtle feedback that would otherwise be unavailable.
Consumer panel	Often used to test new products using the same persons in several tests; a problem is that panel members do not always represent the buying population and may not always give honest answers.
Focus group	Frequently used to gather information from small homogeneous groups; allows the researcher to see how people view a product, intervention, or other issue; serves as a communications bridge between the researcher and the people the researcher is trying to reach; not to be used to persuade, convince, or reach a consensus.

TABLE

9-3

Methods Used to Collect Primary Data

Source: Adapted from S. C. Parks, Research techniques used to support marketing management decisions, in *Research: Successful Approaches,* ed. E. R. Monsen (Chicago: American Dietetic Association, 1992), pp. 308–10. © The American Dietetic Association. Reprinted with permission.

methods that use closed-ended questions, focus groups use a general guide that presents ideas or broad topics for discussion. Participants can respond in their own terms rather than being forced to respond to predetermined categories.

General guidelines for conducting a focus group interview can be summarized as follows:[27]

1. Establish a question guide rather than a questionnaire for the moderator to use in stimulating response and discussion.

2. Phrase the questions so that they will elicit more than merely yes-or-no answers and are directed more to what people do, how they feel, and what they think than to factual responses.

3. Listen to the answers; the way things are said may be as important as the answers themselves in that nuances of expression, mood, and word choice may stimulate new directions for the exchange or reveal richer attitudinal information.

4. Formulate new questions stemming from the responses to stimulate others to react.

5. If participants are reluctant or hesitant, employ the indirect device of asking a question about a third person rather than asking the respondent directly.

6. Tape record the entire discussion so that it can be reviewed to capture gems of insight that may be overlooked during the session.

The general advantages and disadvantages of qualitative and quantitative research are listed in Table 9-5 on page 283. Focus groups, in particular, have several limitations, as listed on the next page.

TABLE
9-4

How to Collect Secondary Marketing Research Data

Source: S. C. Parks, Research techniques used to support marketing management decisions, in *Research: Successful Approaches,* ed. E. R. Monsen (Chicago: American Dietetic Association, 1992), p. 306. © The American Dietetic Association. Reprinted with permission.

1. Start by consulting the most promising guides, i.e., *Reader's Guide to Periodical Literature, The New York Times Index,* the *Business Periodicals Index,* and the *Index to Health Care Literature.* These indexes will provide access to current business literature.
2. Refer to the Standard Industrial Classification (SIC) Manual to obtain SIC codes. These will allow you to access specific statistics for particular industries in both printed and on-line databases.
3. Use free government information sources, e.g., Department of Commerce, Bureau of the Census, Department of Aging, and National Institutes of Health. The federal government prepares three census reports—population, housing, and business. State, county, and local governments have similar statistics.
4. Learn about other government sources. The *American Statistics Index, Statistical Abstract of the United States,* and *Survey of Current Business* are excellent sources of business and general economic statistics.
5. Check state and local (city or county) government sources. Start by writing to the state departments of commerce, development, or libraries. At the local level, try city or county planning offices and the economic development commission; they generally have data on present and future growth plans.
6. Use business and professional associations. The American Dietetic Association, the National Center for Nutrition and Dietetics, and the National Agricultural Library are excellent food and nutrition sources.
7. Check directories, such as *Dun and Bradstreet, Moody's Manuals,* and *Thomas Register.* These sources will provide data on various organizations and businesses in a given market area.
8. Check other sources of commercial printed information. The *Sales Management Annual Survey of Buying Power* provides local information on population, income, retail (including eating and drinking establishments), and an index of market potential. *Restaurants and Institutions* magazine publishes market surveys, generally in the July and October issues. *Gallup Poll* publishes studies about food, eating habits, and health trends on an annual basis.
9. Learn about existing databases and data banks that can provide useful demographic, buyer behavior and psychographic data. There are more than 5000 on-line data banks that have both general and specific information. To access them, check *Directory of On-Line Information Resources* (CSG Press, Rockville, Maryland) and *Database Catalog* (Dialog, Palo Alto, California).
10. Select the right specialist to work with. Information brokers provide such services on a fee basis. Many public and university libraries offer database searches for a minimal fee. Your local library should, at a minimum, be able to tell you where to go to access the information.

Limitations of focus group interviews include:

◆ The small sample size

◆ Potential bias and variability in the skill of the moderator

◆ Possibility of confusing qualitative with quantitative results

◆ Subjectivity in analyzing results

RESEARCH	ADVANTAGES	DISADVANTAGES
◆ Qualitative		
Focus group	Helps understand consumers' perspectives	Not able to generalize to larger populations
Interview/ convenience sample	Taps issues most important to consumers; acquires knowledge of consumers' vocabulary; taps issues unforeseen by investigator	
◆ Quantitative		
Questionnaire/ random sample	Enables generalizations to be made to larger populations	Limits responses to what investigators themselves think important; question wording can lead to respondents' misunderstanding

TABLE

9-5

General Advantages and Disadvantages of Qualitative and Quantitative Research

Source: B. E. Cogswell and coauthors, A method for investigating consumers' perspectives on health care, *Journal of Health Care Marketing* 5 (1985): 56. © American Marketing Association. Used with permission.

◆ ANALYZING THE ENVIRONMENT

The final step in the situational analysis is to identify any external environmental factors or social trends that may influence the needs of the program or organization. Such issues include health care reform, legislative and regulatory changes, shifting demographics, and the competition. For example, a declining birth rate and a growing population of older people are affecting the composition of many communities. Changes in the typical family, including older, first-time parents, the high divorce rate, and increasing numbers of working mothers, also affect the needs of a given community.

The general age of the target area is also influential in determining needed programs. In an area largely inhabited by retirement-age people, classes on prenatal nutrition counseling will have far less impact than, for instance, a class on heart-healthy cooking for one or two. Another significant trend is the maturing of the baby boom generation, which must be considered when developing or expanding any public health program. Figure 9-7 tracks the changing nature of this generation.

◆ ANALYZING THE COMPETITION

Once you have a thorough understanding of your consumers, you must determine how your existing competitors are positioned in the marketplace. What are their strengths and weaknesses (see Table 9-6 on page 286)? What is the attitude of your target market toward the competition?

Your aim is to find a **market niche** for your program or service in which your strengths can be matched with the needs of your particular target market. To satisfy those needs, you must know and understand your target audience so well that your service provides the perfect fit and "sells" itself, setting you apart from other providers in the same market and improving your **competitive edge**.

Market niche The particular area of service or the particular product suited to the specific clients to be reached. The underlying philosophy is that you cannot be all things to all people, so you must find the spot that fits your objectives and goals and enables you to meet a particular unmet need.

Competitive edge An advantage over others in the business, gained through use of business strategies, market research, expert management, new product development, or other sound business techniques.

FIGURE
9-7

Tracking the Baby Boom Generation

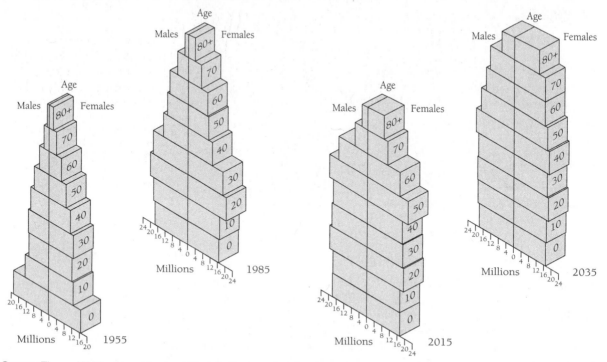

Source: Thomas W. Merrick and Stephen J. Tordella, Demographics: People and Markets, *Population Bulletin* Vol. 43, No. 1 (Washington, D.C.: Population Reference Bureau, Inc., 1988).

Examples of niches include your area of expertise, professional image, size, location, and customer service. You will want your target market to perceive that it can benefit from using your services as opposed to those of your competition.

Marketing Strategy: The Four Ps of Marketing

The marketing process involves four distinct groups of elements traditionally known as the four Ps: product, place, price, and promotion. These four elements make up what is called the marketing mix (see Figure 9-8 on page 287). The marketing mix is involved in any purchase decision. For example, every time you buy a box of "Shredded Wheat" rather than a box of "Cheerios," you purchase it at a competitive price in a grocery store, possibly due to a television advertisement. Such a sale was the result of a marketing strategy made months before by Nabisco Brands regarding the issues of product, price, place, and promotion.

The development of the appropriate marketing mix should result directly from the previous step of the marketing process—the analysis of the consumer,

---

Understanding Baby Boomers

Baby boomers, or the approximately 77 million individuals who were born between 1946 and 1964, represent almost one-third of the U.S. population. By virtue of their large numbers, baby boomers are a driving force for current and future trends. An understanding of their preferences, character, lifestyle, and location is and will continue to be critical to public health marketing. In 1991, the first of this generation turned 45, and in 2029, the last of the baby boomers will turn 65.

Although there are several subsets of baby boomers, some general characteristics can be noted:*

◆ Boomers have the power to change the marketplace. Due to their numbers and affluence, they are able to drive trends, especially as they age. Of importance to nutritionists, these consumers are generally concerned about what is healthful and convenient.

◆ Boomers make decisions based upon personal beliefs and want to be empowered. They prefer programs that offer information and options in a learner-involved format, such as a supermarket tour.

◆ Boomers are constantly pressed for time as they juggle careers, child care, home responsibilities, and leisure activities. Programs need to be practical and convenient and should be presented in an understandable format.

◆ Boomers look for value and quality in their investments and are becoming thriftier with age. They seek information on how to relate market choices to value.

◆ Boomers will not age gracefully. Programs must be upbeat and dynamic for these on-the-go consumers.

◆ Boomers like nostalgia. Nostalgia can be used to reinforce nutrition messages, for example, modifying traditional family recipes and holiday menus to reflect current nutritional advice.

*The Boomer Report 2, no. 4, 5, 6, 7 (1990), and S. T. Borra, Food and nutrition education for baby boomers: Challenges and opportunities, Nutrition News 54 (1991): 5–6.

---

environment, and competition. Once the needs of the target audience have been identified and analyzed, the set of four Ps can be constructed. The primary focus of the four Ps is the identified target market. Successful marketers get the right product, service, or program to the right place at the right time for the right price.[28]

The marketing mix must be adapted for each target market for marketing to be effective. Consider, for example, the community nutritionist in a community health education program who decides to utilize recently received grant money to offer a series of nutrition classes to the public. After thoroughly researching the community's interests and preferences, he develops a series of classes called "Monday Night Nutrition." The series includes the following sessions:

Session 1. How to Separate Nutrition Fact from Fiction

Session 2. Understanding Eating Disorders

Worksheet for Analyzing the Competition

Source: Adapted from C. B. Matthews, Marketing your services: Strategies that work, *ASHA Magazine* 30 (1988): 23.

COMPETITOR	STRENGTHS	WEAKNESSES	MY COMPETITIVE ADVANTAGE
Wellness center	Great location	Large and diverse; no known specialty	I specialize in cardiovascular nutrition counseling.
Sports medicine clinic	Personable staff	Outdated brochures and videos; nearly impossible to find parking	I maintain up-to-date educational resources; I travel to the client in my "Nutritionist-on Wheels" mobile.

Session 3. Eating for the Nineties: Vegetarian Style

Session 4. Eating for Two: Nutrition and Pregnancy

Session 5. Heart-Healthy Nutrition: Where's the Fat?

Session 6. Nutrition for the Weekend Athlete

Session 7. Never Say Diet: Achieving Healthful Body Weight

Session 8. Eating in the Fast Lane: Nutritious Fast Foods

Note that each session addresses a different target market (e.g., vegetarians, session 3; pregnant women, session 4; those with heart disease, session 5; weight-loss seekers, session 7). A different marketing mix strategy will be needed to address the special needs and preferences of each of these target markets. The following sections discuss the points to consider when developing a marketing mix for a particular target market.

Once you have completed your situational analysis and designed a **marketing strategy** (see Table 9-7 on page 288), it is helpful to draw up a position statement about yourself or your product or program that includes the following:[29]

Marketing strategy The selection of a target market, the choice of a competitive position, and the development of an effective marketing mix to reach and serve the chosen customers.

◆ A definition of the target market

◆ A definition of the benefits you provide—both tangible and intangible

◆ A description of what distinguishes your service from the other services available in the same market

◆ PRODUCT

Product Anything offered in the marketplace to be exchanged for money or something of value. It may be either a tangible good or a service.

The term **product** refers to all of the characteristics of the product or service that are to be exchanged with the target market. Characteristics such as style, special features, packaging, quality, brand names, and options must be designed to fit the needs and preferences of the target market. From a marketing standpoint, the product or service—whether it's a new automobile, diet soft drink, or nutrition class for a congregate meal site—is viewed as a collection of tangible and intangible attributes that may be offered to a market to satisfy a want or need.[30]

In community nutrition, the product is often a service to be delivered. These services should be of high quality, tailored to fit the needs of the target market,

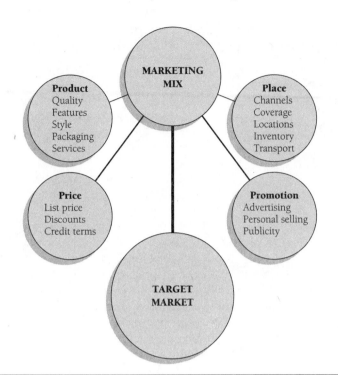

FIGURE

9-8

The Four Ps of the Marketing Mix

Source: Reprinted with permission from M. Ward, *Marketing Strategies: A Resource for Registered Dietitians* (Binghamton, N.Y.: Niles & Phipps, 1984), p. 111.

and adapted to meet the consumers' social characteristics (e.g., culture, ethnicity, language skills). A group of dietitians in private practice delineated their services as including individual counseling for modified diets, weight reduction, sports nutrition, normal nutrition, prenatal diets, and eating disorders; group programs and workshops on nutrition topics; consulting services to schools, health care facilities, supermarkets, health spas, and restaurants; and teaching courses at community colleges and universities.[31]

◆ PLACE

Place refers to the actual location where the exchange takes place. Accessibility, convenience, and comfort for the client are the criteria to consider. Are your hours of operation convenient and flexible? Is parking available?

Place also includes the channels of distribution required to deliver the service or product to the consumer. The distribution channels are the intermediaries—individuals, facilities, or agencies—that control or influence the consumer's choice of service or product.[32] Health providers, employers, school boards, voluntary health organizations, shopping malls, and commercial retailers are a few of the important intermediaries for community nutritionists. They are viewed as channels for reaching identified target markets.

In other instances, distribution channels are more like "gatekeepers"—you cannot reach your target except by going through them. Physicians, parents, media program directors, corporate executives, members of Congress, and insur-

TABLE

9-7

A Marketing Strategy Worksheet

Source: Reprinted with permission from M. Ward, *Marketing Strategies: A Resource for Registered Dietitians* (Binghamton, N.Y.: Niles & Phipps, 1984), p. 111.

MARKETING PROCESS	EXAMPLE
Target market	Individuals with the desire to lose weight
Nutrition services	Weight control and counseling Objectives: ◆ Behavior modification to change eating habits ◆ Increased activity level ◆ Gradual weight loss of 1–2 lb. per week
Price	$30 per hour
Place	Dietitian's office
Promotion	◆ Yellow pages ◆ Newspaper ads ◆ Brochures to doctors' offices ◆ Talks to groups
Competition	◆ Hospital outpatient dietitian ◆ Weight Watchers ◆ Diet Center ◆ TOPS ◆ Health spa

ance company decision makers can all be gatekeepers, depending on the service offering and target audience. The overall marketing strategy may include one approach for the client and a different approach to reach the intermediary or gatekeeper.

Distribution channels vary depending on the target market and service provided. Since third-party reimbursement by insurance companies for nutrition services usually requires a physician referral, a dietitian in private practice may want to target obstetricians, cardiologists, or other medical practice groups identified as distribution channels. Another approach the dietitian might take is to target insurance companies or state legislators in an effort to change the current third-party reimbursement system. A wellness program dietitian might identify corporate executives or employers as distribution channels, since approval for a wellness program usually rests with a company's management.

◆ PRICE

Price includes both tangible costs (fee for service) and intangible commodities (time, effort, inconvenience) that the consumer must bear in the marketing exchange. Once you understand what the consumer perceives as the costs involved in adopting a health behavior or participating in a given program, you have a better chance of influencing the exchange. You may do this by persuading the consumer that the benefits to be received outweigh the perceived costs. Alternatively, incentives (money, groceries, gifts, personal recognition) can be offered to increase motivation and facilitate consumer participation. Likewise, costs can be reduced (less waiting time) or prices discounted to certain groups (senior citizens, students). Any of these tactics can considerably reduce the "price" consumers perceive that they pay for the program or service.

◆ PROMOTION

The last P in the marketing mix—promotion—refers to the agency or organization's informative or persuasive communication with the target market. What do you want to say? To whom do you want to say it? When do you want to say it?[33] The communication messages are designed to have a measurable effect on the knowledge, attitude, and/or behavior of the target market.[34] The medium, message content, and message format are chosen to complement the target market's communication needs.[35]

Promotion has four general objectives:[36]

◆ To inform and educate consumers about the existence of a product (or service) and its capabilities (what the community program has to offer)

◆ To remind present and former users of the product's continuing existence (e.g., prenatal nutrition counseling)

◆ To persuade prospective purchasers that the product is worth buying (improved health status, other benefits)

◆ To inform consumers about where and how to obtain and use the product (accessibility, location, and time)

Although people frequently think that promotion is limited to advertising, promotion actually includes much more than advertising, as shown in Table 9-8. As one author has noted:

> Marketers generally agree that although mass media approaches are appropriate for developing consumer awareness in the short term, face-to-face programs such as workplace encounters are more effective (though not always cost-effective) in chang-

PERSONAL PROMOTION AIDS	MEDIA AND PUBLIC EVENTS	GRAPHIC/PRINT MATERIALS
One-to-one communication	Public relations	Logos
Networking	Publicity	Brochures
Business cards	News releases	Portfolios
Letters	Press kits	Proposals
Résumés	Media interviews	Posters
Letters of reference	News conferences	Banners
Use of a name	Press briefings	Audiovisual aids
	Special events	Computer graphics
	Celebrities	Giveaways (T-shirts,
	Advertising	mugs, tote bags)
	Direct mail	
	Public speaking	
	Writing	

TABLE 9-8

Promotional Tools
Source: Adapted from K. K. Helm and J. C. Rose, *The Competitive Edge: Marketing Strategies for the Registered Dietitian* (Chicago: American Dietetic Association, 1986), p. 45. © The American Dietetic Association. Reprinted with permission.

ing behavior in the long term. In designing any communication policy, the marketer commonly considers the effects that may be achievable through the use of a mix of approaches, capitalizing on the strengths of each.[37]

The four most common promotional tools are advertising, sales promotion, personal selling, and publicity.

Advertising is standardized communication in print or electronic media that is purchased.[38] Examples of advertising media include telephone directory yellow pages, billboards, newspapers, radio, trade and professional journals, and magazines. The role of advertising is to communicate a concise and targeted message that ultimately stimulates action by the carefully defined audience. Advertising can reach large numbers of people in many locations and can help build image. In advertising, you control the nature and timing of the message because you are buying the time or space. Which media you choose will depend on the characteristics of your target market, the size of your budget, and the goals of your advertising campaign. The advantages and limitations of the major media categories are listed in Table 9-9. The boxed insert offers tips for working with the media.

Sales promotion consists of such things as coupons, free samples, point-of-purchase materials, and trade catalogs. The use of these activities as part of the promotion strategy encourages potential consumers to purchase or use a particular product or service.

Personal selling or communication can be done through small group meetings, counseling sessions and nutrition classes, formal presentations to organiza-

Advertising Any paid form of nonpersonal presentation and promotion of ideas, goods, or services by an identified sponsor.

Sales promotion Short-term incentives to encourage purchases or sales of a product or service.

Personal selling/ communication Oral presentation in a conversation with one or more prospective purchasers for the purpose of making sales or building goodwill.

TABLE 9-9

Advantages and Limitations of Major Media Categories

Source: Adapted from P. Kotler and R. N. Clarke, *Marketing for Health Care Organizations* (Englewood Cliffs, N.J.: Prentice-Hall, 1987), p. 451.

MEDIUM	ADVANTAGES	LIMITATIONS
Newspapers	Flexibility; timeliness; good local market coverage; broad acceptance; high believability	Short life; poor reproduction quality; small "pass-along" audience
Television	Combines sight, sound, and motion; appealing to the senses; high attention; high reach	High absolute cost; high clutter; fleeting exposure; less audience selectivity
Direct mail	Audience selectivity; flexibility; no ad competition within the same medium; personalization	Relatively high cost; "junk mail" image
Radio	Mass use; high geographic and demographic selectivity; low cost	Audio presentation only; lower attention than television; nonstandardized rate structures; fleeting exposure
Magazines	High geographic and demographic selectivity; credibility and prestige; high-quality reproduction; long life; good pass-along readership	Long ad purchase lead time; some waste circulation; no guarantee of position
Outdoor	Flexibility; high repeat exposure; low cost; low competition	No audience selectivity; creative limitations

Media Tips

"Chance favors the prepared mind," said Louis Pasteur. When working with the media, always be prepared to provide credible nutrition information. Besides keeping current with the various scientific and trade journals and the popular press, you'll need to consider radio and television news and talk shows as well. (Chapter 2's Professional Focus offered tips for becoming a media monitor.) By doing so, everyone benefits: the media by providing information of value to their audiences, the public by receiving accurate information, and you as a community nutritionist by enhancing your image and visibility as a professional. As you work with the media, consider the following tips:

◆ Be sure that the information you supply is accurate—check and recheck all names, dates, facts, and figures. This helps establish your credibility with the media.

◆ Become familiar with the format and types of coverage of the various media—television and radio news and talk shows, newspapers, newsletters and local publications, and trade publications and magazines. Adapt your messages to the format of the media you choose. Identify how a particular audience will benefit from the information you provide.

◆ Nurture good press relations with the media contact people (reporters, editors, program directors, and producers) in your area. Keep a list of the names, addresses, phone numbers, and deadlines of the media in your community. They are the "gatekeepers" to your target audiences.

◆ Write a "pitch" letter or "news release" about a topic to the medium of your choice. Consider your letter or release to be your personal sales representative. Convince your readers that the information you possess is of value and interest to their audiences. Writers learn to capture their readers' attention with a news "hook" in the first paragraph, followed by answers to the five Ws: who, what, when, where, and why.

◆ Occasionally, you may send an "FYI" (for your information) piece (e.g., a research report or recently published article) to the people on your contact list. This alerts them to potential newsworthy topics or events they may find useful either now or at a later date. Make yourself available to them for follow-up information or assistance.

◆ Be consumer-oriented. Keep your audience in mind as you prepare your media information. Be both an authority on nutrition information and an entertainer, when appropriate. Get the audience interested and involved with your message. Consider using visuals to support your messages.

◆ When working with television or radio, consider your appearance—dress with professional style. Practice your presentation as much as possible beforehand. You'll want your facial expressions, body language, and voice to show enthusiasm and animation for your topic.

*Adapted from G. A. Levey, Communicating with the media, in *Communicating as Professionals,* R. Chernoff, ed. (Chicago: American Dietetic Association, 1986), pp. 57–60; and *The Competitive Edge: Marketing Strategies for the Registered Dietitian* (Chicago: American Dietetic Association, 1986), pp. 54–62.

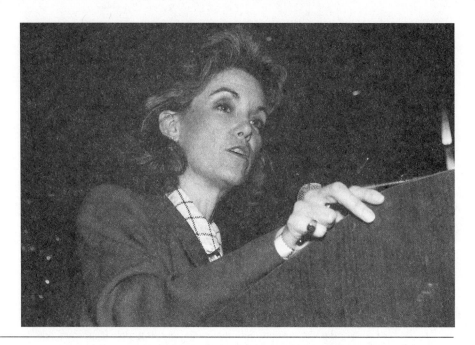

Public speaking can increase your visibility and strengthen your image as an expert with potential clients.

The Professional Focus at the end of Chapter 12 offers numerous tips for effective public speaking.

tions or community groups, displays and booths at health fairs and related conferences, and telephone conversations or personal meetings with the public and other professsionals (e.g., your referral sources). Unlike the standardized message presented in advertising, the message presented in personal selling can be tailored to fit the needs of the particular individual or group. Personal selling also offers other advantages:[39]

♦ Direct contact provides positive feedback to the listener through both the verbal and the nonverbal gestures of the communicator.

♦ The interpersonal contact facilitates the transfer of the message better than alternate methods.

♦ The communicator can ensure comprehension by asking questions and monitoring responses.

♦ The communicator has an opportunity to probe for resistance to change and then is in a position to address each issue.

♦ The listener may believe that someone is now in a position to monitor his behavior and thus hold him accountable for it.

Publicity Nonpersonal stimulation of demand for a product, service, or business unit by planting commercially significant news about it in a published medium or obtaining favorable presentation of it on radio, television, or stage that is not paid for by the sponsor.

Publicity, or public relations, is used to create a positive image of an individual or organization in the mind of the consumer. The American Dietetic Association receives publicity every March during National Nutrition Month activities.

Publicity tools include articles in newsletters or local newspapers, informational brochures and newsletters, radio and television interviews, other forms of public speaking, displays, posters, audiovisual materials, thank you notes, and other tools that present a favorable image of the organization or professional to the target market.

Public service announcements (PSAs) can also be utilized as a form of publicity. They offer the advantage of being free of charge and have the potential of reaching a large audience. PSAs promote programs, activities, and services of federal, state, or local governments and the activities of nonprofit organizations when they are regarded as serving a community interest.[40] A nutrition message can be a PSA with credit given to the organization submitting it. Here are five tips for creating effective PSAs:[41]

♦ Produce announcements of professional quality. One professional PSA is better than several low-quality ones.

♦ Get the audience involved. Sound effects, questions, repetition, and humor are sometimes more effective at grabbing the attention of the audience than the factual approach.

♦ Market the service offered, not just the PSA topic. Offer a brochure, a toll-free information hotline, or a screening service.

♦ Simplify the response action needed. Advertise a local phone number or an easy-to-remember P.O. box number.

♦ Develop and nurture a good rapport with the television and radio public service directors. They may be able to improve the PSA's production quality and increase scheduled air time.

Two additional promotional tools deserve mention: direct mail and word-of-mouth referrals. Many marketers develop brochures, newsletters, fliers, and other promotional items that are mailed to specific targeted groups or geographical areas. Others claim that word-of-mouth referrals—having associates and clients do some of the promoting for you—are one of the most important promotional strategies. A successful program or service will generate its own word-of-mouth publicity because satisfied consumers will tell others about the program and may encourage their participation.

The promotional strategies used by individuals or organizations will vary depending on the populations they are trying to reach, the goals of the program, and the resources available for promoting it. Table 9-10 shows a sample marketing plan for a sports nutrition counseling service and identifies the promotional tools used.

Monitoring and Evaluation

Evaluation is the key to the success of any marketing program. Methods include tracking changes in volume or net profit, referral sources, and customer satisfaction.[42] In this step of the marketing process, you need to ask: Are you accomplishing your goals? Who benefited from the service? What changes in knowledge, attitudes, and practices occurred? What are the actual costs of providing the service? What changes are warranted to make the service more effective in the

Chapter 10 focuses on the essentials of evaluation.

TABLE 9-10	Sports Nutrition Marketing Plan				
POTENTIAL CLIENTS	**SELLING POINTS**	**OBSTACLES**	**TOOLS**	**DATE**	**COST**
Sports medicine clinics					
◆ Dr. Stanford's Clinic	◆ Appeals to athletes	◆ Staff biases	Calls and letters	2 weeks	Time, postage, phone
◆ Greenlief Sports Medicine Center	◆ Individualized	◆ Competition from St. Luke's Hospital	Interviews	ASAP*	Time, travel
◆ Alpine Sports Clinic	◆ Will augment present programs	Sports Medicine (nutritionist)	Proposals Become speaker	ASAP ASAP	Time, travel Varies; some income
◆ Dallas Sports Center	◆ Will generate money ◆ Will give marketing edge in city to their program	◆ Competition from Drs. Green & Brown (exercise physiologists)	at sports conferences Contact local newspapers/media	As needed	Time
	◆ Dietitians' reputation will increase in the area		Develop booklet	6 months	Time, graphics, printing
			Send articles to national magazines	6 months	Time, postage, phone
Health clubs					
◆ President's	◆ Revenue generating for health clubs through individual consults and attract-ing new members	◆ Staff biases ◆ No budget ◆ May want to pay as employee, not consultant	Call managers Interviews Proposals "Brown-bag" talks	2 weeks ASAP As needed ASAP	Time Time, travel, reports Time, travel Time, travel, handouts
◆ Racquet City					
◆ Spa Lady	◆ Gives new compet-itive edge through expanded programs in nutrition and wellness	◆ May want exclu-sive in the area			
◆ Las Colinas					
Sports teams					
◆ Professional sports	◆ Improved athletic performance ◆ Recovery from illness and injury ◆ Ideal athletic weight control	◆ Biases against out-side consultants ◆ Philosophical nutritional differences ◆ Low/no budget	Calls and letters Lectures Menu planning Consulting with coaches	Future development " " "	Time, postage Time, handouts Time, handouts Time, travel
◆ University intercollegiate					
*ASAP = As soon as possible					

Source: K. K. Helm and J. C. Rose, *The Competitive Edge: Marketing Strategies for the Registered Dietitian* (Chicago: American Dietetic Association, 1986), p. 46. © The American Dietetic Association. Reprinted with permission.

future? For example, once you understand the profile of clients who were suc-cessful with a given program, your promotional efforts can be targeted more effectively.

If your marketing plan included a thorough situational analysis and you care-fully translated these results into a marketing mix for your targeted audience, a periodic assessment may be all that is needed. Marketing is an ongoing process, however, and situations change—sometimes affecting your marketing strategy. If so, you may need to reevaluate your objectives and goals. Are they still achiev-able? Do you need to take an alternative direction? Redirect your strategy?

In *Guerilla Marketing,* J. C. Levinson cautions against abandoning one's marketing plan once it begins generating favorable results. Instead he advises an ongoing commitment to your marketing orientation and continued investment in your marketing strategy. He offers "ten truths you must never forget":[43]

1. The market is constantly changing.
2. People forget fast.
3. Your competition isn't quitting.
4. Marketing strengthens your identity.
5. Marketing is essential to survival and growth.
6. Marketing enables you to hold on to your old customers.
7. Marketing maintains morale.
8. Marketing gives you an advantage over competitors who have ceased marketing.
9. Marketing allows your business to continue operating.
10. You have invested money that you stand to lose.

Social Marketing: Community Campaigns for Change

A descendant of commercial marketing, **social marketing** makes a comprehensive effort to influence the acceptability of social ideas in a population, usually for the purpose of changing behavior.[44] Commercial marketing techniques can be applied to social, political, and economic ideas, issues, policies, and programs. In other words, health ideas like cardiovascular fitness, low-fat eating, and hypertension screening can be sold in the same way as presidential candidates or toothpaste.[45] Examples of social marketing include the public service messages produced by electronic and print media such as messages intended to change behavior related to smoking, hypertension, use of seat belts, teenage pregnancy, driving after drinking, drug use, safe sex, suicide, and similar concerns.

Whereas traditional marketing seeks to satisfy the needs and wants of targeted consumers, social marketing aims to change their attitudes and/or behavior. To do so, the marketing process must be followed in its entirety.[46] Marketers identify four types of behavior change, listed here in order of increasing difficulty:

Social marketing The marketing of socially relevant programs, ideas, or behaviors concerned with "the design, implementation, and control of programs seeking to increase the acceptability of a social idea (preventive health behavior) or cause in a target group, and involving considerations of product, planning, pricing, communication, distribution, and marketing research."

◆ **Cognitive change.** A change in knowledge is the easiest to market, but there appears to be little connection between knowledge change and behavior change. Examples include campaigns to explain the nutritional value of different foods or campaigns to expand awareness of government programs like Food Stamps or WIC.

◆ **Action change.** This kind of change is more difficult to achieve than cognitive changes, as the individual must first understand the reason for change and then invest something of value (time, money, energy) to make the change. Screening programs for hypertension, hypercholesterolemia, or breast cancer involve this type of change.

◆ **Behavior change.** This type of change is more difficult to achieve than either cognitive or action changes because it costs the consumer more in terms of personal involvement on a continuing basis—for example, the adoption of a low-fat, high-fiber daily diet or the addition of regular physical exercise to one's lifestyle.

◆ **Value change.** This type of change is the most difficult to market. An example would be population control strategies to persuade families to have fewer children.

The classic example of social marketing programs—family planning initiatives in developing countries—came on the scene in the early 1960s. Notice in Table 9-11 that a comprehensive social marketing campaign—in this case, for breastfeeding promotion—integrates the essentials of marketing:

◆ It begins with market research to define the problem and set realistic goals.

◆ It takes a consumer orientation—focusing on the needs and wants of the consumer.

◆ It adheres to the principles of segmentation and situational analysis to better understand the needs and characteristics of the target market.

TABLE

9-11

Procedures and Activities to Launch and Operate a Comprehensive Social Marketing Program for Breastfeeding Promotion
Source: Adapted from P. F. Basch, *International Health* (London: Oxford University Press, 1990), p. 286.

◆ Establish the need for a local campaign to increase the incidence of breastfeeding among low-income women, and gain approval for this particular breastfeeding promotion program.
◆ Obtain funding for program planning and implementation.
◆ Set up a program: staff, procedures, materials, etc.
◆ Do market research about attitudes toward breastfeeding, acceptability and desirability of breastfeeding, and specific beliefs and infant feeding practices in various ethnic and cultural groups.
◆ Create and test locally comprehensible and socially acceptable advertising messages to promote the desired behavior, taking into account the level of literacy.
◆ Formulate the campaign messages and materials (e.g. training videos).
◆ Get the message to the public through locally appropriate means, such as posters, print advertisements, radio and television, schools, home visits, group instruction, professional contacts, or other means. Enlist the aid of supportive groups.
◆ Assure that the campaign is reaching its target audience.
◆ Deal as appropriate with rumors, myths, misinformation, or similar threats to the program.
◆ Assess results of the program. This may require a case-control study in comparable areas where breastfeeding is, and is not, promoted.

◆ It utilizes qualitative market research on the opinions and desires of the target market and the environment and integrates this information into a full marketing mix with product development, distribution, pricing, and promotion.

◆ Its promotional strategy includes not only all the components of a persuasive communications campaign, but cultural sensitivity as well.

◆ It emphasizes the pretesting of all concepts, messages, and materials for deliberate feedback to improve specificity.

◆ It provides an ongoing means to monitor and evaluate program objectives and results over time.

Social marketing goes beyond advertising. It seeks to bring about changes in the behavior as well as in the attitudes and knowledge of the target audience.[47] Social marketing can be applied to a wide variety of social problems but is particularly appropriate in three situations:[48]

1. When new research data and information on practices need to be disseminated to improve people's lives. Examples include campaigns for cancer prevention, breastfeeding promotion, and childhood immunization.

2. When countermarketing is needed to offset the negative effects of a practice or promotional efforts of companies for products that are potentially harmful—for example, cigarettes, alcoholic beverages, or the promotion of infant formula in developing countries.

3. When activation is needed to move people from intention to action—for example, motivating people to lose weight, exercise, or floss their teeth. Without movement, there is no marketing.[49]

Social Marketing at the Community Level

The Pawtucket Heart Health Program (PHHP) is presented here as an example of how marketing principles can be utilized in the planning, implementation, and evaluation of a community-wide social marketing campaign. The Pawtucket "Know Your Cholesterol" campaign was one of the earliest cholesterol awareness and screening efforts.[50] The following objectives for the campaign were formulated based on national random sampling data of both the general population and physicians:

◆ Physician education

◆ Increased awareness among the general population of blood cholesterol as a risk factor for coronary heart disease

◆ Increased numbers of people knowing their cholesterol level as a result of attending PHHP-sponsored screening, counseling, and referral events (SCOREs)

◆ Large numbers of people showing reductions in their blood cholesterol level at two-month follow-up measurements

In segmenting the community of Pawtucket, Rhode Island, adults were a primary focus since demographics (gender and age) showed that awareness levels were equivalent for men and women in the national sample. Cardiologists, family practice physicians, and physicians in general practice were targeted for direct mail educational packages and grand rounds presentations on blood cholesterol and heart disease at the community hospital. Middle-aged men who had previous contact with the PHHP were also the focus of a direct mail and telemarketing campaign to attend SCOREs during the campaign period.

Early program development steps included a pilot test of a self-help "nutrition kit" on lowering cholesterol levels and pretesting of the SCORE protocol at the community hospital. Promotional tools selected to reach the general and targeted audiences included newspapers; print media distributed through worksites, churches, and schools; direct mail and telemarketing; and SCORE delivery at worksites, churches, and various other community locations. Television and radio were not used to avoid spillover into the control community.

In the marketing mix, SCOREs were initially priced at five dollars per person for both an initial and follow-up measurement. The researchers reasoned that people who had already paid for a second measurement would be more likely to have a follow-up test than if they had to pay for it separately. Price reductions and specials were also offered. Promotional publicity strategies included the "kick-off" SCORE at a St. Patrick's Day parade and six weekly advice columns in the local newspaper.

Results showed that 1439 adults attended 39 SCOREs. Sixty percent were identified as having elevated serum cholesterol levels. Two months after the campaign, 72.3 percent of these persons had returned for a second measurement. Nearly 60 percent of this group had reduced their serum cholesterol levels.

The essential components of the campaign's marketing strategy were integrated into the ongoing activities of the PHHP. During the first two years following the campaign, over 10,000 persons had their blood cholesterol level measured, were given information on dietary management of high serum cholesterol, and were referred to physicians when necessary. A later survey of local physicians showed they were more aggressive in initiating either diet or drug therapy than physicians in the neighboring community or those who had participated in the national survey. The local physicians cited increased patient requests for blood cholesterol measurements and/or nutrition information as the major reason for changing their practice. The researchers concluded that informed consumers had influenced changes in their physicians' treatment of high serum cholesterol levels. Their overall conclusion was that "a well-functioning marketing operation can lead to more effective and efficient use of resources and improved consumer satisfaction. . . . **Health marketing** has the potential of reaching the largest possible group of people at the least cost with the most effective, consumer-satisfying program." [51]

Marketing concepts for community nutrition programs and public health services are gradually maturing. The challenge for the remainder of the decade and the next century will be to utilize the marketing strategies described in this chapter effectively so as to reap the benefits of well-planned nutrition services and programs despite dwindling resources.

Health marketing refers to health promotion programs that are developed to satisfy consumer needs, strategized to meet as broad an audience as is in need of the program, and thereby enhance the organization's ability to effect population-wide changes in targeted risk behaviors.

Marketing tools can be employed in health promotion programs to respond effectively to the needs and wants of consumers and thus greatly enhance the probability of eliciting the desired health behavior. A consumer orientation—understanding what the potential consumer wants and needs—can provide the basis for effective use of resources allocated for public health programs. Development of an effective marketing program spells the difference between success and failure.

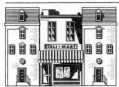 # COMMUNITY LEARNING ACTIVITY

In this Community Learning Activity, you will continue using the target population you selected in Chapter 6 and develop a marketing strategy for your target audience.

1. Identify your consumers: the users, referral sources, and key decision makers within this group. Are there any environmental factors that you need to consider?

2. What sources of data might you use to better understand your target group?

3. Describe each element of your marketing mix: product, place, price, and promotion.

Lighten Up—Be Willing to Make Mistakes and Risk Failure

"When a man knows he is to be hanged in a fortnight, it concentrates his mind wonderfully."

—Samuel Johnson, 1777

If you knew that you had only a few months to live, would you live differently than you do right now? Would you find time to take dancing lessons, learn to rollerblade, snorkel off the Great Barrier Reef, study the stock market, get a pilot's license, or try your hand at papier-mâché? Would you take more chances and worry less about your image?

Most of us would probably answer that last question in the affirmative. We would *choose* to live differently if we knew that only a few grains of sand were left in the hourglass. Nadine Stair, at the age of 85, said the same thing: "If I had my life to live over again, I'd try to make more mistakes next time. I would relax. I would limber up. I would be sillier than I have been this trip. I know of a very few things I would take seriously. I would take more trips. I would climb more mountains, swim more rivers and watch more sunsets. I would do more walking and looking. I would eat more ice cream and less beans. . . . If I had it to do over again, I would go places, do things and travel lighter than I have. . . . I'd pick more daisies."[1]

Notice that the first thing Nadine Stair said she would do differently "next time" was to try to make more mistakes. Most people work hard to *avoid* making mistakes, and few of us are willing to undertake a venture so risky that mistakes are almost guaranteed and the probability of failure looms large. In our culture, these activities are to be avoided at all costs. If you doubt this, go to your local bookstore or library and search for books on failure, making mistakes, and risk taking. You won't find any of the following books: *The Joy of Failing, The Seven Habits of Complete Nincompoops, The One-Minute Mistake Maker, Fit for Failure* or *100 Risk Takers Who Fell Flat on Their Faces*.

◆ SOME PEOPLE DON'T GIVE UP ON THEIR GOALS

Virtually every successful entrepreneur, adventurer, and risk taker *has* made mistakes and *has* failed at some point in his or her struggle to reach a personal or professional goal. In an essay in *Science*, Harold T. Shapiro, president of Princeton University, remarked that "the world too often calls it failure if we do not immediately reach our goals; true failure lies, rather, in giving up on our goals."[2] What would our world be like if the following individuals had given up on their goals?

◆ In 1842, at a time when most young British women of position were concerned mainly with parties and pending marriages, Florence Nightingale felt a "call" to perform some lifework. Although she sensed that her destiny "lay among the miserable of the world," the precise nature of this vocation eluded her for many years. Not until she was in her early thirties did she begin to pursue a career in nursing despite the persistent objections of her mother and sister, a cultural bias against nursing care, and the resistance of the traditional medical establishment. Over a

Continued

lifetime of hard work, her determination and vision radically altered the practice and professionalism of nursing. Nightingale was among the first to document and describe hospital conditions, and she became an expert on sanitation. She reformed the health administration of the British army in response to the brutal mortality of the Crimean War and thereby influenced medical practice for years to come. Her reports on proper hospital construction, the training of nurses, and patient care led to the establishment of sanitary commissions and eventually to the public health service.[3]

◆ Thomas Alva Edison, born in 1847, has been described as "one of the outstanding geniuses in the history of technology."[4] He received very little formal schooling, having been expelled by a schoolmaster as "addled," and was taught history, science, and philosophy primarily by his mother. His fascination with the wireless telegraph as a young boy led to a lifelong enjoyment of experimentation and research. At his death in 1931, he held 1093 patents on such devices as the incandescent electric lamp, the phonograph, the carbon telephone transmitter, and the motion picture projector.

At one point in his career, Edison struggled to develop a storage battery. "I don't think Nature would be so unkind as to withhold the secret of a *good* storage battery if a real earnest hunt for it is made," he said. "I'm going to hunt."[5] This was no mean feat. He knew what was required of a good battery—it must last for years, should not lose capacity when recharged, and needed to be nearly indestructible. He began by testing one chemical after another in a series of experiments that spanned a decade. When 10,000 experiments failed to give the desired results, Edison remarked, ". . . I have not failed. I've just found 10,000 ways that won't work."[6] He eventually succeeded.

◆ When he was a 20-year-old student at Yale University, Fred Smith wrote a term paper that analyzed freight services existing at the time. He concluded that there was a market for a company that moved "high-priority, time-sensitive" goods such as medicines and electronic components. He believed the existing system was cumbersome and failed to respond quickly to consumers' needs. In his paper, he proposed an overnight delivery service based on a "hub-and-spokes" air freight system. His professor was unimpressed with Smith's proposal, citing a restrictive regulatory environment and competition from airlines as major barriers to implementing such a service. The paper earned a grade of C.

Smith did not give up on his idea, although he could not do anything about it for several years. Eventually, at the age of 29, he founded a company, Federal Express, designed to deliver packages "absolutely, positively overnight." In March 1973, his first planes flew over the eastern United States, carrying a total of six packages. One month later the volume had increased to 186 packages. In its first years, the company nearly folded from a lack of capital, concerns about Smith's leadership, and a formal charge of fraud against him. The company—with Smith at its helm—survived this difficult period. By 1983, its earnings were more than $1 billion. By the late 1980s, Federal Express was handling more than 700,000 packages and parcels daily and had altered American business practices substantially.[7]

Continued

◆ PROFESSIONAL FOCUS—*Continued*

◆ THE SECRET OF SUCCESS

Risk takers make mistakes and sometimes fail. If they have a common feature, however, it is their willingness and determination to persevere, sometimes against great odds. In our professional lives, it is impossible to avoid risk and the possibility of failure. The trick is to learn how to minimize risk and capitalize on your mistakes. Here are a few points to keep in mind when you are next faced with undertaking a risky venture:

1. Do your homework. There are risks and there are *calculated* risks. The difference between the two is substantial. To prepare for a calculated risk, talk with people who have undertaken similar ventures. Find out about the unexpected problems they experienced and how they handled them.

2. Write down your options and the potential outcome of each. This activity will help you focus on the option that may stand the best chance for success. Then, write down the worst possible thing that could happen if you proceeded with that option. Is it something you can live with? If not, how can the option be changed to protect you or your employees?

3. Learn from your mistakes or failures. We all make them, but we don't all learn from them. In the business world, bankruptcy is often viewed as the ultimate failure. One entrepreneur commented that "if you hadn't been bankrupt at least once, you hadn't really learned much about business."[8] Although it is certainly painful, business failure can be an opportunity for learning new lessons both personally and professionally. The successful entrepreneur and risk taker has the ability to learn from her experiences and regain control of her destiny.

4. Be committed to your goal. Having a high level of commitment to the work at hand is one element that distinguishes the successful entrepreneur from the also-rans.[9]

◆ WORDS TO WORK BY

In his book of wildlife portraits, the artist Robert Bateman remarked, "A great master teacher once said, 'In order to learn how to draw you have to make two thousand mistakes. Get busy and start making them.'"[10] These are apt words to keep in mind as you begin traveling *your* career path.

1. As cited in R. N. Bolles, *The Three Boxes of Life—And How to Get Out of Them* (Berkeley, Calif.: Ten Speed Press, 1981), p. 377.
2. H. T. Shapiro, The willingness to risk failure, *Science* 250 (1990): 609.
3. C. Woodham-Smith, *Florence Nightingale* (New York: McGraw-Hill, 1951). The quotation in this paragraph was taken from p. 31 of this book.
4. Edison, in *The New Encyclopaedia Britannica: Macropaedia,* vol. 17, 15th ed. (Chicago: Encyclopaedia Britannica, 1985), pp. 1049–51.
5. W. A. Simonds, *Edison—His Life, His Work, His Genius* (London: Kimble & Bradford, 1935), p. 278.
6. As cited by Shapiro, Willingness to risk failure.
7. W. Davis, *The Innovators* (New York: American Management Association, 1987), pp. 361–65.
8. As cited in B. J. Bird, *Entrepreneurial Behavior* (Glenview, Ill.: Scott, Foresman, 1989), pp. 354–55.
9. Bird, *Entrepreneurial Behavior,* pp. 366–67.
10. R. Bateman, *The Art of Robert Bateman* (Ontario: Penguin Books Canada, 1981), p. 19.

NOTES

1. The opening vignette was adapted from E. Clift, Social marketing and communication: Changing health behavior in the Third World, *American Journal of Health Promotion* 3 (1989): 17–24.

2. P. F. Basch, *International Health* (New York: Oxford University Press, 1990), p. 285.

3. S. C. Parks and D. L. Moody, A marketing model: Applications for dietetic professionals, *Journal of the American Dietetic Association* 86 (1986): 37–43.

4. Clift, Social marketing, p. 17. The margin definition was adapted from P. Kotler, *Marketing in Non-profit Organizations,* 2nd ed. (Englewood Cliffs, N.J.: Prentice-Hall, 1982), p. 6.

5. W. Smith, *Social marketing: Two Ways to Improve Health Delivery* (Washington, D.C.: Academy for Educational Development, 1984), as cited by Clift, Social marketing, p. 24.

6. C. B. Matthews, Marketing your services: Strategies that work, *ASHA Magazine* 30 (1988): 21–25.

7. J. G. Keith, Marketing health care: What the recent literature is telling us, *Hospital and Health Services Administration* 2 (1981): 66–91, and G. E. A. Dever, *Community Health Analysis,* 2nd ed. (Gaithersburg, Md.: Aspen Publishers, 1991), p. 249.

8. Dever, *Community Health Analysis,* p. 249.

9. The various orientations described here were adapted from P. Kotler and R. N. Clarke, *Marketing for Health Care Organizations* (Englewood Cliffs, N.J.: Prentice-Hall, 1987), pp. 1–38. The margin definitions are from pp. 29–31 of this book.

10. Parks and Moody, A marketing model, pp. 39–40.

11. S. H. Fine, *The Marketing of Ideas and Social Issues* (New York: Praeger, 1981), as cited by R. C. Lefebvre and J. A. Flora, Social marketing and public health intervention, *Health Education Quarterly* 15 (1988): 299–315.

12. Dever, *Community Health Analysis,* p. 249.

13. W. D. Novelli, "Selling" public health programs. How marketing applies, *Medical Marketing & Media* (May 1989): 36–44.

14. Lefebvre and Flora, Social marketing, p. 301.

15. Dever, *Community Health Analysis,* pp. 252–53.

16. The discussion of the marketing planning process was adapted from Matthews, Marketing your services, pp. 21–25.

17. K. K. Helm and J. C. Rose, *The Competitive Edge: Marketing Strategies for the Registered Dietitian* (Chicago: American Dietetic Association, 1986), pp. 17–18.

18. Matthews, Marketing your services, p. 23.

19. M. Ward, *Marketing Strategies: A Resource for Registered Dietitians* (Binghamton, N.Y.: Niles & Phipps, 1984), p. 63.

20. Ibid.

21. W. Lancaster, T. McIllwain, and J. Lancaster, Health marketing: Implications for health promotion, *Family and Community Health* (February 1983): 47.

22. Ibid., p. 45.

23. Dever, *Community Health Analysis,* pp. 253–64.

24. The section on demographics and psychographics was adapted from Dever, *Community Health Analysis,* pp. 255–77.

25. C. Bryant and D. Bailey, The Use of Focus Group Research in Program Development. Unpublished manuscript, Lexington, KY, 1989; and R. A. Krueger, *Focus Groups: A Practical Guide for Applied Research* (Newbury Park, Calif.: Sage Publications, 1989).

26. M. Griffiths, Designing More Appropriate Breastfeeding Education Programs Through the Use of Focused Group Discussions, Unpublished manuscript (Washington, D.C.: The Manoff Group, 1989).

27. The list of guidelines is from R. K. Manoff, *Social Marketing: New Imperative for Public Health* (New York: Praeger, 1989), p. 126.

28. S. W. Brown and A. P. Morley, Jr., *Marketing Strategies for Physicians: A Guide to Practice Growth* (Oradell, N.J.: Medical Economics Books, 1986).

29. Parks and Moody, A marketing model, p. 40.

30. W. D. Novelli, Health care, politicians, toothpaste: All can be marketed the same way, *Marketing News* 14 (1981): 1, 7.

31. Ward, *Marketing Strategies,* p. 81.

32. Novelli, Health care, p. 7.

33. Matthews, Marketing your services, p. 25.

34. P. Kotler, *Marketing Management* (Englewood Cliffs, N.J.: Prentice-Hall, 1980), Chapter 3.

35. Kotler, *Marketing in Non-profit Organizations,* as cited by Parks and Moody, A marketing model, p. 40.

36. Dever, *Community Health Analysis,* p. 252.

37. J. A. Quelch, Marketing principles and the future of preventive health care, *Millbank Memorial Fund Quarterly/Health and Society* 58 (1980): 317, as cited by Dever, *Community Health Analysis,* p. 283.

38. The section on promotional tools was adapted from Ward, *Marketing Strategies,* pp. 17–22.

39. The list of advantages is from T. Golaszewski and P. Prabhaker, Applying marketing strategies to worksite health promotion efforts, *Occupational Health Nursing* 32 (1984): 188–92.

40. Ward, *Marketing Strategies,* p. 19.

41. The list of five tips was adapted from ibid., pp. 72–73.

42. Matthews, Marketing your services, p. 25.

43. J. C. Levinson, *Guerilla Marketing* (Boston: Houghton Mifflin, 1984), pp. 26–27.

44. The margin definition is from Kotler and Clark, *Marketing for Health Care Organizations.*

45. Novelli, Health care.

46. Dever, *Community Health Analysis,* p. 280.

47. This synopsis of the social marketing process was adapted from Clift, Social marketing, p. 18.

48. The three situations described here are from K. F. Fox and P. Kotler, The marketing of social causes: The first 10 years, *Journal of Marketing* 44 (1980): 24–33.

49. P. E. Smith, Cost-benefit analysis and the marketing of nutrition services, in *Benefits of Nutrition Services: A Costing and Marketing Approach* (Columbus, Ohio: Ross Laboratory, 1987), p. 30.

50. The discussion of the PHHP was adapted from Lefebvre and Flora, Social marketing, pp. 309–11.

51. Ibid., p. 302.

Program Evaluation

However beautiful the strategy, you should occasionally look at the results.
—Winston Churchill

Introduction

◆ Vitamin A deficiency has been linked with childhood morbidity and mortality. In central Java, where vitamin A–deficient children have a higher mortality rate than children with adequate vitamin A stores, a program of vitamin A supplementation was evaluated in several villages. In two treatment villages, children aged 1 to 5 years were given four milliliters of red palm oil; in another treatment village, children from this same age group were given nonfat milk fortified with vitamins A and D. A third village received no treatment, while a fourth received only a placebo. An analysis of the program's effectiveness found significant increases in mean serum retinol levels in the treatment villages compared with the placebo and no-treatment villages. The program evaluators also determined that the fortified nonfat milk was well received, but they recommended that preference be given to locally available sources of vitamin A, such as red palm oil, "elephant ears," and other greens.[1]

◆ The effectiveness of SHAPEDOWN, a family-based, behavior modification program for obese adolescents, was studied by health professionals at the University of Colorado Health Sciences Center in Denver. An evaluation of a variety of physical, metabolic, and behavioral outcomes, including relative weight, body mass index, hemoglobin, serum cholesterol, self-esteem, and depression, showed that the program was effective in improving body image and self-esteem among participants. However, it was not more effective than the standard treatment in promoting long-term weight loss.[2]

◆ Using data from the Longitudinal Study of Growth and Development, conducted by the Institute of Nutrition of Central America and Panama (INCAP) from 1969 to 1971 in four villages in Guatemala, researchers from Cornell University determined that gender bias in food intake existed among Guatemalan preschool children, with males having higher energy and protein intakes than females. This gender bias in food intake had significant effects on subsequent growth and illness rates among children first evaluated at 0 to 23 months of age. It is not clear whether gender bias in food intake continued during the 1980s or whether education and health programs should focus on this issue.[3]

These are just a few examples of the many programs and projects that undergo evaluation. **Evaluation** refers to the use of scientific methods to judge and improve the planning, monitoring, effectiveness, and efficiency of health, nutrition, and other human service programs. The purpose of program evaluation—or evaluation research, as it is sometimes called—is to gather information to be used in making decisions about a program or service. In this sense, evaluation is a managerial activity, for managers use evaluation findings to make decisions about redistributing resources, changing program delivery, or continuing a program.[4] Evaluation research is part of program planning and implementation, and it can be viewed as an aspect of the control process.

In this chapter, we describe the elements of evaluation, including the various types of evaluation and the process by which programs are evaluated.

Evaluation The measurable determination of the value or degree of success in achieving specific objectives.

Questions about Evaluation: Why? How? By Whom?

Managers must distinguish between useful and wasteful programs, efficient and time-consuming processes, and effective and ineffective efforts in delivering community-based nutrition services. They must decide how to correct deficient programs and monitor changes in program delivery. When evaluating their programs, managers begin by asking the following questions:[5]

◆ What are the nature and scope of the problem requiring action?

◆ What interventions may be undertaken to address the problem?

◆ What is the appropriate target population for the intervention?

◆ Is the intervention reaching the target population?

◆ Is the intervention being implemented according to the original program plan?

◆ Is the program effective?

◆ How much does the program cost?

◆ What are the program's costs relative to its effectiveness and benefits?

These questions should be familiar to you, for they have surfaced at other points in this textbook, including the review of the epidemiologic method (Chapter 2) and the description of the program planning process (Chapters 6 and 7). The appearance of these or similar questions throughout the text reveals the importance of evaluation to community nutrition practice and program delivery.

The nature of these questions indicates that evaluations are undertaken for a variety of reasons. Evaluations may be used for administrative purposes: to determine whether some elements of a program should be changed, to identify ways in which the delivery of interventions can be improved, to pinpoint weaknesses in program content, to meet certain accountability requirements of the funding agency or senior management, to ensure that program resources (e.g., supplies, equipment, personnel, facilities) are being used properly, or to assess cost-benefit

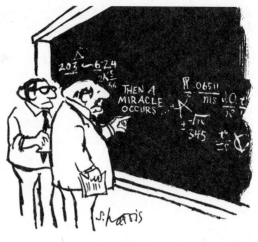

"I THINK YOU SHOULD BE MORE EXPLICIT HERE IN STEP TWO."

©1994 by Sidney Harris

factors. They may be undertaken to test innovative approaches to a nutrition or public health problem, for policy or planning purposes, or to support the advocacy for one program over another. Finally, evaluations may be undertaken to determine whether objectives have been met or whether priorities need to be changed.[6] Consult Table 10-1 for a list of reasons for undertaking evaluations.[7]

Considering the many reasons for conducting evaluations, it isn't surprising that they have many uses as well. As indicated earlier, evaluations are undertaken to help make decisions. Sometimes evaluation findings are used to influence a particular executive or politician who has the authority to distribute resources and shape public policy. For example, the American Dietetic Association (ADA) reviewed the literature on the economic benefits of nutrition services in acute, outpatient, home, long-term, and preventive care and in the care of pregnant women, infants, children, and older adults. It then developed a platform or position statement on the benefits of nutrition services in health care. The platform was used in the ADA's grassroots lobbying campaign of members of Congress and state legislatures.[8] The platform was designed to help policymakers appreciate the importance of nutrition services and *decide* to recognize dietetics professionals as the qualified providers of these services in the final health care reform legislation.[9] In other situations, evaluation findings alert managers and policymakers to the need for expanding or refining programs. The findings of the INCAP study cited at the beginning of this chapter might be used to justify modifying existing health education programs to alleviate gender bias in food intake among Guatemalan children.

Generally, evaluation findings are used at two levels. Not only are they applied to an immediate problem and hence used by the managers and program

Evaluation to Improve Your Program

◆ To improve methods of placing clients in various activity programs
◆ To measure the effect of your program or the extent of client progress in your program
◆ To assess the adequacy of program goals
◆ To identify weaknesses in the program content
◆ To measure staff effectiveness
◆ To identify effective instructional, leadership, or facilitation techniques
◆ To measure the effectiveness of resources (such as materials, supplies, equipment, or facilities)

Evaluation to Justify Your Program or to Show Accountability

◆ To justify the budget or expenditures
◆ To show the need for increased funds
◆ To justify staff, resources, facilities, etc.
◆ To justify program goals and procedures
◆ To account for program practices
◆ To compare program outcomes against program standards

Evaluation to Document Your Program in General

◆ To record client attendance and progress
◆ To document the nature of client involvement and interaction
◆ To record data on clients who drop out and those who complete the program
◆ To document the major program accomplishments
◆ To list program weaknesses expressed by staff or others
◆ To list leader/therapist functions and activities
◆ To describe the context or atmosphere of the treatment setting
◆ To file supportive statements and testimonies about the program

TABLE

10-1

Purposes of Program Evaluation
Source: A. D. Grotelueschen and coauthors, *An Evaluation Planner* (Urbana, Ill.: Office for the Study of Continuing Professional Education, University of Illinois at Urbana-Champaign, 1974). Permission to reprint granted by Arden D. Grotelueschen.

staff who are focused on that problem, but they are also used to shape policies and services beyond the scope of the original problem. In other words, evaluations have many different audiences, some of whom may be directly involved in the program, while others are not involved at all or may be concerned with the program at some future date.

This discussion brings us to the question of who actually carries out evaluations. Depending upon the circumstances, evaluations may be carried out by program staff, other agency staff, or outside consultants. Thus, the evaluator may be intimately familiar with all aspects of a program, because she manages or is involved with it, or she may have a limited knowledge of the program. Regardless, the evaluator is responsible for all aspects of the evaluation from negotiating the evaluation focus to collecting data and preparing the final report. Because evaluations often occur in politically charged atmospheres, where program stakeholders fret about the evaluation's outcome and its ramifications, the evaluator must be sensitive to this environment. In the final analysis, the evaluator must be able to recognize what has to be done, while understanding that she cannot do it all herself.[10]

Classes and Types of Evaluations

The purpose and scope of a specific evaluation depend upon the questions being asked about the program. An evaluation may focus on one particular program component—for example, whether screening every client for high blood cholesterol levels is cost-effective—or it may be comprehensive and examine the design of the program, how it is delivered, and whether it is being utilized properly. In this section, we review the different classes of evaluations—namely, those aimed at program development and design, those involved with program implementation, and those focused on program utility—and the types of evaluation that might be undertaken within each class.[11]

◆ PROGRAM DEVELOPMENT AND DESIGN

Evaluation research is often applied during the program design stage. The organization may need to know, for example, whether community pressures and concerns justify the development of a new program or whether an existing program can be altered to address the issue. The evaluator works, then, with program sponsors, managers, and staff to examine the concept of the proposed program, its scope, and its target population.

The first step in evaluating program design is to assess the program's goals and objectives. Recall from Chapter 6 that objectives are specific statements of achievement that indicate how outcomes will be measured. Direct, well-written objectives provide effective guidance for managers and staff as well as explicit information about program delivery, outcomes, and results that the evaluator can use. Next, the program's proposed intervention is examined to determine whether it can be implemented within the specified time frame. Interventions with low feasibility will not be accepted by managers, policymakers, or other stakeholders. Additional design elements, such as the target population and the components of the delivery system, are also examined. Finally, the evaluator assesses the costs associated with each aspect of the program's design, such as personnel salaries, materials and supplies, fees, and advertising.

Formative evaluation The process of testing and assessing certain elements of a program before it is implemented fully.

Sometimes, it is necessary and prudent to test certain design elements during the development stage. This process, called **formative evaluation**, helps pinpoint and eliminate any kinks in the proposed delivery system or intervention before the program is implemented fully. Formative studies can be either simple or complex and can be as comprehensive as any other type of evaluation. For example, in one three-year program designed to promote increased gardening and consumption of the ivy gourd, a vitamin A–rich food, in northeastern Thailand, formative research was undertaken. First, a baseline survey measured the usual dietary intake of vitamin A and clinical and nonclinical signs of vitamin A deficiency in two regional districts. Physical examinations and tests of serum retinol and dark adaptation were carried out among mothers aged 18 to 35 years and their 2- to 6-year-old children to determine vitamin A status. Focus group surveys and in-depth interviews were conducted to provide data about the behaviors influencing food consumption. This formative evaluation of vitamin A status and behaviors related to consuming vitamin A–rich foods led the program developers to focus their program efforts on promoting good nutrition among children and their mothers.[12]

◆ PROGRAM IMPLEMENTATION

There are many reasons for seeking information about how a program is operating. First, managers must make decisions daily to ensure that their program operates smoothly, uses personnel and supplies efficiently, and delivers services to clients and consumers effectively. Second, the program sponsors and stakeholders want assurance that they got what they paid for and that funds for the program were wisely spent. Such accountability is especially important in today's fiscal and political environment. Third, a program is set up to meet a particular need within the community. It is critical to determine whether, in fact, the program met the needs of the target population. In most cases, regular feedback about program delivery is the best way for managers to document the program's effectiveness, justify the ways staff are employed, provide a rationale for further program support, and defend the program's performance and impact when compared with similar community programs.

Monitoring how a program operates helps managers to answer questions and make decisions about what services to provide, how to provide them, and for whom. This type of evaluation is called **process evaluation** and involves examining program activities in terms of (1) the age, sex, race, occupation, or other demographic variables of the target population; (2) the program's organization, funding, and staffing; and (3) its location and timing.[13] Process evaluation focuses on program *activities* rather than *outcomes*. (Evaluations that focus on program outcomes are called "impact" evaluations; they are discussed in the next section.)

Process evaluation A measure of program activities or efforts—that is, how a program is implemented.

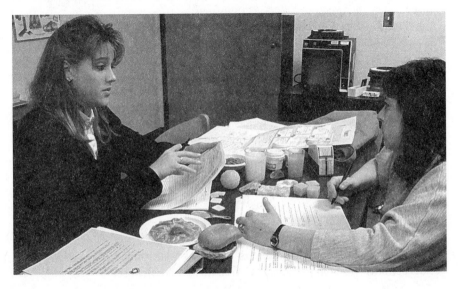

Managers use process evaluation to examine the ways in which a program is delivered, such as determining whether program nutritionists use similar diet counseling techniques and educational materials.

Process evaluation is a fairly new research endeavor, but it is gaining recognition because it can help managers make good decisions. Through process evaluation, managers can systematically exclude the various explanations that may arise for a given outcome. If the program appears to have had no effect, process evaluation can determine which, if any, of the following problems was the reason:[14]

- The program was not properly implemented (meaning that program staff were not fully effective in implementing the program).
- The program could not be implemented properly in some participants (suggesting that compliance with the program protocol was a problem for some participants).
- Some participants had difficulty accessing the program.

Alternatively, if the program has had a beneficial effect on the defined outcomes, process evaluation can determine whether the effect was due, in fact, to the program or to one of the following:

- The greater receptivity of some participants or target groups compared with others
- Competing interventions

Process evaluation focuses on how a program is delivered. In the course of conducting a process evaluation, the evaluator examines the target population to determine how they were attracted to the program and to what extent they participated. In addition, the program is evaluated for bias in terms of how participants were served—that is, whether the target group received too much or too little coverage by the program. Such information can be obtained by examining the records kept on program participants and by conducting surveys of the target population and the program participants. The participant records should reveal which services were used and how often. Surveys help define the characteristics of clients who used the program, compared with those who dropped out or refused to use the program.

Process evaluation deals with activities that are planned to occur. In the example of the ABC Fitness Program, four process objectives were listed (see Table 6-4). We might examine the third process objective listed there—to obtain an estimate of usual fat intake using a 24-hour recall of all participants at the beginning and end of the program—and consider how the planned activity compared with the actual results. If 66 employees entered the program and 24-hour recalls were obtained on 57 of them as planned, we can calculate the percentage of activities attained, using the following formula:

$$\frac{\text{Actual activities}}{\text{Planned activities}} \times 100 = \text{Percentage of activities attained}$$

$$\frac{57}{66} \times 100 = 86.3 \text{ percent}$$

Thus, 86.3 percent of the planned 24-hour recalls were actually obtained during the specified time period. A number of questions arise immediately: Why weren't recalls obtained from all participants? Was there a problem scheduling employees to see the dietitian and, if so, why? Were the instructions to participants unclear? The information obtained through process evaluation signals the program manager that adjustments need to be made at one or more points of the delivery system.

In another example, individuals on the staff of ambulatory nutrition services at Yale–New Haven Hospital in New Haven, Connecticut, developed an index to measure the staff's productivity, so that they could evaluate and improve patient scheduling and define staff activities specifically. By analyzing patient encounter records and the monthly activity reports of the ambulatory dietitians, the individuals developed a patient/time productivity index: [(extended visits $\times$ 2) + (brief visits $\times$ 1) + (weigh-ins $\times$ 0.5) + (telephone consults $\times$ 0.25) + (group class census $\times$ 0.25)] $\div$ number of hours worked. The productivity equation provided staff members with continuous feedback about their performance, and it was eventually incorporated into performance appraisals as an objective measure of their compliance with performance expectations.[15] As you can see, process objectives and evaluations provide many clues about how a program is functioning and whether clients' needs are being met.

◆ PROGRAM UTILITY

Program sponsors, managers, and other stakeholders also want to know the degree to which the program had an impact and what its benefits were in relation to the cost. The former, called **impact** or **outcome evaluation**, is a measure of how effective a program was in changing a particular aspect of nutrition or health status. The determination of the program's benefits relative to its cost is called **fiscal** or **efficiency evaluation**.

Impact or Outcome Evaluation   The purpose of impact evaluation (also referred to as outcome or summative evaluation) is to determine whether the program or intervention had an effect on the target population's health status, food intake, morbidity, mortality, or other outcomes. Impact evaluations are a challenging managerial activity, for they require technical skills in survey design and analysis. The problems associated with impact evaluations arise from the difficulty of determining whether a particular effect was "caused" by the intervention and was not due to some extraneous factor. It is possible that factors beyond the control of the program staff influenced the outcome significantly. Such confounding factors might include secular trends within the community, the occurrence of unexpected events such as a natural catastrophe, or certain characteristics of clients (for example, they tended to "self-select" for the program).

An important aspect of impact evaluation is the choice of the indicator or measure that reflects a condition or problem. Recall from Chapter 7 that an **indicator** is "a quantitative measure that can be used as a guide to monitor and evaluate the quality of important patient care and support service activities."[16] An indicator is not a direct measure of quality, but a "flag" that identifies a specific performance issue that needs further review. In the public health arena, the infant mortality rate has been described as the most common indicator of the general health of a nation's population. Other indicators include longevity, prevalence and incidence rates for diseases, personal characteristics (sex, age, educational level),

Impact or **outcome evaluation** The process of measuring a program's effectiveness in changing one or more aspects of nutrition or health status.

Fiscal or **efficiency evaluation** The process of determining a program's benefits relative to its cost.

Indicator A quantitative measure that can be used as a guide to monitor and evaluate the quality of important client care and support service activities.

lifestyle habits (smoking, drug abuse, eating habits, activity level), social networks (family, friends), environmental factors (exposure to air pollution, work conditions), and quality of life factors (positive attitude, life satisfaction).[17]

Outcome indicator Measures what happens (or does not happen) after a function is performed (or not performed).

There are both outcome and process indicators. An **outcome indicator** measures what happens (or does not happen) after a function is performed (or not performed).[18] For example, participants in a technical workshop on controlling micronutrient malnutrition identified the following outcome indicators for surveillance of micronutrient malnutrition: Bitot's spots, serum retinol, history of night blindness, goiter diagnosed by palpitation, urinary iodine, hematocrit, hemoglobin, and serum ferritin.[19] A **process indicator** measures an important activity that contributes directly or indirectly to client care. Process indicators are concerned with how practitioners carry out their duties.[20] The patient/time productivity index cited in the previous section is a good example of a process indicator.

Process indicator Measures an important activity that contributes directly or indirectly to client care.

Clearly, any number of outcome and process indicators could be selected when undertaking an impact evaluation. Refer to Table 10-2 for a list of the indicators for populations at nutritional risk used by the New York State Nutrition Surveillance Program.[21] The actual indicators chosen for study are dictated by the program's goals and objectives. A list of criteria for choosing the final set of indicators to be used in assessing a program's impact is given in Table 10-3.

The experimental design selected for the impact evaluation depends upon the questions being asked. The standard design is the randomized "true" experiment in which clients are assigned randomly to either a treatment group or a nontreatment group (called the comparison or control group). Most randomized experiments include pre- and post-tests of the outcome indicators. Another type

---

TABLE

10-2

The New York State Nutrition Surveillance Program Indicators for Populations at Nutritional Risk

Source: J. M. Dodds and T. A. Melnick, Development of the New York State Nutrition Surveillance Program, *Public Health Reports* 108 (1993): 232.

Low-income women, infants, and children

Program coverage rates based on an income less than 185% of the poverty level
Low-birth weight rate
Infant mortality rate

Frail elderly

Frailty rate, based on:
◆ Rate of elderly minority group members
◆ Rate of those with income less than 100% of the poverty level
◆ Rate of those older than 85 years
◆ Rate of those older than 75 years and living alone
◆ Rate of discharge with nutrition-related diagnoses
Program coverage rates
Program follow-up, length of program use

Homeless and destitute persons

Emergency food program enumeration to select sites for random samples of monthly monitoring
Annual program census
Program follow-up of food quality

◆ Importance.	Does the measure provide useful and important information on the program that justifies the difficulties in collecting, analyzing, or presenting the data?
◆ Validity.	Does the measure address the aspect of concern? Can changes in the value of the measure be interpreted clearly as desirable or undesirable, and can the changes be attributed directly to the program?
◆ Uniqueness.	Does the information provided by the measure duplicate information provided by another measure?
◆ Accuracy.	Are the likely data sources sufficiently reliable, or are there biases, exaggerations, omissions, or errors that are likely to make the measure inaccurate or misleading?
◆ Timeliness.	Can the data be collected and analyzed in time for the decision?
◆ Privacy and confidentiality.	Are there concerns for privacy or confidentiality that would prevent analysts from obtaining the required information?
◆ Costs of data collection.	Can the resource or cost requirements for data collection be met?
◆ Completeness.	Does the final set of measures cover the major aspects of concern?

TABLE

10-3

Criteria for Choosing a Final Set of Indicators
Source: H. Hatry, L. Blair, D. Fisk, and W. Kimmel, *Program Analysis for State and Local Governments,* 2nd ed. (Washington, D.C.: Urban Institute Press, 1988), p. 41. Used with permission.

of experimental design is the quasi experiment; clients who agree to participate in a program are assigned to the "experimental" group, while clients who do not wish to participate become the "constructed control" group. Obviously, the quasi experiment uses a nonrandom assignment of clients. The time-series design uses periodic measurements of important outcomes to estimate a program's impact over a period of time ranging from several months to several years. This protocol of repeated measurements allows the evaluator to track a trend in the program's impact. In still another design, a cross section of the target population is surveyed to provide an estimate at a single point in time. Clients who received a certain treatment are compared with those who did not in terms of the outcome indicators. Regardless of the design chosen, the evaluator will want to ensure that the impact assessment is both "generalizable," meaning that its results can be applied to the same program implemented in a similar setting, and reproducible, meaning that similar findings would be found by another evaluator using the same design, program elements, and outcome measures. The actual choice of design is influenced by the program objectives, the cost of the impact assessment, and the personnel available to carry it out, among other factors.[22]

Impact evaluations help managers plan for change. Consider the analysis of the nutrition education component of the Title III-C program, which provides for well-balanced, hot meals to be served during the week in congregate settings or homes to maintain the well-being of elderly recipients. The Title III-C program requires that a minimum of two nutrition education sessions per quarter be provided to program participants. An evaluation of this component of the program among Title III-C recipients living in a large county in Arizona found that almost half of the participants were not receiving the mandated nutrition education sessions. The evaluators reported that the elderly participants were "ready and willing" for nutrition education and could benefit from it, especially as a majority of them had low incomes and a limited knowledge of nutrition. These evaluation findings were not meant as an indictment of existing efforts to provide nutrition education, but rather they served as a signal that managers and program administrators need to seek innovative and effective ways of incorporating nutrition education into Title III-C congregate nutrition programs.[23]

Fiscal or Efficiency Evaluation The purpose of fiscal evaluation is to determine how program outcomes compare with their costs. There are two types of efficiency evaluations: cost-benefit analysis and cost-effectiveness analysis.

A cost-benefit analysis requires that managers estimate both the tangible and intangible benefits of a program and the direct and indirect costs of implementing that program, as summarized in Table 10-4 for Nutrition in Action's ABC Fitness Program.[24] Once these have been specified, they must be translated into a common measure, usually a monetary unit. In other words, the cost-benefit analysis examines the program outcomes in terms of money saved or reduced costs. A prenatal program that costs $200 to produce per participant and results in reduced medical costs of $800 can be expressed as a cost-benefit ratio of 1:4. For every one dollar required to produce the program, there is a four dollars savings in medical costs.[25]

Estimating the benefits of a nutrition program, where only a portion of the program benefits can reasonably be given a monetary value, is difficult. As an

TABLE 10-4		
Costs and Benefits Considered in a Cost-Benefit Analysis of Nutrition in Action's ABC Fitness Program		

TYPE	COSTS	BENEFITS
Direct	◆ Salaries of instructors ◆ Telephone ◆ Equipment (e.g., computer) ◆ Travel (e.g., gas and mileage to and from participating worksites) ◆ Postage ◆ Office supplies ◆ Teaching supplies (e.g., slides, overheads, food models, handouts) ◆ Advertising for program ◆ Dues and subscriptions	◆ Revenue from the program
Indirect	◆ Benefits (e.g., health insurance) ◆ Rental of office space ◆ Utilities ◆ Equipment depreciation ◆ Maintenance and repairs ◆ Janitorial services	◆ Increased community exposure for the program ◆ Reduced use of health care services by employees of participating worksites

example, consider a program initiated in a health clinic in a rural area near Beijing, China. The target population consisted of weanling children, aged 6 to 13 months, living in the district; many of them are at high risk of malnutrition, especially iron-deficiency anemia, when they are switched from breast milk to locally available weaning foods.[26] As part of the program, weanling children in the district received a special micronutrient-fortified rusk daily for three months. The outcome indicators were anthropometric measurements (length, weight), hemoglobin concentration, free erythrocyte protoporphyrin in red cells, and plasma ferritin. Some of the benefits and costs of the program are outlined in Table 10-5. In this example, the program manager can readily place a monetary value on the contribution of supplies and personnel to the program's costs. Expressing the benefits in monetary terms is less precise, but it can be estimated. For example, if the program improved the iron, nutrition, and health status of 75 percent of the target population, with the result that they were brought to the health clinic fewer times for the treatment of infections or other conditions, then the manager can estimate this "savings" in the cost of the clinic's primary care personnel treating the infants. Consult the boxed insert for a description of a cost-benefit analysis of the Special Supplemental Food Program for Women, Infants, and Children (WIC).

The second type of efficiency evaluation is cost-effectiveness analysis. Unlike cost-benefit analysis, which reduces a program's benefits and costs to a common monetary unit, cost-effectiveness analysis relates the effectiveness of reaching the program's goals to the monetary value of the resources going into the program. With this type of evaluation, similar programs can be compared to one another or ranked in order of their cost per program goal. A cost-effectiveness analysis

Benefits to Target Population

Improved iron status
Improved nutrition status
Improved health status (as measured by fewer infections and other conditions requiring
　treatment)

Costs of Implementing Program*

Personnel
　Physician
　Nurse
　Nutritionist
　Assistant
Supplies
　Weanling rusks
　Medical supplies
　Laboratory supplies
　General office supplies
Equipment
　Medical
　Laboratory

*This list of the costs associated with the program delivery is not complete. Other costs include utilities, furniture, and the like.

TABLE

10-5

Direct Benefits and Costs of a Weanling Nutrition Program

A Cost-Benefit Analysis of the WIC Program

A cost-benefit analysis helps managers gauge how well a program is meeting its clients' needs and provides data that can be used to influence policymakers. Let's consider an evaluation of prenatal participation in the Special Supplemental Food Program for Women, Infants, and Children (WIC). This cost-benefit analysis was undertaken in North Carolina in 1988.[1] It involved the following steps:[2]

1. **Identify the primary client.** The primary client was the Division of Maternal and Child Health, Department of Environment, Health, and Natural Resources, Raleigh, North Carolina.

2. **Specify the purpose of the evaluation.** The cost-benefit analysis was designed to assess the effect of participation in the prenatal WIC program on low birth weight and Medicaid costs for the medical care of infants born in 1988.

3. **Specify the objectives of the evaluation.** The objectives for the evaluation of WIC prenatal participation in North Carolina in 1988 were to determine:

   ◆ The birth weight of all infants born to WIC mothers.

   ◆ The birth weight of a random sample of infants born to non-WIC mothers.

   ◆ The cost per client of participating in the WIC program.

   ◆ The type and cost of hospital claims for newborn care paid by Medicaid.

4. **Calculate a dollar value for each benefit of the program.** The direct benefits to participants in the WIC program included food and nutrition counseling. Indirect benefits included the birth of infants weighing >2500 grams and reduced costs to Medicaid for the medical management of newborn care. (The dollar value assigned to these benefits was not reported in the published analysis.)

5. **Calculate the costs associated with the program.** Both personnel and material costs were considered. In this analysis, the direct costs included the total value of food vouchers redeemed through the WIC program; administrative costs, estimated at an average of $170 per woman; and the newborn medical care costs paid by Medicaid. Medicaid covered such costs for newborn care as physician services, medications, and inpatient/outpatient care. The direct costs are summarized in Table 10-6, which shows the Medicaid costs for infants whose mothers received WIC prenatal care, Medicaid costs for infants whose mothers did not participate in WIC, and the estimated WIC program costs.

6. **Calculate the total cost per client.** The average cost of the program was $179 per white woman, $164 per black woman, and $170 for both groups.

Continued

would be done, for example, to determine which of two methods of intervention—individual dietary counseling or group nutrition education classes—produces a desired outcome for less cost.

Efficiency evaluation is challenging for planners and policymakers, because it is difficult to determine the point at which a program's costs outweigh its bene-

TABLE 10-6	Average Costs to Medicaid and Average Costs of WIC Services		
	MEDICAID COSTS	**WIC COSTS**[a]	**BENEFIT-TO-COST RATIO**
	WIC	**Non-WIC**		
White	$1778	$2121	$179	1.92
Black	1902	2517	164	3.75
Total	1856	2350	170	2.91

[a]WIC costs include administrative and food costs.

Source: Copyright The American Dietetic Association. Reprinted by permission from *Journal of the American Dietetic Association,* Vol. 93: 1993, p. 166.

7. **Calculate the benefit-to-cost ratio and/or the net savings.** The benefit-to-cost ratio, also shown in Table 10-6, was calculated by subtracting the Medicaid costs for the WIC group (column 1) from the Medicaid costs for the non-WIC group (column 2) and dividing by the WIC costs (column 3). The net savings was the actual dollar difference between the total benefits and the total costs. The estimated net savings was $343 for whites and $615 for blacks (column 1 subtracted from column 2).

The cost-benefit analysis revealed that the savings in Medicaid costs outweighed the costs of WIC services. The benefit-to-cost ratio was 1.92 for white women and 3.75 for black women, meaning that for each dollar spent on WIC, Medicaid saved $1.92 on whites and $3.75 on blacks. In addition, women who received WIC prenatal care gave birth to fewer infants with low and very low birth weights than women who did not participate in WIC.

A cost-benefit analysis undertaken by another state with a different sample of women and infants would likely produce slightly different results in program costs and the benefit-to-cost ratio. Even so, the findings of fiscal evaluations can be used to convince policymakers that money allocated for the WIC program is well spent and that cost savings can be achieved with nutrition intervention.

1. The description of the cost-benefit analysis of the WIC program was adapted from P. A. Buescher and coauthors, Prenatal WIC participation can reduce low birth weight and newborn medical costs: A cost-benefit analysis of WIC participation in North Carolina, *Journal of the American Dietetic Association* 93 (1993): 163–66.
2. The procedure for conducting a cost-benefit analysis was adapted from the Ross Roundtable Report, *Benefits of Nutrition Services: A Costing and Marketing Approach* (Columbus, Ohio: Ross Laboratories, 1987), pp. 24–29.

fits.[27] Nonetheless, efforts to document the economic benefits of nutrition services have increased in recent years, due largely to health care reform and the ADA's drive to have dietetics professionals recognized as the providers of cost-effective prevention services.[28] The ADA has begun documenting the economic costs and benefits of nutrition care for diverse populations, including burn and surgical patients, pregnant women, infants, and adults with chronic diseases such as hypertension, diabetes mellitus, obesity, and atherosclerosis. In some areas, such as prenatal care, there is ample evidence that nutrition programs have a positive economic benefit and cost savings; in other areas, such as providing nutrition education to improve dental health among children, additional data are needed to confirm the value of nutrition services.[29]

The Program Evaluation Process

There is no single procedure for carrying out an evaluation, as each must be tailored for the organization or department in which it is conducted. Nevertheless, the Joint Commission on Accreditation of Healthcare Organizations (JCAHO), the licensing and governing agency for the evaluation of health care services, has developed a 10-step process to help health care organizations monitor and evaluate health outcomes and improve health care. The 10-step process is commonly referred to as quality assurance (QA). **Quality assurance** is a problem-solving approach used to measure and monitor health care to ensure that it is both effective and efficient. The primary goal of a quality assurance program is improving the public's health outcome.[30]

Quality assurance A problem-solving approach used to measure and monitor health care to ensure that it is effective and efficient.

The quality assurance program helps the organization use its resources effectively by focusing on high-priority quality-of-care issues. The quality assurance program has several mandates: it should meet the organization's needs, use available resources, and have achievable goals.[31] Before implementing the JCAHO 10-step process for quality assurance, three issues should be addressed:

Ensuring program effectiveness requires a two-step process. QA is the first step in identifying problems and improving program delivery. The second step, called Improvement of Organizational Performance or IOP, is designed to ensure that the organization uses its resources efficiently and produces services of high quality and at a reasonable cost. The emphasis of IOP is on Continuous Quality Improvement (CQI) through teamwork, training, quality control, and performance review.

◆ First, define the primary client. This step is necessary because many parties will be interested in the evaluation outcome. By determining the primary client at the outset, the evaluator clarifies the party to whom he is accountable and whose mandate guides the evaluation.

◆ Second, formulate the purpose and objectives of the evaluation. A broad statement of purpose guides the evaluator. Is the evaluation designed to assess the need for changing the program delivery? Demonstrate that public monies are being spent appropriately? Contribute to our understanding of community nutrition practice? An evaluation may have more than one purpose. Specific, measurable objectives are also needed. Without objectives, the evaluator cannot be sure that he has assessed precisely what he was supposed to assess.

◆ Third, draw up an administrative agreement between the evaluator and the program manager or other involved parties to ensure that everyone is operating on the same wavelength. The agreement might cover such topics as the scope of the evaluation; details about the plan for conducting the evaluation, the collection and analysis of data, and the research design; the breakdown of expenditures; the responsibilities of program staff in carrying out certain evaluation tasks; the protocol for consulting management about the program delivery; quality control measures; and how the final report will be distributed and publicized.

Once the groundwork for the evaluation has been laid, the JCAHO 10-step process, summarized in Table 10-7, can be followed:[32]

1. Assign responsibility for monitoring and evaluating activities. The personnel responsible for identifying indicators, collecting data, evaluating care, and monitoring the evaluation process should be designated first. In a public health department, the senior public health nutritionist may serve as the quality assurance officer.

2. Delineate the scope of care provided by the organization or department. An inventory should be made of the organization's or department's activities and areas of responsibilities. For example, Nutrition at Work provides counseling and programming related to nutrition, health, and fitness among adults. It does not provide pediatric AIDS counseling.

3. Identify the most important aspects of care provided by the organization or department. These are called functions. Those functions that affect the largest number of clients, pose the greatest risk to client health, or represent an ongoing problem should be given priority. For Nutrition at Work, the important aspects of care might include providing counseling and education for clients, monitoring the survey of executive risk factors, and evaluating risk factor reduction among clients.

4. Identify indicators. The choice of indicators depends upon the purpose and objectives of the evaluation. The indicators, whether outcome or process, should be measurable. For Nutrition at Work, one indicator might be "client comprehension of nutrition education."

5. Establish thresholds (levels, patterns, and trends) for the indicators that trigger an evaluation of care. In other words, for each indicator, there should be an acceptable level and an unacceptable range that signals the need for evaluation. Thresholds can also be thought of as performance standards. Performance or quality standards are a benchmark against which the evaluation outcomes can be measured. The threshold for the

1. Assign responsibility. 2. Delineate the scope of care. 3. Identify the important aspects of care. 4. Identify indicators. 5. Establish thresholds for evaluation. 6. Collect and organize data. 7. Evaluate care. 8. Take action to improve care. 9. Assess actions and document improvements. 10. Communicate findings or outcomes.	**TABLE** **10-7** **The JCAHO 10-Step Process for Quality Assurance**

Source: R. P. Puckett, JCAHO's agenda for change. Copyright The American Dietetic Association. Reprinted by permission from *Journal of the American Dietetic Association,* Vol. 91: 1991, p. 1225.

indicator "client comprehension of nutrition education" might be set at 75 percent, meaning that 75 percent of the clients participating in Nutrition at Work's fitness programs will have a score of "good" or better on a nutrition knowledge test.

6. Monitor the important aspects of care by collecting and organizing the data for each indicator. This step addresses the design of the program evaluation. A program evaluation should be appropriate, yield interpretable results, and be generalizable. A sophisticated design is not needed if a simpler design will serve as well. In our example of Nutrition at Work, the level of client comprehension of nutrition education was estimated by administering a knowledge test based on material presented in individual and group counseling sessions.

7. When thresholds are met, evaluate care to identify opportunities for improvement or to correct problems. Even when the threshold has been met or exceeded, managers should continually look for ways in which overall program performance and delivery can be improved.

8. Take actions to improve care or to correct identified problems. When thresholds are not met within a certain period of time (for example, six months, one year), develop an action plan to identify the problem, what caused it, how it can be corrected, who is responsible for implementing the appropriate change, when the action or change is to occur, and what action is to be taken.

9. Assess the effectiveness of the actions and document the improvement in care. This step addresses the need for constant monitoring of the problem to ensure that it is finally resolved.

10. Communicate the results of the monitoring and evaluation process to relevant individuals, departments, or services and to the quality assurance program. The final report should be comprehensive, kept to a reasonable length, and include specific recommendations for action. (Tips for effectively communicating the evaluation findings appear in the next section.)

Although these procedural steps of program evaluation were developed primarily for health organizations such as hospitals, HMOs, and clinics, they are relevant to other types of organizations. Regardless of the organizational setting, evaluation research should be flexible. In *Designing Evaluations of Educational and Social Programs,* Lee J. Cronbach put it this way: ". . . evaluations should not be cast into a single mold. For any good evaluation many good designs can be proposed, but no perfect ones."[33]

Communicating Evaluation Findings

Because the primary purpose of evaluations is to provide information for decision making, you do not want your findings to go unused. If they are stored away in a filing cabinet or get dumped into the "circular file," a program may continue missing the mark or a success story may go unnoticed. With careful planning and work, you can ensure that the main findings of your evaluation get the attention they deserve.

Even as you begin the actual evaluation, you should be thinking about the final report! As the evaluation progresses, make notes of how problems were handled and which documents or materials were used. Retain copies of survey instruments and computer printouts as reference items or for use in the report's appendix. When you begin preparing your report, keep these three rules in mind:[34]

♦ Communicate the information to the appropriate potential users.

♦ Ensure that the report addresses the issues that the users perceive to be important.

♦ Ensure that the report is delivered in time to be useful and in a form that the intended users can easily understand.

Notice that we come back to the importance of identifying the primary client for your evaluation. In some situations—perhaps, in most—an evaluation will have many potential users. Although you may be preparing your findings for your immediate supervisor, it is likely that they will be reviewed by a much broader audience: senior management, the board of directors, an accrediting or funding agency, policymakers, and so forth. Thus, when preparing your report, tailor your findings for your primary client, but be mindful that they will be examined by other users. From the very beginning, put yourself in the user's place and ask the following questions:[35]

♦ To what extent and in what specific ways is the information *relevant* to the user's problems?

♦ To what extent is the information *practical* from the user's perspective?

♦ To what extent is the information *useful* and immediately applicable to the user's situation?

♦ What information will the user consider *credible?*

♦ To what extent is the information *understandable* to the primary user?

♦ How can reporting practices ensure that the information is delivered in a *timely* fashion so that it can be used in making decisions?

With these questions in mind, prepare your report. Depending upon the purpose and objectives of your evaluation, the report may be either informal (e.g., a short memorandum) or formal (e.g., a full report). In either case, the report should be concise and understandable and should give the user what she needs to make a decision. Our focus in this discussion is on the formal report, which tends to have a particular organization:[36]

1. **Front cover.** The front cover should provide (1) the title of the program and its location; (2) the name of the evaluator(s); (3) the period covered by the report; and (4) the date the report was submitted. The front cover should be neat and formatted attractively.

◆ PROFESSIONAL FOCUS

Introducing Sally P. Temple, M.S., R.D.

◆ HER BACKGROUND . . .

Sally Temple is currently the director of the Division of Cardiovascular Health in the Center for Health Promotion, South Carolina Department of Health and Environmental Control in Columbia, South Carolina. The focus of this position is to assist the district health promotion staff in developing community-based health promotion interventions. She spends a considerable amount of time networking and building partnerships between the state health department and other organizations.

◆ SHE HAS THIS TO SAY ABOUT ENTREPRENEURSHIP . . .

"Being an entrepreneur is critical when working with the community, because the community is constantly changing and evolving. Nutrition fads come and go—what works today may not work tomorrow. The entrepreneurial nutritionist looks for new ways to create healthy communities and is willing to take the risk to work with nontraditional partners who will jointly make a difference in the community environment."

Temple is currently involved in a statewide, community-based health promotion program that charts a new direction for South Carolina. She comments, "Our former clinic-based model sought high-risk individuals living in the community and prescribed a treatment protocol for them. This clinic-based program utilized a variety of health care professionals who often worked in a vacuum. The community-based approach that we currently use is different. It focuses on attacking chronic diseases such as heart disease and cancer *before* symptoms and disease develop. And it requires teamwork and extensive community organization."

"Community organization," notes Temple, "involves developing partnerships, often with nontraditional partners. For example, using parents as advocates for a healthy school environment, including healthy food in the school cafeteria, can be more effective than having a health professional tell the school of the changes that need to be made."

Temple points to policy as another key element of the successful community-based program. She says, "Policies related to the access of healthy foods and nutrition skills development are critical for a supportive environment. Worksites, schools, restaurants, and grocery stores are all potential sites for policies that influence behavior and the environment."

In Temple's view, the growth of community-based programming has implications for the practice of community nutrition. "As nutrition professionals working in community-based programs," she says, "we are catalysts and enablers, equipping the community to take responsibility and action for creating an environment that supports healthy eating patterns. Instead of developing a nutrition plan of action *for* the community, we are working *with* the community to stimulate policy change and cultivate a healthy community."

"The important thing is for community nutritionists to diversify—to see themselves as more than providers of nutrition information. Today, community nutritionists take an active leadership role in creating public and private partnerships, ensuring citizen participation in the process, and promoting policy changes. They work to make sure the community environment supports health."

2. **Summary.** Sometimes called the *executive summary,* this section of the report is a brief overview of the evaluation, explaining why and how it was done and listing its major conclusions and recommendations. Typically, this section is prepared for the individual who does not have time to read the full report. Therefore, it should not be longer than one or two pages. Even though the summary appears first in the report, it should be written *last.*

3. **Background information.** This section places the program in context, describing what the program was designed to do and how it began. The amount of detail provided in this section will depend upon the needs and knowledge of the users. If most readers are unfamiliar with the program, it should be described in some detail; if most readers are involved with the program, this section can be kept short. A typical outline for this section might include the following:

   ◆ Origin of the program

   ◆ Goals of the program

   ◆ Clients involved in the program

   ◆ Characteristics of the program materials, activities, and administrative procedures

   ◆ Staff involved with the program

4. **Description of the evaluation study.** This section states the purpose of the evaluation, including why it was conducted and what it was intended to accomplish. Here you define the scope of the evaluation and describe how it was carried out. This section establishes the credibility of the evaluator and the evaluation findings (much like the "Methods" section of a research paper). Technical information about the study design and analysis is presented here. Technical language should be kept to a minimum, however. Refer readers to appendixes for specific technical information and copies of any instruments used in the evaluation study. A general outline for this section might include the following headings:

   ◆ Purposes of the evaluation

   ◆ Evaluation design

   ◆ Outcome measures

     ◆ Instruments used

     ◆ Data collection and analysis procedures

   ◆ Process measures

     ◆ Instruments used

     ◆ Data collection and analysis procedures

5. **Results.** This section presents the results of the outcome or process evaluation. It is appropriate to present data or summarize findings in tables, figures, graphs, or charts. Before you begin writing this section, you should

have already analyzed the data, tested for statistical significance (if appropriate), and prepared the tables, figures, and other illustrations.

6. **Discussion of results.** The results of the evaluation study are interpreted in this section, which should address two key issues: How certain is it that the program caused the results? How good were the results? The Results section explores some of the reasons why a certain outcome was reached and how the program compares to similar programs. Any strengths and weaknesses of the program are described here.

7. **Conclusions, recommendations, and options.** This section is an influential part of the report, as it outlines the major conclusions that can be drawn from the evaluation and lists a suggested course of action for enhancing the program's strengths and dealing with its deficiencies. The recommendations should address specific aspects of the program and follow logically from your interpretation of the evaluation findings. Preparing a list of recommendations about the program's delivery or impact is especially important when the actual results differ from the predetermined objectives.

Once your report is written, you must decide how best to distribute it. Any number of options are available. You may decide to send the full report to your immediate supervisor, division director, and board of directors and a copy of the executive summary to interested community groups. You may also decide to inform the media by preparing and distributing a press release. In some cases, one or more of these strategies for publishing the evaluation findings will have been specified upfront by the primary client; if not, you may want to suggest the formats you believe will best communicate the findings to the various audiences. Figure 10-1 shows how the findings of the evaluation study might be distributed.

The Challenge of Multicultural Evaluation

Multiculturalism poses some unique and difficult problems for evaluation research, as it brings into focus the conflicts, misunderstandings, confusions, and tensions inherent in multicultural settings. Although this is especially true for evaluators working in foreign countries, it is also the reality for those working in their own culturally diverse communities. Conducting a fair and democratic evaluation in a multicultural environment requires striking a balance between the rights of minority culture groups and the rights of the larger culture—a complex policy issue.

What does multiculturalism mean for the evaluator? First, the evaluator must strive to remain neutral in the face of competing minority interests. This is especially true when stakeholders have strong views about the evaluation outcome, try to influence the outcome, or downplay the possible contribution of the evaluation process.[37] Second, the evaluator must search out and define the views and interests of the minority groups to ensure that their needs are being met. When the minority group is defined as "poor" or "powerless," the evaluator has

Audience/users	Technical report	Executive summary	Technical professional paper	Popular article	News release, press conference	Public meeting	Media appearance	Staff workshop	Brochure	Memorandum	Personal presentation
Program administrators	✓	✓	✓	✓	✓			✓		✓	✓
Board members, trustees, other management staff		✓		✓							
Advisory committees	✓	✓	✓								
Funding agencies	✓	✓									✓
Community groups		✓		✓		✓					
Current clients				✓		✓	✓				
Potential clients								✓			
Political bodies (e.g., city councils, legislatures)		✓		✓							
Program service providers (e.g., nutritionists, health educators)		✓		✓				✓	✓	✓	✓
Organizations interested in the program content			✓	✓							
Media					✓	✓					

FIGURE 10-1

Forms of Communicating Evaluation Findings to Various Audiences

Source: L. L. Morris and coauthors, *How to Communicate Evaluation Findings* (Newbury, Calif.: Sage Publications, 1987), pp. 9–10. Used with permission.

an obligation to recognize the views and interests of this group. Finally, the evaluator must be sensitive to the cultural differences that make implementing the evaluation difficult. The manner in which questions are asked, or the questions themselves, may be barriers to obtaining reliable data about the program's impact. Perhaps the best message about multiculturalism was given by E. R. House at the University of Colorado at Boulder: "Treat minority cultures as you would be treated. Sooner or later, everyone may be a minority."[38]

The Larger Realm of Program Evaluation

Although the immediate purpose of program evaluation is to help managers make decisions about the short- and long-term operation of their programs, evaluations also serve to inform the community at large about a program's successes or failures. When a community-based nutrition program succeeds, nutritionists in other locations across the country want to know how the lessons can be used in their communities. Likewise, when programs fail, community nutritionists want to examine these failures and figure out how to avoid them in the future.

Program evaluations force community nutrition organizers to determine whether they are progressing toward their initial goals and if these goals are still appropriate. They stimulate an examination of a program's strengths and weaknesses, whether its benefits balance its costs, and whether the program should or can be redesigned to improve its effectiveness and efficiency. The finding that a program is not accomplishing its objectives signals a need to consider whether the program is worthwhile or whether its goals can be accomplished in some other fashion.[39] By undertaking systematic, periodic evaluations, managers and other stakeholders are likely to ensure that their program successfully addresses a public health or nutrition problem and improves the community's health.

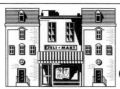 # COMMUNITY LEARNING ACTIVITY

In this Community Learning Activity, you will address some of the evaluation research issues discussed in this chapter. At this point, you should have outlined what your program is designed to accomplish. With that in mind, complete the following activities:

1. Define the primary client for your evaluation. Who are the other stakeholders with an interest in your program?

2. Specify two primary outcome indicators and thresholds.

3. For one of your outcome objectives, specified in Chapter 6's Community Learning Activity, describe how you would collect data to show that your program accomplished what it was supposed to accomplish.

4. Describe one formative study that you would undertake before launching your program.

NOTES

1. A. Gadomski and C. Kjolhede, Vitamin A deficiency and childhood morbidity and mortality: Scientific background and implications for child survival, Occasional Paper No. 4, Johns Hopkins University School of Hygiene and Public Health, Institute for International Programs (Baltimore, Md.: Johns Hopkins University, 1988), pp. 31–34.

2. D. A. Thomas-Dobersen and coauthors, Evaluation of a weight management intervention program in adolescents with insulin-dependent diabetes mellitus, *Journal of the American Dietetic Association* 93 (1993): 535–40.

3. E. A. Frongillo, Jr., and F. Bégin, Gender bias in food intake favors male preschool Guatemalan children, *Journal of Nutrition* 123 (1993): 189–96.

4. P. H. Rossi and H. E. Freeman, *Evaluation—A Systematic Approach* (Beverly Hills, Calif.: Sage Publications, 1985), pp. 19–27.

5. Ibid., p. 18.

6. A. D. Spiegel and H. H. Hyman, *Strategic Health Planning: Methods and Techniques Applied to Marketing and Management* (Norwood, N.J.: Ablex Publishing, 1991), pp. 324–25.

7. A. D. Grotelueschen and coauthors, *An Evaluation Planner* (Urbana, Ill.: Office for the Study of Continuing Professional Education, University of Illinois at Urbana-Champaign, 1974).

8. Health care reform legislative platform: Economic benefits of nutrition services, *Journal of the American Dietetic Association* 93 (1993): 686–90.

9. Grassroots lobbying network in place, *ADA Courier* 32 (1993): 1–2.

10. D. J. Caron, Knowledge required to perform the duties of an evaluator, *Canadian Journal of Program Evaluation* 8 (1993): 59–78.

11. Rossi and Freeman, *Evaluation,* pp. 38–45.

12. S. Smitasiri and coauthors, Participatory action for nutrition education: Social marketing vitamin A–rich foods in Thailand, *Ecology of Food and Nutrition* 28 (1992): 199–210.

13. G. E. A. Dever, *Community Health Analysis—Global Awareness at the Local Level* (Gaithersburg, Md.: Aspen Publishers, 1991), pp. 45–73.

14. J. B. McKinlay, The promotion of health through planned sociopolitical change: Challenges for research and policy, *Social Science and Medicine* 36 (1993): 109–17.

15. L. S. Bell and M. M. Fairchild, Development of a productivity index to increase accountability of ambulatory nutrition services, *Journal of the American Dietetic Association* 89 (1989): 517–19.

16. Characteristics of clinical indicators, *QRB* (November 1989): 330–39.

17. Spiegel and Hyman, *Strategic Health Planning,* pp. 352–69.

18. The definitions of outcome and process indicators were taken from For Your Information, Learning the language of quality care, *Journal of the American Dietetic Association* 93 (1993): 531–32.

19. F. L. Trowbridge and coauthors, Coordinated strategies for controlling micronutrient malnutrition: A technical workshop, *Journal of Nutrition* 123 (1993): 775–87.

20. R. Lehmann, Forum on clinical indicator development: A discussion of the use and development of indicators, *QRB* (July 1989): 223–27.

21. J. M. Dodds and T. A. Melnik, Development of the New York State Nutrition Surveillance Program, *Public Health Reports* 108 (1993): 230–40.

22. Rossi and Freeman, *Evaluation,* pp. 227–319.

23. L. L. Hutchings and A. M. Tinsley, Nutrition education for older adults: How Title III-C program participants perceive their needs, *Journal of Nutrition Education* 23 (1991): 53–58.

24. H. G. Tolpin, Economics of health care, *Journal of the American Dietetic Association* 76 (1980): 217–22.

25. E. Bartlett, Cost-benefit and cost-effectiveness analyses, in *Benefits of Nutrition Services: A Costing and Marketing Approach* (Columbus, Ohio: Ross Laboratories, 1987), p. 20.

26. D-s. Liu and coauthors, Nutritional efficacy of a fortified weaning rusk in a rural area near Beijing, *American Journal of Clinical Nutrition* 57 (1993): 506–11.

27. G. D. Berman and coauthors, Effectiveness research and assessment of clinical outcome: A review of federal government and medical community involvement, *Mayo Clinic Proceedings* 65 (1990): 657–63.

28. Health care reform legislative platform: Economic benefits of nutrition services, *Journal of the American Dietetic Assocation* 93 (1993): 686–90.

29. Specific information about the costs and benefits of nutrition services can be found in D. D. Disbrow, The costs and benefits of nutrition services: A literature review, *Journal of the American Dietetic Association* 89 (1989): S-3–S-66 and P. L. Splett, Effectiveness and cost effectiveness of nutrition care: A critical analysis with recommendations, *Journal of the American Dietetic Association* 91 (1991): S-1–S-53.

30. N. H. Wooldridge and G. Joyner, Quality assurance, in *Call to Action: Better Nutrition for Mothers, Children, and Families,* ed. C. O. Sharbaugh (Washington, D.C.: National Center for Education in Maternal and Child Health, 1991), p. 257.

31. S. F. Edelstein, Using thresholds to monitor dietetic services: The JCAHO 10-step process for quality assurance, *Journal of the American Dietetic Association* 91 (1991): 1261–65.

32. Ibid.

33. L. J. Cronbach, *Designing Evaluations of Educational and Social Programs* (San Francisco: Jossey-Bass, 1982), pp. 1–2.

34. L. L. Morris and coauthors, *How to Communicate Evaluation Findings* (Newbury Park, Calif.: Sage Publications, 1987), pp. 9–10.

35. Ibid., pp. 20–22.

36. Ibid., pp. 77–89.

37. M. O'Brecht, Stakeholder pressures and organizational structure for program evaluation, *Canadian Journal of Program Evaluation* 7 (1992): 139–47.

38. E. R. House, Multicultural evaluation in Canada and the United States, *Canadian Journal of Program Evaluation* 7 (1992): 153.

39. H. J. Rubin and I. S. Rubin, *Community Organizing and Development,* 2nd ed. (New York: Macmillan, 1992), pp. 410–13.

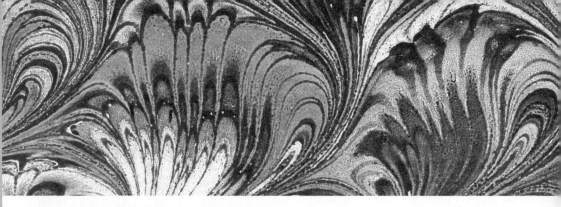

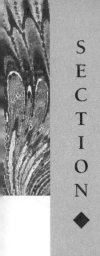

Raising the Roof: Programs for Promoting and Protecting the Public's Health

Putting the roof into place is a critical moment in erecting a home, office, or high-rise building. Suddenly, the structure *looks* like a building. Until the roof goes up, the structure is glaringly incomplete, and workers must toil in sun, wind, and rain. The roof offers protection from the elements for workers who must finish the interior and make the building habitable.

Putting a nutrition program into place in the community is much like raising a roof. The program helps "protect" certain people from the environmental and social elements that place them at risk for disease and poor health. By providing knowledge about how to choose foods for good health, it offers some security to those who have little money to spend on food. It helps control the problems associated with malnutrition, whether those problems arise from too little or too much food.

In this section, we present information about the major food assistance and nutrition programs of the federal government and other noteworthy community-based programs. The section is generally divided along lifecycle lines, with chapters on mothers and infants, children and adolescents, and adults. We include chapters on poverty, food insecurity, and international issues in nutrition, because we believe these areas are increasingly important in a shrinking global community.

We encourage you to draw on the material you have already learned in studying the chapters that follow. By now, you can appreciate the complexities of policy making, goal setting, program design, and human behavior. You know how challenging the process of program development can be. As you review the programs described in these chapters, consider how *you* would change the delivery of community-based nutrition programs and the policies that influence them.

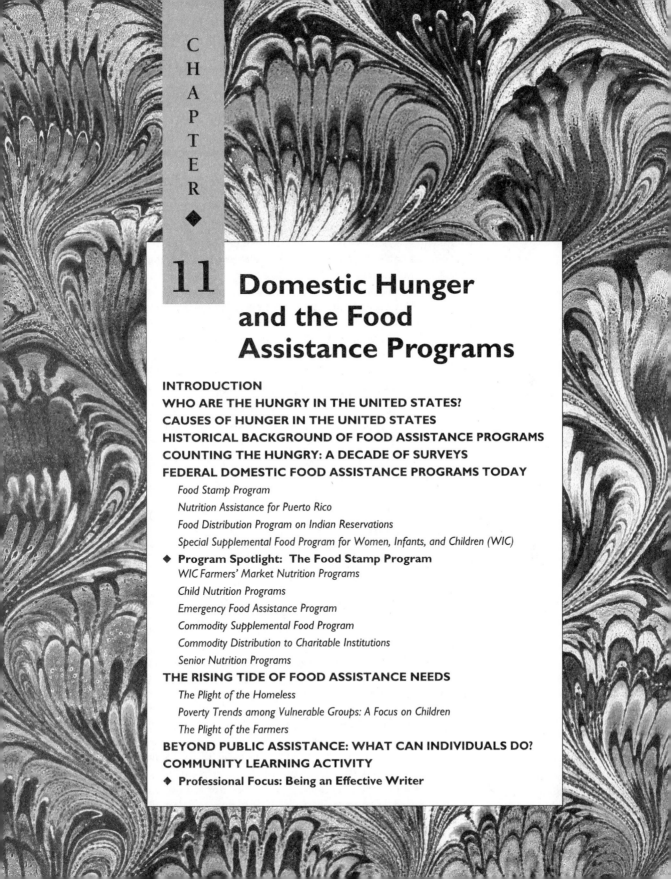

11 Domestic Hunger and the Food Assistance Programs

Something to Think About . . .

The goal of nutrition is to apply scientific knowledge to feed people, to feed them adequately, and to feed them all. . . . It would be a mistake to think of nutrition simply as a group of empirical prescriptions for personal and social behavior. Rather, nutrition is an agenda, the fulfillment of which requires the knowledge of a number of sciences—biochemistry, physiology, pathology, epidemiology, psychology, economics, and sociology. By its nature, nutrition is a set of scientific disciplines whose end is action. . . . Nutritionists, unlike biochemists or physiologists, but like cardiologists and pediatricians, have to see their science as one whose goal is the benefit of mankind. Action often has to be taken on a reasonable presumption of health benefit without obvious health costs. As researchers, nutritionists have made amazing strides over an extremely short period in the history of science. I have every confidence we will continue to do so. But studying the metabolism of vitamin B-12 in the laboratory rat or the pathology of aging in the gerbil is not enough. While research continues in nutrition and agriculture, we must provide for the people who are here now, in America and the world. It is my hope that the new generation of nutritionists, trained in the sciences that form the basis of nutrition, will also keep this goal clearly in mind.

—Jean Mayer

Introduction

The problems of overnutrition—obesity, heart disease, cancer, and others—have guided the nutrition and health objectives and recommendations of the economically developed nations, for these are the diseases of our society. Not everyone shares these problems, though. People in developing nations, as well as people in the less-privileged parts of developed nations, suffer the problems of **undernutrition**, which is characterized by chronic debilitating hunger and **malnutrition**. These conditions are most visible in times of **famine**, but they are widespread and persistent even when famine does not occur. They have been with us throughout history, and despite numerous development and assistance programs, they are not disappearing; the number of hungry and malnourished people continues to grow. Hunger and malnutrition can be found among people of both sexes and all ages and nationalities. Even so, these problems hit some groups harder than others.

Everyone has known the uncomfortable feeling of hunger that signals "time to eat" and passes with the eating of the next meal. But many people know hunger more intimately because a meal does not follow to quiet the signal. For them, hunger is a constant companion bringing ceaseless discomfort, weakness,

Undernutrition As used in this chapter, a continuous lack of the food energy and nutrients necessary to achieve and maintain health and protection from disease; both a domestic and a world problem.

Malnutrition The impairment of health resulting from a relative deficiency or excess of food energy and specific nutrients necessary for health.

and pain—the continuous lack of food and nutrients. People who live with chronic hunger either have too little food to eat or do not receive an adequate intake of the essential nutrients from the foods available to them—either way, malnutrition ensues. One person in the developing world described hunger as follows:

> For hunger is a curious thing: at first it is with you all the time, waking and sleeping and in your dreams, and your belly cries out insistently, and there is a gnawing and a pain as if your very vitals were being devoured, and you must stop it at any cost, and you buy a moment's respite even while you know and fear the sequel. Then the pain is no longer sharp but dull, and this too is with you always, so that you think of food many times a day and each time a terrible sickness assails you, and because you know this you try to avoid the thought, but you cannot, it is with you. Then that too is gone, all pain, all desire, only a great emptiness is left, like the sky, like a well in drought, and it is now that the strength drains from your limbs, and you try to rise and you cannot, or to swallow and your throat is powerless, and both the swallow and the effort of retaining the liquid tax you to the uttermost.[1]

Today the phenomenon of hunger is being discussed in terms of food security or insecurity. **Food security** means that all people at all times have access to enough food for an active, healthy life. At a minimum, it includes the following: (1) the ready availability of nutritionally adequate and safe foods and (2) the ability to acquire personally acceptable foods in a socially acceptable way.[2] A writer in Boston describes **food insecurity** in more personal terms:[3]

> I've had no income and I've paid no rent for many months. My landlord let me stay. He felt sorry for me because I had no money. The Friday before Christmas he gave me ten dollars. For days I have had nothing but water. I knew I needed food; I tried to go out but I was too weak to walk to the store. I felt as if I were dying. I saw the mailman and told him I thought I was starving. He brought me food and then he made some phone calls and that's when they began delivering these lunches. But I had already lost so much weight that five meals a week are not enough to keep me going.
>
> I just pray to God I can survive. I keep praying I have the will to save some of my food so I can divide it up and make it last. It's hard to save because I am so hungry that I want to eat it right away. On Friday, I held over two peas from the lunch. I ate one pea on Saturday morning. Then I got into bed with the taste of food in my mouth and I waited as long as I could. Later on in the day I ate the other pea.
>
> Today I saved the container that the mashed potatoes were in and tonight, before bed, I'll lick the sides of the container. When there are bones I keep them. I know this is going to be hard for you to believe and I am almost ashamed to tell you, but these days I boil the bones until they're soft and then I eat them. Today there were no bones.[4]

This chapter examines the extent of hunger and malnutrition in the United States; Chapter 15 examines the incidence of hunger around the world. Both chapters offer suggestions for personal involvement with the issues presented. As you read, challenge yourself with the following questions: What problems would you attack first in solving the problem of hunger and food insecurity? Should we solve our own hunger problems before tackling problems related to international hunger? These issues are complex and often overwhelming from an individual's

Famine Widespread lack of access to food due to natural disasters, political factors, or war; characterized by a large number of deaths due to starvation and malnutrition.

Food security Access by all people at all times to enough food through normal channels for an active, healthy life.

Food insecurity The inability to acquire or consume an adequate quality or sufficient quantity of food in socially acceptable ways, or the uncertainty that one will be able to do so.

standpoint. Remember, however, as you read, that it is better to light one small candle than to curse the darkness.

Who Are the Hungry in the United States?

The United States is one of the wealthiest nations in the world, consumes 40 percent of the world's resources, and is home to only 6 percent of the world's people.[5] Still, it does not meet the food needs of its poor.

Through the late 1960s, hunger was evident among the chronic poor: migrant workers, Native Americans, southern blacks, unemployed minorities, and some of the elderly. These groups were hungry during the 1970s and 1980s as well, as were the newly unemployed blue-collar workers. Now, hunger is reaching into other segments of the population without regard for age, marital status, previous employment or successes, family ties, or efforts to change the situation. The U.S. farm economy has been burdened by chronic price-depressing surpluses, and available resources are failing to reach many groups. One person in 12 goes hungry at least two days a month. The millions who experience hunger today in the United States include the following:

◆ **The young.** One in five U.S. children lives in poverty.[6]

◆ **The new poor.** Changes in the nation's economy during the 1980s have hurt millions of people who were once members of the middle class—displaced farm families and former blue-collar workers forced out of manufacturing (oil, natural gas, steel, and mining) into the service sector (maintenance and the hotel and restaurant industry). The auto industry, for example, has laid off some 40 percent of its workers since 1980. Only a third of them find jobs that pay as well as their old ones. A job that pays the minimum wage does not lift a family above the federal poverty line, and many such jobs fail to provide fringe benefits to help meet rising health care costs. A minority of the poor in the United States are on welfare; most are working people.

◆ **The elderly.** Social Security and other programs have pulled many older people out of poverty, but large numbers of older people who cannot work and have no savings or families to turn to are facing rising bills for housing, utilities, food, and health care.

◆ **The homeless.** As many as 3 million people may now be living on the streets. More than half of the homeless are single mothers with children; many of the homeless are former residents of psychiatric institutions.

◆ **Low-income women.** Many women live in poverty, struggling to provide child care while working for the minimum wage.

◆ **Ethnic minorities.** Although the majority of the poor in America are white, the median income of African American and Hispanic families is lower than that of white families.

Poverty The state of having too little money to meet minimum needs for food, clothing, and shelter. As of 1994, the U.S. Department of Health and Human Services defined a poverty-level income as $14,800 annually for a family of four.

The most compelling single reason for this hunger is **poverty**.

Causes of Hunger in the United States

Poverty and hunger are interdependent. Most studies conducted since 1980 attribute the increases in hunger throughout the country to worsening economic conditions among the poor. Table 11-1 shows how poverty has increased among a number of population groups. Why are these increases in poverty occurring? For one thing, federal spending for antipoverty programs was significantly reduced during the 1980s (see Figure 11-1). Between 1982 and 1985, federal expenditures for human services programs were cut by $110 billion in an attempt to reduce the national debt. Programs were eliminated, eligibility requirements were tightened, no adjustments for inflation were allowed, and budgets for the remaining programs were slashed. Some of the most severe reductions came in programs directly affecting those deepest in poverty, including Aid to Families with Dependent Children (AFDC), food stamps, low-income housing assistance, and child nutrition. Funding for the school lunch program was cut by one-third.[7] Cuts in college financial aid effectively blocked a pathway out of poverty taken by many in the past.

While poverty is the major cause of hunger in the United States, other problems also contribute:

◆ Alcoholism and chronic substance abuse, which often contribute to increased poverty and malnutrition among not only the afflicted individuals, but their families as well.

◆ Mental illness, loneliness, isolation, depression, and despair, which may result in people ceasing to be concerned for their own physical well-being.

◆ The reluctance of people, particularly the elderly, to accept what they perceive as "welfare" or "charity."

◆ Delays in receiving requested food stamps and other public assistance benefits.

◆ An increase in the number of single mothers without the means to care for their children.

◆ Poor management of limited family financial resources.

CATEGORY	NATIONAL RATE OF POVERTY INCREASE
Infants and children under six years old	+63%
The "working poor"*	+56%
Poor married couples (two-parent families)	+47%
Young adults living independently	+13%
Single-parent families (usually headed by women)	+10%
The elderly	−3%

*Families who receive 75% of their income from jobs, as opposed to public assistance benefits.

TABLE

11-1

Increases in U.S. Poverty during the 1980s
Source: U.S. Bureau of the Census, *Statistical Updates* (Washington, D.C.: U.S. Government Printing Office, 1989).

FIGURE

11-1

U.S. Federal Budget Increases and Decreases, 1980–1990*

Source: Adapted from Bread for the World Institute, *Hunger 1990: A Report on the State of World Hunger* (Washington, D.C.: Bread for the World Institute, 1990), p. 98. Reprinted by permission.

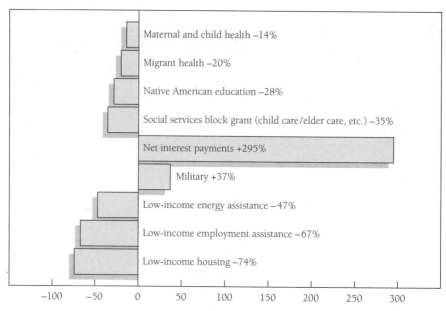

Maternal and child health –14%
Migrant health –20%
Native American education –28%
Social services block grant (child care/elder care, etc.) –35%
Net interest payments +295%
Military +37%
Low-income energy assistance –47%
Low-income employment assistance –67%
Low-income housing –74%

*All figures are adjusted for inflation. Military figures are from 1980–1990; low-income figures are from fiscal years 1981–1990.

♦ Health problems of old age, precipitating an inability to purchase and prepare food.

♦ Lack of nutritional adequacy and balance in the food available to hungry people through emergency feeding programs and food assistance organizations, which take what they can get and pass it on to hungry people.

♦ Lack of access to assistance programs because of intimidation, ineligibility, complicated paperwork, and other reasons.

♦ Insufficient community food resources for the hungry.

♦ Insufficient community transportation systems to deliver food to hungry people who have no transportation.[8]

Health experts saw similar situations back in the 1930s and 1960s. Let us first look at how programs were developed to handle the problems of hunger and poverty in those times and then at how those programs are working now.

Historical Background of Food Assistance Programs

During the Great Depression of the 1930s, concern about the plight of farmers who were losing their farms and the economic problems facing U.S. families in general led Congress to enact legislation giving the federal government the authority to buy and distribute excess food commodities. A few years later, Congress initiated an experimental Food Stamp Program to enable low-income people to buy food. Then in 1946, it passed the National School Lunch Act in response to testimony from the surgeon general that "70 percent of the boys who had poor nutrition 10 to 12 years ago were rejected by the draft." Despite these programs, in the 1960s, large numbers of people were still going hungry in the United States, and some of them suffered seriously from malnutrition as a result.

As evidence accumulated during the 1960s and 1970s showing that hunger was prevalent in the United States, poverty and hunger became national priorities. Old programs were revised and new programs were developed in an attempt to prevent malnutrition in those people found to be at greatest risk. The Food Stamp Program was expanded to serve more people. School lunch and breakfast programs were enlarged to support children nutritionally while they learned. Feeding programs were started to reach senior citizens. To provide food and nutrition education during the years when nutrition has the most crucial impact on growth, development, and future health, a supplemental food and nutrition program (WIC) was established for low-income pregnant and breastfeeding women, infants, and children who were nutritionally at risk. These and other events in the history of U.S. federal efforts to address domestic hunger are highlighted in the boxed insert.

As a result of these efforts, hunger diminished as a serious problem for the United States. Several studies, including comparative observations made 10 years apart, documented the difference the food assistance programs had made. In a baseline study in the late 1960s, a Field Foundation report stated:

> Wherever we went and wherever we looked we saw children in significant numbers who were hungry and sick, children for whom hunger is a daily fact of life, and sickness in many forms, an inevitability. The children we saw were . . . hungry, weak, apathetic . . . visibly and predictably losing their health, their energy, their spirits . . . suffering from hunger and disease, and . . . dying from them.

Ten years later, in 1977, the same group reported:

> Our first and overwhelming impression is that there are far fewer grossly malnourished people in this country today than there were ten years ago. . . . This change does not appear to be due to an overall improvement in living standards or to a decrease in joblessness in those areas . . . . But in the area of food there is a difference. The Food Stamp program, school lunch and breakfast programs, and the Women-Infant-Children programs have made the difference.[9]

Now, however, hunger is on the rise due to growing poverty and cuts in government aid. By the end of the 1980s, as shown in Figure 11-2 on page 340, 31.5 million people in the United States lived on incomes below the official poverty line ($13,400 for a family of four in 1990); 12.5 million of them lived on incomes of less than half of the poverty line.[10] The number of people living in poverty rose to 33.6 million (13.5 percent of the population) in 1990, the first year the poverty rate had increased since 1982–1983. The national trends in poverty are shown in Table 11-2 on page 341. A later section of the chapter takes a closer look at the U.S. food assistance programs to explain why federal budget cuts exacerbate the problem of hunger in this country.

The History of U.S. Federal Policies Addressing Hunger: An Overview

1930	The USDA and Federal Emergency Relief Administration distribute surplus agricultural commodities as food relief.
1933	Congress creates the Agricultural Adjustment Administration to control farm prices and production and the Federal Surplus Relief Corporation to distribute surplus farm products to needy families.
1935–1942	Congress provides for continued operation of the Federal Surplus Commodities Corporation, which, under the USDA, purchases commodities for distribution to state welfare agencies.
1936–1942	Amendments to the Agricultural Act permit food donations to school lunches.
1939–1943	The Federal Surplus Commodities Corporation initiates an experimental food stamp program.
1946	The National School Lunch Program is established.
1954	The Special Milk Program is established.
1955	The USDA determines that the average low-income family spends one-third of its after-tax income on food.
1961	President John F. Kennedy expands the use of surplus foods for needy people at home and abroad and announces eight pilot food stamp programs.
1964	Congress establishes the national Food Stamp Program. The Social Security Administration establishes the poverty line at three times the cost of the USDA's lowest-cost Economy Food Plan. Since 1969, values have been adjusted according to the Consumer Price Index.
1966	The Child Nutrition Act passes. It initiates the School Breakfast Program, which becomes permanent in 1975. President Lyndon B. Johnson outlines the Food for Freedom program.
1968–1977	The Senate establishes the Select Committee on Nutrition and Human Needs to lead the nation's antihunger efforts.
1968–1970	The Ten-State and Preschool Nutrition Surveys and *Hunger, U.S.A.* report evidence of malnutrition among children in poverty.
1969	President Richard M. Nixon announces a "war on hunger" and holds the White House Conference on Food, Nutrition, and Health. The USDA establishes the Food and Nutrition Service to administer federal food assistance programs.
1971	Results of the Ten-State Survey released to Congress indicate high risk of malnutrition among low-income groups.
1972	Congress authorizes the Special Supplemental Food Program for Women, Infants, and Children (WIC). The Older Americans Act authorizes the Nutrition Program for Older Americans.
1973	Amendments to the Older Americans Act establish congregate and home-delivered meals programs.

Continued

—Continued

1977	The Food and Agricultural Act and Child Nutrition and National School Lunch Amendments are passed.
1981	The USDA establishes a small demonstration project for commodity distribution, the Special Supplemental Dairy Distribution Program, which becomes institutionalized as the Temporary Emergency Food Assistance Program (TEFAP) in 1983.
1981–1982	Congress passes the Omnibus Budget Reconciliation Acts, Omnibus Farm Bill, and Tax Equity and Fiscal Responsibility Act, which eliminate, restrict, and reduce food and income benefits.
1984	The President's Task Force on Food Assistance finds little evidence of widespread or increasing undernutrition but concludes that hunger exists and is intolerable in the United States.
1986	The General Accounting Office finds that methodologic flaws discredit findings of the Physician Task Force on Hunger that hunger is prevalent in counties with low food stamp participation rates.
1988	The DHHS publishes the *Surgeon General's Report on Nutrition and Health,* which states that lack of access to an appropriate diet should not be a health problem for any American. Congress passes the Hunger Prevention Act increasing eligibility and benefits for Food Stamps, Child Care, and TEFAP programs.
1989	The House Select Committee on Hunger holds hearings on food security in the United States.
1991	The Mickey Leland Childhood Hunger Relief Act (HR-1202, S-757) is introduced.

Source: M. Nestle and S. Guttmacher, Hunger in the United States: Rationale, methods, and policy implications of state hunger surveys. Reprinted with permission, *Journal of Nutrition Education* 24 (1992): 22S, Society for Nutrition Education.

Counting the Hungry: A Decade of Surveys

We can get a sense of the number of people who are too poor to feed themselves adequately by looking at the group officially counted as poor by the U.S. Bureau of the Census. Data collected by the National Nutrition Monitoring System and state and local surveys also provide information about the prevalence of hunger.

The poverty line was developed in 1965 by taking the cost of an emergency short-term diet—called the Thrifty Food Plan—and multiplying it by 3.3. (The factor of 3.3 was used because a 1955 survey had shown that low-income people spent about one-third of their incomes on food.) This figure became the "poverty line," and it has been adjusted every year since then, based on changes in the Consumer Price Index (see Table 11-3 on page 342). Besides being out of date, the food budget used in the 1965 calculation reflects a diet that is just barely ade-

FIGURE

11-2

Total U.S. Population in Poverty (Millions), 1980–1992

Source: Adapted from Bread for the World Institute, *Hunger 1994: Transforming the Politics of Hunger* (Washington, D.C.: Bread for the World Institute, 1993). Reprinted by permission.

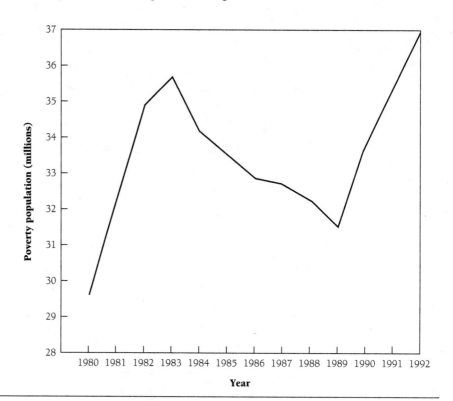

quate—one designed for short-term use when funds are extremely low. This means that everyone whose income is below the poverty line has less money than is needed to buy even a short-term, emergency diet.

Despite its inadequacies, the official poverty line defines eligibility for most federal assistance programs. Needy individuals with incomes a certain amount above the poverty line are automatically ineligible for programs like food stamps or free and reduced-price school meals. Such criteria mean that the programs now in place do not reach all people in need and do not provide enough to allow those they do reach to escape poverty.

Since the early 1980s, numerous studies on hunger have been conducted throughout the United States.* Almost without exception, these studies find hunger to be a serious and rapidly growing problem. Approximately 20 million people in the United States—12 million children and 8 million adults—are suffering from chronic hunger, and the problem is getting worse in all regions of the country. A recent analysis of 28 state hunger surveys found consistent results across all surveys and evidence for several broad conclusions listed on the next page.[11]

*Studies have been conducted by the U.S. Conference of Mayors, the Center on Hunger, Poverty, and Nutrition Policy at Tufts University, the National Council of Churches, the Citizens' Commission on Hunger in New England, Bread for the World Institute, the President's Task Force on Food Assistance, the Physician Task Force on Hunger, and the Food Research and Action Center, among others.

TABLE
11-2   **National Trends in Poverty, 1970–1991**

	1970	1980	1982	1984	1986	1987	1988	1989	1990	1991
Population in millions	205.1	227.8	232.5	237.0	241.6	243.9	246.3	248.3	248.7	252.2
Total poverty rate (%)	12.6	13.0	15.0	14.4	13.6	13.4	13.1	12.8	13.5	14.2
White poverty rate (%)	9.9	10.2	12.0	11.5	11.0	10.4	10.1	10.0	10.7	11.3
Black poverty rate (%)	33.5	32.5	35.6	33.8	31.1	32.6	31.6	30.7	31.9	32.7
Hispanic poverty rate	—	25.7	29.9	28.4	27.3	28.1	26.8	26.2	28.1	28.7
Elderly poverty rate (%)	24.6	15.7	14.6	12.4	12.4	12.5	12.0	11.4	12.2	12.4
Total child poverty rate (%)	15.1	18.3	21.9	21.5	20.5	20.5	19.7	19.6	20.6	21.1
White child poverty rate (%)	—	13.9	17.0	16.7	16.1	15.4	14.6	14.8	15.9	16.1
Black child poverty rate (%)	—	42.3	47.6	46.6	43.1	45.6	44.2	43.7	44.8	45.6
Hispanic child poverty rate (%)	—	39.7	33.2	39.5	39.2	37.7	39.6	37.9	36.2	39.8
Poverty rate of people in female-headed households (%)	38.1	36.7	40.6	38.4	38.3	38.3	37.2	32.2	33.4	39.7
Percentage of federal budget spent on food assistance	0.5	2.4	2.1	2.1	1.9	1.9	1.9	1.9	1.9	2.0
Total infant mortality rate	20.0	12.6	11.5	10.8	10.4	10.1	10.0	10.0	9.1	8.9
White infant mortality rate	17.8	11.0	10.1	9.4	8.9	8.6	8.5	8.5	7.7	—
Black infant mortality rate	32.6	21.4	19.6	18.4	18.0	17.9	17.6	17.6	17.0	—
Unemployment rate (%)	4.9	7.1	9.7	7.5	7.0	6.2	5.5	5.3	5.5	6.7

Source: Adapted from Bread for the World Institute, *Hunger 1994: Transforming the Politics of Hunger* (Washington, D.C.: Bread for the World Institute, 1993), p. 170.

◆ Food insufficiency has become a chronic problem in the United States.

◆ Food insufficiency is not due to food shortages. Hunger results from unequal distribution of economic resources—poverty.

◆ People who lack access to a variety of resources—not just food—are most at risk of hunger. When income is inadequate to meet the costs of housing, utilities, health care, and other fixed expenses, these items compete with and may take precedence over food.

◆ The federal poverty level is an inappropriate index of hunger, since it is based on a formula that fails to account for changes in the cost of living, regional variations in costs, or unusual expenses that may be required.

◆ The U.S. social welfare system does not provide an adequate safety net.

◆ Private charity cannot solve the hunger problem. Voluntary activities are limited in expertise, time, and resources and are likely to require government support in order to continue.

◆ Hunger is inextricably linked to poverty, which in turn is inextricably linked to underemployment and the costs of housing and other basic needs.

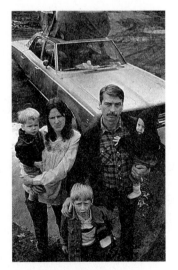

Many families with incomes at or below the minimum wage do not know where their next meal is coming from.

The National Nutrition Monitoring System (NNMS), as discussed in Chapter 5, is a valuable tool for assessing the needs of hungry people nationwide and

TABLE

11-3

Annual Poverty Guidelines, 1994

Source: Adapted from Community Nutrition Institute, *Nutrition Week,* March 11, 1994, p. 8.

HOUSEHOLD SIZE	POVERTY GUIDELINE[a] (100% POVERTY)[b]
1	$ 7,360
2	9,840
3	12,320
4	14,800
5	17,280
6	19,760
7	22,240
8	24,720

For each additional family member, add $2,480.

[a]The poverty guideline for Alaska starts at $9200 and rises by increments of $3100, and that for Hawaii starts at $8470 and rises by $2850.
[b]This table shows income levels equal to the poverty line (100% of the poverty line). Programs sometimes set program income eligibility at some point above the poverty line. For example, if a program sets income eligibility at 130% of the poverty line, then the cutoff for a family of two living in the 48 contiguous states is $9190 × 130% = $11,947.

gaining support for public policies to end hunger.[12] The NNMS has proposed using indicators of food security or insecurity as a necessary component of the measurement of nutrition status of individuals, communities, and nations.[13] Accordingly, for the third NHANES, questions were developed that focus on the individual experience of food insecurity (see Table 11-4).[14] These questions enable the NNMS to relate food security or insecurity to measurements of nutrition and health status.[15] State and local surveys can also use the questions in comparing local population data to the national data collected by NHANES III. Surveys such as NHANES and the Nationwide Food Consumption Survey (NFCS) also provide information about population characteristics that can be useful in designing interventions for target populations.[16]

Federal Domestic Food Assistance Programs Today

The Food and Nutrition Service (FNS) administers the 14 U.S. Department of Agriculture (USDA) food assistance programs. The agency's goals are to provide needy people with access to a more nutritious diet, to improve the eating habits of the nation's children, and to stabilize farm prices through the distribution of surplus foods.[17]

The FNS administers all its programs in partnership with the states. The individual states determine most details regarding distribution of food benefits and eligibility of participants, and the FNS provides funding to cover most of these administrative costs.

Congress appropriated $35.9 billion for the FNS to operate the food assistance programs in 1993—up from $32.7 billion in 1992 and $1.1 billion in 1969,

Food sufficiency questions in the NHANES III Family Questionnaire administered during the household interview

◆ Which one of the following statements *best* describes the food eaten by (you/your family)? Do you have *enough* food to eat, *sometimes not enough* to eat, or *often not enough* to eat?

◆ Thinking about the past month, how many days did (you/your family) have no food or money to buy food?

◆ Which of the following reasons explain why your family has had this problem?
   a. You did not have transportation?
   b. You did not have working appliances for storing or preparing foods (such as stove, refrigerator)?
   c. You did not have enough money, food stamps, or WIC vouchers to buy food or beverages?
   d. Any other reason?

Food sufficiency questions asked of individuals during the private dietary interview in NHANES III

◆ Thinking about the past month, how many days did you have no food or money to buy food?

◆ Is that because there wasn't enough money to buy food or is there another reason?

◆ During the past month did you skip any meals because there wasn't enough food or money to buy food?

◆ How many days in the month did you skip any meals because there wasn't enough food or money to buy food?

◆ Did you skip any meals yesterday because there wasn't enough food or money to buy food?

◆ During the past month, were there any days when you did not eat at all because there wasn't enough food or money to buy food?

◆ In the past month, how many days were there when you didn't eat at all?

TABLE

11-4

Third National Health and Nutrition Examination Survey's Food Insecurity Measures
Source: Adapted from R. R. Briefel and C. E. Woteki, Development of food sufficiency questions for the third National Health and Nutrition Examination Survey. Reprinted with permission, *Journal of Nutrition Education* 24 (1992): 24S–28S, Society for Nutrition Education.

the first year of the agency's operation. As shown in Figure 11-3, the Food Stamp Program accounts for the majority of these funds.

Other food assistance programs for seniors (Congregate Meals and Home-Delivered Meals) are administered by the Administration on Aging of the Department of Health and Human Services (DHHS). Each food assistance program is discussed in turn in the sections that follow.[18]

◆ FOOD STAMP PROGRAM

The Food Stamp Program (FSP) is designed to improve the diets of people with low incomes by providing coupons to cover part or all of their household's food budget. The FSP is an entitlement program, meaning that anyone who meets eligibility standards is entitled to receive benefits. Eligibility and allotments are based on income, household size, assets, housing costs, work requirements, and other factors. Most households must have gross monthly incomes below 130 per-

The Food Stamp Program is currently authorized by the Food Stamp Act of 1977 (P.L. 95–113).

Work requirements: At the time of application and once every 12 months, all able-bodied household members between 18 and 60 years of age and 16- and 17-year-old heads of households who are not in school must register to work. Many adult recipients must participate in employment and training programs.

FIGURE

11-3

Food Program Costs, 1977–1990

Source: Reprinted with permission from Community Nutrition Institute, *Nutrition Week,* June 14, 1991.

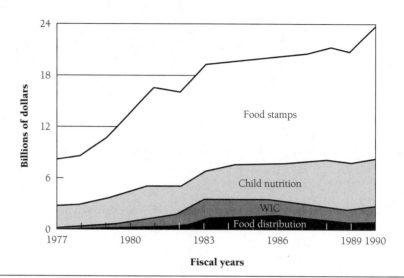

Net income is all the household's income that counts in figuring food stamps minus the deductions for which the household is eligible. Most households may have up to $2000 in countable resources (cash, bank accounts, car, stocks/bonds, and so forth). Households may have $3000 if at least one person is age 60 years or older.

cent of the poverty line and net monthly income at or below 100 percent of the poverty guidelines for their household size (see Table 11-5 for both standards). Households with elderly or persons with disabilities are subject only to the net income test. The majority of food stamp households have gross incomes below the poverty line; over 40 percent have gross incomes below half the poverty line. At least 60 percent of all food stamp recipients are children (50 percent) or elderly (10 percent).

The USDA issues food stamp coupons through state welfare or human services agencies to households—people who buy and prepare food together. The number of stamps a household receives varies according to its size and income (see Figure 11-4). Food stamp benefits average fifty-seven cents per meal, with a maximum benefit of about ninety cents. Recipients may use the coupons like cash to purchase food and seeds at stores authorized to accept them. They cannot buy ready-to-eat hot foods, vitamins or medicines, pet foods, tobacco, cleaning items, alcohol, or nonfood items (except seeds and garden plants) with coupons.

◆ NUTRITION ASSISTANCE FOR PUERTO RICO

The Food Stamp Program in Puerto Rico was replaced in 1982 by a block grant program (P.L. 97–35). The territory now provides cash and coupons to eligible participants rather than food stamps or food commodities. The grant can also be used to pay up to 50 percent of administrative costs for special projects related to food production and distribution. For example, a special cattle tick eradication program was funded in 1992. The program served approximately 1.5 million people monthly throughout 1992, providing monthly benefits of $54.76 per person.

GROSS MONTHLY INCOME ELIGIBILITY STANDARDS (130% OF POVERTY LINE)			
Household Size	48 States*	Alaska	Hawaii
1	$ 797	$ 997	$ 918
2	1066	1333	1226
3	1335	1668	1535
4	1603	2004	1844
5	1872	2340	2153
6	2141	2676	2461
7	2409	3012	2770
8	2678	3348	3079
Each additional member	+269	+336	+309

NET MONTHLY INCOME ELIGIBILITY STANDARDS (100% OF POVERTY LINE)			
Household Size	48 States*	Alaska	Hawaii
1	$ 613	$ 767	$ 706
2	820	1025	943
3	1027	1283	1180
4	1233	1541	1417
5	1440	1799	1655
6	1647	2057	1893
7	1853	2315	2131
8	2060	2573	2368
Each additional member	+207	+258	+238

*Includes District of Columbia, Guam, and Virgin Islands.

TABLE

11-5

The Food Stamp Program's Monthly Income Eligibility Guidelines (Gross and Net), 1994
Source: These figures have been adapted from Community Nutrition Institute, *Nutrition Week,* March 11, 1994, p. 8.

◆ FOOD DISTRIBUTION PROGRAM ON INDIAN RESERVATIONS

Also known as the Needy Family Program, the Food Distribution Program on Indian Reservations (FDPIR), is the oldest of the FNS programs—dating back to the Great Depression of the 1930s (P.L. 74–320). It was the main form of food assistance for all low-income people in the United States until the Food Stamp Program was expanded in the early 1970s. The FDPIR provides monthly packages of commodity foods to low-income Native American households living on or near reservations. The USDA commodities include canned meats and fish products; vegetables, fruits, and juices; dried beans; peanuts or peanut butter; milk, butter, and cheese; pasta, flour, or grains; adult cereals; corn syrup or honey; and vegetable oil and shortening. A nutrition education plan is currently underway to help participants make more nutritious use of the foods they receive.

Participants may choose from month to month whether they will participate in the Food Stamp Program or the food distribution program. Many who do not

FIGURE

11-4

Food Stamp Allotments Based on the Thrifty Food Plan, 1993

Source: Adapted from B. Shollenberger and B. Howell, *Underfunded and underfed: Food programs and hunger in America,* Background Paper No. 75 (Washington, D.C.: Bread for the World Institute, 1984), and Food Research and Action Center, *Fact Sheets on the Federal Food Assistance Programs* (Washington, D.C.: FRAC, 1993), p. 4.

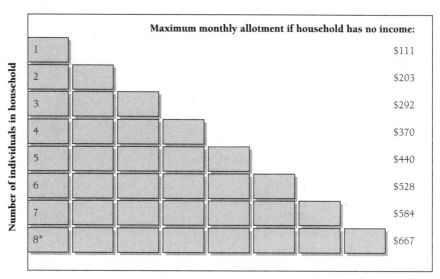

Number of individuals in household

	Maximum monthly allotment if household has no income:
1	$111
2	$203
3	$292
4	$370
5	$440
6	$528
7	$584
8*	$667

*For each additional person, add $83

Subtract 30% of available monthly income from the maximum food stamp allotment to determine the coupon allotment. For example, a 4-person household with $400 in available income would receive $250 in food stamps. 30% of income = $120. Maximum monthly allotment for a family of 4 = $370 − $120 = $250 food stamp allotment.

have easy access to grocery stores prefer the FDPIR. An average of 119,000 participants were served monthly in 1992; monthly packages were valued at $36.64 per person.

◆ SPECIAL SUPPLEMENTAL FOOD PROGRAM FOR WOMEN, INFANTS, AND CHILDREN (WIC)

WIC, authorized in 1974, is a cost-effective program of grants to state and local health agencies. WIC provides supplemental foods to infants, children up to age five, and pregnant, breastfeeding, and non-breastfeeding postpartum women who qualify financially and are at nutritional risk. Financial eligibility is determined by income (between 100 percent and 185 percent of the poverty line or below) or by participation in the AFDC, Food Stamp, or Medicaid programs. Nutritional risks, determined by a health professional, may include one of three types: medically-based risks (anemia, underweight, maternal age, history of high-risk pregnancies); diet-based risks (inadequate dietary pattern); or conditions that make the applicant predisposed to medically-based or diet-based risks, such as alcoholism or drug addiction. As of 1993, homelessness and migrancy are considered nutritional risks for purposes of WIC.

Authorization for WIC: Congress created a pilot WIC project in 1972 (P.L. 92–433) and authorized WIC as a national program as part of the National School Lunch and Child Nutrition Act Amendments of 1975 (P.L. 94–105).

The WIC program serves both a remedial and a preventive role. Its services include the following:

◆ Food packages or vouchers for supplemental food to provide specific nutrients (protein, calcium, iron, and vitamins A and C) known to be lacking in the diets of the target population.

[This discussion continues on page 349.]

◆ *The Food Stamp Program*

The Food Stamp Program (FSP) dates back to the food assistance programs of the Great Depression—a time when farmers were burdened with surplus crops they could not sell while thousands stood in breadlines, waiting for something to eat.[1] To help both farmers and consumers, the government began distributing the surplus farm foods to hungry citizens. Today, food stamp coupons enable recipients to buy food in grocery stores.

Nutrition surveys in the United States have demonstrated consistently that the lower a family's income, the less adequate its nutrition status.[2] Few low-income families obtain an adequate intake of nutrients. The problem is not that people with low incomes don't know how to shop, but that they are unable to buy sufficient amounts of nourishing foods. Some families with low incomes who receive food stamps are probably as skilled as, or even more skilled than, others at food shopping.[3] Thus, income apparently confers the ability to obtain a nutritionally adequate diet, and indeed, the number of households that meet or exceed the RDA rise and fall with income. Table 5-7 in Chapter 5 showed typical findings for six nutrients. People with lower incomes had lower intakes of five of them (iron intakes were low for all income levels).

The stated objective of the FSP is to "improve the diets of low-income households by increasing their food purchasing ability." Unfortunately, the ability of the FSP to achieve its objective has been questioned.[4] Although the program potentially increases a household's ability to purchase nourishing foods, food stamps may be used to buy most available human foods. The effect of the food stamp purchases on nutrient intakes of participants will vary depending on the nutritional composition of the foods they select.

One of two major problems with the FSP is that benefit allotments are insufficient to meet needs. Many households receiving food stamps still need emergency food by the end of the month because their stamps rarely last the entire month. In a study of 1,922 households, monthly food expenditures of FSP participants, including cash, food stamps, and WIC benefits, averaged just under 80 percent of the value of the Thrifty Food Plan.[5] Results from the Nationwide Food Consumption Surveys have shown that only 12 percent of people purchasing food valued at 100 percent of the Thrifty Food Plan were eating nutritionally adequate diets, indicating that the FSP households spending only 80 percent of the value of the Thrifty Food Plan may be at nutritional risk.[6]

The second major problem is that many households who are eligible for the FSP and in need do not participate. In 1993, an estimated 50 million people were living at income levels at or near the poverty line. These people were all potentially eligible to receive food stamps, yet only 27 million people participated in the program.[7] Reasons for nonparticipation include embarrassment about receiving assistance, complex rules and requirements, confusing paperwork, caseworker hostility, and lack of public information about eligibility requirements. Figure 11-5 shows the gap between eligibility and participation in the FSP in selected states.

Continued

PROGRAM SPOTLIGHT

FIGURE

11-5

Poverty and Food Stamp Assistance in Selected States, 1988–1989

Source: Reprinted by permission of Bread for the World Institute, *Hunger 1990: A Report on the State of World Hunger* (Washington, D.C.: Bread for the World Institute, 1990), p. 97.

—Continued

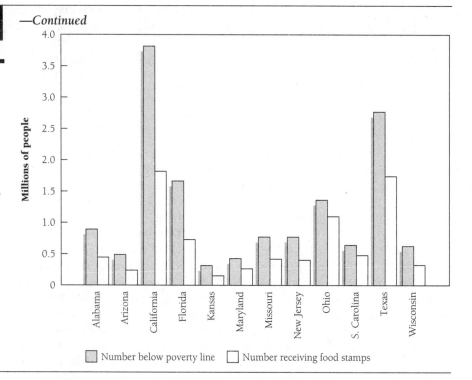

The USDA is currently trying to improve participation rates by eligibles through a number of outreach efforts targeted at low-participation groups, such as persons who are elderly, working poor, non-English speaking, homeless, or living in rural areas. Outreach efforts include training community workers and volunteers to refer families to food stamp offices, community education and mass media campaigns, and individualized client assistance.[8]

To improve the FSP's ability to meet the needs of low-income households, the following steps are recommended:[9]

◆ Improve and expand outreach about the FSP.

◆ Lower administrative barriers to participation in the FSP.

◆ Increase food stamp benefits so that families can afford to eat a nutritionally adequate diet throughout each month.

◆ Provide nutrition education materials to food stamp households.

1. Food and Nutrition Service, *Food Program Facts* (Washington, D.C.: USDA, 1992), p. 11.
2. B. B. Peterkin, R. L. Kerr, and M. Y. Hama, Nutritional adequacy of diets of low-income households, *Journal of Nutrition Education* 14 (1982): 102–4.

Continued

—Continued

3. B. B. Peterkin and M. Y. Hama, Food shopping skills of the rich and the poor, *Family Economics Review* 3 (1983): 8–12.
4. J. Allen and K. Gadson, Food consumption and nutritional status of low-income households, *National Food Review* 26 (1984): 27–31.
5. Food Research and Action Center, *Community Childhood Hunger Identification Project* (Washington, D.C.: FRAC, 1991), p. 42.
6. Peterkin, Kerr, and Hama, Nutritional adequacy.
7. Bread for the World Institute, *Hunger 1994: Transforming the Politics of Hunger* (Washington, D.C.: Bread for the World Institute, 1993), p. 151.
8. Community Nutrition Institute, *Nutrition Week,* January 22, 1993, p. 6.
9. Food Research and Action Center, *Community Childhood Hunger,* pp. 80–81.

PROGRAM SPOTLIGHT

◆ Nutrition education.

◆ Referrals to health care services.

Unlike most of the other food assistance programs, WIC is not an entitlement program. Approximately 5.4 million women, infants, and children received monthly WIC benefits in 1992, with the average monthly food package costing $30 per person. Due to caps on allocated federal funds, WIC currently reaches only about 60 percent of eligible persons.

More about WIC appears in Chapter 12.

◆ WIC FARMERS' MARKET NUTRITION PROGRAM

The WIC Farmers' Market Nutrition Program (FMNP) was created to accomplish two goals:

◆ To provide fresh, nutritious fruits and vegetables to WIC participants

◆ To expand the awareness and use of farmers' markets by consumers

Under the program, coupons ranging from $10 to $20 per year are issued to eligible recipients. States may also use their own matching funds to issue FMNP coupons to other groups, such as elderly persons, older children, the homeless, or other low-income people.

Congress created a pilot FMNP through the Hunger Prevention Act of 1988 (P.L. 100–435) and awarded grants to 10 states (Connecticut, Iowa, Maryland, Massachusetts, Michigan, New York, Pennsylvania, Texas, Vermont, and Washington). The FMNP was authorized in 1992 (P.L. 102–314) as a national program through an amendment to the Child Nutrition Act of 1966.

◆ CHILD NUTRITION PROGRAMS

Many federal programs address the special nutritional needs of children. The following sections describe the USDA's child nutrition programs. Chapter 13 provides more detail about the USDA programs as well as other major federal and private nutrition programs for children and adolescents.

National School Lunch and Breakfast Programs   The National School Lunch Program (NSLP) and the School Breakfast Program provide financial assistance to schools so that every student can receive a nutritious lunch, breakfast, or both. Participating schools get cash payments on the basis of the number of meals served in the free, reduced-price, and full-price categories and also receive food commodities. Program schools must serve meals meeting specified nutritional

The NSLP was authorized in 1946 by the National School Lunch Act (P.L. 79–396). The School Breakfast Program was authorized by the Child Nutrition Act of 1966 (P.L. 89–642).

guidelines and must offer free or reduced-price meals to eligible students. These programs enable students in households with incomes at or below 130 percent of the poverty line to receive meals at no cost and allow students from households with incomes between 130 and 185 percent of the poverty line to receive a reduced-price meal. Children whose families participate in the AFDC or Food Stamp Program are automatically eligible for free school meals.

Nationally, the USDA runs the programs; on the state level, the programs are run by the state Department of Education. They usually can be implemented with little cost to the school district. The income eligibility guidelines for the NSLP, School Breakfast Program, Child and Adult Care Food Program, Summer Food Service Program, and Special Milk Program are listed in Table 11-6. In 1992, more than 24 million children participated in the NSLP at more than 92,000 schools and residential institutions. Half of these children received their meal free or at a reduced price. Approximately 4.9 million participated in the School Breakfast Program, which is offered in some 46,000 schools and institutions.

The SFSP was authorized in 1975 as an amendment to the National School Lunch Act (P.L. 94–105).

Summer Food Service Program for Children   The Summer Food Service Program (SFSP) funds meals and snacks for eligible children during school vacation periods. The program operates in areas where half or more of the children are from households with incomes at or below 185 percent of the poverty level. Sponsors of the program include local schools, government units (e.g., parks and recreation departments), summer camps, community action agencies, and other nonprofit organizations. The SFSP offers meals that meet the same nutritional standards as those provided by the School Lunch Program at no cost to all children, up to age 18, who attend the program site. Approximately 2 million children participated in the SFSP in 1992.

The SMP was incorporated into the Child Nutrition Act of 1966 (P.L. 89–642).

Special Milk Program   The Special Milk Program (SMP) provides cash reimbursement for each half-pint of milk served to children in schools that are not participating in the National School Lunch Program. Nearly 192 million half-pints of milk were served in 1992.

TABLE

11-6

Income Eligibility Standards for the Federal Child Nutrition Programs

Source: These figures have been adapted from Community Nutrition Institute, *Nutrition Week*, March 11, 1994, p. 8.

Household Size	Federal Poverty Guideline (100% of Poverty)	Free-Meal Eligibility (130% of Poverty)	Reduced-Price Meal Eligibility (185% of Poverty)
1	$ 7,360	$ 9,568	$13,616
2	9,840	12,792	18,204
3	12,320	16,016	22,792
4	14,800	19,240	27,380
5	17,280	22,464	31,968
6	19,760	25,688	36,556
7	22,240	28,912	41,144
8	24,720	32,136	45,732
For each additional family member, add:	+2,480	+3,224	+4,588

Child and Adult Care Food Program　The Child and Adult Care Food Program (CACFP) is designed to help public and private nonresidential child and adult day care programs provide nutritious meals for children up to age 12, the elderly, and certain people with disabilities. The program provides cash reimbursements for two meals and one snack per child per day plus one additional meal or snack for children in care for eight or more hours. Sponsors may also receive USDA commodity foods. The CACFP served over 1.7 million participants every day in 1992.

The CACFP was permanently authorized in 1978 (P.L. 94–105). The 1987 amendments to the Older Americans Act authorized the Child Care Food Program to change its name and expand its service to include the elderly and persons with disabilities.

◆ EMERGENCY FOOD ASSISTANCE PROGRAM

The Emergency Food Assistance Program, which was formerly known as the "Temporary" Emergency Food Assistance Program and retains the acronym TEFAP, has operated now for over a decade. The TEFAP was designed to reduce the level of government-held surplus commodities by distributing them to low-income households to supplement the recipients' purchased food. Most states set eligibility criteria at between 130 and 150 percent of the poverty line. In many states, AFDC and food stamp participants are automatically eligible for the TEFAP. Most commodities distributed prior to 1988 were surplus foods such as packaged dairy products, flour, rice, honey, and cornmeal. In the Hunger Prevention Act of 1988 (P.L. 100–435), Congress authorized the purchase of additional commodities to enhance the amount and variety distributed. Additional items have since included canned meat, canned and dried fruit, peanut butter, dried potatoes, citrus juice, and legumes.

The TEFAP was authorized by the Temporary Emergency Food Assistance Act of 1983 (P.L. 98–8). The 1990 Farm Bill (P.L. 101–624) reauthorized TEFAP for five more years and dropped the word "Temporary" from the program's name.

◆ COMMODITY SUPPLEMENTAL FOOD PROGRAM

The Commodity Supplemental Food Program (CSFP), currently available in approximately 13 states, is a direct food distribution program providing supplemental foods and nutrition education. The CSFP serves a target population similar to WIC and persons 60 years of age and older as well. Recipients may not participate in both WIC and the CSFP. Food packages are designed to suit the nutritional needs of participants and may include canned fruit juice, canned fruits and vegetables, hot cereal, nonfat dry milk, evaporated milk, egg mix, dry beans, peanut butter, canned meat or poultry, dehydrated potatoes, pasta, rice, cheese, butter, honey, and infant cereal and formula. Distribution sites make packages available on a monthly basis. Monthly participation through 1992 was 336,000 (65 percent women, infants, and children and 35 percent elderly).

The CSFP was authorized by the Agriculture and Consumer Protection Act of 1973.

◆ COMMODITY DISTRIBUTION TO CHARITABLE INSTITUTIONS

Food commodities are distributed to nonprofit, charitable institutions that serve meals to low-income people on a regular basis. These include homes for the elderly, hospitals, soup kitchens, food banks, meals-on-wheels programs, temporary shelters, and summer camps or orphanages not participating in any federal child nutrition program.

◆ SENIOR NUTRITION PROGRAMS

The federal Nutrition Program for Older Americans (Title III) is intended to improve older people's nutrition status and enable them to avoid medical problems, continue living in communities of their own choice, and stay out of institutions. Its specific goals are to provide the following:

- ◆ Low-cost, nutritious meals
- ◆ Opportunities for social interaction
- ◆ Nutrition education and shopping assistance
- ◆ Counseling and referral to other social services
- ◆ Transportation services

The Congregate Meals Program and the Home-Delivered Meals Program were authorized by the Older Americans Act of 1965 (P.L. 89–73).

One of the Title III efforts is the Congregate Meals Program. Administrators try to select sites for congregate meals that will attract as many of the eligible elderly as possible. Through the Home-Delivered Meals Program, meals are also delivered to those who are homebound either permanently or temporarily. The home-delivery program ensures nutrition, but its recipients miss out on the social benefit of the congregate meal sites; every effort is made to persuade them to come to the shared meals if they can. The DHHS's Administration on Aging administers these programs.

All persons 60 years and older are eligible to receive meals from these programs, regardless of their income level. Priority is given to those who are economically and socially needy.

Another program for the elderly is the USDA's Nutrition Program for the Elderly (NPE). The NPE provides cash and commodity foods to local senior citizen centers for use in the Congregate and Home-Delivered Meals Programs. Over 247 million meals were served in 1992. Chapter 14 provides additional information about these programs.

The Rising Tide of Food Assistance Needs

Emergency food services:
- ◆ *Soup kitchens*
- ◆ *Church charities*
- ◆ *Surplus food giveaways*
- ◆ *Food banks*
- ◆ *Food pantries*
- ◆ *Prepared and perishable food programs*

Despite all of these federal food assistance programs, hunger and the public demand for emergency food assistance have increased in every region of the United States since 1980. The country has become a soup kitchen society to an extent unmatched since the breadlines of the Great Depression. The demand for emergency food assistance increased by 22 percent between 1989 and 1990, and then by another 26 percent between 1990 and 1991.[19] The worsening economic conditions of the poor are attributed to the federal economic policies of the 1980s. Much of the increased public demand for food assistance is coming from the "new poor"—those who, until recently, had been employed, productive, and financially stable. Many seeking emergency food assistance are families with children, who find that food stamps are unable to meet their food needs.

Second Harvest A national network to which the majority of food banks belong.

To help fill the gaps in the federal programs, concerned citizens are working through community programs and churches to provide meals to the hungry. **Second Harvest,** the nation's largest supplier of surplus food, distributed over

476.4 million pounds of food (up 18 percent from 1989) to nearly 200 **food banks** and some 50,000 agencies for direct distribution around the nation in 1990 (see Figure 11-6).[20] However, even the dramatic increases in the number of food banks, **food pantries, soup kitchens, prepared and perishable food programs**, and other emergency food assistance programs cannot keep pace with the growing number of hungry people seeking food assistance. Each day's supply of meals lasts only for that day, leaving the problem of poverty unsolved; moreover, one out of every five needy people is not even receiving meals. These people must scavenge garbage, steal food or money to buy food, or continue to starve.

◆ THE PLIGHT OF THE HOMELESS

Estimates of the number of homeless range from 600,000 to 3 million. In addition, nearly 3 million people spend more than 70 percent of their income on rent and are at risk of becoming homeless.[21]

The U.S. Conference of Mayors surveyed 28 major cities to assess the status of hunger and homelessness in the urban United States during 1992.* Lack of food, inadequate diets, poor nutrition status, and nutrition-related health problems—stunted growth, failure to thrive, low birth weight babies, infant mortality, anemia, and compromised immune systems—are common among homeless persons.[22] Increasing numbers of people living with the HIV virus are homeless due to the high costs of health care or lack of supportive housing.[23] Tuberculosis is spreading at alarming rates among homeless persons because of the close sleeping arrangements in shelters and on the streets.

The lack of affordable housing leads the list of causes of homelessness identified by the mayors. Without adequate low-income housing, many poor people are forced to choose between shelter and food. Other causes include unemployment, underemployment, poverty, inadequate public assistance benefits, the high cost of health care, substance abuse and lack of needed services, and mental illness and lack of needed services. Figure 11-7 shows the average composition of the survey cities' homeless population. Children accounted for 24 percent of the homeless in these cities.[24]

Although low-income, homeless people may qualify for any of the USDA's 14 food assistance programs, homeless people who try to receive public assistance face many barriers. For example, transportation to agency offices may not be affordable or accessible. The homeless may also lack the documentation required to apply for the various benefits programs.

Several steps are necessary to end homelessness in the United States. Local communities need to focus on outreach efforts to inform homeless persons of existing services and help them obtain benefits. More 24-hour shelters with programs such as literacy classes, medical services, nutrition education, drug and alcohol rehabilitation, job training and placement, and child care, as well as food and shelter, must be established. Longer-term solutions include improving the

Food banks Nonprofit community organizations that collect surplus commodities from the government and edible but often unmarketable foods from private industry for use by nonprofit charities, institutions, and feeding programs at nominal cost.

Food pantries Usually attached to existing nonprofit agencies, these pantries distribute bags or boxes of groceries to people experiencing food emergencies. Distributed foods are prepared and consumed elsewhere. Pantries often require referrals or proof of need. There are roughly two food pantries to every soup kitchen.

Soup kitchen Small feeding operations attached to existing organizations, such as churches, civic groups, or nonprofit agencies, that serve prepared meals that are consumed on-site. Soup kitchens generally do not require clients to prove need or show identification.

Prepared and perishable food programs (PPFPs) Nonprofit programs that help to feed people in need by linking sources of unused, unserved cooked and fresh food—like caterers, restaurants, hotel kitchens, and cafeterias—with social service agencies that serve meals to people who would otherwise go hungry. *Foodchain* is a national network of over 125 community-based PPFPs in 41 states and Canada.

*The 28 cities surveyed were Alexandria, Boston, Charleston, Charlotte, Chicago, Cleveland, Denver, Hartford, Kansas City, Los Angeles, Louisville, Miami, Minneapolis, Nashville, New Orleans, New York City, Norfolk, Philadelphia, Phoenix, Portland, St. Paul, Salt Lake City, San Antonio, San Diego, San Francisco, Santa Monica, Seattle, and Trenton.

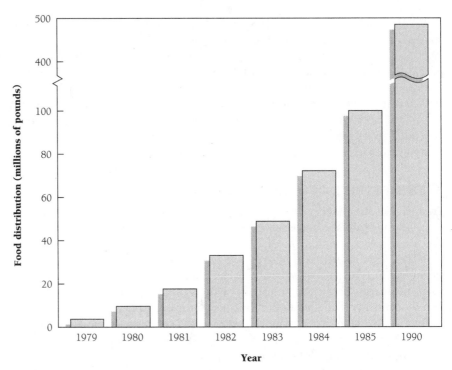

FIGURE

11-6

Demand for Emergency Food Assistance
Source: Adapted and updated from J. Larry Brown, "Hunger in the U.S." *Scientific American* 256 (1987): 40.

Food distributed by the Second Harvest network rose from 2.5 million pounds in 1979 to 100 million pounds in 1985 and then to well over 475 million pounds in 1990, reflecting the efforts of private organizations to cope with the rise in hunger. Second Harvest services state food banks.

The Hunger Prevention Act of 1988 requires states to help eligible homeless women, infants, and children to enroll in WIC.

economy and creating jobs that pay adequately. Improving the Food Stamp Program and increasing funding for it and for WIC are other necessary measures. Other steps cited by the Conference of Mayors as crucial for ending homelessness include making more housing available at affordable prices and providing comprehensive services to vulnerable populations.

◆ POVERTY TRENDS AMONG VULNERABLE GROUPS: A FOCUS ON CHILDREN

Poverty and hunger affect certain socioeconomic, geographic, and demographic groups more than others. According to one report, those most at risk of hunger are female-headed households, children, the rural poor, farmworkers, the homeless, and older people.[25] African-American, Hispanic, and Native American peoples in all these groups have consistently been vulnerable to hunger.[26]

The hunger surveys of the 1980s reported an increasing demand for emergency food by families with young children. As a result, the Food Research and Action Center (FRAC) designed the Community Childhood Hunger Identification Project (CCHIP) to document the prevalence of hunger in children. CCHIP has implemented a number of surveys across the nation among low-

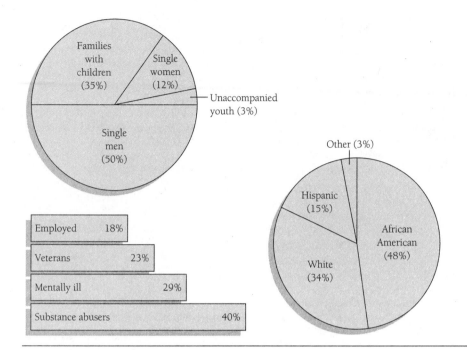

FIGURE

11-7

Demographics of the Homeless Population in 28 Survey Cities
Source: Adapted from The U.S. Conference of Mayors, *A Status Report on Hunger and Homelessness in America's Cities: 1992* (Washington, D.C.: U.S. Conference of Mayors, 1992).

income families (with incomes at or below 185 percent of the federal poverty line) with at least one child under the age of 12. The studies document conditions such as participation in food assistance programs, finances, and children's health.[27]

CCHIP documents hunger using a hunger index—a scale of eight questions (see Table 11-7) that indicate whether a household is affected by food insecurity, food shortages, perceived food insufficiency, or altered food intake due to resource constraints.[28] Families are asked whether lack of money in the past 12 months caused them to cut food portions, skip meals, limit the number of foods served, or send children to bed hungry. Families answering affirmatively to five or more of eight such questions are considered hungry. A score of one to four indicates that the family is at risk of hunger due to the presence of at least one food shortage problem.[29] The CCHIP conceptual model (see Figure 11-8 on page 359) shows the large number of interrelated factors associated with hunger and poverty.

As a result of the ongoing CCHIP surveys, FRAC estimates that one in eight children—between 6.6 million and 10.6 million children—under 12 years of age is hungry and every fifth child is vulnerable to hunger as a result of their families' inadequate incomes.[30] Children in minority groups are particularly at risk for hunger. By the end of the 1980s, half of African-American children and 40 percent of Hispanic children under six lived in poverty.[31]

◆ THE PLIGHT OF THE FARMERS

Changes in the domestic economy are proving adverse for producers as well as for consumers. U.S. farmers today lack significant control over the products they

TABLE
11-7

Community Childhood Hunger Identification Project's Hunger Scale*

Source: Adapted from C. A. Wehler, R. I. Scott, and J. J. Anderson, The Community Childhood Hunger Identification Project: A model of domestic hunger—demonstration project in Seattle, Washington. Reprinted with permission, *Journal of Nutrition Education* 24 (1992): 29S–35S, Society for Nutrition Education.

1. Does your household ever run out of money to buy food to make a meal?
2. Do you or members of your household ever eat less than you feel you should because there is not enough money for food?
3. Do you or members of your household ever cut the size of meals or skip meals because there is not enough money for food?
4. Do your children ever eat less than you feel they should because there is not enough money for food?
5. Do you ever cut the size of your children's meals or do they ever skip meals because there is not enough money for food?
6. Do your children ever say they are hungry because there is not enough food in the house?
7. Do you ever rely on a limited number of foods to feed your children because you are running out of money to buy food for a meal?
8. Do any of your children ever go to bed hungry because there is not enough money to buy food?

*Hunger criterion: five positive responses out of eight.

produce, the prices they must pay for supplies, and the prices they receive in return for their commodities. Just prior to 1980, the USDA urged farmers to produce more corn and soybeans for export. Accordingly, farmers borrowed heavily to expand their production capabilities. Since that time, their costs for seed, fertilizer, equipment, and loans have steadily risen while crop prices have declined. Today, thousands of U.S. farmers are hungry, frustrated, and desperate about their debt.[32]

The number of hungry farm families is not known, but agencies that provide aid to the rural poor say the demand for food assistance is increasing. Ironically, farm families generally do not grow fruits, vegetables, and other crops and animals to feed themselves. With modern practices aimed at efficiency, most farmers raise two or three crops—for example, feed corn, sorghum, and wheat—and buy most of their food from the grocery store. As a result, when crop prices drop, farmers struggle to survive under the sagging prices and realize no significant profits. Eventually, the farmers go out of business from lack of profits, just as would happen to any other type of business in the United States.

Beyond Public Assistance: What Can Individuals Do?

Solutions to the hunger problem depend on the willingness of people to take action and work together. A national coalition of organizations concerned with domestic hunger has launched a campaign to end hunger in the United States and significantly reduce poverty by the year 2000. The coalition issued the *Medford Declaration* in 1992. This declaration (in the boxed insert) states that adequate

The Medford Declaration
Ending Domestic Hunger: A Statement of Commitment

We can end hunger in America, and we can end it now. Three decades ago a new president challenged our nation with two goals: to reach the moon, and to end domestic hunger. We have reached only one of these goals. It is time to achieve the other. Hunger has no place in the new world tomorrow brings. It is a form of economic suicide. Hunger is also inconsistent with our conscience. If anything is un-American, it is hunger.

We believe Americans have reached a consensus on ending hunger. We come to this consensus from many points of view. Many of us are moved by the belief that the United States is losing its economic leadership, and that we must invest more in our children and families to insure national productivity in a more competitive world. Others are moved by enlightened self-interest, point out that we either pay now or pay later for preventable problems. Still other citizens address domestic hunger out of strong moral or religious convictions. And many in the fields of education and medicine are moved by the crippling impact of hunger on the health and learning capacity of our children. From many walks of life, we are one people—a people who agree that we can eradicate hunger in our country. A people who believe we must do so.

Abolishing hunger at home will require two steps. In the short term we must use existing channels to see that food is available to the hungry on an adequate and consistent basis. If we fully utilize existing public programs—in conjunction with the heroic efforts of voluntary food providers in local communities—we can end hunger very soon. But we must move as a nation to end the causes of hunger as well. Many things can be done to increase the purchasing power of American households, and to fulfill the desire for independence and self-reliance which so characterizes our people. We can achieve this two-step goal before the start of the new century.

We can begin with children . . . and we can virtually eliminate domestic hunger by 1995.

Programs exist to insure that all Americans have enough to eat by 1995. Within months we can meet emergency needs by moving surplus foodstuffs into the communities of the nation as quickly as we ship goods to feed our military personnel overseas. Within two years we can fully use existing federal food programs to prevent hunger.

We must begin with children. We can reach every needy child with the school lunch and breakfast program. We can start with the six million poor youngsters who often begin their school day with no food. We can fully use the highly effective WIC program to help insure that poor mothers do not give birth to undernourished babies . . . protecting four million more youngsters who presently are at risk. We can expand the benefits of food stamps which help unemployed households make it through economically difficult times. And we can insure that no elderly citizen goes without the nutrients provided by Meals on Wheels and congregate feeding. These steps alone can virtually wipe out domestic hunger by mid-decade.

We can achieve economic self-reliance for most American households by the year 2000.

Promoting adequate purchasing power is the way to achieve the goal of a hunger-free United States. This nation will have defeated chronic hunger when its people achieve "food security"—regular access to an adequate diet through normal means.

Continued

—Continued

A variety of steps can be taken this decade to accomplish this end: market-based employment and training programs to build skills and expand jobs; making sure child care is available so parents can work; expanding concepts such as earned income tax credits and children's allowances so that the tax system strengthens families. The goal is to increase the purchasing power of employed heads-of-household so that work raises families out of poverty.

The current window of world peace now gives us the opportunity to abolish domestic hunger. We can increase the competitiveness of our work force and protect the vital energies of our young. And we can assist emerging democracies of the world with pride because all Americans will enjoy the most basic fruit of our own democracy—freedom and family security.

We stand at a special moment in history. Perhaps for the first time, our desire to end hunger is converging with the opportunity to do so. We have moved from ability to consensus. We now need the political leadership to achieve the long-held goal of an America free of hunger.

*For further information, contact: World Hunger Year, Food Research and Action Center, Center on Hunger, Poverty, and Nutrition Policy, or End Hunger Network (see Appendix B for addresses). Reprinted by permission, *Journal of Nutrition Education* 24 (1992): 89S, Society for Nutrition Education.

---

funding of federal domestic food assistance programs, such as WIC and food stamps, could quickly eliminate outright hunger in the United States. The declaration also calls for long-term efforts to address the causes of hunger, especially by increasing the purchasing power of low-income households.

Can we realistically hope to end hunger in the United States by the year 2000? Professor Larry Brown of Tufts University provides our response:

> The chief answer to those who question whether we can eliminate hunger lies in the fact that we virtually did so in our recent past. The programs created by the nation in the late 1960s and early 1970s worked. The evidence indicates that hunger significantly declined in the face of a national commitment expressed through the vehicles of school meals, food stamps, WIC, and elderly feeding programs. By fully utilizing these existing programs, we could again end hunger.
>
> The larger question—the truly complicated one—is how to eliminate the cause of hunger: poverty. The United States pays a high price for poverty, and hunger is only one part of it. From a public health perspective it is the height of folly to permit such a significant risk factor for illness and premature mortality to persist. From a moral perspective the prevalence of poverty in the world's wealthiest nation is yet another matter.
>
> Our nation has the ability to end hunger in a matter of months once we determine to do so. The larger issue is whether we will address poverty and, in doing so, not only eliminate hunger but prevent much untimely disease and death as well.[33]

Regardless of the type and level of involvement a person chooses, each person can make a difference. The government programs described in this chapter need people's support in a number of ways. Individual people can do all of the following:

**FIGURE
11-8**

CCHIP Conceptual Model of Factors Associated with Hunger and Its Outcomes

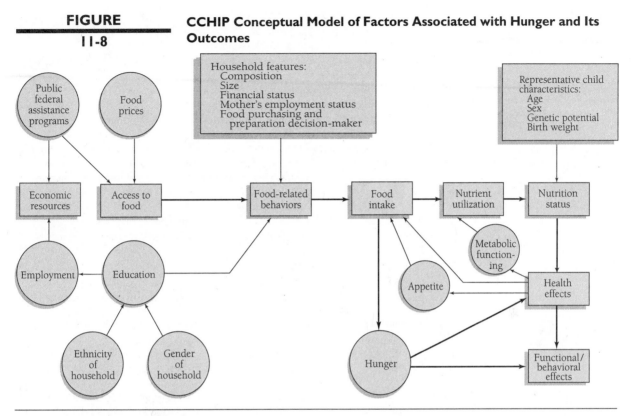

Source: Adapted from C. A. Wehler, R. I. Scott, and J. J. Anderson, The Community Childhood Hunger Identification Project: A model of domestic hunger—demonstration project in Seattle, Washington. Reprinted with permission, *Journal of Nutrition Education* 24 (1992): 32S, Society for Nutrition Education.

◆ Assist in these programs as volunteers. Community nutritionists can educate providers about the nutritional needs of various population groups, identify the most effective means of providing the needed nutrients from limited resources, and teach participants how to shop for the most economical nutritious foods.

◆ Help develop means of informing low-income people about food-related services and programs for which they are eligible.

◆ Help increase the accessibility of existing programs and services to those who need them.

◆ Document the needs that exist in their own communities (see the Community Learning Activity at the end of this chapter).

◆ Join with others in the community who have similar interests. The former House Select Committee on Hunger developed a set of "hunger-free" criteria (listed in Table 11-8) as guidelines for implementing comprehensive food assistance networks. The criteria are meant to provide a useful means of evaluating local antihunger networks.

TABLE

11-8

Hunger-Free Criteria
Source: Reprinted with permission from Community Nutrition Institute, *Nutrition Week*, April 3, 1992, p. 3.

"Hunger-free communities" must meet 14 criteria that should be implemented "in order to comprehensively address local hunger problems":

1. Communities should develop a system for providing information on local food services and donors.
2. There should be coordinated efforts to collect information on the extent of food insecurity existing in the community.
3. A group of residents should gather information detailing the needs of the community to help develop a plan for responding to existing gaps in services.
4. Residents of the community should be educated about the food assistance programs and work with their local officials and private sponsors.
5. Steps should be taken to establish partnerships through which the public and private sectors work together to solve local food insecurity problems.
6. Communities should sponsor forums for educating residents about local food insecurity and encourage their involvement in activities to combat hunger.
7. Emergency food program sponsors should be familiar with support programs so that they can refer needy persons to broader and longer-term support.
8. Projects should be developed to improve the supply of low-cost, nutritious foods to residents of the community.
9. Efforts should be made to target services to those groups who are particularly vulnerable to food insecurity problems.
10. Steps should be taken to establish a reliable system for transporting food to programs that provide meals services for low-income households.
11. Communities should establish easily accessible food delivery sites.
12. Communities should secure public transit routes to provide direct access to public assistance services and food outlets.
13. Nutrition classes should be offered to inform consumers about the relationship between diet and health and to enhance food-buying and preparation skills.
14. Communities should establish programs for collecting and channeling wholesome food otherwise going to waste.

◆ Follow current hunger legislation; call and write legislators about hunger issues; lobby to draw political attention to the need for more job opportunities and a higher minimum wage.

Besides individual actions, all persons who are concerned about the problems of poverty and undernutrition in the United States can exercise their right to affect the political process. Anyone can decide what local, state, and national governments should do to help, and communicate these ideas to elected officials for needed legislative changes. Individuals who volunteer their efforts and express their convictions to improve food assistance programs can also make a difference. Consider the following words, spoken over a hundred years ago:

> I am only one,
> But still I am one.
> I cannot do everything,
> But still I can do something;
> And because I cannot do everything
> I will not refuse to do the something that I can do.[34]

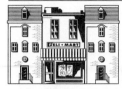

COMMUNITY LEARNING ACTIVITY

Through this activity, you will become familiar with the basic steps for documenting hunger in a community. Your documentation should give you a sense of the food insecurity in your own community. Your hunger documentation may also be useful for informing and/or influencing the decisions of local, state, and federal legislators regarding food security issues.

Four steps are required to provide a basic profile of food security in a community. In this activity, we ask you to focus on Steps 1 and 3.[35]

1. Estimate the size of the group at risk of hunger. Check the most recent U.S. Census of Population and Housing. Track statistics for those listed as "poor" and "near-poor" by age, sex, race, and type of family. These books of statistics from the Bureau of the Census are available in most libraries.

2. Estimate the amount of help available through government food programs and welfare assistance. For example, if 7500 people are classified as living in poverty-level households, how many of these people receive food stamps? Cash welfare such as AFDC and Supplemental Security Income (SSI)? Free or reduced-price meals for their children? WIC benefits? Congregate or home-delivered meals if they are over age 60? Sources of information would be the director or agency staff of the various food assistance and welfare programs.

3. Learn how emergency food needs have changed (increased or decreased) in the community. Talk with the staff of local soup kitchens, food banks, and food pantries to determine whether they are providing more emergency food and if so, how much. Note how many emergency food agencies there are in the community.

4. Determine whether there are indications that overall health status is being affected. You can do this by examining basic health indicators for the community: infant mortality rates, the incidence of low birth weight, the incidence of "failure-to-thrive" among children, and, if possible, the number of hospitalizations in which malnutrition is listed as one of the precipitating causes of treatment. You would need to check vital statistics at local and county health departments and local hospital records for this step. You could also check with the health planning agency for your state to see if a "health status report" has been prepared. Much of this information is documented in these state reports for health planning purposes.

It is recommended that you collect this information for three consecutive years, so that you'll have a sense of whether the situation is improving or getting worse (see Table 11-9).

TABLE

11-9

Basic Facts for Documenting Hunger in a Community
Source: Adapted from Food Research and Action Center, *How to Document Hunger in Your Community* (Washington, D.C.: FRAC, 1983), pp. 5–6.

SAMPLE

for _____, _____ (_____ County)
      City   State

1. Population and Poverty Count

   POPULATION   NUMBER IN POVERTY   POOR PLUS NEAR-POOR

   _____   _____   _____

   Of those below the poverty line:

          OVER 65   UNDER 18

          _____   _____

	1994	1995	1996
2. Receiving Help from Government			
Food Assistance			
Food Stamps	____	____	____
School Lunch	____	____	____
School Breakfast	____	____	____
WIC	____	____	____
CCFP	____	____	____
Nutrition for Elderly	____	____	____
Cash Welfare			
AFDC	____	____	____
SSI	____	____	____
3. Emergency Assistance			
Number of Providers			
Soup Kitchens	____	____	____
Food Pantries	____	____	____
Food Bank	____	____	____
Other	____	____	____
Serving	____	____	____
(number of people served or number of meals served)			
4. Health Indicators			
Infant mortality rate	____	____	____
LBW incidence	____	____	____
Failure-to-thrive incidence	____	____	____
Hospitalizations related to malnutrition	____	____	____

◆ PROFESSIONAL FOCUS

Being an Effective Writer

The written word, Rudyard Kipling once observed, is "the most powerful drug used by mankind." It inspires, educates, moves, and engages us. Because it is so powerful, we want to be sure that we can express ourselves well, regardless of the audience for whom we are writing or the topic being discussed.

But how do you become a good writer? Any number of strategies, some of which are described here, can help you improve your writing skills, but one of the most important steps you can take is to practice. To learn to express yourself clearly and concisely, you must practice, practice, practice. Fortunately, most of us have ample opportunity to practice our craft, for our jobs or schooling require us to write many types of documents: business letters, informal memos, reports, study proposals, scientific articles, fact sheets for the general public, and project updates, to name just a few. Mastering the basic principles of grammar and syntax is also important. Knowing how to use these tools properly will serve you well in all writing situations.

◆ THREE BASIC RULES OF WRITING

Although there are different types of writing—for example, professional and business writing versus writing copy for an advertisement—several basic principles apply:

1. **Know what you want to say**. A well-known fiction writer once remarked, "I don't find writing particularly difficult, it's figuring out what I want to say that's so hard!" If you don't know what you want to tell the reader, your writing will meander around and leave the reader bewildered and unsatisfied. Your first step then is to decide what point or points you want to make. Jot them down before you begin to write your article or report. Once you clarify in your own mind precisely what it is that you want to say, the writing itself will flow more smoothly, and the reader will follow your thinking more easily.

2. **Eliminate clutter**. "The secret of good writing is to strip every sentence to its cleanest components."[1] Every word in every sentence must serve a useful purpose. If it doesn't, mark it out. Consider the approach used by Franklin D. Roosevelt to convert a federal government memo into plain English. The original blackout memo read:[2]

   > Such preparations shall be made as will completely obscure all Federal buildings and non-Federal buildings occupied by the Federal government during an air raid for any period of time from visibility by reason of internal or external illumination.

   "Tell them," Roosevelt said, "that in buildings where they have to keep the work going to put something across the windows."

   By changing gobbledygook into plain English, Roosevelt made the memo simple and direct—and comprehensible. This strategy is important in all types of writing. Consider this statement from one computer company's "customer bulletin": "Management is given enhanced decision participation in key areas of information

Continued

system resources." What on earth does that mean? It might mean "The more you know about your system, the better it will work," or it could mean something else.[3] The wording is so jumbled that the customer can't be sure what the company is trying to tell her and will probably take her business elsewhere as a result.

Whenever possible, eliminate clutter and jargon. To free your writing from clutter, clear your head of clutter. Clear writing comes from clear thinking.

3. **Edit, edit, edit.** A well-written piece does not occur by accident. It is crafted through diligent editing. Writers often edit their manuscripts eight, nine, ten, or more times. Editing pares the piece to the bare bones. It makes the writing stronger, tighter, and more precise. The paragraph shown in Figure 11-9 is an example of an edited manuscript. This particular paragraph was taken from William Zinsser's book, *On Writing Well*. What you see in the figure is a draft that had already been edited four or five times. Zinsser says that he is "always amazed at how much clutter can still be profitably cut."[4]

◆ DIFFERENT STROKES FOR DIFFERENT FOLKS

Not all writing assignments are the same. Some require the formal language of the scientific method, while others are meant to entertain (*and* inform). Choose the style, format, and tone of voice appropriate for the piece you are writing.

1. **Writing for the general public.** Writing for the general public is an important part of the community nutritionist's job. Newspaper and magazine articles, fact sheets, brochures, pamphlets, and posters can all be used to teach and inform consumers. In addition to the basic writing principles outlined in the previous section, two things are important to bear in mind when writing for the general public:

   ◆ The most important sentence in any piece is the first one. If it doesn't engage the reader and induce him to read further, your article or brochure is dead. Therefore, the lead sentence must capture the reader immediately. Consider this lead to an article about designer tomatoes: "Strap on your goggles, consumers, this one's getting messy."[5] The reader wonders instantly why tomatoes should be stirring up trouble. Or this lead from an article about dieting: "Dieters are a diverse group, but they share one common goal: to make their current diet their last one. Unfortunately, lasting results aren't what most get. In fact, the odds are overwhelming—9 to 1—that people who've lost weight will gain it back."[6] Anyone who has tried to lose weight will find this lead enticing. In addition to capturing the reader's attention, the lead must do some work. It must provide a few details that tell the reader why the article was written and why she ought to read it.

   ◆ Know when to close. Choosing an endpoint is as important as choosing a lead. A closing sentence works well when it surprises the reader or makes him think about the article's topic. An article about the challenge of change concluded with this comment, made by a man who participated in Dean Ornish's lifestyle program for high-risk heart disease patients: "What Ornish has given me is that opening and an understanding of what members of the group have said many times: A longer life may be important, but a better life is of the essence."[7] This closing remark works because it is personal and thought-provoking.

Continued

◆ **PROFESSIONAL FOCUS**—*Continued*

This carelessness can take any number of ~~different~~ forms. Perhaps a sentence is so excessively ~~long and~~ cluttered that the reader, hacking his way through ~~all~~ the verbiage, simply doesn't know what ~~the writer~~ *it* means. Perhaps a sentence has been so shoddily constructed that the reader could read it in any of ~~two or three different~~ *several* ways. ~~He thinks he knows what the writer is trying to say, but he's not sure.~~ Perhaps the writer has switched pronouns in mid-sentence, or ~~perhaps he~~ switched tenses, so the reader loses track of who is talking ~~to whom~~ or ~~exactly~~ when the action took place. Perhaps Sentence B is not a logical sequel to Sentence A -- the writer, in whose head the connection is ~~perfectly~~ clear, has not ~~given enough thought to providing~~ *bothered to provide* the missing link. Perhaps the writer has used an important word incorrectly by not taking the trouble to look it up ~~and make sure~~. He may think that "sanguine" and "sanguinary" mean the same thing, but ~~I can assure you that~~ the difference is a bloody big one ~~to the reader.~~ *The reader* He can only ~~try to~~ infer ~~as to~~ (speaking of big differences) what the writer is trying to imply.

FIGURE 11-9

An Example of an Edited Manuscript

Source: Copyright © 1976, 1980, 1985, 1988, 1990 by William K. Zinsser. From *On Writing Well,* 4th ed., published by HarperCollins.

2. **Writing for professional audiences.** Materials written for professional groups must conform to a more rigorous, traditional format and style than those aimed at consumers. Scientific articles, for example, have specific subheadings and a formal tone (refer to the Professional Focus for Chapter 2). The best way to learn how to write these types of documents is to study published articles. Once again, editing is important. When possible, ask your colleagues to review your manuscripts. Their comments will help you identify places where your meaning is unclear.

◆ **READING AND WRITING**

Russell Baker, who won the Pulitzer Prize for his book *Growing Up,* was asked to write a piece about punctuation as part of a series on writing published by the International Paper Company. Baker began his piece by saying, "When you write, you make a sound in the reader's head. It can be a dull mumble—that's why so much government prose makes you sleepy—or it can be a joyful noise, a sly whisper, a throb of passion." He went on to speak of the importance of punctuation in letting your voice speak to the reader. "Punctuation,"

Continued

he wrote, "plays the role of body language. It helps readers hear you the way you want to be heard."[8]

How can you learn to master the rules of punctuation and the principles of writing? Read. The more you read, the better you write. The better you write, the better you communicate. The better you communicate, the better you inform, inspire, and educate. To improve your writing skills, consider adding one or more of the following resources to your professional library:

◆ *On Writing Well* by W. Zinsser

◆ *The Elements of Style* by W. Strunk, Jr., and E. B. White

◆ *The Chicago Manual of Style,* by the University of Chicago Press

◆ *The Elements of Grammar* by M. Shertzer

◆ *Fowler's Modern English Usage* by H. W. Fowler

NOTES

1. W. Zinsser, *On Writing Well* (New York: Harper & Row, 1988), p. 7.
2. Ibid., p. 8.
3. Ibid., p. 153.
4. Ibid., p. 10.
5. B. Carey, Tasty tomatoes: Now there's a concept, *Health* 7 (1993): 24.
6. C. Simon, The triumphant dieter, *Psychology Today,* June 1989, p. 48.
7. G. Leonard, A change of heart, *In Health* 5 (1992): 51.
8. The quotation by Russell Baker was taken from an advertisement that appeared in *Discover,* April 1987, pp. 30–31.

NOTES

1. K. Markandaya, *Nectar in a Sieve,* 2nd American ed. (New York: John Day, 1955), pp. 121–22.
2. C. C. Campbell, Food insecurity: A nutritional outcome or a predictor variable? *Journal of Nutrition* 121 (1991): 408–15.
3. The margin definition of food insecurity was adapted from K. Radimer and coauthors, Understanding hunger and developing indicators to assess it in women and children, *Journal of Nutrition Education* 24 (1992): 36S–45S.
4. L. Schwartz-Nobel, *Starving in the Shadow of Plenty* (New York: Putnam, 1981), pp. 35–36.
5. This section was adapted from E. Whitney, E. Hamilton, and M. Boyle, *Understanding Nutrition,* 4th ed. (St. Paul, Minn.: West Publishing Company, 1987), pp. 561–62, 565–69.
6. Physician Task Force on Hunger in America, *Hunger in America: The Growing Epidemic* (Middletown, Conn.: Wesleyan University Press, 1985), p. 17.
7. Ibid.
8. Department of Health and Rehabilitative Services and the Florida Task Force on Hunger, *Hunger in Florida: A Report to the Legislature* (Tallahassee, Fla.: Department of Health and Rehabilitative Services, April 1986), pp. 32–33.
9. N. Kotz, *Hunger in America: The Federal Response* (New York: Field Foundation, 1979), p. 17.
10. Bread for the World Institute, *Hunger 1994: Transforming the Politics of Hunger* (Washington, D.C.: Bread for the World Institute, 1993), pp. 151–56.
11. M. Nestle and S. Guttmacher, Hunger in the United States: Rationale, methods, and policy implications of

state hunger surveys, *Journal of Nutrition Education* 24 (1992): 20S–22S.

12. U.S. begins Nutrition Monitoring: BFW was key supporter, *Bread for the World Newsletter* 4 (1992): 5.

13. Campbell, Food insecurity, p. 408.

14. Ibid., p. 411.

15. R. Briefel and C. Woteki, Development of food sufficiency questions for the third National Health and Nutrition Examination Survey, *Journal of Nutrition Education* 24 (1992): 24S–28S.

16. J. P. Habicht and L. D. Meyers, Principles for effective surveys of hunger and malnutrition in the United States, *Journal of Nutrition* 121 (1991): 403–7.

17. Food and Nutrition Service, *Food Program Facts* (Alexandria, Va.: U.S. Department of Agriculture, 1992), p. 1.

18. The discussions of the food assistance programs were adapted from Food Research and Action Center, *Fact Sheets on the Federal Food Programs* (Washington, D.C.: FRAC, 1991), pp. 1–3; Food and Nutrition Service, *Food Assistance Programs* (Alexandria, Va.: USDA, 1992), pp. 1–73; and *1993 Catalog of Federal Domestic Assistance* (Washington, D.C.: U.S. Government Printing Office, 1993), pp. 69–86, 952–58.

19. Bread for the World Institute, *Hunger 1992: Second Annual Report of the State of World Hunger* (Washington, D.C.: Bread for the World Institute, 1991), pp. 12–19, and Hunger and undernutrition in America, *Dairy Council Digest* 63 (1992): 7–12.

20. Bread for the World Institute, *Hunger 1992*, p. 15. The margin definitions were adapted from *SEEDS (Sprouts Edition)* 14 (1992): 2.

21. Bread for the World Institute, *Hunger 1993: Uprooted People* (Washington, D.C.: Bread for the World Institute, 1992), p. 107.

22. J. L. Wiecha, J. T. Dwyer, and M. Dunn-Strohecker, Nutrition and health services needs among the homeless, *Public Health Reports* 106 (1991): 364–74.

23. The discussion of homelessness and the steps to end it was adapted from Bread for the World Institute, *Hunger 1993*, pp. 108–9.

24. U.S. Conference of Mayors, *A Status Report on Hunger and Homelessness in America's Cities: 1992* (Washington, D.C.: U.S. Conference of Mayors, 1992).

25. Bread for the World Institute, *Hunger 1990* (Washington, D.C.: Bread for the World Institute, 1990), pp. 88–99.

26. Ibid., p. 91.

27. Community Nutrition Institute, Utah shows one in five children are hungry, *Nutrition Week*, February 26, 1993, p. 6.

28. C. A. Wehler, R. I. Scott, and J. J. Anderson, The Community Childhood Hunger Identification Project: A model of domestic hunger—demonstration project in Seattle, Washington, *Journal of Nutrition Education* 24 (1992): 29S–35S.

29. Ibid., p. 30S.

30. Hunger and undernutrition in America, p. 7.

31. Bread for the World Institute, *Hunger 1990*, p. 91.

32. Select Committee on Hunger, *Farm Crisis: Growing Poverty and Hunger among America's Food Producers* (Washington, D.C.: U.S. Government Printing Office, 1987), p. 163.

33. J. L. Brown and D. Allen, Hunger in America, *Annual Reviews in Public Health* 9 (1988): 503–26.

34. The quotation is by Edward Everett Hale (1822–1909), *For the Lend-a-Hand Society*.

35. This activity was adapted from *How to Document Hunger in Your Community* (Washington, D.C.: Food Research and Action Center, 1983), pp. 3–21.

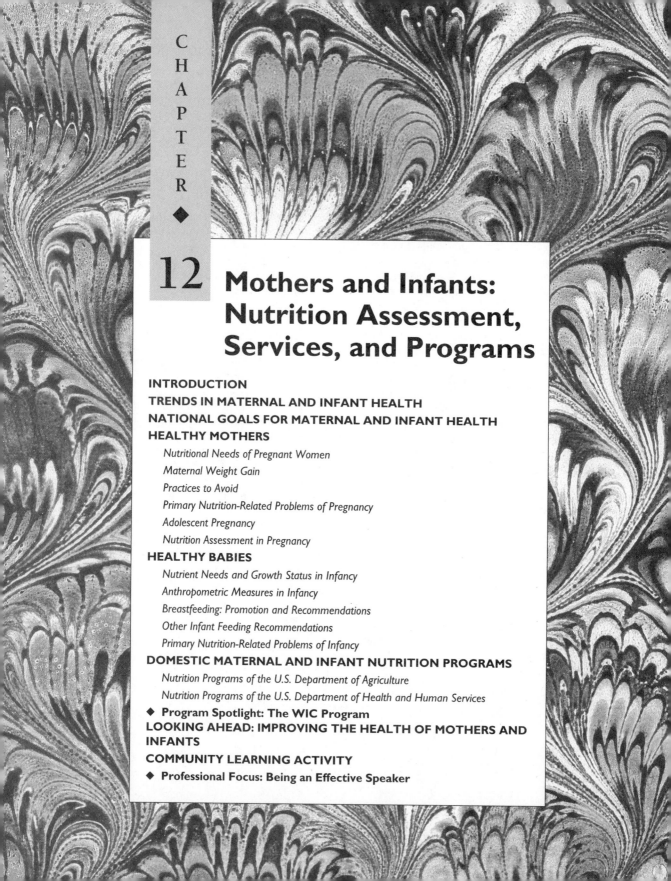

12 Mothers and Infants: Nutrition Assessment, Services, and Programs

Something to Think About . . .

There is no finer investment for any country than putting milk into babies.
                                                          —Winston Churchill

Introduction

The effects of nutrition extend from one generation to the next, and this is particularly evident during pregnancy. Research has demonstrated that the poor nutrition of a woman during her early pregnancy can impair the health of her *grand-
child,* even after that child has become an adult.[1] For example, if a mother's
nutrient stores are inadequate early in pregnancy when the placenta is developing, the fetus will develop poorly, no matter how well the mother eats later. After
getting such a poor start on life, the female child may grow up poorly equipped to
support a normal pregnancy, and she, too, may bear a poorly developed infant.

Infants born of malnourished mothers are more likely than healthy women's
infants to become ill, to have birth defects, and to suffer retarded mental or physical development. This remains true even if they later receive abundant, nourishing food. The many growth-retarded Korean orphans adopted by U.S. families
after the Korean War, for example, experienced several years of catch-up growth,
which did not completely remedy the growth deficits caused by early malnutrition.[2] Malnutrition in the prenatal and early postnatal periods also affects learning ability and behavior. Clearly, it is critical to provide the best nutrition possible at the early stages of life. This chapter focuses on the particular nutrient
requirements and nutrition-related problems of pregnancy, lactation, and infancy
and examines the nutrition programs and services that target pregnant women
and their infants.

Trends in Maternal and Infant Health

The health of a nation is often judged by the health status of its mothers and
infants. One of the best indicators of a nation's health, according to epidemiologists, is the **infant mortality rate (IMR)**. Although the United States spends more
money on health care than most other countries, its IMR of 8.9 is considerably
higher than several industrialized countries'—for example, 4.8 and 5.8 for Japan

Infant mortality rate (IMR)
Infant deaths under one year of
age, expressed as a rate per
1000 live births.

369

TABLE
12-1

A Comparison of Infant Mortality Rates Worldwide, 1991

Japan	4.8
Sweden	5.8
Denmark	6.1
Finland	6.1
Norway	6.1
Switzerland	6.8
Canada	7.2
Australia	7.4
Netherlands	7.5
France	7.7
Germany	8.1
Belgium	8.4
Ireland	8.4
United Kingdom	8.4
United States	8.9
Spain	9.2
Austria	9.2
Italy	9.4
New Zealand	9.4
Israel	10.1

Source: Adapted from UNICEF, *The State of the World's Children* (Oxford: Oxford University Press, 1992), and *The State of World Population* (New York: U.N. Fund for Population Activities, 1992).

and Sweden, respectively (see Table 12-1). Although the U.S. IMR is at an all-time low, important measures of increased risk of death, such as incidence of low birth weight and receipt of prenatal care, show no recent improvement.[3] In addition, disparities in IMRs persist between ethnic groups and between poor and nonpoor infants, as shown in Figure 12-1. The IMR for black infants remains about twice as high as that for white infants. The failure to further improve the IMR in the United States has been attributed to the number of infants born with low birth weights.

If the pregnant woman does not receive adequate nourishment and does not gain the recommended amount of weight, she may give birth to a baby of **low birth weight (LBW)**. Not all small babies are unhealthy, but birth weight and length of gestation are the primary indicators of the infant's future health status. An LBW baby is more likely to experience complications during delivery than a normal-weight baby and has a statistically greater chance of having physical and mental birth defects, contracting diseases, and dying early in life. Low birth weight in full-term infants is a major contributing factor to infant mortality.[4] Clearly, a key to reducing infant mortality is reducing the incidence of LBW babies. To do so, several factors need to be addressed: poverty, minority status, lack of access to health care, inability to pay for health care, poor nutrition, low level of educational achievement, unsanitary living conditions, and unhealthful habits such as smoking, drinking, and drug use. Figure 12-2 depicts the percentage of LBW infants by race in the United States.

Improving the health and nutrition status of pregnant women and infants remains a national challenge. Although **maternal mortality rates** have decreased significantly during the last four decades from a high of 83.3 per 100,000 live births in the 1950s to a low of 6.6 in 1987, black women still have a three times greater risk of dying than white women.[5]

National Goals for Maternal and Infant Health

Maternal mortality rate
Number of women's deaths assigned to causes related to pregnancy, expressed as a rate per 100,000 live births.

Within the past decade a number of research reports, such as the *Surgeon General's Report* and *Healthy People 2000,* have established goals and recommendations designed to improve the nutrition and health status of mothers and infants.[6] The Institute of Medicine's Committee on Nutritional Status During Pregnancy and Lactation provides the most recent findings on the unique role of nutrition in the outcome of pregnancy and lactation.[7] In order for the United States to achieve further reductions in infant mortality and eliminate racial and ethnic differences in pregnancy outcome, health care professionals must focus on changing the behaviors and outcomes that affect pregnancy outcomes.[8] For example, health problems and behaviors such as smoking, substance abuse, and poor nutrition need to be addressed prior to conception. A summary of selected objectives to improve maternal and infant health by the year 2000 are listed in Table 12-2.

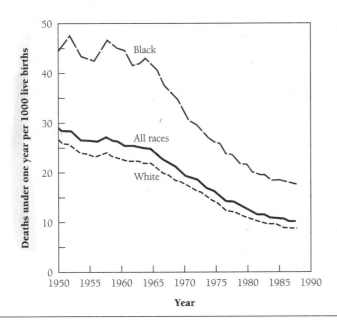

FIGURE

12-1

**U.S. Infant Mortality
Rates by Race, 1950–1988**
Source: Office of Maternal and
Child Health, Public Health Service,
U.S. Department of Health and
Human Services, *Child Health USA
'90* (Washington, D.C.: U.S.
Department of Health and Human
Services, 1990), p. 16.

Healthy Mothers

A number of factors contribute to maternal and infant health. Genetic, environmental, and behavioral factors affect risk and the outcome of pregnancy. A woman's nutrition prior to and throughout pregnancy is crucial to both her health and the growth, development, and health of the infant she conceives. Ideally, a woman starts pregnancy at a healthful weight, with filled nutrient stores and the firmly established habit of eating a balanced and varied diet. In this section, we discuss the nutritional needs of pregnant women, nutrition-related health problems associated with pregnancy, and the nutrition assessment methods important to this population.

◆ NUTRITIONAL NEEDS OF PREGNANT WOMEN

For most women, nutrient needs during pregnancy and lactation are higher than at any other time in their adult life and are greater for certain nutrients than for others (see Figure 12-3 on page 374). Notice that although nutrient needs are much higher than usual, energy needs are not. An increase of only 15 percent of maintenance calories is recommended to support the metabolic demands of pregnancy and fetal development. The 1989 RDA for energy is an additional 300 calories per day during the second and third trimesters.

As shown in Table 12-3, increased amounts of nearly all nutrients are recommended during pregnancy and lactation.[9] The Subcommittee on Dietary Intake

Low birth weight (LBW) A birth weight of 5 1/2 lb (2500 g) or less, used as a predictor of poor health in the newborn and as a probable indicator of poor nutrition status of the mother during and/or before pregnancy. Normal birth weight for a full-term baby is 6 1/2 to 8 3/4 lb (about 3000 to 4000 g). LBW infants are of two different types. Some are premature; they are born early (prior to 38 weeks of gestation) and are the right size for their gestational age. Others have suffered growth failure in the uterus; they may or may not be born early, but they are small for gestational age (small-for-date).

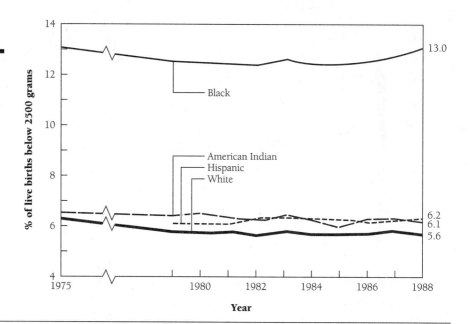

FIGURE

12-2

Percentage of Low-Birth Weight Infants by Race in the United States, 1975–1988

Source: Office of Maternal and Child Health, Public Health Service, U.S. Department of Health and Human Services, *Child Health USA '90* (Washington, D.C.: U.S. Department of Health and Human Services, 1990), p. 18.

and Nutrient Supplementation of the Institute of Medicine believes that the nutrient needs of pregnancy are best met by the routine intake of a variety of foods (see Table 12-4 on page 376) and advises against routine supplementation of all pregnant women with the exception of iron.[10] The advice is based in part on two observations:[11]

◆ Food supplies energy and other essential nutrients not necessarily provided by supplements.

◆ Nutrient supplements have the potential for inadvertent overuse, which may compromise nutrition status and be toxic to the fetus—especially early in pregnancy.

Based on a review of several studies, the subcommittee concluded that protein, folate, iron, zinc, calcium, and vitamins known to be toxic in excess amounts deserved special attention in the diets of pregnant women.[12]

The pregnancy RDA for protein is 60 grams—an additional 10 to 16 grams per day over nonpregnant requirements. Most women are already eating enough protein to cover the increased demand of pregnancy.

The pregnant woman's recommended folate intake is more than twice that of the nonpregnant woman due to the large increase in her blood volume and the rapid growth of the fetus. Certain studies have shown that folate supplements given around the time of conception reduce the recurrence of **neural-tube defects** such as spina bifida in the infants of women who previously have had such births.[13] However, it is possible to obtain the recommended amount of folate, without supplements, from a diet that includes fruits, juices, whole-grain or forti-

Neural-tube defects Any of a number of birth defects in the orderly formation of the neural tube during early gestation. Both the brain and the spinal cord develop from the neural tube; defects result in various central nervous system disorders.

TABLE

12-2

***Healthy People 2000*
Objectives to Improve
Maternal and Infant
Health**

Source: U.S. Department of Health
and Human Services, Public Health
Service, *Healthy People 2000:
National Health Promotion and Disease
Prevention Objectives* (Washington,
D.C.: Department of Health and
Human Services, DHHS Pub. No.
91–50212, 1990).

Health Status Objectives

◆ Reduce the infant mortality rate to no more than 7 per 1000 live births. (Baseline: 10.1 per 1000 live births in 1987)
  ◆ Among blacks: 11/1000 live births. (Baseline: 17.9 in 1987)
  ◆ Among Native Americans and Alaska natives: 8.5/1000 live births. (Baseline: 12.5 in 1984)
  ◆ Among Hispanics: 8/1000 live births. (Baseline: 12.9 for Puerto Ricans in 1984)
◆ Reduce the maternal mortality rate to no more than 3.3 per 100,000 live births. (Baseline: 6.6 per 100,000 in 1987)
◆ Reduce the incidence of fetal alcohol syndrome to no more than 0.12 per 1000 live births. (Baseline: 0.22 per 1000 live births in 1987)

Risk Reduction Objectives

◆ Reduce low birth weight to an incidence of no more than 5% of live births. (Baseline: 6.9% in 1987) Among blacks: 9% of live births. (Baseline: 12.7% in 1987)
◆ Increase to at least 85% the proportion of mothers who achieve the minimum recommended weight gain during their pregnancies. (Baseline: 67% of married women in 1987)
◆ Increase to at least 75% the proportion of mothers who breastfeed their babies in the early postpartum period and to at least 50% the proportion who continue breastfeeding until their babies are 5 to 6 months old. (Baseline: 54% at discharge from birth site and 21% at 5 to 6 months in 1988)
◆ Increase abstinence from tobacco use by pregnant women to at least 90% and increase abstinence from alcohol, cocaine, and marijuana by pregnant women by at least 20%. (Baseline: 75% of pregnant women abstained from tobacco use in 1985)
◆ Increase calcium intake so at least 50% of pregnant and lactating women consume three or more servings daily of foods rich in calcium. (Baseline: 24% of pregnant and lactating women in 1985–1986)
◆ Reduce iron deficiency to less than 3% among women of childbearing age. (Baseline: 5% for women aged 20 to 44 years in 1976–1980)

fied cereals, and green vegetables.* Therefore, the routine use of a folate supplement is not recommended unless the physician has reason to believe the pregnant woman's folate intake is low. In those instances, a supplement of 300 micrograms of folate per day is recommended.

The RDA for iron during pregnancy is an additional 15 milligrams of iron per day to meet maternal and fetal needs. Iron-deficiency anemia is a common prob-

*To lower the risk of neural tube birth defects, women are advised to consume the recommended 400 micrograms of folate a day for pregnancy *before* becoming pregnant. Recently the Food and Drug Administration (FDA) has proposed rules that will require manufacturers to add folate to enriched flours, breads, rolls, buns, corn grits, corn meal, farina, rice, macaroni, and noodle products. FDA also proposes that the labels of folate-containing supplements and foods be allowed to describe the vitamin's effect on birth defects. Such labels must also state that regular daily consumption of folate should not exceed 1.0 milligram from all sources. (**Source:** FDA proposes adding folic acid to grains, *FDA Consumer* 27 (1993): 2, and *Federal Register* (October 14, 1993): 58 FR 53254–53317.)

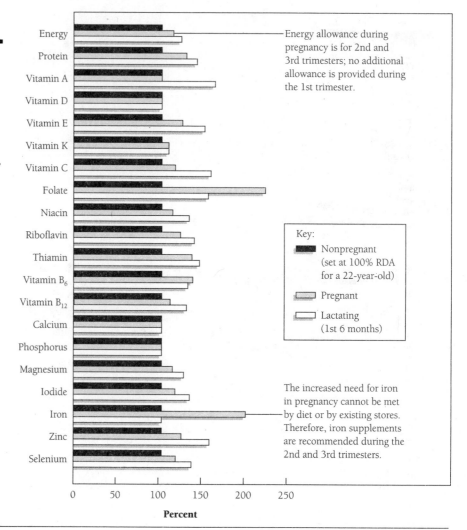

FIGURE 12-3

Comparison of Nutrient Needs of Nonpregnant, Pregnant, and Lactating Women

Energy allowance during pregnancy is for 2nd and 3rd trimesters; no additional allowance is provided during the 1st trimester.

Key:
- Nonpregnant (set at 100% RDA for a 22-year-old)
- Pregnant
- Lactating (1st 6 months)

The increased need for iron in pregnancy cannot be met by diet or by existing stores. Therefore, iron supplements are recommended during the 2nd and 3rd trimesters.

lem among nonpregnant women, and as a result, many women begin pregnancy with diminished iron stores. For this reason, an iron supplement of 30 milligrams of ferrous iron daily during the second and third trimesters is recommended. To facilitate iron absorption from the supplement, it should be taken between meals with vitamin C–rich fruit juices or at bedtime on an empty stomach. Since supplemental doses of iron greater than 30 milligrams can interfere with zinc absorption, pregnant women are encouraged to include good sources of zinc in their daily diets.

The RDA for calcium in pregnancy is 1200 milligrams, a 50 percent increase over adult values—the same amount recommended for females up to the age of 24 years. During the last trimester of pregnancy when fetal skeletal growth is maximum and teeth are being formed, the fetus draws approximately 300 mil-

NUTRIENT	NONPREGNANT WOMEN 15–25+ YEARS	PREGNANCY	LACTATION First 6 months	LACTATION Second 6 months
Energy (kcal)	2200	+300 *	+500	+500
Protein (g)	44–50	60	65	62
Vitamin A (µg RE)	800	800	1300	1200
Vitamin D (µg)	10–5	10	10	10
Vitamin E (mg α-TE)	8	10	12	11
Vitamin K (µg)	55–65	65	65	65
Vitamin C (mg)	60	70	95	90
Thiamin (mg)	1.1	1.5	1.6	1.6
Riboflavin (mg)	1.3	1.6	1.8	1.7
Niacin (mg NE)	15	17	20	20
Vitamin B_6 (mg)	1.5–1.6	2.2	2.1	2.1
Folate (µg)	180	400	280	260
Vitamin B_{12} (µg)	2.0	2.2	2.6	2.6
Calcium (mg)	1200–800	1200	1200	1200
Phosphorus (mg)	1200–800	1200	1200	1200
Magnesium (mg)	300–280	320	355	340
Iron (mg)	15	30	15	15
Zinc (mg)	12	15	19	16
Iodine (µg)	150	175	200	200
Selenium (µg)	50–55	65	75	75

*during the 2nd and 3rd trimesters

TABLE 12-3

Recommended Dietary Allowances for Pregnant and Lactating Women

Source: Food and Nutrition Board, National Research Council, National Academy of Sciences, *Recommended Dietary Allowances,* 10th ed. (Washington, D.C.: National Academy Press, 1989). Used with permission.

ligrams per day from the maternal blood supply.[14] Dairy products are recommended because they are also sources of vitamin D and riboflavin. However, in cases where lactose intolerance is a problem, a calcium supplement should be considered. This is particularly important for women under 25 years of age whose bone mineral density is still increasing. In such cases, a 600-milligram supplement of calcium per day during pregnancy is recommended if the woman normally consumes less than 600 milligrams of calcium a day.

Routine supplementation with vitamins during pregnancy is not advised, and excess intakes of certain vitamins, notably vitamins A and D, can cause fetal malformations.[15] Nutrient supplementation may be appropriate in certain circumstances, however. For example, supplements of vitamin D (10 micrograms per day) and vitamin B_{12} (2 micrograms per day) may be recommended for vegans, or a low-dose multivitamin-mineral supplement beginning in the second trimester may be appropriate for women who do not ordinarily consume an adequate diet or are in high-risk categories, such as women carrying more than one fetus, heavy cigarette smokers, and alcohol and drug abusers.[16] A summary of the Food and Nutrition Board's guidelines is provided in the boxed insert.

◆ MATERNAL WEIGHT GAIN

Normal weight gain and adequate nutrition support the health of the mother and the development of the fetus. The National Academy of Sciences' Committee rec-

FOOD	NUMBER OF SERVINGS	
	Nonpregnant Woman	Pregnant or Lactating Woman[a]
Protein foods	2 to 3	3 (3+)
Milk and milk products	2	3 to 4 (4+)
Enriched or whole-grain breads and cereals	6 to 11	7 to 11 (7+)
Vitamin C–rich fruits and vegetables	1	1 (1+)
Vitamin A–rich fruits and vegetables	1	1
Other fruits and vegetables	3 to 5	4 to 6 (4+)

[a]Numbers in parentheses indicate numbers of servings recommended for the pregnant teenager.

ommendations for weight gain take into account a mother's prepregnancy weight-for-height or body mass index (BMI), as shown in Table 12-5. The committee recommends that a woman who begins pregnancy at a healthful weight should gain between 25 and 35 pounds. Women pregnant with twins need to gain 35 to 45 pounds. An underweight woman needs to gain between 28 and 40 pounds; an overweight woman, between 15 and 25 pounds. Weight gains at the upper end of the range are recommended for pregnant teenagers and black women because of their increased risk of low weight gains and delivery of LBW infants.

Low weight gain in pregnancy is associated with increased risk of delivering an LBW infant; these infants have high mortality rates. Excessive weight gain in pregnancy increases the risk of complications during labor and delivery, as well as postpartum obesity.[17] Obese women (greater than 135 percent of the standard weight-for-height) also have an increased risk for complications during pregnancy, including hypertension and gestational diabetes.

The infant at birth will weigh only about 6 to 8 pounds, but the body tissues the mother builds (blood, blood vessels, muscle, fat stores, and others) to provide a healthful environment for the fetus's development weigh more than 20 pounds (see Table 12-6 on page 379). Weight gain should be lowest during the first trimester—2 to 4 pounds for the trimester—followed by a steady gain of about a pound per week thereafter, as shown in Figure 12-4 on page 380. If a woman gains more than the recommended amount of weight early in pregnancy, she should not try to diet in the last weeks. Dieting during pregnancy is not recommended. A *sudden* large weight gain, however, may indicate the onset of pregnancy-induced hypertension, discussed later; a woman experiencing this type of weight gain should see her health care provider.

Some of the weight a woman gains in pregnancy is lost at delivery. A woman who has gained the recommended 25 to 35 pounds generally loses the remainder within a few months as her blood volume returns to normal and she loses the fluids she has accumulated.

◆ PRACTICES TO AVOID

Optimal pregnancy outcome is influenced by maternal nutrient intake, but can also be affected by maternal use of nonfood substances, excess caffeine, low-calorie

Nutrient Supplementation in Pregnancy

◆ Dietary supplements should not replace dietary counseling or a well-balanced diet; improvement of diet quality through use of nutritious foods is preferred to supplementation.

◆ To meet the increased need for iron during the second and third trimesters of pregnancy, a low-dose iron supplement (30 milligrams of ferrous iron daily) is advised.

◆ If therapeutic levels of iron (more than 30 milligrams daily) are given to treat anemia, supplementation with 15 milligrams of zinc and 2 milligrams of copper is recommended because the iron may interfere with the absorption and utilization of these trace elements.

◆ Pregnant women can meet the physiologic requirements for folate from diet; it is prudent to supplement the diet with low doses (300 micrograms a day) of folate if there is any question about the adequacy of intake of this nutrient.

◆ Because of accumulating data that excessive vitamin A consumption poses a teratogenic risk, supplementation with preformed vitamin A should be avoided during the first trimester unless there is specific evidence of a deficiency. Carotene intake need not be restricted.

◆ For pregnant women who do not ordinarily consume an adequate diet and for those in high-risk categories, such as women carrying more than one fetus, heavy cigarette smokers, and alcohol and drug abusers, a multivitamin-mineral supplement is recommended. The supplement should be taken between meals or at bedtime to facilitate absorption, and it should contain:

Iron 30 mg	Vitamin B_6 2 mg
Zinc 15 mg	Folate 300 µg
Copper 2 mg	Vitamin C 50 mg
Calcium 250 mg	Vitamin D 5 µg

◆ A 10-microgram (400 IU) supplement of vitamin D is recommended for vegans and others with a low intake of vitamin D–fortified milk. A vitamin B_{12} supplement of 2.0 micrograms daily is recommended for vegans.

◆ A calcium supplement of 600 milligrams daily is recommended for women under age 25 whose daily dietary calcium intake is less than 600 milligrams. To enhance absorption and limit interaction with iron supplements, the calcium should be taken at mealtimes.

Source: Food and Nutrition Board, Institute of Medicine, National Academy of Sciences, *Nutrition During Pregnancy* (Washington, D.C.: National Academy Press, 1990).

diets, tobacco, alcohol, and illicit drugs. **Pica** refers to the craving of nonfood items having little or no nutritional value. Pica of pregnancy typically involves the consumption of dirt, clay, or laundry starch, but episodes of pica have included compulsive ingestion of such things as ice, paper, and coffee grounds.[18] The medical consequences of pica can include malnutrition, as nonfood items replace nutritious foods in the diet; obesity, from overconsumption of items such as starch; the

Pica The craving of nonfood items such as clay, ice, and cornstarch. Pica does not appear to be limited to any particular geographic area, race, sex, culture, or social status.

TABLE 12-5	Recommended Weight Gain for Pregnant Women Based on Body Mass Index

WEIGHT CATEGORY BASED ON BMI[a]	TOTAL WEIGHT GAIN[b]		FIRST TRIMESTER GAIN		SECOND AND THIRD TRIMESTER WEEKLY GAIN	
	lb	kg	lb	kg	lb	kg
Underweight (BMI <19.8)	28–40	12.5–18	5	2.3	1.07	0.49
Normal weight (BMI 19.8–26)	25–35	11.5–16	3.5	1.6	0.97	0.44
Overweight (BMI >26–29)	15–25	7–11.5	2	0.9	0.67	0.3
Obese (BMI >29)	at least 15	6				

[a]BMI = body mass index = weight (kg)/height (m)^2.
[b]Young adolescents and black women should strive for gains at the upper end of the recommended range. Short women (<62 in or <157 cm) should strive for gains at the lower end of the range.

Source: Reprinted with permission from B. S. Worthington-Roberts, Nutrition during pregnancy and lactation, in *Krause's Food, Nutrition and Diet Therapy,* ed. L. K. Mahan and M. Arlin (Philadelphia: W. B. Saunders, 1992), p. 153.

ingestion of toxic compounds; or intestinal obstruction, from consuming large amounts of clay or starch.[19]

The Food and Drug Administration has advised pregnant women to avoid unnecessary consumption of caffeine because animal studies suggest that it causes birth defects.[20] Studies in humans have generally failed to show that caffeine use has a negative effect on pregnancy outcome, although limited evidence has shown that moderate-to-heavy use may contribute to lower infant birth weight.[21] Women who choose to use caffeine during pregnancy are generally advised to do so in moderation, if at all—the equivalent of a cup of coffee or two 12-ounce cola beverages a day.

Some practices are truly harmful, and their potential impact on pregnancy outcome is too great to risk. Low-carbohydrate or low-calorie diets that cause ketosis deprive the fetus's brain of needed glucose and cause congenital deformity. The invisible effects may be even more serious. For example, carbohydrate metabolism may be rendered permanently defective, or the infant's brain may be permanently damaged. Protein deprivation can cause children's height and head circumference to diminish markedly and irreversibly.

Another harmful maternal practice is smoking, which restricts the blood supply to the growing fetus, thereby limiting the delivery of nutrients and removal of wastes. Smoking stunts growth, thus increasing the risk of premature delivery, low infant birth weight, retarded development, and complications at birth. Smoking is responsible for 20 to 30 percent of all LBW deliveries in the United States.[22] Sudden infant death syndrome (SIDS) has been linked to a mother's smoking during pregnancy as well.[23]

During the past 15 years, research has confirmed that excessive consumption of alcohol adversely affects fetal development.[24] Even as few as 1 or 2 drinks daily can cause **fetal alcohol syndrome (FAS)**—irreversible brain damage and mental and physical retardation in the fetus. The most severe impact of maternal drinking is likely to be in the first month, before the woman even is sure she is pregnant. This preventable condition (FAS) is estimated to occur in approximately one to two infants per 1000 live births and is the leading known cause of mental retardation in the United States.[25] Birth defects, low birth weight, and spontaneous abortions occur more often in pregnancies of women who drink even as little as 2 ounces of alcohol daily during pregnancy. Accumulating evidence that even one drink may be too much has led the surgeon general to take the position that women should stop drinking as soon as they *plan* to become pregnant.[26]

◆ PRIMARY NUTRITION-RELATED PROBLEMS OF PREGNANCY

Common physical problems in pregnancy include "morning" sickness and, later, constipation. The nausea of morning sickness seems unavoidable because it arises from the hormonal changes taking place early in pregnancy, but it can sometimes be alleviated. A suggested strategy is to start the day with a few sips of water and a soda cracker or other bland carbohydrate food to get something into the stomach before getting out of bed.

Later during pregnancy, as the hormones of pregnancy alter her muscle tone and the growing fetus crowds her intestinal organs, an expectant mother may complain of constipation. A high-fiber diet, plentiful fluid intake, and moderate exercise will help to relieve this condition.

More serious problems needing control during pregnancy include hypertension and diabetes:

◆ **Hypertension.** Preeclampsia and eclampsia are hypertensive conditions induced by pregnancy (see Table 12-7). Preeclampsia is characterized by high blood pressure, protein in the urine, and generalized edema that may cause sudden, large weight gain from retained water. Fluid retention alone, which is quite common in pregnant women, is not sufficient to diagnose preeclampsia.[27] Warning signs of preeclampsia include severe and constant headaches, sudden weight gain (1 pound a day), swelling, dizziness, and blurred vision. Eclampsia, the most severe form of this pregnancy-induced hypertension (PIH), is characterized by convulsions that may lead to coma. Both conditions present serious health risks to mother and fetus. PIH can retard fetal growth and cause the placenta to separate from the uterus, resulting in stillbirth. The former practice of restricting salt and prescribing diuretics for the edema of PIH is not recommended, and pregnant women are advised to use salt to taste. Pregnant women who consume calcium supplements of 1500 to 2000 milligrams per day may be at lower risk of PIH.[28]

◆ **Diabetes.** Infants born to women with diabetes are at greater risk for prematurity, congenital defects, excessively high birth weight, and respirato-

TABLE

12-6

An Example of the Pregnant Woman's Weight Gain

DEVELOP-MENT	WEIGHT GAIN (LB)
Infant at birth	$7\frac{1}{2}$
Placenta	1
Increase in mother's blood volume to supply placenta	4
Increase in size of mother's uterus and the muscles to support it	$2\frac{1}{2}$
Increase in size of mother's breasts	3
Fluid to surround infant in amniotic sac	2
Mother's fat stores	5–10
Total	25–30

Note: The pattern of gain should be about a pound a month for the first three months and a pound a week thereafter. Different patterns of weight gain are suggested for underweight, normal-weight, and overweight women, described by E. McCarthy, Report of a Montreal Diet Dispensary experience, *Journal of the Canadian Dietetic Association* 44 (1983): 71–75.

Fetal alcohol syndrome (FAS) The cluster of symptoms seen in an infant or child whose mother consumed excess alcohol during pregnancy, including retarded growth, impaired development of the central nervous system, and facial malformations.

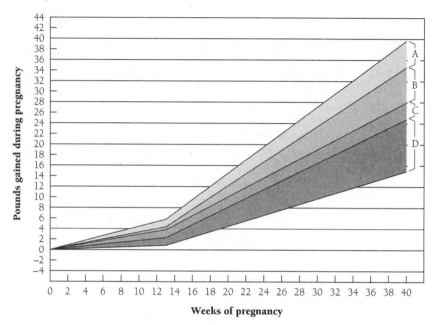

FIGURE
12-4

Desirable Weight Gains during Pregnancy

Source: Courtesy of National Dairy Council, *Great Beginnings: The Weighting Game Graph* (Rosemont, Ill.: National Dairy Council, 1991); adapted from Food and Nutrition Board, Institute of Medicine, National Academy of Sciences, *Nutrition During Pregnancy* (Washington, D.C.: National Academy Press, 1990).

The woman who is of normal weight prior to pregnancy should gain in the B–C range, 25 to 35 lb during the pregnancy. The underweight woman should gain in the A–B range, 28 to 40 lb. The woman who is overweight prior to pregnancy should gain in the D range, 15 to 25 lb.

ry distress syndrome.[29] Metabolic control of diabetes before and throughout pregnancy is critical. In some women, pregnancy can alter carbohydrate metabolism and precipitate a condition known as gestational diabetes. The abnormal blood glucose levels seen during pregnancy return to normal postpartum for about two-thirds of women diagnosed with the condition. Risk factors include age 35 or older, previous history of gestational diabetes, obesity, and a family history of diabetes.

Some women with gestational diabetes have the classic symptoms of diabetes—increased thirst, hunger, urination, weakness—but other women have no warning symptoms of the condition. For this reason, all pregnant women today are screened for gestational diabetes between the 24th and 28th weeks of gestation (see Table 12-8).[30]

◆ ADOLESCENT PREGNANCY

More than a million teenagers become pregnant in the United States each year—one out of every five babies is born to a teenager—and more than a tenth of these mothers are under age 15. The complex social, emotional, and physical factors involved make teen pregnancy one of the most challenging situations for nutrition counseling. According to a position paper from the American Dietetic Association, pregnant adolescents are nutritionally at risk and require intervention early and throughout pregnancy.[31] Medical and nutritional risks are particularly high when the teenager is within two years of menarche (usually 15 years of

CONDITION	CHARACTERISTICS
Preeclampsia	Hypertension with proteinuria and/or edema developing after the twentieth week of pregnancy: almost exclusive incidence in primigravidae and affects women at reproductive age extremes (under 20 or over 35 years). *Hypertension:* 140/90 or increase of 30 mm Hg systolic or 15 mm Hg diastolic above woman's usual baseline; at least two observations 6 or more hours apart. *Proteinuria:* 500 mg or more in 24-hour urine collection or random 2+ protein; develops late in course of PIH. *Edema:* significant; usually in face and hands.
Severe preeclampsia	One or more of following symptoms: systolic pressure 160 mm Hg or diastolic 110 mm Hg on two observations 6 or more hours apart at bed rest; proteinuria at least 5 g/24 hours or random 3 to 4+; blurred vision, headache, altered consciousness; pulmonary edema. *Advancing disease:* epigastric or upper quadrant pain, impaired liver function, thrombocytopenia.
Eclampsia	Extension of preeclampsia with grand mal seizure, occurring near time of labor.

TABLE

12-7

Pregnancy-Induced Hypertension (PIH)

Source: B. Worthington-Roberts and S. R. Williams, *Nutrition in Pregnancy and Lactation,* 5th ed. (St. Louis: Times Mirror/Mosby, 1993), p. 245. Adapted from S. E. Willis, *American Journal of Nursing* 82 (1982): 792, in N. F. Gant and R. J. Worley, *Hypertension in Pregnancy: Concepts and Management* (New York: Appleton-Century-Crofts, 1980).

age or younger).[32] Risks include higher rates of PIH, iron-deficiency anemia, premature birth, stillbirths, LBW infants, and prolonged labor in pregnant teens than in older women. In addition, mothers under 15 years of age bear more babies who die within the first year than do any other age group.[33]

The increased energy and nutrient demands of pregnancy place adolescent girls, who are already at risk for nutritional problems, at even greater risk. To support the needs of both mother and infant, adolescents are encouraged to strive for pregnancy weight gains at the upper end of the ranges recommended for pregnant women (see Table 12-5). Those who gain between 30 and 35 pounds during pregnancy have lower risks of delivering LBW infants.[34] Adequate nutrition can substantially improve the course and outcome of adolescent pregnancy.[35]

◆ NUTRITION ASSESSMENT IN PREGNANCY

Nutrition assessment and monitoring during pregnancy can be divided into three categories: preconception care, the initial prenatal visit, and subsequent prenatal visits.[36] Since a woman's nutrition status and lifestyle habits prior to pregnancy can influence the outcome of pregnancy, these are important factors to consider prior to pregnancy. Nutritional risk factors that may be present at the start of pregnancy are listed in Table 12-9. Preconception care should ideally be available to all women. It should include nutrition assessment, nutrition counseling, and appropriate supplementation and referral to correct nutritional problems existing prior to conception. Prepregnancy weight-for-height should be categorized using BMI so that appropriate weight gain can be recommended for pregnancy (refer to Table 12-5 on page 378).

TABLE

12-8

Screening and Diagnosis of Gestational Diabetes

Source: Adapted from *Diabetes* 34 (1985): 123–26, and M. Powers, *Handbook of Diabetes Nutritional Management* (Rockville, Md.: Aspen Publishers, 1987), p. 342.

◆ **Protocol for one-hour glucose screen:**
1. Who/when
   A. Early pregnancy
      ◆ Fasting glucosuria × 2
      ◆ Family history of diabetes
      ◆ Previous large baby with birth weight over 9 lb (4000 g)
      ◆ Maternal obesity
      ◆ Advanced maternal age (> 35 years)
      ◆ High parity (≥ 5)
      ◆ Previous unexplained stillbirth, neonatal death, or malformation
   B. All women at 24–28 weeks of gestation
2. Procedure
   ◆ Draw blood sugar (fasting or after meal).
   ◆ Drink 50 g oral glucose load.
   ◆ Measure venous plasma glucose 1 hour later.
   ◆ A value of ≥140 mg/dL indicates the need for a full diagnostic glucose tolerance test (GTT). (See Diagnosis of gestational diabetes mellitus below.)
3. Follow-up
   ◆ If early pregnancy screen is normal and woman is in high-risk group, repeat test at 24–28 weeks gestation.
   ◆ If screen is abnormal, perform 3-hour GTT.
◆ **Diagnosis of gestational diabetes mellitus:**
1. Administer a 100 g oral glucose load in the morning after overnight (8 hr) fast.
2. Measure fasting venous plasma glucose at 1, 2, and 3 hours.
3. Two or more of the following venous plasma concentrations must be met or exceeded for positive diagnosis:
   ◆ Fasting, 105 mg/dL
   ◆ 1 hr, 190 mg/dL
   ◆ 2 hr, 165 mg/dL
   ◆ 3 hr, 145 mg/dL

Assessment of pregnant teens follows the general pattern for assessment of older pregnant women (see Table 12-10). Assessment issues include acceptance of the pregnancy, food resources and food preparation facilities, body image, living situation, relationship with the father of the infant, peer relationships, nutrition status, prenatal care, nutrition attitude and knowledge, preparation for child feeding, financial resources, continuation of education, day care, and knowledge and attitudes of infant feeding methods.[37] Frequent snacking by teens in general on foods high in fat and sugar results in lower-than-recommended intakes of calcium, iron, zinc, folate, and vitamins B$_6$, A, and C—nutrients needing special attention in the diet of the pregnant teen. Recommended servings of foods for the pregnant adolescent are shown in Table 12-4 on page 376.

The nutrition status of all women should be assessed at their initial prenatal visit. This assessment should include the following components:[38]

◆ **Dietary measures.** Diet history, including food habits, attitudes, and folklore; allergies; use of vitamin and mineral supplements; and lifestyles (e.g., substance abuse; existence of pica).

◆ **Age.** Teenage, especially 15 years or younger, or 35 years or older.

◆ **Number of pregnancies.** Frequent pregnancies with short intervals between pregnancies.

◆ **Pregnancy outcome.** History of poor outcome.

◆ **Socioeconomic status.** Poverty, low level of education, or lack of support from family.

◆ **Lifestyle habits.** Smoking, alcohol, or other drug use.

◆ **Maternal weight.** Less than 85% of standard weight-for-height or more than 120% of standard weight.

◆ **Maternal nutrition.** Bizarre or faddist food habits, nutrient deficiencies or toxicities.

◆ **Maternal health.** Chronic disorders: high blood pressure; diabetes; heart, respiratory, and kidney disease; certain genetic disorders (e.g., PKU); use of therapeutic diets and drugs.

TABLE

12-9

Nutritional Risk Factors Present at the Onset of Pregnancy

Source: Adapted with permission from B. Worthington-Roberts and S. R. Williams, *Nutrition in Pregnancy and Lactation,* 5th ed. (St. Louis: Times Mirror/Mosby, 1993), p. 208.

◆ **Clinical measures.** Obstetric history, including outcome of previous pregnancies, interval between pregnancies, and history of problems during course of previous pregnancies (PIH, gestational diabetes, iron-deficiency anemia, inadequate or excessive weight gain pattern).

◆ **Anthropometric measures.** Measurement of weight-for-height; the weight should be recorded and plotted on a weight gain grid (refer back to Figure 12-4). Skinfold measures are not recommended for routine assessment.[39]

◆ **Laboratory values.** Screening for anemia by hematocrit and/or hemoglobin (see Table 12-11). A urine analysis for ketones, glucose, and protein spillage may be ordered for women with gestational diabetes or preeclampsia.

During each subsequent prenatal visit, weight gain should be monitored and the pattern of weight gain evaluated, as indicated in Table 12-11. Screening for anemia should be repeated on at least one other occasion during pregnancy. Routine assessment of dietary practices is recommended for all women so that their need for an improved diet or vitamin or mineral supplementation can be evaluated. The nutrition status of women in high-risk categories (see Table 12-12) should be reevaluated at each visit.

Poor dietary practices should be improved by appropriate interventions. These may include general nutrition education, individualized diet counseling, and referral to food assistance programs (e.g., Special Supplemental Food Program for Women, Infants, and Children [WIC] and Food Stamps) or to programs that promote improved food acquisition or preparation practices (e.g., the Expanded Food and Nutrition Education Program—EFNEP).[40]

Healthy Babies

The growth of infants directly reflects their nutritional well-being and is the major indicator of their nutrition status. A baby grows faster during the first year

TABLE

12-10

Protocol for Nutrition Assessment in Pregnancy

Source: Adapted with permission from L. K. Mahan and J. M. Rees, *Nutrition in Adolescence* (St. Louis: Times Mirror/Mosby, 1984).

◆ Initial evaluation
Review clinical data:
   Height and weight
   Gynecological age (adolescents)
   Physical signs of health
   Expected delivery date
Review laboratory data:
   Hematocrit or hemoglobin
   Urinalysis
Assess attitude about and acceptance of prepregnancy weight and feelings about weight gain during pregnancy.
Assess intake patterns using dietary methodology best suited to client and professional.
Make preliminary assessment of food resources and refer to supportive agencies if necessary.
Check for nausea and vomiting and suggest possible remedy.
Discuss supplemental vitamins and minerals.
Make initial plan that sets priorities for issues.
Determine client's understanding of relation between nutrition and health.

◆ Second visit
Check on referrals to other agencies.
Discuss results of initial evaluation and suggest any changes necessary in dietary patterns (use printed materials as appropriate).
Do any further investigations when necessary:
   Laboratory studies
      For specific diagnosis of anemia:
      ◆ Protoporphyrin heme or serum ferritin
      ◆ Serum or red cell folate
      ◆ Serum vitamin B_{12}
Further probing of dietary habits if necessary
Monitor weight gain; discuss projected weight gain for following visit and total for gestation.
Assess and address issues affecting nutrition status in order of priority for the individual:
   ◆ Activity level
   ◆ Appetite changes
   ◆ Pica, food cravings, and aversions
   ◆ Allergies/food intolerances
   ◆ Supplementation practices

◆ Subsequent visits
Monitor and support appropriate weight gain: include discussion of fitness and encourage safe exercise.
Continue to address issues affecting nutrition status.
Check for heartburn, small food-intake capacity, and elimination problems; suggest dietary interventions.
Begin preliminary discussion and comparison of advantages/disadvantages of breastfeeding and formula feeding.

◆ Final prenatal visit(s)
Discuss infant feeding.
If breastfeeding is chosen, provide preliminary guidance about breastfeeding practices.
If formula feeding is chosen, discuss product selection and preparation; define important details about feeding techniques.

◆ Postpartum visits
Help client to understand safe methods of managing weight following delivery.
Review infant feeding practices and infant growth; provide assistance when problems are identified.

of life than ever again; its birth weight doubles during the first four to six months and triples by the end of the first year. Adequate nutrition during infancy is critical to support this rapid rate of growth and development. Clearly, from the point of view of nutrition, the first year is the most important year of a person's life. This section provides a brief overview of nutrient requirements, current recommendations and health objectives for feeding healthy infants, and the relationship between infant feeding and selected pediatric nutrition issues.

◆ NUTRIENT NEEDS AND GROWTH STATUS IN INFANCY

The infant's rapid growth and metabolism demand an adequate supply of all essential nutrients. Because of their small size, infants need smaller total amounts of the nutrients than adults do, but based on body weight, infants need over twice as much of many of the nutrients. Figure 12-5 compares a five-month-old baby's needs with those of an adult man; as you can see, some of the differences are extraordinary. After six months, energy needs increase less rapidly as the growth rate begins to slow down, but some of the energy saved by slower growth is spent on increased activity.

◆ ANTHROPOMETRIC MEASURES IN INFANCY

Anthropometric measurements that are routinely obtained in the examination of infants include length, weight, and head circumference. These measures assess physical size and growth.

TABLE

12-11

Nutritional Risk Factors Occurring during Pregnancy

Low hemoglobin and/or hematocrit:
  Hemoglobin less than 12.0 g/100 ml
  Hematocrit less than 35.0%
Inadequate weight gain:
  Any weight loss
  Weight gain of less than 2 lb (1 kg) per month after the first trimester
Excessive weight gain:
  Weight gain greater than 2 lb (1 kg) per week after the first trimester

Source: Adapted with permission from B. Worthington-Roberts and S. R. Williams, *Nutrition in Pregnancy and Lactation,* 5th ed. (St. Louis: Times Mirror/Mosby, 1993), p. 208.

TABLE

12-12

High-Risk Pregnancies

PERSONAL CHARACTERISTICS (CANNOT CHANGE)	PERSONAL HABITS, LIVING SITUATION (SEEK TO CHANGE)	CHRONIC PREEXISTING MATERNAL MEDICAL PROBLEMS (SCREEN, TREAT)	OBSTETRIC HISTORY (SCREEN, PREVENT)	CURRENT/POTENTIAL PREGNANCY-INDUCED PROBLEMS (SCREEN, PREVENT, TREAT)
Sex	Smoking	Hypertension	Low birth weight	Anemia
Age	Alcohol/drug use	IDDM	Macrosomia	Iron deficiency
Adolescent	Poor diet	NIDDM	Stillbirth	Folate deficiency
Older woman	Malnutrition	Heart disease	Abortion	PIH
Family history	Obesity	Pulmonary disease	Fetal anomalies	Gestational diabetes
Diabetes	Underweight	Renal disease	High parity	
Heart disease	Sedentary lifestyle	MPKU	Multipara	
Hypertension				
PKU				

Source: Adapted with permission from B. Worthington-Roberts and S. R. Williams, *Nutrition in Pregnancy and Lactation,* 5th ed. (St. Louis: Times Mirror/Mosby, 1993) p. 240.

FIGURE

12-5

Nutrient RDA of a Five-Month-Old Infant and an Adult Male Compared on the Basis of Body Weight
Source: Reprinted by permission from *Understanding Nutrition*, 6th ed., by E. N. Whitney and S. R. Rolfes. Copyright © 1993 by West Publishing Company. All rights reserved.

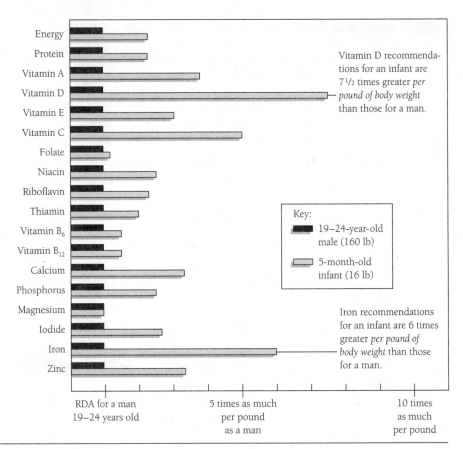

Vitamin D recommendations for an infant are 7 1/2 times greater *per pound of body weight* than those for a man.

Key:
▨ 19–24-year-old male (160 lb)
▢ 5-month-old infant (16 lb)

Iron recommendations for an infant are 6 times greater *per pound of body weight* than those for a man.

RDA for a man 19–24 years old   5 times as much per pound as a man   10 times as much per pound

Infants should be weighed nude, using a table model beam scale that allows the infant to lie or sit. Length should be measured in the recumbent position on a measuring board that has a fixed headboard and movable footboard attached at right angles to the surface.[41]

Head circumference measures can confirm that growth is proceeding normally or help detect protein-energy malnutrition (PEM) and evaluate the extent of its impact on brain size. To measure head circumference, a nonstretchable tape is placed around the largest part of the infant's head: just above the eyebrow ridges, just above the point where the ears attach, and around the occipital prominence at the back of the head.[42] The head circumference percentile should be similar to the infant's weight and length percentiles.

The National Center for Health Statistics (NCHS) growth charts, such as those shown in Figure 12-6, are used to analyze measures of growth status in infants. A single plotting is used to assess how an infant ranks in comparison to other infants of the same age and sex in the United States. If a measurement is less than the 10th percentile, it should be checked for accuracy and further evaluated. Height-for-age less than the 5th percentile reflects chronic undernutrition. Weight-for-height (length) less than the 5th percentile may reflect acute malnu-

FIGURE 12-6   Examples of Growth Charts

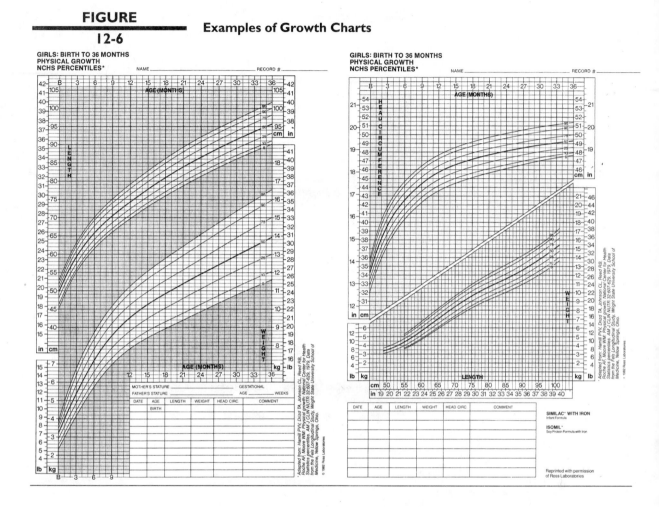

trition. Excessive weight-for-length (above the 95th percentile) indicates over-weight.[43] Under normal conditions, the growth rate usually varies within two percentiles. Greater variation indicates the possibility of inadequate nutrition and needs to be evaluated further.

The two charts shown above are used for girls from birth to 36 months. The first chart gives percentiles for length and weight for age; the other, percentiles for head circumference for age and weight for length.

◆ BREASTFEEDING: PROMOTION AND RECOMMENDATIONS

Breastfeeding offers both emotional and physical health advantages. Emotional bonding is facilitated by many events and behaviors of mother and infant during the early months and years; one of the first can be breastfeeding.

During the first two or three days of lactation, the breasts produce colostrum, a premilk substance containing antibodies and white cells from the mother's blood. Colostrum and breast milk both contain the bifidus factor that favors the growth of the "friendly" bacteria *Lactobacillus bifidus* in the infant's digestive tract so that other, harmful bacteria cannot grow there. Breast milk also contains the powerful antibacterial agent, lactoferrin, and other factors including several enzymes, several hormones (including thyroid hormone and prostaglandins), and lipids that help protect the infant against infection.

Breast milk is also tailor-made to meet the nutrient needs of the young infant. Breastfed infants usually require no nutrient supplements except for vitamin D and fluoride (see Table 12-13). At four to six months, infants may require an iron supplement, depending on food intake.

Breastfeeding provides other benefits as well. It protects against allergy development during the vulnerable first few weeks; the act of suckling favors normal tooth and jaw alignment; and breastfed babies are less likely to be obese because they are less likely to be overfed. A woman who wants to breastfeed can derive justification and satisfaction from all these advantages.

These attributes, along with the convenience and lower cost of breastfeeding, have led many organizations and medical experts to encourage breastfeeding for all normal full-term infants.[44] Despite the health benefits, however, the incidence of breastfeeding has declined since the early 1980s (see Figure 12-7).[45] Analysis of data from the Ross Laboratories Mothers Survey indicates that breastfeeding rates continue to be the highest among women who are older, well-educated, relatively affluent, and/or living in the western United States. Among those least likely to breastfeed are women who are low income, black, less than age 20, and/or living in the southeastern United States.[46]

A number of barriers to achieving the nation's health objective of increasing the incidence of breastfeeding have been identified. These include lack of knowledge, an absence of work policies and facilities that support lactating women (e.g., extended maternity leave, part-time employment, facilities for pumping

TABLE 12-13 **Supplements for Full-Term Infants**	VITAMIN D[a]	IRON[b]	FLUORIDE[c]
Breastfed infants:			
Birth to six months of age	✓		✓
Six months to one year	✓	✓	✓
Formula-fed infants:			
Birth to six months of age			✓
Six months to one year		✓	✓

[a]Vitamin D supplements are recommended only for as long as breast milk is the major milk the infant consumes.
[b]Infants four to six months of age need additional iron, preferably in the form of iron-fortified cereal for both breastfed and formula-fed infants and iron-fortified infant formula for formula-fed infants.
[c]The Committee on Nutrition of the American Academy of Pediatrics recommends initiating fluoride supplements for breastfed infants, formula-fed infants who receive ready-to-use formulas (these are prepared with water low in fluoride), or those who receive formula mixed with water that contains little or no fluoride (less than 0.3 ppm).

Source: E. Whitney and S. Rolfes, *Understanding Nutrition,* 6th ed. (St. Paul, Minn.: West Publishing, 1993). Adapted from Committee on Nutrition, American Academy of Pediatrics, Vitamin and mineral supplement needs of normal children in the United States, in *Pediatric Nutrition Handbook,* 2nd ed., ed. G. B. Forbes and C. W. Woodruff (Elk Grove Village, Ill.: American Academy of Pediatrics, 1985), pp. 37–48.

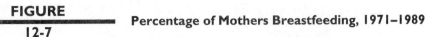

FIGURE 12-7   **Percentage of Mothers Breastfeeding, 1971–1989**

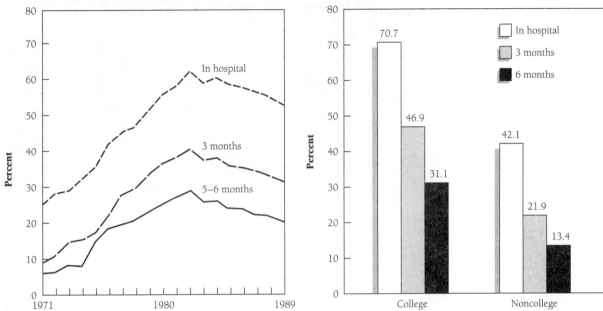

Percentage breastfeeding: 1971–1989 all races

Percentage breastfeeding by education: 1989

Source: Office of Maternal and Child Health, Public Health Service, U.S. Department of Health and Human Services, *Child Health USA '89* (Washington, D.C.: U.S. Department of Health and Human Services, 1989).

breast milk or breastfeeding, and on-site child care); the portrayal of bottle feeding rather than breastfeeding as the norm in American society; and the lack of breastfeeding incentives and support for low-income women.

One example of a successful approach to increasing breastfeeding rates in low-income, urban populations is the peer counseling method promoted by the La Leche League International.[47] The WIC program has initiated breastfeeding promotion projects among low-income women using the peer counselor method.[48] With this approach, peer support counselors are trained to provide culturally appropriate interventions for initiating and maintaining breastfeeding in their communities. The peer counselor is paired with an expectant or new mother for individual assistance and informal discussions in their neighborhood. Results of similar grassroots approaches to breastfeeding promotion are encouraging, with both the rate and duration of breastfeeding among the women in the programs showing significant increases.[49]

Focus groups can be useful in designing breastfeeding promotion projects. For example, the project "Best Start: Breastfeeding for Healthy Mothers, Healthy Babies" was organized in the southeastern United States by a coalition of nutrition and public health officials concerned about declining rates of breastfeeding in the region.[50] Focus groups were especially helpful in exploring topics related to breastfeeding among participants who were ambivalent or undecided. Research

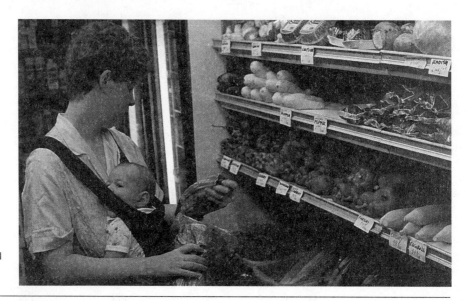

A nutritious diet supports successful lactation which offers many health advantages to the newborn infant.

findings pointed to the need for a carefully coordinated campaign that utilized a combination of strategies to improve the image of breastfeeding and help women overcome the barriers they perceived to breastfeeding. Based on information generated from the focus group interviews, guidelines were formulated for program development (see the boxed insert for the guidelines).

◆ OTHER INFANT FEEDING RECOMMENDATIONS

Like the breastfeeding mother, the mother who offers formula to her baby has reasons for making her choice, and her feelings should be honored. Infant formulas are manufactured to approximate the nutrient composition of breast milk. The immunologic protection of breast milk, however, cannot be duplicated.

Many mothers breastfeed at first and then wean within the first one to six months. When a woman chooses to wean her infant during the first six months of life, it is imperative that she shift to *formula,* not to plain milk of any kind— whole, low-fat, or nonfat. Only formula contains enough iron (to name but one of many factors) to support normal development in the baby's first months of life. National and international standards have been set for the nutrient content of infant formulas.

For infants with special problems, many variations of infant formulas are available. Special formulas based on soy protein are available for infants allergic to milk protein, and formulas with the lactose replaced can be used for infants with lactose intolerance.

Whole cow's milk is not recommended during the first year of life, according to the American Academy of Pediatrics (AAP).[51] This recommendation replaces an earlier one suggesting that once the baby was obtaining at least a third of the total daily food energy from a balanced mixture of cereal, vegetables, fruits, and

Using Focus Group Findings

Using comments made by women participating in focus groups, planners of the Best Start breastfeeding promotion project formulated the following guidelines:

- ◆ **Campaign tone.** The tone should be emotional to reflect the strong feelings women attach to their aspirations for their children and themselves as mothers.

- ◆ **Message design.** Educational messages should be succinct and easily understood to counteract the mistaken belief that breastfeeding is complicated and requires major lifestyle changes. Promotional messages should emphasize confidence and the pride breastfeeding mothers gain from nursing.

- ◆ **Spokespersons.** Celebrities are not perceived as credible sources of advice on infant feeding. Also, most focus group respondents find it difficult to identify with wealthy women featured on many of the pamphlets, posters, and other breastfeeding promotion materials used in health departments. Whenever possible, women featured in the materials should be of the same economic, ethnic, and age groups as those targeted or should not have a clear class affiliation. Visual images in print and broadcast materials should communicate modernity and confidence.

- ◆ **Educational approaches.** Educational strategies and materials need to be redesigned so that they no longer reinforce women's perceptions of breastfeeding as difficult. The emphasis on being healthy and relaxed and following special dietary guidelines needs to be replaced with reassurance that most women produce sufficient quantities of highly nutritious breast milk despite variations in diet, stress levels, and health status.

- ◆ **Professional training.** Motivational and training materials are needed to counter professionals' mistaken belief that their economically disadvantaged clients are not interested in breastfeeding and do not value health professionals' advice. Counseling strategies need to be redesigned to address the special needs of low-income women. Of special concern are recommendations for overcoming clients' lack of confidence and enabling them to realize their aspirations as women and mothers.

- ◆ **Program activities/components.** A variety of mutually reinforcing activities are needed to reach social network members who influence women's infant feeding decisions and create hospital, home, and community environments conducive to lactation.

Source: Adapted from C. Bryant and D. Bailey, The use of focus group research in program development. Unpublished manuscript, Lexington, Ky, 1989.

other foods (usually after six months of age), whole cow's milk fortified with vitamins A and D was acceptable as an accompanying beverage.[52]

Solid foods should normally be added to a breastfed baby's diet when the baby is between six months and one year of age. A baby who is formula fed might be started on solid foods between three and four months, depending on readiness. Indicators of readiness are listed on the next page.

◆ The infant's birth weight has doubled.

◆ The infant consumes 8 ounces of formula in less than four hours and still is hungry.

◆ The infant is consuming 32 ounces of formula a day and wants more.

◆ The infant is six months old.

Solids should not be introduced too early, because infants are more likely to develop allergies to them in the early months. But all babies are different, and the program of additions should depend on the individual baby, not on any rigid schedule. Table 12-14 presents a suggested sequence for feeding infants.

◆ PRIMARY NUTRITION-RELATED PROBLEMS OF INFANCY

Iron deficiency and food allergies are two of the most significant nutrition-related problems of infants.

Iron Deficiency   Iron deficiency remains a prevalent nutritional problem in infancy, although it has declined in recent years due in large part to the increasing use of iron-fortified formulas.[53] The use of cow's milk earlier than recommended in infancy can cause iron deficiency due to its poor iron content and the potential to cause gastrointestinal blood loss in susceptible infants.[54] Other factors contributing to iron deficiency in infancy include breastfeeding for more than six months without providing supplemental iron, feeding infant formula not fortified with iron, the infant's rapid rate of growth, low birth weight, and low socioeconomic status.[55] To prevent iron deficiency, the AAP recommends that infants be fed breast milk or iron-fortified formula for the first year of life, with appropriate foods added between the ages of four and six months as shown in Table 12-14.

Food Allergies   Genetics is probably the most significant factor affecting an infant's susceptibility to food allergies.[56] Nevertheless, food allergies are much

---

TABLE

12-14

First Foods for the Infant

Source: Reprinted by permission from *Personal Nutrition,* 2nd ed. by M. A. Boyle and G. Zyla. Copyright © 1992 by West Publishing Company. All rights reserved.

AGE (MONTHS)	ADDITION
4 to 6	Iron-fortified rice cereal, followed by other cereals (for iron; baby can swallow and can digest starch now)[a]
5 to 7	Strained vegetables and/or fruits and their juices,[b] one by one (perhaps vegetables before fruits, so the baby will learn to like their less sweet flavors)
6 to 8	Protein foods (cheese, yogurt, tofu, cooked beans, meat, fish, chicken, egg yolk)
9	Finely chopped meat (the baby can chew now), toast, teething crackers (for emerging teeth)
10 to 12	Whole egg (allergies are less likely now), whole milk

[a]Later other cereals can be introduced, but they should still be iron-fortified varieties.
[b]All baby juices are fortified with vitamin C. Orange juice may cause allergies; apple juice may be a better juice to feed first. Dilute juices with water and offer in a cup to prevent nursing bottle syndrome.

less prevalent in breastfed babies than in formula-fed infants. At-risk infants can be identified from elevated cord blood levels of Immunoglobulin E (IgE) or by a family history. Breast milk is recommended for infants allergic to cow's milk protein and is preferable to soy or goat's milk formulas, since infants are sometimes intolerant of these proteins as well. To reduce the risk of food sensitivity or allergic reactions to other foods, new foods should be introduced singly to facilitate prompt detection of allergies. For example, if a cereal causes irritability due to skin rash, digestive upset, or respiratory discomfort, discontinue its use before going on to the next food. Several days should elapse between the introduction of each new food to allow time for clinical symptoms to appear.

Domestic Maternal and Infant Nutrition Programs

Nutrition plays a vital role in the outcome of pregnancy as well as the growth and development of infants. A stable base of essential programs and services is required to meet maternal and infant health care needs. This section describes the nutrition programs and related services available to meet the demands of the vulnerable lifecycle periods of pregnancy and infancy.

◆ NUTRITION PROGRAMS OF THE U.S. DEPARTMENT OF AGRICULTURE

Several programs of the U.S. Department of Agriculture (USDA) directly or indirectly provide nutrition support during pregnancy and infancy.

Food Stamp Program   The Food Stamp Program (FSP) is designed to improve the diets of people with low incomes by providing coupons to cover part or all of their household's food budget. Chapter 11 provided an overview of this program. As explained previously, program participants can use the food stamp coupons to buy food in any retail store that has been approved by the Food and Nutrition Service to accept and redeem them. For many economically disadvantaged women, the FSP is the major means by which they are able to purchase adequate diets for their families. The Select Panel for the Promotion of Child Health reported that food stamp users purchase more nutritious foods per dollar spent on food than eligible households that do not participate in the program.[57]

WIC Farmers' Market Nutrition Program   The WIC Farmers' Market Nutrition Program (FMNP) was created to provide fresh, nutritious fruits and vegetables to WIC participants, and to expand the awareness and use of farmers' markets by consumers.

Eligible recipients receive FMNP coupons in the range of $10 to $20 per year. A study reported by the Food Research and Action Center showed that WIC women who received FMNP coupons increased both fruit and vegetable consumption by about 5 percent compared to WIC women who did not receive coupons. The FMNP participants also patronized farmers' markets more than nonrecipients, even after they were no longer eligible for WIC.

Food Distribution Program The Food Distribution Program is designed to reduce the level of government-held surplus commodities by distributing them to low-income households to supplement recipients' purchased food. Most states set eligibility criteria at between 130 and 150 percent of the poverty line. In many states, participants in the Aid to Families with Dependent Children (AFDC) and Food Stamp programs are automatically eligible. Most foods distributed prior to 1988 were surplus commodities such as packaged dairy products, flour, rice, honey, and cornmeal. Through the Hunger Prevention Act of 1988 (P.L. 100–435), Congress authorized the purchase of additional commodities to enhance the amount and variety distributed. Additional items have since included canned meat, canned and dried fruit, peanut butter, dried potatoes, citrus juice, and legumes. Commodities are distributed to needy families through local food banks, charitable institutions, and local government agencies. The Food Distribution Program on Indian reservations provides Native Americans living on or near reservations with access to donated foods (see Chapter 11).

Commodity Supplemental Food Program The Commodity Supplemental Food Program (CSFP) is a direct food distribution program providing supplemental foods and nutrition education. The CSFP provides supplemental foods to infants and children and to pregnant, postpartum, and breastfeeding women with low incomes who are vulnerable to malnutrition and live in approved project areas. Recipients may not participate in both WIC and CSFP. The USDA purchases the foods for distribution through state agencies on a monthly basis.

Expanded Food and Nutrition Education Program (EFNEP) The Expanded Food and Nutrition Education Program (EFNEP) is one of two federally funded programs designed specifically for nutrition education. (The other is the Nutrition Education and Training [NET] program, described in Chapter 13.) The EFNEP is directed at low-income families and is administered by the USDA Extension Service. It was authorized in 1968 to provide food and nutrition education to homemakers with young children. The program is implemented by trained nutrition aides from the local community under the supervision of county Cooperative Extension Home Economists. These paraprofessionals work to develop a one-to-one relationship with disadvantaged homemakers enrolled in the program. In recent years, multimedia strategies have been tested to expand the scope of nutrition education for this population.[58]

◆ NUTRITION PROGRAMS OF THE U.S. DEPARTMENT OF HEALTH AND HUMAN SERVICES

The U.S. Department of Health and Human Services (DHHS) also sponsors several programs that are concerned with health and nutrition status during pregnancy and infancy.

Title V Maternal and Child Health Program Enacted in 1935, Title V of the Social Security Act is the only federal program concerned exclusively with the health of mothers, infants, and children. It provides federal support to the states to enhance their ability to "promote, improve, and deliver" maternal, infant, and

[This discussion continues on page 399.]

◆ *The WIC Program*

In 1969, the White House Conference on Food, Nutrition, and Health recommended that special attention be given to the nutritional needs of pregnant and breastfeeding women, infants, and preschool children. As a result, WIC was authorized in 1972 by P.L. 92–433 as an amendment to the Child Nutrition Act of 1966. The legislation states that the WIC program is to ". . . serve as an adjunct to good health care, during critical times of growth and development. . . ." To encourage earlier and more frequent utilization of health services, federal regulations mandate that local agencies may qualify as WIC sponsors only if they can make health care services available to WIC enrollees.[1]

The WIC program is based on two assumptions. One is that inadequate nutritional intakes and health behaviors of low-income women, infants, and children make them vulnerable to adverse health outcomes. The other is that nutrition intervention at critical periods of growth and development will prevent health problems and improve the health status of participants.

WIC is federally funded but administered by the states. Cash grants are made to authorized agencies of each state and to officially recognized Indian tribes or councils, which then provide WIC services through local service sites. Priority for the creation of local programs is given to areas whose populations need benefits most, based on high rates of infant mortality, low birth weight, and low income.

WIC began as a two-year pilot project for each of fiscal years 1973 and 1974 to provide supplemental foods to infants, children up to age five, and pregnant, breastfeeding, and non-breastfeeding postpartum women who qualify financially and are considered by competent professionals to be at nutritional risk because of inadequate nutrition and inadequate income.[2] Competent professionals include physicians, nutritionists, nurses, and other health officials. Financial eligibility is determined by income (between 100 percent and 185 percent of the poverty line or below) or by participation in the AFDC, Food Stamp, or Medicaid programs. Nutritional risks, determined by a health professional, may include one of three types: medically-based risks (anemia, underweight, maternal age, history of high-risk pregnancies); diet-based risks (inadequate dietary pattern); or conditions that make the applicant predisposed to medically based or diet-based risks, such as alcoholism or drug addiction.

The WIC program serves both a remedial and a preventive role. Services provided include the following:

◆ Food packages or vouchers for food packages to provide specific nutrients (protein, calcium, iron, and vitamins A and C) known to be lacking in the diets of the target population. WIC foods include iron-fortified infant formula and infant cereal, iron-fortified breakfast cereal, vitamin C–rich fruit or vegetable juice, eggs, milk, cheese, and peanut butter or dried beans and peas.

Continued

Continued

◆ Nutrition education including individual nutrition counseling and group nutrition classes.

◆ Referral to health care services including immunizations, prenatal care, family planning, or substance-abuse treatment.

The provision of nutritious supplemental foods to needy pregnant women is expected to improve the outcome of pregnancy. For infants and children, the food supplements are intended to reduce the incidence of anemia and to improve physical and mental development. Some states distribute food directly, but most provide vouchers or checks that participants can use at authorized food stores. The food voucher lists the quantities of specific foods, including brand names, that can be purchased with the voucher or check.

The combination of supplementary food, nutrition education, and preventive health care distinguishes WIC from other federal food assistance programs. Some of the potential impacts of program participation are summarized in Figure 12-8. Program benefits include improved dietary quality, more efficient food purchasing, better use of health services, and improved maternal, fetal, and child health and development.[3]

WIC has been described as one of the most efficient programs undertaken by the federal government. Over the years, the program has expanded significantly; the 1.9 million women and children served in 1980 at a cost of $725 million had grown by 1991 to more than 5.2 million women, infants, and children served at a cost of $2.3 billion (the average monthly food package costs $32 per person). The dramatic growth in WIC since 1972 has caused policymakers to focus attention on quantifying the program's benefits.[4] To date, the program's proven benefits include the following:[5]

◆ In 1984, the General Accounting Office reviewed all previous WIC studies and concluded that WIC reduces the incidence of low birth weight by 16 to 20 percent.

◆ The 1986 National WIC Evaluation released by the USDA found that WIC has contributed to a reduction of 20 to 33 percent in fetal mortality and that the head size of infants whose mothers received WIC during pregnancy increased measurably.[6]

◆ In 1990, a USDA study of the health records of more than 100,000 mothers and babies found that the program increased birth weight significantly.

◆ Women who participate in WIC have longer pregnancies leading to fewer premature births. This not only benefits the infants, but it saves millions of dollars in Medicaid bills that would otherwise have been required for neonatal intensive care. It is estimated that every dollar spent on WIC for pregnant women can save as much as $4.21 in Medicaid costs.[7]

Continued

Continued

FIGURE 12-8   **WIC Benefits and Potential Program Impacts**

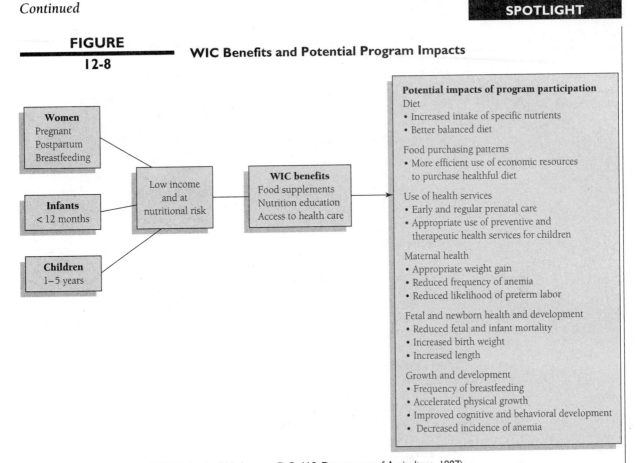

Source: D. Rush, *The National WIC Evaluation* (Washington, D.C.: U.S. Department of Agriculture, 1987).

◆ A Yale University School of Medicine study found a remarkable decrease in the prevalence of anemia among low-income children in New Haven since the early 1970s. The researchers concluded: "The marked improvement can most probably be attributed to the nutritional supplementation with iron-fortified foods provided by the WIC program."[8]

◆ WIC also appears to lead to better mental performance. WIC children whose mothers participated in WIC during pregnancy had better vocabulary and memory test scores than nonparticipants.

Continued

PROGRAM SPOTLIGHT

Continued

EXHIBIT

12-1

Source: Mathematica Policy Research, Inc.

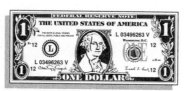

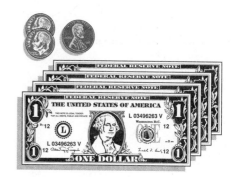

Every $1.00 spent on WIC prenatal care saves up to $4.21 in Medicaid costs.

◆ WIC participation is associated with regular use of health care services; WIC children are more likely than not to receive some form of immunization against infectious diseases.

Unlike most of the other food assistance programs, WIC is not an entitlement program and therefore can serve only as many people as its annual appropriation from Congress permits. Under federal regulations, once a local agency has reached its maximum caseload, vacancies must be filled in the following order of priority to assure that program resources are allocated to those at greatest nutritional risk:

1. Pregnant women, breastfeeding women, and infants determined to be at nutritional risk by a blood test, anthropometric measures, or other documentation of a nutrition-related medical condition.

2. Infants, up to six months of age, whose mothers were at nutritional risk during pregnancy.

3. Children at nutritional risk as determined by a blood test, anthropometric measures, or documentation of a nutrition-related medical condition.

4. Pregnant or breastfeeding women and infants at nutritional risk because of an inadequate dietary pattern.

5. Children at nutritional risk because of an inadequate dietary pattern.

6. Non-breastfeeding, postpartum women at nutritional risk.

Due to the caps placed on allocated federal funds, WIC currently reaches about 60 percent of eligible persons. Barriers to participation in WIC include limited government funding, lack of transportation, insufficient time or money to travel to the clinic, insufficient outreach to potential WIC recipients, the absence or expense of child care, inconvenient clinic hours, and understaffing of WIC facilities.

Continued

Continued

Overall, research evaluating WIC's effectiveness finds positive outcomes for WIC participants compared to nonparticipants.[9] The following measures would help lower the barriers to program participation and improve the nutrition status and health care of women, infants, and children even further:

◆ Increase congressional funding for the program to enable more eligible women, infants, and children to receive WIC benefits.

◆ Improve the coordination between WIC and programs providing or financing maternal and child health care services.

◆ Implement outreach activities to increase access to WIC program benefits by all who are eligible.

1. Select Panel for the Promotion of Child Health, WIC: The Special Supplemental Food Program for Women, Infants, and Children, in *Better Health for Our Children: A National Strategy*, 2 vols. (Washington, D.C.: U.S. Department of Health and Human Services, 1981), 2:57–68.
2. J. E. Austin and C. Hitt, *Nutrition Intervention in the United States: Cases and Concepts* (Cambridge, Mass.: Ballinger, 1979), p. 37.
3. D. Rush and coauthors, The national WIC evaluation: Evaluation of the Special Supplemental Food Program for Women, Infants, and Children, *American Journal of Clinical Nutrition* 48 (1988): 389–93.
4. B. Devaney, The Special Supplemental Food Program for Women, Infants, and Children (WIC), *Contemporary Nutrition* 16 (1991).
5. J. L. Brown, S. N. Gershoff, and J. T. Cook, The politics of hunger: When science and ideology clash, *International Journal of Health Services* 22 (1992): 221–37.
6. Rush, The national WIC evaluation, p. 412.
7. Mathematica Policy Research, *The Savings in Medicaid Costs for Newborns and Their Mothers from Prenatal Participation in the WIC Program,* Report prepared for the U.S. Department of Agriculture, Food and Nutrition Service, Office of Analysis and Evaluation, Washington, D.C., 1990.
8. WIC reform means more mothers and children served, *Nutrition Forum Newsletter* (February 1988): 9–11.
9. Devaney, The Special Supplemental Food Program, and P. A. Buescher and coauthors, Prenatal WIC participation can reduce low birth weight and newborn medical costs: A cost-benefit analysis of WIC participation in North Carolina, *Journal of the American Dietetic Association* 93 (1993): 163–66.

child health (MCH) care and programs for children with special health care needs (CSHCN), especially in rural areas and regions experiencing severe economic stress. The aim of Congress in passing this legislation was to improve the health of mothers, infants, and children in areas where the need was greatest.

The states are allocated Title V MCH funds to be used for (1) services and programs to reduce infant mortality and improve child and maternal health; and (2) services, programs, and facilities to locate, diagnose, and treat children who have special health care needs (e.g., chronic medical conditions) or are at risk of

The state programs for Children with Special Health Care Needs (CSHCN) were formerly known as Crippled Children's Services (CC).

physical or developmental disabilities.[59] The Title V MCH program provides for nutrition assessment, dietary counseling, nutrition education, and referral to food assistance programs for infants, preschool and school-aged children, children with special health care needs, adolescents, and women of childbearing age. It also supports training in nutrition for health and nutrition professionals who are involved in developing nutrition services.[60]

On several occasions, significant amendments have been added to the original law:

◆ **1963.** A series of amendments authorized grants to state and local health departments for Maternal and Infant Care (MIC) projects aimed mainly at reducing mental retardation and infant mortality through improved prenatal, perinatal, and postpartum care.

◆ **1965.** Amendments authorized special project grants to provide comprehensive health services to children and youth through state and local health agencies and other public or nonprofit organizations.

◆ **1967.** An amendment provided for special grants for dental services for children. Other amendments linked CSHCN programs and Medicaid in the provision of Early Periodic Screening, Diagnosis, and Treatment (EPSDT), described below.

The Title V MCH program is administered federally by the Bureau of Maternal and Child Health and Resources Development in the Health Resources and Services Administration of the Public Health Service (refer to the organizational chart of the DHHS in Figure 1-2). Administration of the MCH program is the responsibility of the MCH unit within each state's health agency. Most of the CSHCN programs are also administered through state health agencies; some, however, are delivered through other state agencies, such as welfare departments, social service agencies, or state universities. Under the law, each state is required to operate a "program of projects" in each of five areas: (1) maternity and infant care, (2) intensive infant care, (3) family planning, (4) health care for children and youth, and (5) dental care for children.[61]

States have varying degrees of control over local use of Title V funds. Most state MCH funds are used to support well-child checkups, immunization programs, vision and hearing screenings, and school health services, as well as other programs. CSHCN program funds are used to provide direct services to children with special health care needs through local clinics and/or fee-for-service arrangements with physicians in private practice. Regardless of the method of delivering CSHCN programs, a multidisciplinary approach to providing health care is used by nearly all states.[62]

The Select Panel for the Promotion of Child Health reported that Title V program efforts have resulted in significant improvements in maternal and child health. The program is believed to have contributed to the decline in infant and maternal mortality, the reduction of disability in handicapped children, and a general improvement in the health status of children.[63]

Medicaid and EPSDT Congress created the Medicaid program in 1965 to ensure financial access to health care for the economically disadvantaged. It was enacted through Title XIX of the Social Security Act. The Medicaid program is an entitlement program built upon the welfare model. It is constructed as a state-administered medical assistance program that reimburses providers for specific services delivered to eligible recipients. Under amendments enacted in 1967, the states are required to provide EPSDT as a mandatory Medicaid service. As outlined by Congress, the purpose of EPSDT is to improve the health status of children from low-income families by providing health services not typically found under the current Medicaid program. EPSDT requires an assessment of the nutrition status of eligible children and their referral for treatment.[64] Whereas Medicaid is mainly a provider payment program for medical services, EPSDT regulations stipulate that states must develop protocols for identifying eligible children, informing them of the EPSDT program, and ensuring that referral, preventive, and treatment services are made available to participants.

The federal administration of Medicaid is the responsibility of the Health Care Financing Administration (HCFA) within the DHHS. The HCFA's Office of Child Health administers EPSDT at the federal level.

Medicaid and EPSDT have been credited with increasing the access of low-income women, infants, and children to health care services. EPSDT, by virtue of its aggressive preventive strategy, has been effective in improving child health. However, strict eligibility requirements and federal statutory policies have to some extent limited the ability of these programs to reach their full potential.[65]

Community Health Centers   The Community Health Centers program was initiated by the Office of Economic Opportunity in 1966 and authorized by the Public Health Service Act. It is designed to provide health services and related training in medically underserviced areas. The primary program focus is on comprehensive primary care services through community health centers, including migrant health centers, Appalachian Health Demonstration projects, the Rural Health Initiative project, and the Urban Health Initiative project.[66] Preventive services are also offered through Community Health Centers, including well-child care, nutrition assessment, and health education. The program is administered federally by the Bureau of Community Health Services within the Health Resources and Services Administration of the Public Health Service.[67]

Looking Ahead: Improving the Health of Mothers and Infants

Many of the existing health care programs do not have nutrition counseling or education available within their own sites. Often, these programs refer their clients to the WIC program for nutrition services. The heavy caseloads in many WIC programs, however, limit the amount of personalized nutrition counseling they can offer. Clearly, more must be done to assure that quality nutrition counseling is available and accessible for pregnant women and their infants.

A few states have been successful in providing reimbursable nutrition counseling services to maternal and child health programs. The South Carolina High

Risk Channeling Project provides nutrition services, reimbursable by Medicaid, to all participants. The Kentucky Department for Health Services uses some of its MCH Block Grant funds to hire public health nutritionists specifically to provide nutrition counseling for high-risk clients in the local maternal and child health care programs.[68]

Some voluntary health organizations such as local chapters of the La Leche League International and the March of Dimes Birth Defects Foundation offer classes that are helpful to particular groups or can provide appropriate nutrition education materials helpful to the community nutritionist working with maternal-child populations.

The increasing numbers of working women, including those planning families or with young infants, along with the growth in worksite health promotion programs have implications for community nutritionists in providing nutrition education and related services to this population. Some worksites have included components designed for pregnant and lactating women (e.g., breastfeeding promotion and prenatal education programs) in their overall health promotion programs.[69]

Where adolescents are concerned, a variety of comprehensive community programs exist to assist the pregnant teen with her educational, social, medical, and nutritional needs. Most of these programs include three common components: (1) early and consistent prenatal care, (2) continuing education on a classroom basis, and (3) counseling on an individual or group basis.[70] The importance of these programs in improving maternal and child health is well recognized. Since teen pregnancy is usually unplanned, efforts should be made to improve the nutrition and health status of all adolescents through nutrition education and counseling in the classroom as well as in physicians' offices.[71]

To assure that all pregnant women have access to satisfactory prenatal services in the future, efforts are needed to convince policymakers of the importance of the following recommendations:[72]

◆ Food supplementation and nutrition education should be available to all pregnant women with low incomes.

◆ Additional federal funds should be appropriated to WIC to make it available to all pregnant low-income women.

◆ Nutrition counseling and education should be provided to all pregnant women whose care is financed by Medicaid.

◆ State Medicaid programs should be required to include nutrition counseling and education as reimbursable services.

◆ Federal and state funds should be provided to health department clinics and community health centers to allow for employment of public health nutritionists to offer nutrition counseling to all pregnant women who attend these facilities.

◆ Health insurance policies should include prenatal nutrition counseling as a reimbursable service for all pregnant women living in the United States.

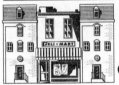

COMMUNITY LEARNING ACTIVITY

As mentioned in the chapter, WIC is not an entitlement program. Due to the caps placed on allocated federal funds, WIC currently reaches about 60 percent of eligible persons. We ask that you describe the benefits of participation in the WIC program by searching the relevant nutrition literature. Next, draft a letter to your legislator, requesting increased funding for WIC to make it a fully funded program.

◆ PROFESSIONAL FOCUS

Being an Effective Speaker

Public speaking ranks Number One on most people's list of most-dreaded activities. It causes churning stomachs, sweaty palms, dry mouths, and outright fear among many competent professional women and men. Many people would sooner have a root canal than give a 30-minute speech at a convention! If you feel this way about public speaking, take heart. You are not alone. More importantly, you *can* master the art of public speaking.

Tips for making an effective presentation are outlined below. These basic principles apply to many different situations, from a formal presentation at a scientific meeting to an informal update for your colleagues at a staff meeting. They also apply to many teaching situations.

◆ THINGS TO DO BEFORE YOUR PRESENTATION

Public speaking is a skill just like any other skill. Even so, you may find that you expect more of yourself when it comes to public speaking than you would in other settings. If you are learning to downhill ski, you don't expect to be skiing the double-black diamond trails and moguls at the end of your first season. If you are learning to speak Spanish, you don't expect to converse fluently after only a few lessons. So, why should you expect to be a first-rate public speaker after a handful of presentations? In the same way that you acquire any skill, public speaking requires practice, evaluation, and more practice and evaluation. It is an ongoing process. Even when you become skilled at public speaking, there will be room for improvement. In the beginning, try to remove a little pressure by remembering that you are working toward acquiring a skill that can only be acquired by doing. You *will* improve over time. To accelerate your competency curve, follow these rules:

◆ Organize your presentation around this basic principle of effective speaking: First, tell your audience what you are going to tell them; then, tell them what you want to tell them; and finally, tell them what you told them! This strategy lets your audience know precisely what your presentation will cover and helps them remember the main points.

◆ Prepare your visual aids so that they present your ideas effectively. Here are few suggestions on preparing slides from the Federation of American Societies for Experimental Biology (FASEB):[1]

1. **Clear purpose.** An effective slide should have a main point or central theme.

2. **Readily understood.** The slide's main point should be readily understood by the audience. If it is not, the audience will be trying to figure out what the slide has to say and will not be listening to the speaker.

3. **Simple format.** The slide should be simple and uncluttered. Avoid slides that present large amounts of data such as columns of numbers.

4. **Free of nonessential information.** Information not directly related to the slide's main point should be omitted.

5. **Digestible.** The audience is capable of assimilating only so much information from a slide. It is better to have only a small amount of information (even just one sentence) than to cram numerous points onto a single slide.

Continued

6. **Graphic format.** Some information is best presented graphically. In addition, the use of graphs and charts provides a visual change from slides containing only text.[2]

7. **Visible.** Because most meeting rooms were not designed for projection, some people sitting in the back of the room may not be able to view the slides over the heads of those in front. For this reason, horizontal slides are more appropriate than vertical slides.

8. **Legible.** Studies of projected image size and legibility show that the best slide template is about 42 spaces wide (9 cm) by 14 single space lines (6 cm). The best type size for slides is at least 5 millimeters or 14 points.

9. **Thumbspot slides.** Hold the slide as it reads correctly to you. Then, write a sequence or other identifying number on the lower left corner of the mount. This spot tells the projectionist the correct corner to grasp when placing the slide in a carousel tray.

10. **Integrated with verbal text.** Slides should support and reinforce the verbal text. Conversely, the verbal text should lay a proper foundation for the slide.

Similar principles apply to preparing overheads. Keep the information simple and limit the amount of information provided. To improve legibility, type the master copy in large type. Like slides, overheads should be integrated with your text.

Rehearse your presentation several times—you would do no less for a piano recital! If the presentation is formal, use a table or desk as a podium. Time the presentation from start to finish, including your opening and closing remarks, and adjust your presentation as needed. A general rule of thumb is that you should plan to spend about one minute per slide or overhead. If the presentation is informal, write down the key points you want to make and practice saying them. Rehearsing your presentation ensures that you know your material and how you want to present it.

Use mental imaging to boost your self-confidence. What is mental imaging? Mental imaging is a technique used by many successful business people, politicians, actors, and athletes to develop and strengthen a positive mental picture of their performance. It is a way to relieve stress and reduce anxiety about speaking in public. It sounds hokey—but it works.

Picture Nadia Comaneci at the height of her athletic career as a gymnast. She is preparing to do her routine on the uneven bars in an Olympic competition watched by millions of spectators worldwide. She stands ready to begin her mount. What is going through her head during those few seconds before she launches into her routine? Is she thinking, "Oh, no, there's one spot where I always mess up. I'll never do it right. My coach, family, and country will be humiliated." It isn't remotely possible that Nadia Comaneci's thought processes took this tack. You can be sure that when Nadia Comaneci stood poised to begin her routine in the Olympic competition, she pictured every move from the beginning to the dismount, all done flawlessly. It is an image she worked to cultivate both mentally and physically. The result was a perfect performance.

You can use mental imaging to boost your performance and quell those butterflies in your stomach. On several occasions before your presentation, walk yourself mentally through the speech from beginning to end. Picture being introduced, standing up and

Continued

walking to the podium, adjusting the microphone, smiling, giving your opening remarks, asking for the first slide, and so on, right down to the very end of your presentation. Picture giving your presentation and handling questions at the end with complete confidence. The key to using mental imaging successfully is to use it *whenever* a negative thought about your presentation intrudes. If a mental picture of you passing out behind the podium surfaces suddenly, use mental imaging to squash the picture. Instead, force yourself to picture a confident, in-control YOU. Allow no negative thoughts about your presentation to take form. Encourage only positive thoughts. Mental imaging takes a little practice, but it is worth the effort. You will find that because you *think* you are more confident, you *are* more confident.

◆ THINGS TO DO DURING YOUR PRESENTATION

Use the following techniques to ensure that you give a first-rate presentation:

◆ **Smile.** A smile will go a long way toward helping you relax and making you appear user-friendly to your audience. This is especially important when dealing with the general public.

◆ **Use eye contact.** Regardless of the size of the audience, select one person with whom to establish eye contact. Let your eyes dwell on this one individual a few moments and then move on to another person. This gives the appearance of a one-on-one interactive discussion, which engages the audience in your presentation and helps ensure that they are listening to you.

◆ **Use gestures.** Gestures give energy to your presentation and provide additional emphasis for key points. Practice making them during your rehearsals. Exercise a little common sense here—wild arm movements and pirouettes will detract from your presentation.

◆ **Control the pace.** While a steady pace will ensure that you complete your speech on time, it may make your audience sleepy. Vary the pace to keep the audience interested in what you are saying.

◆ **Use pauses.** Pauses, like gestures, can be used for emphasis. A well-timed pause keeps your audience engaged and allows them a moment to process what you've just said.

◆ **Vary the volume and pitch.** Changing the volume and pitch of your voice has more auditory appeal for the audience than listening to a monotone voice.

Finally, two other points deserve mention. First, remember that the purpose of your presentation is to share information with your audience. The people in your audience will generally be much less critical of your performance than you are. Being an effective speaker means that your audience is listening to your messages and absorbing the material you present. Second, despite all the tips and techniques listed here, you will want to develop your own style. Learn to be yourself *and* a relaxed, confident speaker.

1. The suggestions for preparing good slides were taken from the FASEB Call for Papers for the 1993 Annual Meeting, pp. 30–31.
2. J. W. King and J. Rupnow, A primer on using visuals in technical presentations, *Food Technology* 46 (1992): 157–70.

NOTES

1. E. Hackman and coauthors, Maternal birthweight and subsequent pregnancy outcome, *Journal of the American Medical Association* 250 (1983): 2016–19.

2. N. M. Lien, K. K. Meyer, and M. Winick, Early malnutrition and "late" adoption: A study of the effects of the development of Korean orphans adopted into American families, *American Journal of Clinical Nutrition* 30 (1977): 1734–39.

3. U.S. Department of Health and Human Services, Public Health Service, *Healthy People 2000: National Health Promotion and Disease Prevention Objectives* (Washington, D.C.: U.S. Department of Health and Human Services, DHHS Pub. No. 91–50212, 1990), pp. 366–90.

4. U.S. Department of Health and Human Services, *Healthy People 2000.*

5. R. W. Rochat and coauthors, Maternal mortality in the United States: Report from the maternal mortality collaborative, *Obstetrics and Gynecology* 72 (1988): 91–97.

6. U.S. Department of Health and Human Services, Public Health Service, *The Surgeon General's Report on Nutrition and Health* (Washington, D.C.: U.S. Government Printing Office, DHHS Pub. No. 88–50210, 1988), pp. 540–93.

7. Food and Nutrition Board, Institute of Medicine, National Academy of Sciences, *Nutrition During Pregnancy* (Washington, D.C.: National Academy Press, 1990); Food and Nutrition Board, Institute of Medicine, National Academy of Sciences, *Nutrition During Lactation* (Washington, D.C.: National Academy Press, 1991).

8. U.S. Department of Health and Human Services, *Healthy People 2000,* p. 366.

9. Food and Nutrition Board, National Research Council, National Academy of Sciences, *Recommended Dietary Allowances,* 10th ed. (Washington, D.C.: National Academy Press, 1989).

10. Food and Nutrition Board, *Nutrition During Pregnancy,* p. 17.

11. Ibid.

12. Nutrition during pregnancy and lactation, *Dairy Council Digest* 62 (1991): 13–18.

13. Folate supplements prevent recurrence of neural tube defects, *Nutrition Reviews* 50 (1992): 22–26.

14. B. Worthington-Roberts and R. M. Pitkin, Women's nutrition for optimal reproductive health, in *Call to Action: Better Nutrition for Mothers, Children, and Families,* ed. C. O. Sharbaugh (Washington, D.C.:

National Center for Education in Maternal and Child Health, 1991), p. 124.

15. Food and Nutrition Board, *Nutrition During Pregnancy;* C. W. Suitor and J. D. Gardner, Supplement use among a culturally diverse group of low-income pregnant women, *Journal of the American Dietetic Association* 90 (1990): 268.

16. Food and Nutrition Board, *Nutrition During Pregnancy,* 1990.

17. Ibid.

18. B. Worthington-Roberts and S. R. Williams, *Nutrition in Pregnancy and Lactation,* 4th ed. (St. Louis: Times Mirror/Mosby, 1989), pp. 118–20.

19. Ibid., p. 119.

20. B. Worthington-Roberts, Nutritional support of successful reproduction: An update, *Journal of Nutrition Education* 19 (1987): 1–10.

21. Food and Nutrition Board, *Nutrition During Pregnancy,* pp. 397–99.

22. U.S. Department of Health and Human Services, *Healthy People 2000.*

23. M. G. Bulterys, S. Greenland, and J. F. Kraus, Chronic fetal hypoxia and sudden infant death syndrome: Interaction between maternal smoking and low hematocrit during pregnancy, *Pediatrics* 86 (1990): 535–40.

24. Worthington-Roberts and Pitkin, Women's nutrition for optimal reproductive health, pp. 113–36.

25. Ibid., p. 129.

26. U.S. Department of Health and Human Services, *Surgeon General's Report.*

27. J. C. King and J. Weininger, Pregnancy and lactation, in *Present Knowledge in Nutrition,* 6th ed., ed. M. L. Brown (Washington, D.C.: International Life Sciences Institute—Nutrition Foundation, 1990), pp. 314–19.

28. J. M. Belizan and coauthors, Calcium supplementation to prevent hypertensive disorders of pregnancy, *New England Journal of Medicine* 325 (1991): 1399–1405.

29. U.S. Department of Health and Human Services, *Surgeon General's Report,* pp. 56–57.

30. L. Heggen and coauthors, Gestational diabetes, *Diabetes Forecast* (June 1987): 28–31.

31. Position of the American Dietetic Association: Nutrition management of adolescent pregnancy, *Journal of the American Dietetic Association* 89 (1989): 104–9.

32. M. Story and I. Alton, Nutrition and the pregnant adolescent, *Contemporary Nutrition* 17 (1992): 1–2.

33. E. Whitney and S. Rolfes, *Understanding Nutrition,* 6th ed. (St. Paul, Minn.: West Publishing, 1993), p. 491.

34. M. L. Hediger and coauthors, Rate and amount of weight gain during adolescent pregnancy: Associations with maternal weight-for-height and birth weight, *American Journal of Clinical Nutrition* 52 (1990): 793–99.

35. Position of the American Dietetic Association: Nutrition management of adolescent pregnancy, p. 104.

36. Worthington-Roberts and Pitkin, Women's nutrition, pp. 132–33.

37. Position of the American Dietetic Association: Nutrition management of adolescent pregnancy, pp. 106–7.

38. B. Worthington-Roberts and L. Klerman, Maternal nutrition, in *New Perspectives in Prenatal Care,* ed. I. R. Merkatz, J. E. Thompson, and R. Goldenberg (New York: Elsevier Science Publishing Co., 1990).

39. Ibid.

40. Food and Nutrition Board, *Nutrition During Pregnancy.*

41. E. Whitney, C. Cataldo, and S. Rolfes, *Understanding Normal and Clinical Nutrition,* 3rd ed. (St. Paul, Minn.: West Publishing, 1991), pp. 614–16.

42. The description of head circumference measurement was taken from Whitney, Cataldo, and Rolfes, *Understanding Normal and Clinical Nutrition,* p. 616.

43. J. E. Brown, Nutrition services for pregnant women, infants, children, and adolescents, *Clinical Nutrition* 3 (1984): 100–108.

44. Food and Nutrition Board, *Nutrition During Lactation.*

45. Ibid.

46. U.S. Department of Health and Human Services, *Healthy People 2000,* pp. 379–80.

47. La Leche League International, Breastfeeding Peer Counselor Program, personal communication, November 1993.

48. Food and Nutrition Services, *Promoting Breastfeeding in WIC: A Compendium of Practical Approaches* (Arlington, Va.: U.S. Department of Agriculture, 1988), pp. 1–6.

49. B. J. Solem, K. F. Norr, and A. M. Gallo, Infant feeding practices of low-income mothers, *Journal of Pediatric Health Care* 6 (1992): 54–59.

50. The discussion of focus group findings was taken from C. Bryant and D. Bailey, The use of focus group research in program development. Unpublished manuscript, Lexington, Ky, 1989.

51. American Academy of Pediatrics, Committee on Nutrition, The use of whole cow's milk in infancy, *Pediatrics* 89 (1992): 1105.

52. American Academy of Pediatrics, Committee on Nutrition, The use of whole cow's milk in infancy, *Pediatrics* 72 (1983): 253–55.

53. Whitney and Rolfes, *Understanding Nutrition,* p. 502.

54. E. E. Ziegler, S. J. Fomon, and S. E. Nelson, Cow milk feeding in infancy: Further observations on blood loss from the gastrointestinal tract, *Journal of Pediatrics* 116 (1990): 11.

55. M. Irigoyen and coauthors, Randomized placebo-controlled trial of iron supplementation in infants with low hemoglobin levels fed iron-fortified formulas, *Pediatrics* 88 (1991): 320.

56. The discussion of food allergies was adapted from Infant nutrition in the 1990s, *Dairy Council Digest* 63 (1992): 31–36.

57. Select Panel for the Promotion of Child Health, *Better Health for Our Children: A National Strategy,* 2 vols. (Washington, D.C.: U.S. Department of Health and Human Services, 1981), 1:168.

58. Ibid., 1:156.

59. Ibid., 2:18, and C. Garza and C. Cowell, Infant nutrition, in *Call to Action: Better Nutrition for Mothers, Children, and Families,* ed. C. Sharbaugh (Washington, D.C.: National Center for Education in Maternal and Child Health, 1991), pp. 135–150.

60. U.S. Department of Health and Human Services, *Surgeon General's Report,* p. 544.

61. Select Panel for the Promotion of Child Health, *Better Health,* 2:17–22.

62. Ibid., 2:20.

63. Ibid., 2:21.

64. U.S. Department of Health and Human Services, *Surgeon General's Report,* p. 544.

65. Select Panel for the Promotion of Child Health, *Better Health,* 2:44.

66. Ibid., 1:165.

67. Ibid., 2:101.

68. R. E. Brennan and M. N. Traylor, Components of nutrition services, in *Call to Action: Better Nutrition for Mothers, Children, and Families,* ed. C. Sharbaugh (Washington, D.C.: National Center for Education in Maternal and Child Health, 1991), pp. 243–55.

69. B. Barber-Madden and coauthors, Nutrition for pregnant and lactating women: Implication for worksite health promotion, *Journal of Nutrition Education* 18 (1986): S72–S75.

70. Worthington-Roberts and Williams, *Nutrition in Pregnancy and Lactation,* pp. 239–40.

71. Story and Alton, Nutrition and the pregnant adolescent.

72. The list of recommendations was adapted from Worthington-Roberts and Pitkin, Women's nutrition, p. 133.

Children and Adolescents: Nutrition Assessment, Services, and Programs

C hildren are one-third of our population and all of our future.
—Select Panel for the Promotion of Child Health, 1981

Introduction

The health profile of children and adolescents in the United States has changed dramatically over the past century. Widespread immunization, improved sanitation, public education on nutrition and health, and the discovery of antibiotics have dramatically reduced the rates of child morbidity and mortality due to infectious diseases. Unfortunately, the status of this group today is far from satisfactory, and new perils have arisen in the past few decades: motor vehicle accidents; violence due to suicide, homicide, and abuse; sexually transmitted diseases; substance abuse; and exposure to environmental pollutants.[1] Despite advances in clinical and preventive medicine, children and adolescents in the United States have significant health and nutritional concerns that deserve attention; and there is a sense that policymakers and health practitioners are still falling short of doing what most people believe is necessary to promote the health of all children in the United States.

This chapter approaches child and adolescent health from two perspectives. First, because good nutrition is important to good health, this chapter reviews the nutrient requirements of children and adolescents, their current nutrition-related problems, and basic nutrition screening and assessment methods used with child and adolescent populations. Second, it examines the nutrition programs that target children and teenagers. These programs have the common objective of improving child and adolescent nutrition and, ultimately, enhancing health.

For our purposes, children are generally categorized as ages 1 to 12 years and adolescents as ages 13 to 19 years. Other age categories appear in this chapter, however, because the literature is not entirely consistent on the ages that constitute childhood and adolescence.

National Nutrition Objectives

More than 20 years ago, delegates to the 1970 White House Conference on Children outlined a multidisciplinary strategy for addressing the health, social, physical, educational, and environmental needs of children. Concerned about the widespread neglect of children and the lack of a comprehensive system for delivering health and other services, the delegates called for "a reordering of priorities at all levels of American society so that children and families come first."[2] In the nutrition arena, the delegates recommended that existing food programs be expanded and that all children receive quality nutrition education in school. A separate White House Conference on Youth held in 1971 likewise called for improved nutrition education and services for all young people in need.[3]

Child advocates hoped that the White House Conferences would bring a renewed commitment to improving the health and nutrition status of children (among other objectives). While the conferences may not have fulfilled their ambitious agendas entirely, they did set the stage for major policy developments. Recall from Chapter 1 that the U.S. Department of Health and Human Services (DHHS) began an intensive effort to develop and establish a national public health agenda in the 1970s. In 1979, the Surgeon General issued the first federal report, *Healthy People: The Surgeon General's Report on Health Promotion and Disease Prevention,* which called for increased efforts to reduce death and disabilities from preventable diseases in the general population. The report identified five broad health goals, two of which related to children and adolescents, and 15 broad areas to be given priority attention. Listed for priority were areas where health promotion and disease prevention efforts might be expected to have a positive effect. Nutrition objectives for the year 1990 that focused on children and adolescents, together with their final attainment status, are shown in Table 13-1.[4] Note that most objectives were unmet.

The DHHS also outlined specific nutrition objectives for children and adolescents in its publication *Healthy People 2000: National Health Promotion and Disease Prevention Objectives,* as shown in Table 13-2.[5] Growth retardation, iron-deficiency anemia, dental caries, and obesity are among the priority nutrition concerns. Physical activity and fitness feature prominently in the age-related objectives. Some of the nutrition objectives developed for the general population, especially those related to overweight, dietary fat and fiber intakes, and physical activity, are considered appropriate for children and adolescents as well as adults.

Children

Childhood is a critical time in human development. Children typically grow taller by 2 to 3 inches and heavier by 5 or more pounds each year between the age of one and adolescence.[6] They master fine motor skills (including those related to eating and drinking), become increasingly independent, and learn to express themselves appropriately. Nutrition plays a critical role in the development and growth of children. In this section, we describe the nutrient requirements and primary nutritional problems of U.S. children and the key nutrition assessment methods for this population.

◆ NUTRIENT NEEDS

During the preschool period, children's appetites diminish and their rate of growth slows. The energy requirements of children are determined by their indi-

TABLE

13-1

National Nutrition Objectives for 1990 and Their Final Attainment Status

Source: U.S. Department of Health and Human Services, *Health United States 1991 and Prevention Profile* (Washington, D.C.: U.S. Department of Health and Human Services, 1992), pp. 78–80, 93–98.

1990 GOAL	ATTAINMENT STATUS
Improved Nutrition	
◆ By 1990, growth retardation of infants and children caused by inadequate diets should have been eliminated in the United States as a public health problem.	In 1972–1973, 10 to 15% of infants and children in selected low-income groups were estimated to suffer diet-related growth retardation; in 1983, estimates ranged from 11 to 24%. This objective was not met.*
◆ By 1990, the mean serum cholesterol level in children 1–14 years of age should be at or below 150 mg/dL.	In 1971–1974, for children aged 1 to 17 years, the mean serum cholesterol level was 176 mg/dL. The status of this objective is uncertain due to insufficient data and concerns that the goal is inappropriate for children under 2 years.*
Improved Services and Protection	
By 1990, all states should include nutrition education as part of required comprehensive school health education at elementary and secondary levels.	In 1979, only 10 states mandated nutrition as a core content area in school health education. In 1989, 19 states had mandated nutrition as a core content area in school health education. This objective was not met.
Improved Dental Health	
◆ By 1990, the proportion of 9-year-old children who have experienced dental caries in their permanent teeth should decrease to 60%. (In 1971–74, 71% of 9-year-old children had dental caries.)	In 1979, 49.4% of children 9 years of age had dental caries. In 1986–1987, 34.5% of 9-year-old children had dental caries. This objective was met.
◆ By 1990, at least 50% of schoolchildren living in fluoride-deficient areas that do not have community water systems should be served by an optimally fluoridated school water supply.	Over the past several years, the number of schools with fluoridated water systems has declined, mainly due to their incorporation into public water systems.

*M. Nestle, Promoting health and preventing disease: National nutrition objectives for 1990 and 2000, *Journal of Food Technology* (February 1988): 105.

vidual basal metabolic rates, activity patterns, and rates of growth. Toddlers (ages 1 to 3 years) need about 1300 kcal/day or 102 kcal/kg. By the age of 10 years, children need about 2000 kcal/day or 70 kcal/kg. Although children's total energy needs increase slightly as they grow older, their energy needs per kilogram of body weight actually decrease. (From birth through 10 years, no distinction in energy requirements is made between the sexes.) Children generally become leaner between the ages of 6 months and 6 years; after that time, fat thickness gradually increases in both males and females until puberty is reached. Females have a greater body fat content than males at all stages of development.[7]

Between the ages of 1 and 11 years, children's requirements for protein, vitamins, and minerals generally increase. (Nutrient and energy intake recommendations for children are given in the RDA table on the inside front cover.) Two

Nutrition

◆ Reduce growth retardation among low-income children aged 5 and younger to less than 10%.

◆ Reduce iron deficiency to less than 3% among children aged 1 through 4.

◆ Reduce dietary fat intake to an average of 30% of calories or less and average saturated fat intake to less than 10% of calories among people aged 2 and older.

◆ Reduce overweight to a prevalence of no more than 15% among adolescents aged 12 through 19.

◆ Increase to at least 50% the proportion of overweight people aged 12 and older who have adopted sound dietary practices combined with regular physical activity to attain an appropriate body weight.

◆ Increase calcium intake so at least 50% of youth aged 12 through 24 consume 3 or more servings daily of foods rich in calcium.

◆ Increase to at least 90% the proportion of school lunch and breakfast services and child care food services with menus that are consistent with the nutrition principles in the *Dietary Guidelines for Americans*.

◆ Increase to at least 75% the proportion of the nation's schools that provide nutrition education from preschool through 12th grade, preferably as part of quality school health education.

Oral Health

Reduce dental caries so that the proportion of children with one or more caries (in permanent or primary teeth) is no more than 35% among children aged 6 through 8 and no more than 60% among adolescents aged 15.

Fitness and Physical Activity

◆ Increase to at least 30% the proportion of people aged 6 and older who engage regularly, preferably daily, in light to moderate physical activity for at least 30 minutes per day.

◆ Increase to at least 50% the proportion of children and adolescents in 1st through 12th grade who participate in daily school physical education.

TABLE

13-2

Healthy People 2000 **Nutrition Objectives for Children and Adolescents**
Source: U.S. Department of Health and Human Services, Public Health Service, *Healthy People 2000: National Health Promotion and Disease Prevention Objectives* (Washington, D.C.: 1990), pp. 564–69.

nutrients—calcium and iron—deserve further comment. The allowance of 800 milligrams of calcium per day for children aged 1 to 10 years is somewhat arbitrary, as precise data on the calcium requirements of children are lacking.[8] The lack of information about children's calcium requirement is cause for concern, because children (and adolescents) whose calcium intake is not sufficient to support optimum bone mineralization are at risk of developing osteoporosis later in life.[9] Because iron is needed for growth and development, children's iron requirements are slightly higher than those of adult men.[10]

◆ PRIMARY NUTRITION-RELATED PROBLEMS

Although most children in the United States are well nourished, malnutrition does occur in this population. Malnutrition can take one of two forms: primary malnutrition, which is due to a lack, excess, or imbalance of a nutrient or nutrients in the diet; and secondary malnutrition, which occurs as a result of a disease or illness that affects dietary intake, nutrient needs, or metabolism and hence affects nutrition status.

Undernutrition is a problem for some children in the United States, especially those from low-income and migrant families or certain ethnic and racial minority groups (e.g., blacks, Asians).[11] Children in foster care, many of whom live in poverty, and homeless children are also at risk for undernutrition.[12] More than 20 percent of U.S. children are considered poor.[13]

The most common nutrition-related problems occurring among U.S. children include obesity, iron-deficiency anemia, dental caries, and high blood cholesterol levels:

◆ **Obesity.** Overnutrition is one of the most widespread nutrition disorders among children in the United States. Prevalence estimates for childhood obesity range from 10 to 30 percent, depending upon how obesity is defined.[14] Recent data from the National Health and Nutrition Examination Survey (NHANES) indicate that the prevalence of obesity among 6- to 11-year-old U.S. children increased 54 percent in the past 15 to 20 years.[15] Data from the Hispanic HANES indicate that between 20 and 25 percent of Mexican-American girls and boys aged two to five years are moderately overweight or obese.[16] Childhood obesity is associated with hyperinsulinemia, hypertriglyceridemia, and reduced HDL-cholesterol concentrations and is considered a risk factor for obesity in adulthood.[17] According to recent studies, second to prior obesity, the strongest predictor of subsequent obesity in children is television viewing.[18]

◆ **Iron-deficiency anemia.** Iron deficiency is the most common cause of anemia among children in the United States. Anemia is defined as either a low hemoglobin or a low hematocrit or both, compared with normal concentrations.[19] Based on data from the NHANES II, conducted between 1976 and 1980, the prevalence estimates of impaired iron status for children are 9.3 percent for children aged 1–2 years, 4.3 percent for those aged 3–4 years, and 3.9 percent for those aged 5–10 years.[20] Data from the Pediatric Nutrition Surveillance System survey (PedNSS), which monitors the general health and nutrition status of low-income U.S. children who participate in public health programs, reveal a prevalence of anemia of 20 to 30 percent in the PedNSS population. This figure is much higher than the national average, reflecting the greater risk for iron-deficiency anemia among low-income children.[21] Black children consistently have lower hemoglobin and hematocrit values than white children.[22] In general, the prevalence of anemia has been decreasing in all ethnic groups over the last decade.[23]

◆ **Dental caries.** Dental caries affect 98 percent of all U.S. children, making this condition a widespread public health problem.[24] Data collected in 1986–1987 by the Centers for Disease Control and Prevention (CDC) indicate that about 34 percent of 9-year-old children and 58 percent of 12-year-old children have dental caries, and the number of decayed, missing, and filled permanent teeth increases steadily with age.[25] In 1980, the average child had at least one carious lesion in a permanent tooth by the age of 8 years. By the age of 12 years, the average child had 4 carious lesions; by 17 years of age, 11 lesions. Fortunately, the incidence of dental caries in children has decreased by as much as 30 to 50 percent over the last two decades due, in part, to fluoridation of public drinking water, improved dental hygiene, and the use of fluoride in toothpastes and mouthwashes.[26]

◆ **High blood cholesterol.** There is considerable evidence that atherosclerosis begins in childhood and that this process is related to high blood cholesterol levels. When compared with children in other countries, children and adolescents in the United States have higher blood cholesterol levels and higher dietary intakes of saturated fat and cholesterol. Mean serum cholesterol levels for children reported by the Lipid Research Clinics Prevalence Study are shown in Table 13-3.[27]

◆ ASSESSMENT OF NUTRITION STATUS

Nutrition status can be assessed through anthropometric measurements, biochemical measurements, a clinical assessment, and various diet assessment methods.

Anthropometric Assessment   Anthropometric measurements are of two types: growth and body composition measurements. Growth measurements include recumbent length, height, weight, head circumference, and indices derived from height and weight. Body composition measurements include triceps skinfold and mid-arm circumference.[28]

Age (yr)	Number	Overall Mean	5	10	25	50	75	90	95
MALES									
0–4	238	159	117	129	141	156	176	192	209
5–9	1253	165	125	134	147	164	180	197	209
10–14	2278	162	123	131	144	160	178	196	208
15–19	1980	154	116	124	136	150	170	188	203
FEMALES									
0–4	186	161	115	124	143	161	177	195	206
5–9	1118	169	130	138	150	168	184	201	211
10–14	2087	164	128	135	148	163	179	196	207
15–19	2079	162	124	131	144	160	177	197	209

*All values have been converted from plasma to serum. Plasma value × 1.03 = serum value.

TABLE 13-3

Serum Total Cholesterol Levels in U.S. Children and Adolescents (mg/dL)*

Source: National Heart, Lung, and Blood Institute, *The Lipid Research Clinics Population Studies Data Book: Volume I—The Prevalence Study* (Bethesda, Md.: U.S. Department of Health and Human Services, Public Health Service, National Institutes of Health, NIH Pub. No. 80-1527, July 1980).

◆ Growth measurements.

    ◆ **Recumbent length.** Recumbent length is the appropriate measure of stature for infants and children less than two years of age. Refer to Chapter 12 for a description of the proper method for measuring recumbent length.

    ◆ **Height.** Children over two years of age are measured in a standing position using a stadiometer, portable anthropometer, or a flat wall. When measuring a child's height, have the subject stand straight with the head positioned so that the **Frankfurt plane** is horizontal, as shown in Figure 13-1. The child's feet are together; knees are straight in front; and heels, buttocks, and shoulder blades are in contact with the vertical surface of the stadiometer, anthropometer, or wall. The child should wear a minimal amount of clothing and no shoes. When measuring height against a wall, the assessor uses a book, block, or other rigid object to ensure that the top of the child's head is measured at a right angle to the wall. When using a stadiometer or anthropometer, the movable headboard is lowered gently until it touches the crown of the head. Care must be taken to ensure that the headboard is flat and not angled either up or down. Although the movable headboard is widely used, it can contribute to measurement errors because it is unsteady. Take three height measurements and record the average in either inches or centimeters.

Frankfurt plane A conceptual plane that passes through the auditory meatus (the small flap of skin on the forward edge of the ear) and the tops of the lower bones of the eye sockets immediately below the eye.

FIGURE
13-1

Positioning of the Child for Height Measurement

Source: Reprinted from Robbins, G. E. and Trowbridge, F. L., Anthropometric Techniques and Their Application, in *Nutrition Assessment: A Comprehensive Guide for Planning Intervention,* M. D. Simko, C. Cowell, and J. A. Gilbride, eds., p. 77, with permission of Aspen Publishers, Inc., © 1984.

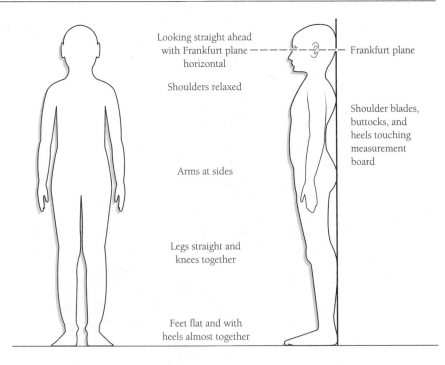

Looking straight ahead with Frankfurt plane horizontal

Frankfurt plane

Shoulders relaxed

Shoulder blades, buttocks, and heels touching measurement board

Arms at sides

Legs straight and knees together

Feet flat and with heels almost together

◆ **Weight.** In field surveys, a toddler's weight can be measured using a weighing sling, as shown in Figure 13-2A. Before the weight is recorded, the assessor must ensure that the toddler is quiet and not fidgeting or moving about. In clinical settings, it is preferable to weigh a preschool child using an electronic scale or beam balance (see Figure 13-2B). The child, in the nude or wearing light underclothing, should stand quietly and unassisted with his arms hanging at his side. The assessor records the weight in pounds or kilograms.

◆ **Head circumference.** To measure head circumference, a flexible, non-stretch tape about 0.6 centimeters wide is used. The child stands in a relaxed position facing the assessor, looking straight ahead so that the Frankfurt plane is in a horizontal position (see Figure 13-3). The tape is placed just above the eyebrows where the head has its maximum circumference. Care must be taken to ensure that the tape is pulled tightly against the head and that it is level on each side. The measurement is recorded to the nearest millimeter.

◆ **Indices derived from growth measurements.** Several indices for assessing growth are derived from a child's height, weight, and age. The actual values for height, weight, and age are plotted on a nomogram or growth chart, which makes it possible to compare a particular child's height and weight for age with a national standard. The anthropometric reference

(A)

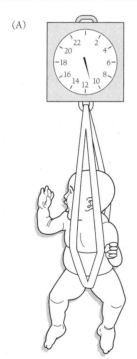

(B)

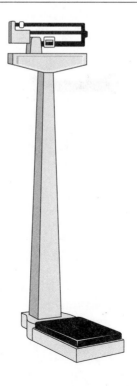

FIGURE

13-2

Methods of Weighing Toddlers and Children

Source: Reproduced with permission from Gibson, R. S. *Principles of Nutritional Assessment,* p. 169 and p. 170, 1990.

FIGURE
13-3

Measuring Head Circumference

Source: Reproduced with permission from Gibson, R. S. *Principles of Nutritional Assessment*, p. 164, 1990.

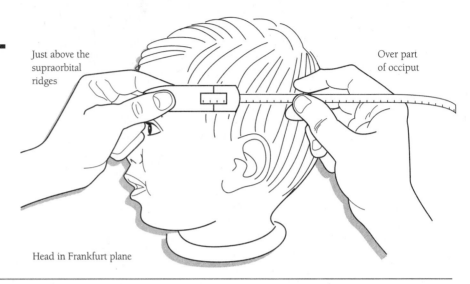

Just above the supraorbital ridges

Over part of occiput

Head in Frankfurt plane

data used in the United States for assessing physical growth are based on a large, nationally representative sample of children from birth to 18 years of age. The percentile curves (e.g., 5th, 10th, 25th, 50th, 75th, 90th, and 95th) for this reference population are displayed on growth charts developed by the National Center for Health Statistics (NCHS). A sample growth chart is shown in Figure 13-4. For a complete set of growth charts for infants and toddlers aged birth to 36 months and children aged 2 to 18 years, see Appendix E, which also contains reference data from the Hispanic HANES for Mexican-American children.

Growth stunting A slowing of skeletal growth and stature.

◆ **Height-for-age.** Low height-for-age is defined as a height-for-age value below the 5th percentile or the –1.65 Z-score of the NCHS-CDC height reference. (Refer to the boxed insert on page 420 for a description of Z-scores.) In other words, low height-for-age reflects a child's failure to achieve for a given age group a distribution of height that conforms to standards established for a well-nourished, healthy population of children.[29] Low height-for-age is sometimes referred to as **growth stunting**, which may be the consequence of poor nutrition, a high frequency of infections, or both.[30] Stunting refers to a slowing of skeletal growth and stature, the "end result of a reduced rate of linear growth."[31]

Although shortness in an individual child may be a normal reflection of the child's genetic heritage, a high prevalence rate of growth stunting reflects poor socioeconomic conditions. In some developing countries, the prevalence rate is as high as 60 to 70 percent. In developed countries, the rate is about 2 to 5 percent.[32] The prevalence of stunting is highest during the second or third year of life.[33]

◆ **Weight-for-height.** Low weight-for-height, or thinness, is defined as a weight-for-height value below the 5th percentile.[34] This indicator is a

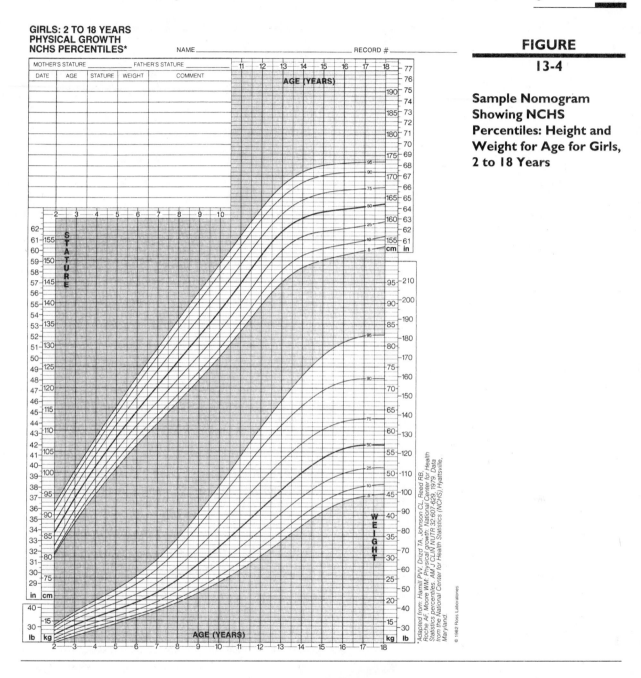

GIRLS: 2 TO 18 YEARS
PHYSICAL GROWTH
NCHS PERCENTILES*

*Adapted from: Hamill PVV, Drizd TA, Johnson CL, Reed RB, Roche AF, Moore WM: Physical growth: National Center for Health Statistics percentiles. AM J CLIN NUTR 32:607-629, 1979. Data from the National Center for Health Statistics (NCHS), Hyattsville, Maryland.

© 1982 Ross Laboratories

FIGURE

13-4

Sample Nomogram Showing NCHS Percentiles: Height and Weight for Age for Girls, 2 to 18 Years

sensitive index of current nutrition status and is often associated with recent severe disease. Between the ages of 1 and 10 years, the indicator is relatively independent of age. In addition, it is relatively independent of ethnic group, particularly among children aged one to five years.[35]

Understanding Z-Scores

Growth indices can be expressed in percentile values or as standard deviation values or Z-scores. The Z-score of each growth index for each child is calculated by the following formula:

$$Z = \frac{\text{Observed value} - \text{Reference mean value}}{\text{Reference standard deviation value}}$$

The relationship of Z-scores to percentile values is shown on the distribution curve in the figure. Note that a Z-score of 0.0 corresponds to the 50th percentile on the distribution curve.*

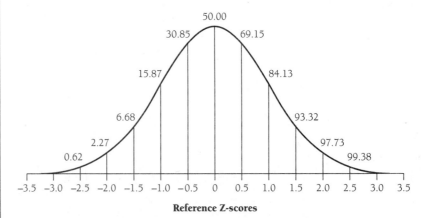

*R. Yip and coauthors, Pediatric Nutrition Surveillance System—United States, 1980–1991, *Morbidity and Mortality Weekly Report* 41/No. SS–7 (November 27, 1992): 8.

Weight-for-height differentiates between nutritional stunting, when a child's weight may be appropriate for her height, and wasting, when weight is very low for height due to reductions in both tissue and fat mass. In developing countries, thinness indicates acute malnutrition, due mainly to starvation, repeated episodes of diarrhea, or both. The prevalence of low weight-for-height is usually less than 5 percent except during periods of famine, war, or other extreme conditions. A prevalence rate greater than 5 percent indicates the presence of serious nutritional problems.

At the other end of the spectrum, a high weight-for-height (a value greater than the 95th percentile) correlates well with obesity and typically indicates excess food consumption, low activity levels, or both.

♦ **Weight-for-age.** Weight-for-age is a composite index of height-for-age and weight-for-height. In children aged six months to about seven years, weight-for-age is an indicator of acute malnutrition. It is widely used to assess protein-energy malnutrition and overnutrition. However, one limitation of using weight-for-age as an indicator of protein-energy malnutrition is that it does not consider height differences. For example, a child who has low weight-for-age may be genetically short with proportionally low height and low weight rather than too thin with a low weight for height. As a result, the prevalence of protein-energy malnutrition in small children may be overestimated if only this indicator is used.[36] Weight-for-age is most useful in clinical settings where repeated measurements of the indicator are used to evaluate children who are not gaining weight.[37]

◆ **Velocity growth curves.** The nomograms for assessing growth are based on cross-sectional data, meaning that measurements were made once on many children of different ages. Sometimes, however, it is useful to determine how a child's growth is changing over time. In this case, cross-sectional data are inappropriate, and longitudinal data are needed, meaning that the same children are measured at specific ages over a period of many years. The velocity growth curves for boys and girls aged 2 to 18 years are shown in Figure 13-5.[38]

◆ **Weight/height ratios.** Weight/height ratios measure body weight corrected for height. The underlying assumption of this calculation is that the ratios are correlated with obesity. For this reason, these ratios are often called obesity or body mass indices. Several such indices exist. The two ratios most commonly used in large-scale population and field studies are Quetelet's index and the ponderal index:

$$\text{Quetelet's index} = \frac{\text{Weight in kg}}{\text{Height in m}^2}$$

$$\text{Ponderal index} = \frac{\text{Height}}{\sqrt[3]{\text{Weight}}}$$

Quetelet's index is sometimes referred to as the body mass index (BMI). The question of whether BMI is an appropriate index for measuring body composition in children and adolescents has not been fully resolved. Some researchers believe that BMI is a good measure of body size for growing children when the child's biological age, which measures the year of peak height velocity, rather than his chronological age is computed.[39] Others maintain that Quetelet's index is appropriate only for the *adult* population. Canada, for example, does not consider Quetelet's index a valid index for individuals under the age of 20 or over 65 years or for women who are pregnant or lactating.[40] Part of the problem with measuring body fat in children is the lack of reference data for this population subgroup. A nomogram for estimating BMI is given in Appendix E (see Figure E5-1).

◆ **Body composition measurements.**

   ◆ **Triceps skinfold.** Skinfold measurements provide an estimate of the body's subcutaneous or storage fat, which in turn provides an estimate of total body fat.[41] Skinfold thickness is measured using a pincer-type caliper that meets the specifications of the Food and Nutrition Board of the National Research Council.[42] Obtaining reliable skinfold measurements requires a trained examiner.

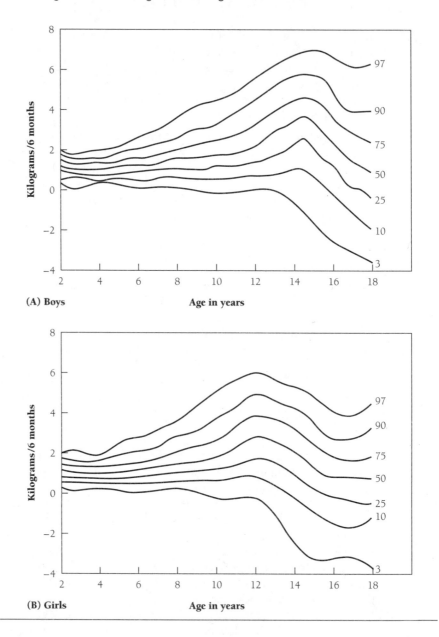

FIGURE

13-5

Percentile Velocity Growth Curves for Boys and Girls, Aged 2 to 18 Years

Source: Reproduced with permission from Abelin, T. et al. *Measurement in Health Promotion and Protection.* Copenhagen, WHO Regional Office for Europe, 1987.

(A) Boys

(B) Girls

While there is no single best measurement of body composition, the triceps skinfold measurement is the most widely used indirect measure of body fat among children. The triceps skinfold is measured at the midpoint of the back of the upper left arm, as shown in Figure 13-6. The triceps skinfold percentiles are given in Appendix E, along with the median triceps skinfold thickness values for Mexican-American, white, and black children aged 1 to 19 years.

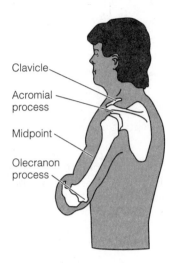

Clavicle

Acromial process

Midpoint

Olecranon process

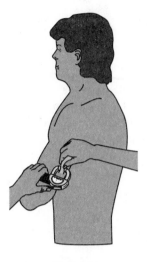

FIGURE

13-6

Measurement of Triceps Skinfold Using a Harpenden Caliper
Source: Reprinted by permission from *Understanding Nutrition* by E. N. Whitney and S. R. Rolfes. Copyright © 1993 by West Publishing Company. All rights reserved.

A. Find the midpoint of the arm:

1. Ask the subject to bend his or her arm at the elbow and lay the hand across the stomach. (If the subject is right-handed, measure the left arm, and vice versa.)

2. Feel the shoulder to locate the acromial process. It helps to slide your fingers along the clavicle to find the acromial process. The olecranon process is the tip of the elbow.

3. Place a measuring tape from the acromial process to the tip of the elbow. Divide this measurement by 2, and mark the midpoint of the arm with a pen.

B. Measure the fatfold:

1. Ask the subject to let his or her arm hang loosely to the side.

2. Grasp a fold of skin and subcutaneous fat between the thumb and forefinger slightly above the midpoint mark. Gently pull the skin away from the underlying muscle. (This step takes a lot of practice. If you want to be sure you don't have muscle as well as fat, ask the subject to contract and relax the muscle. You should be able to feel if you are pinching muscle.)

3. Place the calipers over the fatfold at the midpoint mark, and read the measurement to the nearest millimeter in two to three seconds. (If using plastic calipers, align pressure lines, and read the measurement to the nearest millimeter in two to three seconds.)

4. Repeat Steps 2 and 3 twice more. Add the three readings, and then divide by 3 to find the average.

◆ **Mid-arm circumference.** Because the arm contains both muscle and subcutaneous fat, a decrease in the mid-arm circumference may reflect a reduction in muscle tissue, a reduction in subcutaneous fat, or both. Changes in the mid-arm circumference can be used to monitor progress during nutritional therapy or to diagnose protein-energy malnutrition or starvation. Changes in arm circumference are easy to detect. The measurement is made with a flexible, nonstretch tape and requires little time.[43] The mid-arm circumference percentiles are given in Appendix E.

Biochemical Assessment A variety of biochemical measurements are used routinely in assessing nutrition status, as shown in Table 13-4. Where children are concerned, three measurements are important: iron status, blood cholesterol level, and blood lead level:

◆ **Iron status.** In the clinical setting, two common screening tests for anemia are the hematocrit (Hct) value, which measures the proportion of blood that is composed of red blood cells, and the hemoglobin (Hb)

TABLE

13-4

Biochemical Tests Useful for Assessing Nutrition Status

Source: Adapted from A. Grant and S. DeHoog, *Nutritional Assessment and Support,* 4th ed., 1991 (available from Anne Grant and Susan DeHoog, Box 25057, Northgate Station, Seattle, WA 98125). Used with permission.

NUTRIENT	ASSESSMENT TESTS
Protein	Urinary creatinine excretion, serum albumin, serum prealbumin, serum transferrin, retinol-binding protein, total lymphocyte count, nitrogen balance
Vitamins	
Vitamin A	Retinol-binding protein, serum carotene
Thiamin	Erythrocyte (red blood cell) transketolase activity, urinary thiamin
Riboflavin	Erythrocyte glutathione reductase activity, urinary riboflavin
Vitamin B_6	Urinary xanthurenic acid excretion after tryptophan load test, urinary vitamin B_6, erythrocyte transaminase activity
Niacin	Urinary metabolites NMN (N-methyl nicotinamide) or 2-pyridone, or preferably both expressed as a ratio
Folate	Free folate in the blood, erythrocyte folate (reflects liver stores), urinary formiminoglutamic acid (FIGLU), vitamin B_{12} status (because folate assessment tests alone do not distinguish between the two deficiencies)
Vitamin B_{12}	Serum vitamin B_{12}, erythrocyte vitamin B_{12}, urinary methylmalonic acid synthesis or DUMP test (from the abbreviation of the chemical name of DNA's raw material, deoxyuridine monophosphate)
Biotin	Serum biotin, urinary biotin
Vitamin C	Serum or plasma vitamin C,* leukocyte vitamin C, urinary vitamin C
Vitamin D	Serum alkaline phosphatase
Vitamin E	Serum tocopherol, erythrocyte hemolysis
Vitamin K	Blood clotting time (prothrombin time)
Minerals	
Potassium	Serum potassium
Magnesium	Serum magnesium
Iron	Hemoglobin, hematocrit, serum ferritin, total iron-binding capacity (TIBC), transferrin saturation, erythrocyte protoporphyrin, serum ferritin, mean corpuscular volume (MCV), serum iron
Iodine	Serum protein-bound iodine, radioiodine uptake
Zinc	Plasma zinc, hair zinc

*Vitamin C shifts unpredictably between the plasma and the white blood cells known as leukocytes; thus a plasma or serum determination may not accurately reflect the body's pool. The appropriate clinical test may be a measurement of leukocyte vitamin C. A combination of both tests may be more reliable than either one alone.

value, which represents the number of grams of Hb in 100 milliliters (ml) of whole blood. The following are the specific indicators for detecting poor iron status:[44]

♦ The percentage of children and youths within a population group who are at or below traditional cutoff values for low Hb or Hct for age and sex.

♦ The percentage of children and youths within a population group who have Hb or Hct values below the 5th percentile for the U.S. population for age and sex.

Table 13-5 shows the recommended reference cutoff values for anemia based on the CDC's criteria.[45] Although hemoglobin and hematocrit measurements are commonly used as screening indicators for anemia, they are not ideal measures. Hemoglobin concentration is a relatively insensitive measure of iron status, because its concentration falls only during the third stage of iron deficiency, as shown in Figure 13-7. Hematocrit likewise falls only in the third stage of iron deficiency and for this reason is not considered a sensitive indicator of iron status. Thus, a combination of laboratory values is considered essential for accurately determining iron status. In addition to hemoglobin concentration, serum ferritin, transferrin saturation, and erythrocyte protoporphyrin values are needed for estimating iron status and determining the presence of iron-deficiency anemia.[46]

♦ **Blood cholesterol level.** The Expert Panel on Blood Cholesterol Levels in Children and Adolescents of the National Cholesterol Education Program (NCEP) classifies a total blood cholesterol level of ≥200 mg/dL (≥5.17 mmol/L) or an LDL-cholesterol level of ≥130 mg/dL (≥3.36 mmol/L) as high, when associated with a family or parental history of hypercholes-

AGE (YEARS)/SEX	Hb (g/dL)	Hct (%)
Both sexes		
1–1.9	11.0	33.0
2–4.9	11.2	34.0
5–7.9	11.4	34.5
8–11.9	11.6	35.0
Female		
12–14.9	11.8	35.5
15–17.9	12.0	36.0
≥18	12.0	36.0
Male		
12–14.9	12.3	37.0
15–17.9	12.6	38.0
≥18	13.6	41.0

*Based on the 5th percentile values from the Second National Health and Nutrition Examination Survey, after excluding persons with a higher likelihood of iron deficiency.

TABLE

13-5

Hemoglobin (Hb) and Hematocrit (Hct) Cutoff Values for Children, Nonpregnant Women, and Men*

Source: Centers for Disease Control and Prevention, CDC criteria for anemia in children and childbearing-aged women, *Morbidity and Mortality Weekly Report* 38 (1989): 401.

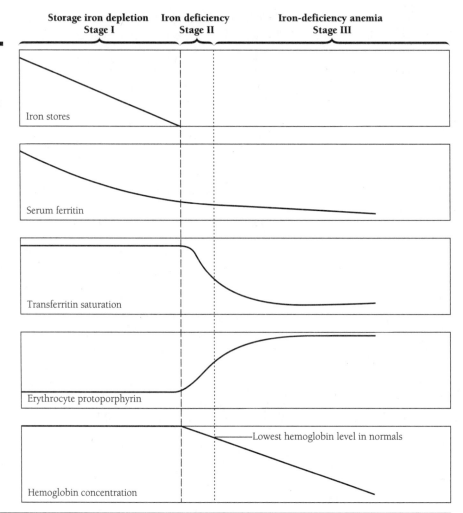

FIGURE

13-7

Changes in Iron Indices During the Development of Iron Deficiency
Source: National Live Stock and Meat Board, *Iron in Human Nutrition* (Chicago: National Live Stock and Meat Board, 1990). Used with permission from the National Live Stock and Meat Board.

terolemia.* Refer to Table 13-6 for the NCEP classification of total and LDL-cholesterol levels in children and adolescents. The panel recommends that children and youths with high blood cholesterol be evaluated further and receive diet therapy, if appropriate. Drug therapy is recommended only for children over 10 years of age whose blood cholesterol level has not responded to an adequate trial of diet therapy lasting from six months to one year.[47]

◆ **Blood lead level.** An elevated blood lead level is defined as a blood lead level high enough to warrant further medical evaluation for the possibility of adverse mental, behavioral, physical, or biochemical effects. The CDC

*To convert milligrams (mg) of cholesterol per deciliter (dL) of blood to millimoles (mmol) per liter (L), multiply by a factor of 0.02586.

CATEGORY	TOTAL CHOLESTEROL (mg/dL)	LDL-CHOLESTEROL (mg/dL)
Acceptable	<170	<110
Borderline	170–199	110–129
High	≥200	≥130

TABLE

13-6

Classification of Total and LDL-Cholesterol Levels in Children and Adolescents from Families with Hypercholesterolemia or Premature Cardiovascular Disease

Source: National Cholesterol Education Program, *Report of the Expert Panel on Blood Cholesterol Levels in Children and Adolescents* (Washington, D.C.: U.S. Department of Health and Human Services, Public Health Service, National Institutes of Health, NIH Pub. No. 91–2732, 1991), p. 5.

recommends that children with blood lead levels exceeding 10 µg/dL be evaluated and referred for treatment.

The Agency for Toxic Substances and Disease Registry estimates that between 3 and 4 million U.S. children under six years of age have blood lead levels about 15 µg/dL, a level associated with some detectable adverse effects. In one survey of a suburban area, 20 percent of children were found to have blood lead levels of 10 µg/dL or above. Data from NHANES II indicate that black children are six times as likely as white children to have blood lead levels greater than 30 µg/dL.[48]

Clinical Assessment   Recall from Chapter 7 that the clinical assessment of health consists of a medical history and a physical examination to detect physical signs and symptoms associated with malnutrition. In assessing a child's nutrition status, clinicians rely on parents or caregivers to provide detailed information about weight changes, food allergies, chronic illnesses, and other conditions that may affect the child's food intake. Table 13-7 lists some of the physical signs associated with health and malnutrition in children.[49]

Diet Assessment   The diet assessment methods described in Chapter 2 are used most often with adults, who are capable of providing information about their dietary patterns on their own. These methods can be adapted for use with children, although the parent or caregiver must provide the information about the child's meal and snack patterns, foods eaten, how foods were prepared, and so forth. Many of the problems inherent in obtaining accurate dietary information from adults apply to diet assessment in children. Parents or caregivers may not recall the child's usual diet accurately and may be influenced by perceptions of "good" and "bad" dietary patterns and current eating habits.[50] Electronic methods of diet assessment (for example, telephones and tape recorders) have been used successfully to obtain dietary intake information directly from pre-adolescent children.[51]

◆ CHILDREN WITH SPECIAL HEALTH CARE NEEDS

A variety of terms and classifications have been used in describing the population with special needs, including developmental disabilities, developmental social

TABLE

13-7

Physical Signs of Health and Malnutrition in Children

	HEALTHY	MALNOURISHED
Hair	Shiny, firm in the scalp	Dull, brittle, dry, loose; falls out
Eyes	Bright, clear pink membranes; adjust easily to darkness	Pale membranes, spots; redness; adjust slowly to darkness
Teeth and Gums	No pain or cavities, gums firm, teeth bright	Missing, discolored, decayed teeth; gums bleed easily and are swollen and spongy
Face	Good complexion	Off-color, scaly, flaky, cracked skin
Glands	No lumps	Swollen at front of neck and cheeks
Tongue	Red, bumpy, rough	Sore, smooth, purplish, swollen
Skin	Smooth, firm, good color	Dry, rough, spotty; "sandpaper" feel or sores; lack of fat under skin
Nails	Firm, pink	Spoon-shaped, brittle, ridged
Behavior	Alert, attentive, cheerful	Irritable, apathetic, inattentive, hyperactive
Internal Systems	Heart rate, heart rhythm, and blood pressure normal; normal digestive function; reflexes and psychological development normal	Heart rate, heart rhythm, or blood pressure abnormal; liver and spleen enlarged; abnormal digestion; mental irritability, confusion; burning, tingling of hands and feet; loss of balance and coordination
Muscles and Bones	Good muscle tone and posture; long bones straight	"Wasted" appearance of muscles; swollen bumps on skull or ends of bones; small bumps on ribs; bowed legs or knock-knees

Note: The physical signs shown here are consistent with malnutrition but not diagnostic of it.

needs, handicapping conditions, chronic disorders, and chronic illnesses.[52] This book uses the relatively new term "special health care needs," which encompasses the definition of developmental disabilities given in the Developmental Disabilities Assistance and Bill of Rights Act of 1990 (P.L. 101–496) and applies to a broad spectrum of handicapping conditions and mental and physical impairments.*

*The Developmental Disabilities Assistance and Bill of Rights Act of 1990 states: "The term 'developmental disability' means a severe chronic disability of a person 5 years of age or older which is attributable to a mental or physical impairment or combination of mental and physical impairments; is manifested before the person attains age twenty-two; is likely to continue indefinitely; results in substantial functional limitations in three or more of the following areas of major life activity: (i) self-care, (ii) receptive and expressive language, (iii) learning, (iv) mobility, (v) self-direction, (vi) capacity for independent living, and (vii) economic sufficiency; and reflects the person's need for a combination and sequence of special, interdisciplinary, or generic care, treatment, or other services which are of lifelong or extended duration and are individually planned and coordinated, except that such term, when applied to infants and young children means individuals from birth to age 5, inclusive, who have substantial developmental delay or specific congenital or acquired conditions with a high probability of resulting in developmental disabilities if services are not provided." (As cited in *Journal of the American Dietetic Association* 92 [1992]: 613.)

Children with special health care needs are at increased nutritional risk because of feeding problems, metabolic aberrations, drug/nutrient interactions, decreased mobility, and alterations in growth patterns. An interdisciplinary approach to managing children with special health care needs is recommended. The interdisciplinary team may include a physician, nurse, psychologist, dentist, dietitian, and occupational, physical, and speech therapists. The components of a basic interdisciplinary team assessment of children with special health care needs are listed in Table 13-8.[53]

Adolescents

Adolescence is a time of change. Between the ages of about 10 to 18 years in girls and 12 to 20 years in boys, there are marked changes in physical, intellectual, and emotional growth and development. The maturation process is initiated and controlled by a variety of hormones, including growth hormone, prolactin, estrogen, testosterone, and the thyroid hormones, among others.[54] Many aspects of the maturation process are influenced by dietary intake and nutrition status. In this section, we review the nutrient requirements and nutrition status of U.S. adolescents, and we examine the nutrition assessment methods for this population. Bear in mind that the adolescent population has been understudied and underserved. Few studies have examined their specific nutrient needs, and few programs and services target the nutrition-related problems of teenagers exclusively.

◆ NUTRIENT NEEDS

The dramatic changes in body composition and the rate of growth that occur during early adolescence give rise to the familiar phrase "the adolescent growth spurt." The magnitude of these changes is such that the linear growth increments during adolescence can contribute about 15 to 25 percent of adult stature. The rate of weight gain can contribute anywhere from 40 to 50 percent of the adult body mass. This remarkable growth rate requires adequate intakes of energy and nutrients.[55]

There is no universally applicable formula for expressing the energy demands of adolescents. The individual teenager's energy need is influenced by body size, activity levels, and biological factors affecting growth. For many nutrients, especially vitamins and minerals, there are few data based specifically on measurements in adolescents. Recommended nutrient intakes for adolescents are based on extrapolations from studies conducted among either adults or children, with a safety factor built in.[56] Consult the RDA table on the inside front cover for the nutrient intake recommendations for adolescents.

◆ PRIMARY NUTRITION-RELATED PROBLEMS

Most adolescents in the United States are perceived as "healthy." Nevertheless, many U.S. adolescents experience a variety of health and nutritional problems,

TABLE
13-8

Interdisciplinary Assessment of Children With Special Health Care Needs

Source: L. A. Wodarski, An interdisciplinary nutrition assessment and intervention protocol for children with disabilities. Copyright The American Dietetic Association. Reprinted by permission from *Journal of the American Dietetic Association,* Vol. 90: 1990, p. 1564.

◆ **Dietary history**
Methods of feeding (e.g., breast, bottle, gavage, spoon, cup); gavage, bottle, and breast weaning
Type of food, order of introduction, and child's age at introduction of solid foods and present intake of solid foods
Foods that cause aspiration or gagging
Current and past special diet orders, including texture modifications
Use of nutritional supplements and vitamin/mineral supplements
Food intolerances/allergies
Current and past medications and noted side effects
Pica or inappropriate food consumption
Appetite, regularity of meals
Fluid preferences and intake pattern
Fad, cultural, or religious diet preferences
Nutrition knowledge and attitude of caregiver regarding meal planning and diet of child
Use of food as reinforcer/pacifier
Where and with whom food is consumed
Participation in school/child care breakfast and/or lunch programs

◆ **Medical history**
Chronic/metabolic disorders
Records of any substance abuse
Incidence of vomiting, nausea, diarrhea, or constipation
Acute or recurring illnesses and/or infections
Obvious manifestation of nutritional deficiencies
Physical activity
Dental screening
Socioeconomic data, including home environment, adequacy of resources, educational status of primary caregiver, social/economic habits, parenting skills, support system for caregiver, and influential sources of information

◆ **Anthropometric assessment**
Height/length
Weight
Mid-arm muscle circumference
Triceps skinfold

◆ **Feeding assessment**
Neurological dysfunction or mechanical obstructions reflected in inefficient sucking and swallowing, bite reflex, strong or hypoactive gag reflex, tongue thrust, protrusion reflex, poor lip control, impaired chewing, malocclusion and high arched palate, and lack of head and trunk control
Dysphagia caused by gross congenital anatomical defects of the tongue, palate, mandible, pharynx, larynx, esophagus, and thorax; neuromuscular causes, such as delayed maturation, cerebral palsy, muscular dystrophy, various syndromes, and bacterial and viral infections; and acute infective conditions, such as stomatitis
Particular problems associated with feeding difficulties, such as delayed introduction of solid foods, delays in self-feeding, mealtime tantrums or disruptive behavior, coercive or manipulative interactive patterns between child and caregiver, and inappropriate uses of rewards/punishment for eating/mealtime

◆ **Clinical assessment**
Skeleton, musculature, and general appearance
Hair, skin, eyes, nails, face
Lips, teeth, gums, and tongue

some related to their risk-seeking behaviors and inability to deal with abstract notions such as "good health" and the link between current behaviors and long-

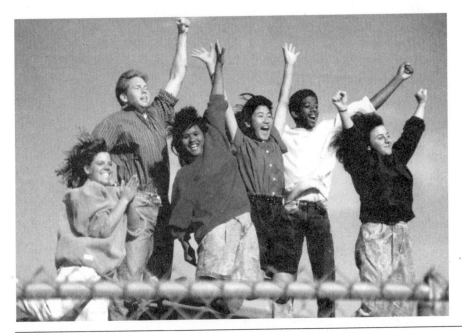

Successful nutrition education activities for teenagers focus on their interests and the relationship of good eating and physical activity to health.

term health. In general, the nutritional health of U.S. teenagers is better today than ever before. Overt nutrient deficiencies, with the exception of iron deficiency, are not the public health problems they once were.[57] Specific nutrition-related problems among U.S. adolescents include undernutrition, obesity, iron-deficiency anemia, high blood cholesterol levels, dental caries, and eating disorders:

◆ **Undernutrition.** Some groups of adolescents are at risk for reduced energy and food intakes. Adolescents from low-income families and those who have run away from home or abuse alcohol or drugs are at risk nutritionally. In 1987, 15.9 percent of youth aged 14 to 21 years lived below the poverty line. Black or Hispanic teenagers are nearly three times more likely to live in poverty than are white youth. Juveniles who live on the street tend to have a host of health problems, including substance abuse and malnutrition. Irregular meal patterns, combined with a high rate of use of substances such as alcohol, marijuana, cocaine, and amphetamines, contribute to low nutrient and energy intakes among street youth.[58] Chronic dieters are also at risk. Thirteen percent of the 17,354 females in grades 7 through 12 who were interviewed in the Minnesota Adolescent Survey reported being chronic dieters, defined as always on a diet or having been on a diet for 10 of the previous 12 months.[59]

◆ **Obesity.** An analysis of recent NHANES data revealed that the prevalence of obesity among 12- to 17-year-olds in the United States increased by 39 percent in the past 15 to 20 years.[60] Data from the Hispanic HANES indicate that about 20 percent of Hispanic girls aged 12 to 18 years exceed the 85th percentile of U.S. standards for BMI. In general, Hispanic children living in the United States carry significantly greater amounts of body fat than do their non-Hispanic counterparts.[61] Given that childhood obesity can lead to adult obesity and that approximately 25 to 30 percent of the adult population is overweight, obesity among teenagers is cause for concern. Genetic susceptibility to obesity, lifestyle, family eating patterns, lack of positive role models, and inactivity all contribute to overweight and obesity in this population. Obese teenagers are also at risk for hypertension and diabetes mellitus, among other disorders.[62]

♦ **Iron-deficiency anemia.** Iron needs increase during adolescence, especially for females. In boys, the requirements for absorbed iron increase from about 1.0 to 2.5 mg/day. This increase reflects the expanding blood volume and rise in hemoglobin concentration that accompanies sexual maturation. (After the adolescent growth spurt, the need for iron falls off.)[63] A relatively recent analysis of iron requirements in menstruating women suggests that 95 percent of menstruating teenage girls require an intake of 3.21 mg absorbed iron/day. For a U.S.-type diet with a bioavailability figure of 16.6 percent (meaning that about 16.6 percent of dietary iron is available for absorption), the dietary iron requirement is 19.3 mg for teenage girls.[64] Whereas most males have an adequate iron intake during adolescence, many females do not. Data from the Nationwide Food Consumption Survey indicate that females between 12 and 22 years of age have iron intakes below the RDA.[65]

♦ **High blood cholesterol levels.** Teenagers have many of the same risk factors for high blood cholesterol as adults: family history of coronary heart disease; diets high in total fat, saturated fat, and cholesterol; hypertension; low activity levels; and smoking. Although the process of atherosclerosis is not completely understood, it is believed that the fatty streaks that develop in young people progress to the fibrous plaques of adulthood.[66]

♦ **Dental caries.** Dental caries are a significant public health problem among teenagers, with about 78 percent of adolescents having one or more caries in permanent or primary teeth.[67] Dental caries are more prevalent among adolescents than among children. A National Dental Research Survey found that only 22 percent of 15-year-olds were caries-free, compared with 56 percent of 10-year-olds. Some population subgroups, such as American Indians, Alaskan Natives, blacks, and Hispanics, are at greater risk of dental caries than other groups because they lack access to or do not avail themselves of dental services.[68]

♦ **Eating disorders.** Eating disorders have become serious health problems in recent years. The most common eating disorders are anorexia nervosa and bulimia nervosa. A constellation of individual, familial, sociocultural, and biological factors contribute to these disorders, which threaten physical health and psychological well-being. Some individuals are more predisposed to develop an eating disorder than others. For example, about 90 percent of people with eating disorders are female. Most are Caucasian, with few cases seen among blacks and other minority groups. Finally, most individuals who develop eating disorders are adolescents or young adults, who typically begin experiencing food-related and self image problems between the ages of 14 and 30 years. Because these syndromes are surrounded by secrecy, their prevalence is not known with certainty, although it has increased dramatically within the past two decades. Estimates of the prevalence in the general population range from 1 percent for anorexia nervosa to 1–5 percent for bulimia nervosa. These types of eating disorders are often seen in adolescent athletes, many of whom compete in sports such as gymnastics, wrestling, distance running, diving, horse racing, and swimming that demand a rigid control of body weight.[69]

◆ ASSESSMENT OF NUTRITION STATUS

As with children, anthropometric measurements, biochemical indicators, a clinical assessment, and a dietary assessment are used in assessing nutrition status in adolescents:

◆ **Anthropometric assessment.** Height, weight, triceps skinfold, and mid-arm circumference measurements are appropriate for evaluating adolescents' growth and development. Refer to the previous section on children for a description of anthropometric methodology and to Appendix E for standard reference data.

◆ **Biochemical assessment.** Because adolescents, especially girls, are at risk of iron-deficiency anemia, it is appropriate to measure hemoglobin and hematocrit values. Recall that there is no single biochemical indicator for assessing iron status in the general population.

Teenagers who are at risk of coronary heart disease should have a lipoprotein analysis to determine their blood lipid profile. Teenagers at risk of CHD include those whose parents or grandparents were found to have arteriosclerosis at the age of 55 years or less, had a myocardial infarction at the age of 55 years or less, or had a blood cholesterol level of 240 mg/dL (6.21 mmol/L) or higher.[70]

◆ **Clinical assessment.** The basic principles of clinical assessment apply to teenagers. An additional factor in the clinical management of adolescents is good communication. Practitioners who know how to engage their teenage clients in a discussion of their problems and health care are likely to be effective. A part of building strong communication links with teenagers is respecting their privacy and desire to make their own decisions.[71]

◆ **Dietary assessment.** The diet assessment methods used with adults can be used with adolescents, with the caveat that issues of validity and reliability apply to both groups. For example, underreporting of food and energy intakes is a problem for adults and teenagers alike. One study of 27 obese adolescents and 28 nonobese teenagers found that although both groups underreported their daily energy intake, the underreporting was more significant among the obese teenagers. In this study, the magnitude of the recording errors tended to increase with increasing body size, suggesting that the more overweight the teenager, the more likely he or she

◆ ENTREPRENEUR IN ACTION

Introducing Rebecca M. Mullis, Ph.D., R.D.

◆ HER BACKGROUND . . .

Becky Mullis has spent a considerable part of her career as an "intrapreneur" in the traditional academic setting. At the University of Minnesota School of Public Health, she was the Director of Nutrition Education for the Minnesota Heart Health Program and co-project director for the Diet and Cancer Community Intervention Trial, among other projects. Her research focused on community-based nutrition interventions for all types of populations. She is currently Assistant Director for Program Development, Nutrition Division, at the Centers for Disease Control and Prevention in Atlanta, Georgia.

◆ SHE HAS THIS TO SAY ABOUT ENTREPRENEURSHIP . . .

"Entrepreneurship is a new idea in community nutrition. Actually, I think of it as 'social entrepreneurship'—engineering the environment and the opportunities for clients and the population as a whole so they can make sound choices within that environment. I see social entrepreneurship being directed toward the public good in a way that differs from traditional entrepreneurship, which focuses on profitability."

Speaking of innovation in community nutrition, Mullis says, "Our job as community nutritionists is not to narrow the market to only healthy choices. Our job is to ensure that the healthy choices are available and that the public knows about those healthy choices. We need to get away from telling people what to do and move toward enabling them to make healthy choices on their own."

Influencing consumers has been a major theme in Mullis's work. "Community nutritionists must be aware of the food environment," she says. "The food environment includes new products in the marketplace, health claims on food labels, and television and magazine advertising. Plus, all of the things people see in restaurants and grocery stores. Consumers need help sorting through this material. And we must do more work with hard-to-reach populations: inner-city consumers, Hispanics, the homeless."

Mullis believes that community nutritionists need to think differently about the environment. "In Minnesota, we developed a grocery store labeling program that led to in-store demonstrations and then to in-store videos for consumers. That experience taught me that no one idea is going to work. We must always be asking ourselves how to apply what we know about nutrition to the context of life. And the context of life is always changing."

"We need to recognize that nutritionists are not experts in everything. If you are working with grocery stores, for example, then remember that grocery store owners are experts in their needs and their business. We bring *our* expertise in nutrition to *their* environment and work with them to apply our nutrition messages to their situations."

"If we just talk to ourselves all of the time, we pool our ignorance," Mullis says. "We are not trained in how to operate a grocery store or get an ordinance passed. There are people, however, who know how to do these things. What we have to do is get these other people to take on our agenda and help us achieve our vision. That's how we can make a difference for people."

was to underreport energy intake.[72] Problems with accurately recording and recalling food and beverage intake are inherently part of diet assessment methodology, but they can be minimized when the client receives proper training and support.

Domestic Child and Adolescent Nutrition Programs

Federal programs addressing the nutritional needs of children and adolescents have existed since the beginning of this century. The Children's Bureau, at one time part of the U.S. Department of Labor, issued dietary advice to parents and teachers and conducted nutrition surveys of low-income children. School feeding programs, augmented by the financial support of local school districts, philanthropic organizations, and private donors, likewise began in the early 1900s. Federal involvement in school food programs increased during the 1930s with the passage of an amendment to the Agricultural Act of 1933, which established a fund to purchase surplus agricultural commodities for donation to needy families and child nutrition programs, including school lunch programs. The Social Security Act of 1935 authorized grants to the states for health services for children and mothers and formulated a national program of nutrition services that included assessment, counseling, referral, and follow-up for this population.

In 1946, the National School Lunch Act, which authorized permanent grants-in-aid to the states, was enacted. To receive cash and commodity assistance under the statute, states had to operate school lunch programs on a nonprofit basis, serve free or reduced-price lunches for needy children, and provide lunches that met certain federal standards. Twenty years later, in 1966, the Child Nutrition Act was passed. It expanded federal efforts to improve child nutrition by establishing numerous programs of year-round food assistance to children of all ages. These programs led to the authorization of the Special Supplemental Food Program for Women, Infants and Children (WIC) in 1972. Many of the programs and policies developed during the 1960s and 1970s still exist today, although most have been modified over the years. This section describes the major domestic nutrition programs for children and adolescents.[73]

◆ NUTRITION PROGRAMS OF THE U.S. DEPARTMENT OF AGRICULTURE

The Food and Nutrition Service was established in 1969 to administer the food assistance programs of the U.S. Department of Agriculture (USDA). The primary aim of this agency is to make food assistance available to people who need it. Other goals include improving the eating habits of U.S. children and stabilizing farm prices through the distribution of surplus foods. In this section, we examine two of the agency's largest food assistance programs for children, the School Breakfast Program and the National School Lunch Program. Refer to Table 13-9

TABLE

13-9

USDA Food Assistance Programs Specifically for Children

PROGRAM	PURPOSE(S)	TYPE OF ASSISTANCE	ELIGIBILITY REQUIREMENTS
National School Lunch Program	Assist states in providing nutritious free or reduced-price lunches to eligible children and encourage the domestic consumption of nutritious agricultural commodities	Formula grants to states	1. All students attending schools where the lunch program is available may participate. 2. Children from families with incomes at or below 130% of the poverty level are eligible for free meals. 3. Children from families with incomes between 130 and 185% of the poverty level are eligible for reduced-price meals. 4. Children from families with incomes over 185% of the poverty level pay full price.
School Breakfast Program	Assist states in providing nutritious, nonprofit breakfasts for children in public and nonprofit private schools of high school grade and under and in residential child care institutions	Formula grants to states	Eligibility requirements are the same as for the School Lunch Program.

Continued

for a brief description of the programs designed specifically for children and to Table 13-10 for an outline of programs that benefit children by assisting their families. These programs were also described in Chapters 11 and 12.

Formula grants A type of funding mechanism in which the funding agency distributes funds to states on the basis of a "formula" that takes into account any number of factors, such as the number of breakfasts or lunches served to eligible children, the number of breakfasts or lunches served free or at a reduced price, and the national average payment for the program.

◆ **School Breakfast Program.** The School Breakfast Program was authorized by the Child Nutrition Act of 1966 (as amended, P.L. 89–642, P.L. 94–105, P.L. 95–627). The program was initially introduced as a two-year pilot project in 1966 and then was made permanent and extended to all public and nonprofit private schools of high school grade or under in 1975. The program is administered in the same manner as the School Lunch Program. Through **formula grants**, the program helps states provide a nutritious, nonprofit breakfast for students. Participating schools must follow standard meal patterns in which breakfasts provide one-fourth of the RDA over time. The breakfast can be either hot or cold, but it must include the foods shown in Table 13-11 on page 440. All students attending a school where the program is offered are eligible to participate. Breakfast is served free or at a reduced price to students from households with incomes

TABLE 13-9		**USDA Food Assistance Programs Specifically for Children—Continued**	

PROGRAM	PURPOSE(S)	TYPE OF ASSISTANCE	ELIGIBILITY REQUIREMENTS
Special Milk Program for Children	Provide cash reimbursement to schools and institutions to encourage the consumption of fluid milk by children	Formula grants to states	1. Eligible schools include public and private nonprofit schools of high school grade and under, and nonprofit residential or nonresidential child care institutions (provided they do not participate in other federal meal service programs). 2. The program is available to all children in participating schools, regardless of their family income (except in those schools operating the program solely for kindergarten children).
Summer Food Service Program for Children	Assist states in conducting nonprofit food service programs that provide meals and snacks for children in needy areas when school is not in session during the summer and at other times, when area schools are closed for vacation	Formula grants to states	Any child under the age of 18 years or any person over the age of 18 years who is handicapped and who participates in a program established for the mentally or physically handicapped may participate.

Source: *1993 Catalog of Federal Domestic Assistance* (Washington, D.C.: U.S. General Services Administration, 1993) and *Food Assistance Programs—Food Program Facts* (Alexandria, Va.: Food and Nutrition Service, U.S. Department of Agriculture, Public Information Staff/News Branch, May 1993).

at or below the income eligibility guidelines. In 1992, 772 million breakfasts were served, 87.2 percent to needy children, through this program.

◆ **National School Lunch Program.** School lunch programs began informally and unofficially in 1935 with the donation of commodity foods to schools. The National School Lunch Program became official in 1946 with the passage of the National School Lunch Act (as amended, P.L. 79–396). Through formula grants, the program helps states make lunches available to schoolchildren and encourages the consumption of domestic agricultural commodities. The program is administered at the federal level by the USDA's Food and Nutrition Service, at the state level through state agencies, and at the local level through school boards. More than 92,000 schools and residential child care institutions take part in this program. In 1992, an estimated 4.09 billion lunches were served; the projected figure for 1993 is 4.2 billion. Read the Program Spotlight for a detailed description of the School Lunch Program.

TABLE 13-10   **Other USDA Food Assistance Programs That Benefit Children**

PROGRAM	PURPOSE(S)	TYPE OF ASSISTANCE	ELIGIBILITY REQUIREMENTS
Special Supplemental Food Program for Women, Infants, and Children	Provide, at no cost, supplemental, nutritious foods, nutrition education, and referrals to health care to low-income pregnant, breastfeeding and postpartum women, infants, and children to 5 years of age who are determined to be at nutritional risk	Formula grants to states	Pregnant, breastfeeding and postpartum women, infants, and children up to 5 years of age are eligible if they are individually determined by a competent professional to be in need of the special supplemental foods provided by the program because they are nutritionally at risk, and they meet an income standard.
WIC Farmers' Market Nutrition Program	Allow WIC participants to purchase fresh produce at authorized farmers' markets	Formula grants to states	Same as those of the WIC program
Child and Adult Care Food Program	Provide federal funds and USDA-donated foods to nonresidential child care and adult day care facilities and to family day care homes for children	Formula grants to states; plus the sale, exchange, or donation of foods	Eligible institutions include licensed or approved nonresidential, public or private, nonprofit child care centers; Head Start centers; settlement houses; neighborhood centers; some for-profit child care centers; and licensed or approved private homes providing day care for a small group of children.
Food Distribution Program	Improve the diets of preschool and school children, and elderly, and other persons in need of food assistance and increase the market for domestically produced foods acquired under surplus removal or price support operations	Sale, exchange, or donation of property and goods	1. Eligibility of individual households is based on state requirements. 2. All children in schools, child care institutions, and summer camps that participate in the program are eligible for food donations.

Continued

◆ NUTRITION PROGRAMS OF THE U.S. DEPARTMENT OF HEALTH AND HUMAN SERVICES

Recall from Chapter 12 that several DHHS programs include a child care component: Title V Maternal and Child Health Program; Medicaid and the Early and Periodic Screening, Diagnosis, and Treatment (EPSDT) programs; and the primary care programs of Community Health Centers. Another DHHS program that benefits children is the Head Start Program.

Initiated in 1965 by the Office of Economic Opportunity, Head Start was authorized by the Economic Opportunity and Community Partnership Act of 1967 (P.L. 93–644, as amended in 1974). The program is coordinated by the

TABLE 13-10	Other USDA Food Assistance Programs That Benefit Children— *Continued*		
PROGRAM	**PURPOSE(S)**	**TYPE OF ASSISTANCE**	**ELIGIBILITY REQUIREMENTS**
Food Stamps	Improve the diets of low-income households by increasing their food purchasing ability	Direct payments in the form of coupons for specified use	Household eligibility and allotments are based on household size, income, assets, housing costs, work requirements, and other factors.
Commodity Supplemental Food Program	Improve the health and nutrition status of low-income pregnant, postpartum and breastfeeding women, infants, and children up to 6 years of age, and elderly persons through the donation of supplemental foods	Formula grants to states; plus, the sale, exchange, or donation of foods	Eligible persons must meet age and income requirements and be determined at nutritional risk by a competent health professional at the local agency.
Food Distribution Program on Indian Reservations	Improve the diets of needy persons living on or near Indian reservations and increase the market for domestically produced foods acquired under surplus removal or price support operations	Project grants; plus, sale, exchange, or donation of foods	Eligible households must be living on or near an Indian reservation that offers the program and must meet certain income and resource guidelines as determined by local authorities.
Temporary Emergency Food Assistance	Make food commodities available to states for distribution to needy persons	Formula grants to states	Needy individuals, including those who are low income or unemployed or receive welfare benefits
Commodity Distribution to Charitable Institutions	Make food commodities available to nonprofit, charitable institutions that serve meals to low-income persons on a regular basis	Formula grants to states	Institutions eligible for this program include homes for the elderly, hospitals, soup kitchens, food banks, meals-on-wheels programs, temporary shelters, and summer camps or orphanages not participating in any federal child nutrition program.

Source: *1993 Catalog of Federal Domestic Assistance* (Washington, D.C.: U.S. General Services Administration, 1993) and *Food Assistance Programs—Food Program Facts* (Alexandria, Va.: Food and Nutrition Service, U.S. Department of Agriculture, Public Information Staff/News Branch, May 1993).

Administration for Children, Youth, and Families in the Office of Human Development Services in the DHHS. It has been described as one of the most successful federal government programs for child development. Head Start provides 3- to 5-year-old children from low-income families with comprehensive education, social, health, and nutrition services. Parental involvement in the program planning and operation is emphasized. Head Start projects provide meals and snacks as well as nutrition assessment and education for children and their parents. The nutrition services are meant to complement the health and education components of the program. The Select Panel for the Promotion of Child Health reported that Head Start has been shown to improve children's health. Children participating in

TABLE 13-11 **Foods Required for Breakfasts Provided under the School Breakfast Program**	◆ ½ pt of fluid milk as a beverage, on cereal, or both—one serving; AND ◆ ½ c serving fruit OR ½ c full-strength fruit or vegetable juice—one serving; AND ◆ bread or bread-alternate (one slice whole-grain or enriched bread, or an equivalent serving of cornbread, biscuits, rolls, muffins, etc.; or ¾ c or 1 oz serving of cereal)—two servings; OR ◆ meat or meat-alternate (one serving of protein-rich foods such as an egg; or a 1 oz serving of meat, poultry, fish, or cheese; or 2 tbsp of peanut butter)—two servings; OR ◆ one bread AND one meat.

Source: *Fact Sheets on the Federal Food Assistance Programs* (Washington, D.C.: Food Research and Action Center, May 1993), pp. 11–12. Used with permission from the Food Research and Action Center.

Head Start have a lower incidence of anemia, receive more immunizations, and have better nutrition and improved overall health compared with children who do not participate.[74]

◆ PROGRAMS FOR CHILDREN WITH SPECIAL HEALTH CARE NEEDS

In the early 1970s, the U.S. courts began to accord greater recognition to the rights of handicapped children. In 1975, the growing advocacy for handicapped children resulted in the passage of P.L. 94–142, the Education for All Handicapped Children Act. This statute requires states to provide a "free appropriate public education" for all handicapped children aged 3 to 21 years. For handicapped children who require special education because of their impairments, states must provide individualized instruction designed to meet their special needs and any related or supportive services that will enable the children to benefit from the education program. Related services include school health services, counseling services, and parent counseling and training.[75]

In 1986, Congress passed the Education of the Handicapped Act Amendments (P.L. 99–457) to provide added incentives to the states to expand public education for children between 3 and 5 years of age.[76] This legislation mandates the provision of comprehensive services, including nutrition services, to children with special health care needs, using a community-based approach that focuses on the family.[77] The legislation also recognizes nutritionists as the health professionals qualified to provide developmental services to children with special health care needs.

Surveys reveal some deficiencies in delivering these services. For example, in the southeastern and southwestern United States in 1983 and 1984, there were only seven full-time equivalent nutrition positions in the State Programs for Children with Special Health Care Needs for more than 200,000 children. A survey of these programs conducted in 1986 found that fewer than 25 state programs had full-time nutrition consultants.[78] In some instances, children with special health care needs are served by dietitians or nutritionists in WIC programs,

[This discussion continues on page 444.]

◆ *National School Lunch Program*

When Congress passed the National School Lunch Act in 1946, it had the following policy objectives:

> It is hereby declared to be the policy of Congress, as a measure of national security, to safeguard the health and well-being of the Nation's children and to encourage the domestic consumption of nutritious agricultural commodities and other food, by assisting the states, through grants-in-aid and other means in providing an adequate supply of foods and other facilities for the establishment, maintenance, operation, and expansion of non-profit school lunch programs.[1]

The statute requires schools to serve lunches free or at a reduced price to students *who are determined by local authorities* to be unable to pay full price because they come from low-income families.[2] The income guidelines for children participating in child nutrition programs are shown in Chapter 11 (Table 11-6).

Schools that elect to participate in the program get cash subsidies and donated commodities from the USDA for each meal served. In return, the lunches they serve must meet federal requirements and must be offered free or at reduced price to eligible children. Specifically, the lunches must include the following:

◆ 8 ounces fluid milk

◆ 2 ounces protein (meat, fish, cheese, two eggs, four tablespoons peanut butter, or one cup dried beans or peas)

◆ 3/4 cup serving consisting of two or more vegetables or fruits or both (juice can meet half of this requirement)

◆ 8 servings bread, pasta or grain per week

The law requires school districts to prepare and publish a statement of the criteria used for free and reduced-price lunches. The officials responsible for determining a child's eligibility must be identified and the procedural steps used in reaching eligibility decisions specified. A system for appeals in individual cases must exist. The names of children who receive free or reduced-price lunches cannot be "published, posted, or announced in any manner to other children," nor can children who participate in the program be required to use a separate lunchroom, lunchtime, serving line, cafeteria entrance, or medium of exchange.[3]

Problems with Participation

The passage of the National School Lunch Act brought federal recognition to the importance of nutrition to learning and growth. Senator George McGovern, chairman of the Senate Select Committee on Nutrition and Human Needs, observed in 1970 that "the need for adequate food during the school day stands as an obvious one. A child cannot learn if he is hungry—that is a simple and undeniable fact. Hunger makes him restless, lethargic, and physically ill. Without

Continued

—Continued

at least one nutritious meal during his 4- to 7-hour stay at the school, no child can benefit from the tremendous educational opportunities offered in American schools today."[4]

Almost from the very beginning, however, there were problems with participation in the program. A survey conducted in 1967 by Their Daily Bread, a women's organization, showed that two out of three children did not participate in the program.[5] Another survey carried out in 1968 confirmed this finding. Of some 50 million eligible schoolchildren, only 18 million children (36 percent) took part in the program. Only about 55 percent of schools participated in the program in 1968.

A number of reasons were cited for the low participation rates during the late 1960s. First, many parents objected to the manner in which school officials determined which children were eligible. Parents were ashamed to sign an affidavit verifying their low income and thus effectively prevented their children from participating. To make matters worse, schools sometimes failed to protect the identity of low-income families. Also, the lack of uniform national standards for eligibility led to inequities. Without uniform guidelines, for example, a child's deportment or attendance record could influence the decision of local officials. Second, some schools refused to participate because they perceived the administrative tasks as being too demanding. Many communities chose not to participate and, instead, elected to reinforce the concept of the local school where children went home for lunch. Finally, some states diverted school lunch funds meant for needy children to other foodservice purposes or to programs for middle-income children.

Some of these concerns have been addressed over the last two decades. For example, in 1989 the law was changed so that schools can "directly certify as eligible" those children whose families participate in food stamp or Aid for Families with Dependent Children programs. Efforts to reduce paperwork and the demands on staff time have resulted in increased program participation. In 1992, 92,300 schools and residential child care institutions offered a school lunch. This figure represents about 95 percent of all public schools. About 59 percent of all public schoolchildren participate in the program. Of the 24.6 million children who ate a school lunch, 11.1 million received a free lunch, 1.8 million received a reduced-price lunch, and 11.7 received a "paid" lunch.

Does the Program Work?

In 1977, the U.S. General Accounting Office considered whether the school lunch program was working. Although the program had been operating for more than 30 years, no major studies of its effectiveness had been undertaken. The results of one study, published in 1984, showed that participating children from families at all income levels had superior nutrient intakes at lunch and higher total daily intakes than children who did not participate. In addition, the quality of the food

Continued

—Continued

was higher for program participants than for children who purchased their lunch from other vendors or brought their lunch from home. These findings have been confirmed by other researchers.[6]

Although evaluations have consistently shown that the National School Lunch Program makes a significant contribution to the daily nutrient and food intakes of participating children, there are concerns that school lunch meals are not as healthy as they might be. A recent USDA survey of 545 schools and 3,350 students found that 38 percent of calories in the average USDA school lunch came from fat, 15 percent of calories came from saturated fat, and the typical lunch contained 1,479 milligrams of salt. These intakes exceeded the USDA's recommendation that children consume no more than 30 percent of calories from fat, 10 percent of calories from saturated fat, and 800 milligrams of salt at lunch. On the positive side, the survey found that students who consumed the USDA school lunch exceeded the target goal of one-third the RDA for all vitamins and minerals. The typical school lunch also provided 95 percent of the RDA for protein. These findings led the USDA to call for a reduction in the amount of fat, saturated fat, and sodium in school lunches.[7]

Making a Good Program Better

The University of Minnesota School of Public Health, in cooperation with the Child Nutrition Section of the Minnesota Department of Education and foodservice directors from four school districts in Minnesota, developed a collaborative project designed to reduce the fat and sodium content of school lunch program lunches. Thirty-four elementary schools participated in the LUNCHPOWER! Healthy School Lunch program. The program materials included a manual for foodservice directors and a training video on rinsing ground beef. A variety of promotional materials were developed for the program, including the LUNCHPOWER! logo, shown at right. Participating schools significantly reduced the amount of total fat in their lunch menus, served lower-fat and lower-sodium meals, and retained students for the program. The LUNCHPOWER! school lunch program is now available from the Beef Industry Council.[8]

Toward a Universal School Lunch Program

In 1970, Senator McGovern and other policymakers argued that schools had the responsibility to provide food during the day in much the same way as they provide classroom facilities, free bus rides, and free textbooks. Their idea was to move the nation toward a universal school lunch program that would be available to all schoolchildren, regardless of income level. In 1975, Senator Hubert Humphrey introduced S. 3123, a bill to establish such a program. The proposal recognized schools as the proper delivery system for ensuring that all children have proper and adequate nourishment during the school day.[9]

Although no universal program exists today, nutritionists remain interested in the concept, according to the Food Research and Action Center. Indeed, mem-

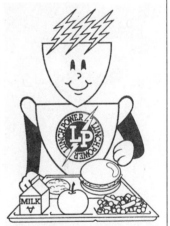

Guide to
LUNCHPOWER!
Healthy School Lunches

Courtesy of the Beef Industry Council.

Continued

—Continued

bers of the American School Food Service Association lobbied Congress to pass a bill that would allow all students to receive a free breakfast and lunch, regardless of their family income. The Universal Student Nutrition Act of 1993 (H.R. 11), introduced by Representative George Miller (D, California), would give schools the option of offering free meals to all students. Under this "universal" system, schools would not have to verify family income, thus reducing administrative work. If the bill is passed by Congress, the universal program would not be implemented fully until July 2000.[10]

1. The quotation was cited in J. E. Austin and C. Hitt, *Nutrition Intervention in the United States* (Cambridge, Mass.: Ballinger, 1979), p. 93.
2. *Food Assistance Programs—Food Program Facts* (Alexandria, Va.: Food and Nutrition Service, U.S. Department of Agriculture, Public Information Staff/News Branch, May 1993); *1993 Catalog of Federal Domestic Assistance* (Washington, D.C.: U.S. General Services Administration, 1993); and *Fact Sheets on the Federal Food Assistance Programs* (Washington, D.C.: Food Research and Action Center, May 1993).
3. Hearings before the Select Committee on Nutrition and Human Needs of the United States Senate, Part 8—Review of the National School Lunch Act (Washington, D.C.: U.S. Government Printing Office, October 13, 1970), pp. 2166–67.
4. Austin and Hitt, *Nutrition Intervention,* p. 91.
5. The description of the survey by Their Daily Bread was taken from the Senate Hearings, Part 8, p. 2121.
6. The description of the effectiveness of the School Lunch Program was adapted from Chapter III: Impact of hunger and malnutrition on student achievement, *School Food Service Research Review* 13 (1989): 17–21.
7. USDA uses school food report to blast meals' excessive fat, sodium, *Nutrition Week* 23 (October 29, 1993): 1, 3.
8. Some details related to the LUNCHPOWER! program were taken from M. P. Snyder and coauthors, Reducing fat and sodium in school lunch programs: The LUNCH-POWER! Intervention Study, *Journal of the American Dietetic Association* 92 (1992): 1087–91, and from personal communication with the senior author, M. Patricia Snyder, M.A., R.D. The Beef Industry Council is located in Chicago, IL.
9. Austin and Hitt, *Nutrition Intervention,* p. 119.
10. Meeting in Washington, school food advocates push for universal meals, *Nutrition Week* 23 (February 26, 1993): 1.

Head Start, public health departments, private clinics, university-based programs, or group homes.

Fortunately, nutrition care for these children has improved in recent years due to new legislation, increased involvement of various agencies, improved delivery of community-based programs, and better home health care. The dietetics community is committed to helping families and communities provide needed nutrition services for children with special health care needs. The American Dietetic Association outlined its position on the importance of providing nutrition services to persons with developmental disabilities, as shown at the top of the next page.

FIGURE

13-8

American Heart
Association's Doctor
Truso

Source: Reproduced with permission. © "The Case of the Sudden
Sickness! A Mystery for Doctor
Truso," 1977. Copyright American
Heart Association.

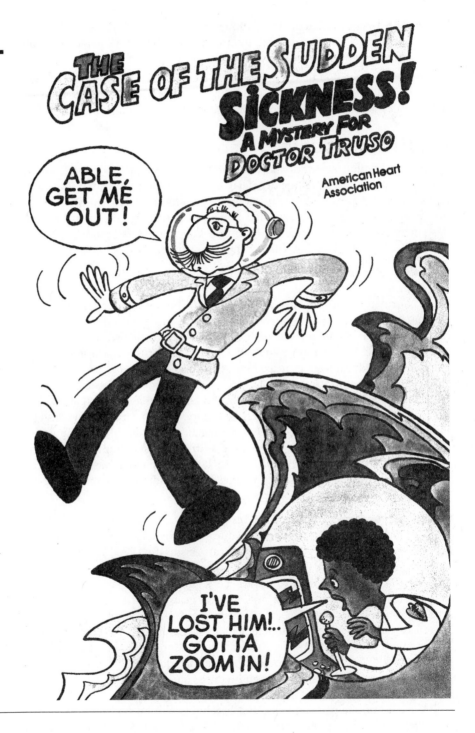

◆ The American Dietetic Association encourages and supports nutrition services which are coordinated, interdisciplinary, family centered, and community based for children with special health care needs.[79]

◆ It is the position of The American Dietetic Association that persons with developmental disabilities should receive comprehensive nutrition services as part of all health care, vocational, and educational programs.[80]

◆ NUTRITION EDUCATION PROGRAMS

Nutrition education strategies aimed at children or their caregivers are found in both the public and private sectors. They strive to increase nutrition knowledge and skills and improve eating patterns among children. Public nutrition education programs include the Expanded Food and Nutrition Education Program, described in Chapter 12, and the Nutrition Education and Training program, which is described here along with various private initiatives.

Nutrition Education and Training   The Nutrition Education and Training (NET) program was established in 1977 by P.L. 95–166, an amendment to the Child Nutrition Act of 1966; it is administered by the USDA's Food and Nutrition Service. NET's purpose is to disseminate scientifically valid information about diet and health to children participating or eligible to participate in school lunch and related child nutrition programs. NET funds are distributed through formula grants to state educational agencies for use by local schools and districts in providing nutrition-related training for teachers and school foodservice personnel. NET funds are also used to conduct nutrition education activities that use both the classroom and the school's foodservice facility. The NET program is designed to help children learn to apply the basic principles of healthful eating and good nutrition to their daily lives and to acquire a firm understanding of the relationship of good nutrition to good health. In 1992, 95,368 school foodservice personnel, 144,665 teachers, and nearly 7 million schoolchildren participated in NET-funded programs in 56 states and territories.

Nutrition Education in the Private Sector   Some voluntary, nonprofit health organizations have developed nutrition education programs or materials for children or their caregivers. The American Heart Association (AHA), for example, has a variety of Schoolsite Program modules for children in kindergarten through grade 12. Each module comes with a teacher's guide, learning and kickoff activities, videotape, and handouts for students, all geared to the appropriate grade level.[81] Figure 13-8 shows Doctor Truso in the AHA's comic book series. The American Cancer Society developed "Changing the Course," a comprehensive nutrition education program for students in kindergarten through grade 12. Changing the Course uses a video, together with handouts and overheads, to help students develop good eating habits and reduce cancer risk by eating more fruits and vegetables and less fat.[82]

A variety of books, pamphlets, and brochures written for children or their caregivers are available from the American Dietetic Association, the American Academy of Pediatrics, and other organizations. "Heart-Healthy Lessons for Children," for example, was developed by a registered dietitian for the Arizona

Heart Institute and Foundation. The lessons are designed to introduce elementary schoolchildren to easy lifestyle changes that reduce CHD risk; the lessons include games, puzzles, and a teacher's guide.[83]

Trade organizations likewise direct some of their nutrition education strategies to children. Brochures or booklets that describe good child feeding practices, outline tips for nutritious snacks, or answer questions about foods or ingredients are available from the National Live Stock and Meat Board, the National Dairy Council, and the Sugar Association, among others. An example of a classroom activity for schoolchildren, developed by the National Dairy Council, is shown in Figure 13-9. Puzzles, posters, and games designed to interest children in foods and nutrition can be purchased from such companies as NCES (Nutrition

---

Snacks give you energy to . . . ?

Color the picture and find out!

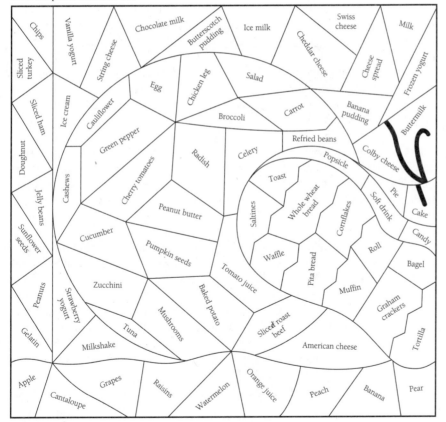

Coloring instructions:

Milk group snacks . . . . blue	Fruit group snacks . . . . green
Meat group snacks . . . . red	Grain group snacks . . . . . . brown
Vegetable group snacks . . . . orange	"Others" category snacks . . . don't color

FIGURE

13-9

An Example of a Classroom Nutrition Education Activity for Schoolchildren
Source: *Nutrition News,* Vol. 56, No. 2, Courtesy of NATIONAL DAIRY COUNCIL®.

Counseling and Education Services) and Nasco Nutrition Teaching Aids. McDonald's "FOOD FUNdamentals" is an example of a child-oriented nutrition education campaign launched by a food company.[84]

Keeping Children and Adolescents Healthy

Programs and services designed to keep children and adolescents healthy can have a lasting effect on the nation's public health. Healthy children and adolescents mean healthy communities. Children and youth who learn good eating habits, exercise regularly, refrain from smoking, learn to manage stress, and develop a strong sense of self are less likely to turn to drugs and alcohol to solve problems and more likely to know how to live constructively.

Successful, effective programs or services for children and youth recognize the stresses of life in the late twentieth century and the mixed media messages about products and values. Programs and services founded on basic health promotion principles must consider the urgent health issues facing today's young people: suicide, child abuse, teen pregnancy, eating disorders, substance abuse, and others. Positive nutrition messages support and expand on other health promotion concepts.

What types of programs work? Health educators in hospitals have found, for example, that programming for children and adolescents succeeds when it is fun and informative. One such program is the "Children's Story Hour and Super Snacks," sponsored by the Bay Hospital Medical Center in Chula Vista, California. Children participating in this program develop stories around food and prepare their own nutritious snacks.[85] Programs work best when they are geared to a specific health or nutritional objective, such as weight loss, improved eating patterns, or increased activity levels. Involving children and adolescents in the planning and implementation of a program increases its effectiveness, as does using peer support to help the participants make decisions about their health. Effective programs also employ trained staff who work well with these populations.

In the final analysis, developing programs and services that meet the needs of our nation's children and youth means recognizing that as today's children grow, they have to perform increasingly complex tasks in a world of constant technological and environmental change. Improving the health of today's young people will enhance the quality of their lives in the immediate future and expand their potential for contributing to our nation's future as adults. In promoting the health and well-being of children and youth, we are recognizing "that children matter for themselves, that childhood has its own intrinsic value, and that society has an obligation to enhance the lives of children today."[86]

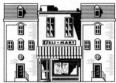

COMMUNITY LEARNING ACTIVITY

Let's assume that you are responsible for evaluating either the School Breakfast Program or Head Start (choose one).

1. What is the first step you would take in evaluating the program's effectiveness? Why did you begin at this point?

2. Describe the outcomes and indicators you would select to determine whether the program meets the needs of its clients. Why did you select these particular outcomes and indicators?

3. Let's assume that the program is *not* meeting the needs of its participants or the target population. What steps would you take to correct the situation as it relates to the following areas?

    a. Program delivery

    b. Policy

4. Describe one marketing strategy you would undertake to enhance program participation.

NOTES

1. P. A. Colón and A. R. Colón, The health of America's children, in *Caring for America's Children*, ed. F. J. Macchiarola and A. Gartner (New York: Academy of Political Science, 1989), pp. 45–57.

2. Report to the President, *White House Conference on Children* (Washington, D.C., 1970), p. 11.

3. U.S. Department of Health and Human Services, Public Health Service, *The Surgeon General's Report on Nutrition and Health* (Washington, D.C.: U.S. Government Printing Office, DHHS Pub. No. 88–50210, 1988), pp. 539–93.

4. U.S. Department of Health and Human Services, *Health United States 1991 and Prevention Profile* (Hyattsville, Md.: U.S. Department of Health and Human Services, 1992), pp. 78–80 and 93–98 and U.S. Department of Health and Human Services, Public Health Service, *Healthy People: The Surgeon General's Report on Health Promotion and Disease Prevention* (Washington, D.C.: U.S. Government Printing Office, PHS Pub. No. 79–55071, 1979).

5. U.S. Department of Health and Human Services, Public Health Service, *Healthy People 2000: National Health Promotion and Disease Prevention Objectives*

(Washington, D.C., 1990), pp. 114–34.

6. The general descriptions of child growth and development and nutrition assessment methods were adapted from E. N. Whitney and S. R. Rolfes, *Understanding Nutrition*, 6th ed. (St. Paul, Minn.: West Publishing Company, 1993), pp. 514–30 and E-1 to E-37.

7. Food and Nutrition Board, National Research Council, *Recommended Dietary Allowances*, 10th ed. (Washington, D.C.: National Academy Press, 1989), pp. 24–38.

8. Ibid., pp. 174–84.

9. M. Peacock, Calcium absorption efficiency and calcium requirements in children and adolescents, *American Journal of Clinical Nutrition* 54 (1991): 261S–65S.

10. Food and Nutrition Board, *Recommended Dietary Allowances*, pp. 195–205.

11. R. Yip and coauthors, Pediatric Nutrition Surveillance System—United States, 1980–1991, *Morbidity and Mortality Weekly Report* 41/No. SS–7 (November 27, 1992): 1–24.

12. P. C. DuRousseau and coauthors, Children in foster care: Are they at nutritional risk? *Journal of the American Dietetic Association* 91 (1991): 83–85, and M. L. Taylor and S. A. Koblinsky, Dietary intake and growth status of

young homeless children, *Journal of the American Dietetic Association* 93 (1993): 464–66.

13. ADA Reports, Position of The American Dietetic Association: Domestic hunger and inadequate access to food, *Journal of the American Dietetic Association* 90 (1990): 1437–41.

14. J. Dwyer and J. Arent, Child nutrition, in *Call to Action: Better Nutrition for Mothers, Children, and Families*, ed. C. O. Sharbaugh (Washington, D.C.: National Center for Education in Maternal and Child Health, 1991), pp. 151–68.

15. G. Kolata, Obese children: A growing problem, *Science* 232 (1986): 20–21.

16. I. G. Pawson and coauthors, Prevalence of overweight and obesity in US Hispanic populations, *American Journal of Clinical Nutrition* 53 (1991): 1522S–28S.

17. M. Knip and O. Nuutinen, Long-term effects of weight reduction on serum lipids and plasma insulin in obese children, *American Journal of Clinical Nutrition* 57 (1993): 490–93, and W. H. Dietz, Prevention of childhood obesity, *Pediatric Clinics of North America* 33 (1986): 823–33.

18. R. A. Behrens and M. E. Longe, *Hospital-Based Health Promotion Programs for Children and Youth* (Chicago: American Hospital Publishing, 1987), pp. 16–17.

19. Yip and coauthors, Pediatric Nutrition Surveillance System.

20. U.S. Department of Health and Human Services, Public Health Service, *Surgeon General's Report*, pp. 465–489.

21. Yip and coauthors, Pediatric Nutrition Surveillance System.

22. C. A. Miller and coauthors, *Monitoring Children's Health: Key Indicators* (Washington, D.C.: American Public Health Association, 1989), pp. 134–43.

23. F. L. Trowbridge and coauthors, Methodological issues in nutrition surveillance: The CDC experience, *Journal of Nutrition* 120 (1990): 1512–18.

24. Dwyer and Arent, Child nutrition.

25. U.S. Department of Health and Human Services, *Health United States 1991*, p. 78.

26. U.S. Department of Health and Human Services, Public Health Service, *Surgeon General's Report*, pp. 345–80.

27. National Cholesterol Education Program, *Report of the Expert Panel on Blood Cholesterol Levels in Children and Adolescents* (Washington, D.C.: U.S. Department of Health and Human Services, Public Health Service, National Institutes of Health, NIH Pub. No. 91-2732, 1991), pp. 1–22.

28. The description of anthropometric assessments of growth and body composition and the margin definitions were adapted from R. S. Gibson, *Principles of Nutritional Assessment* (New York: Oxford University Press, 1990), pp. 163–262.

29. Miller and coauthors, *Monitoring Children's Health*, pp. 70–77.

30. Yip and coauthors, Pediatric Nutrition Surveillance System.

31. As cited in Gibson, *Principles*, p. 175.

32. Yip and coauthors, Pediatric Nutrition Surveillance System.

33. Gibson, *Principles*, pp. 175–76.

34. Yip and coauthors, Pediatric Nutrition Surveillance System.

35. Gibson, *Principles*, pp. 173–74.

36. Ibid., pp. 172–73.

37. Yip and coauthors, Pediatric Nutrition Surveillance System.

38. F. Falkner, Measurement of health, in *Measurement in Health Promotion and Protection*, ed. T. Abelin, Z. J. Brzezinski, and V. D. L. Carstairs (Copenhagen: World Health Organization, 1987), pp. 109–22.

39. V. A. Casey and coauthors, Body mass index from childhood to middle age: A 50-y follow-up, *American Journal of Clinical Nutrition* 56 (1992): 14–18.

40. Health and Welfare Canada, *Canadian Guidelines for Healthy Weights* (Ottawa: Health Services and Promotion Branch, Health and Welfare Canada, 1988).

41. Gibson, *Principles*, pp. 189–93.

42. Sports and Cardiovascular Nutritionists, *Sports Nutrition: A Guide for the Professional Working with Active People* (Chicago: American Dietetic Association, 1986), pp. 3–33.

43. Gibson, *Principles*, pp. 200–202.

44. Miller and coauthors, *Monitoring Children's Health*, pp. 134–35.

45. Centers for Disease Control, CDC criteria for anemia in children and childbearing-aged women, *Morbidity and Mortality Weekly Report* 38 (1989): 400–404.

46. C. A. Finch and J. D. Cook, Iron deficiency, *American Journal of Clinical Nutrition* 39 (1984): 471–77.

47. National Cholesterol Education Program, *Report of the Expert Panel*.

48. The discussion of lead poisoning was adapted from Committee on Environmental Health, Lead poisoning: From screening to primary prevention, *Pediatrics* 92 (1993): 176–83; J. T. Kirchner and B. A. Kelley, Pediatric lead screening in a suburban family practice setting, *Journal of Family Practice* 32 (1991): 397–400; and Miller and coauthors, *Monitoring Children's Health*, pp. 78–88.

49. Whitney and Rolfes, *Understanding Nutrition*, p. 519.

50. J. T. Dwyer and coauthors, The problem of memory in

nutritional epidemiology research, *Journal of the American Dietetic Association* 87 (1987): 1509–12.

51. L. V. Van Horn and coauthors, Dietary assessment in children using electronic methods: Telephones and tape recorders, *Journal of the American Dietetic Association* 90 (1990): 412–16.

52. ADA Reports, Position of The American Dietetic Association: Nutrition services for children with special health care needs, *Journal of the American Dietetic Association* 89 (1989): 1133–37.

53. L. A. Wodarski, An interdisciplinary nutrition assessment and intervention protocol for children with disabilities, *Journal of the American Dietetic Association* 90 (1990): 1563–68.

54. C. N. Bianculli, Physical growth and development in adolescents, in *Health of Adolescents and Youths in the Americas* (Washington, D.C.: Pan American Health Organization, Scientific Pub. No. 489, 1985), pp. 45–50.

55. F. P. Heald, Nutrition in adolescence, in *Health of Adolescents and Youths in the Americas* (Washington, D.C.: Pan American Health Organization, Scientific Pub. No. 489, 1985), pp. 51–61.

56. M. Story and coauthors, Adolescent nutrition: Trends and critical issues for the 1990s, in *Call to Action: Better Nutrition for Mothers, Children, and Families,* ed. C. O. Sharbaugh (Washington, D.C.: National Center for Education in Maternal and Child Health, 1991), pp. 169–89.

57. L. W. Green and D. Horton, Adolescent health: Issues and challenges, in *Promoting Adolescent Health: A Dialog on Research and Practice,* ed. T. J. Coates, A. C. Petersen, and C. Perry (New York: Academic Press, 1982), pp. 23–43.

58. D. J. Sherman, The neglected health care needs of street youth, *Public Health Reports* 107 (1992): 433–40.

59. Story and coauthors, Adolescent nutrition.

60. Kolata, Obese children.

61. I. G. Pawson and coauthors, Prevalence of overweight and obesity in US Hispanic populations, *American Journal of Clinical Nutrition* 53 (1991): 1522S–28S.

62. U.S. Department of Health and Human Services, Public Health Service, *Surgeon General's Report,* pp. 539–93.

63. L. Brabin and B. J. Brabin, The cost of successful adolescent growth and development in girls in relation to iron and vitamin A status, *American Journal of Clinical Nutrition* 55 (1992): 955–58.

64. L. Hallberg and L. Rossander-Hultén, Iron requirements in menstruating women, *American Journal of Clinical Nutrition* 54 (1991): 1047–58.

65. Nutrition Monitoring Division, Human Nutrition Information Service, U.S. Department of Agriculture,

Nationwide Food Consumption Survey (Hyattsville, Md.: U.S. Department of Agriculture, Report No. 1–2, 85–3, and 86–1, 1977–1986).

66. National Cholesterol Education Program, *Report of the Expert Panel.*

67. U.S. Department of Health and Human Services, Public Health Service, *Healthy People 2000,* pp. 571–78.

68. Story and coauthors, Adolescent nutrition.

69. R. A. Thompson and R. T. Sherman, *Helping Athletes with Eating Disorders* (Champaign, Ill.: Human Kinetics Publishers, 1993).

70. National Cholesterol Education Program, *Report of the Expert Panel.*

71. T. J. Silber, Communicating with the adolescent patient, in *Health of Adolescents and Youths in the Americas* (Washington, D.C.: Pan American Health Organization, Scientific Pub. No. 489, 1985), pp. 37–44.

72. L. G. Bandini and coauthors, Validity of reported energy intake in obese and nonobese adolescents, *American Journal of Clinical Nutrition* 52 (1990): 421–25.

73. Information about specific nutrition programs, including participating levels, legislation, and participant eligibility, was adapted from *Food Assistance Programs—Food Program Facts* (Alexandria, Va.: Food and Nutrition Service, U.S. Department of Agriculture, Public Information Staff/News Branch, May 1993); *1993 Catalog of Federal Domestic Assistance* (Washington, D.C.: U.S. General Services Administration, 1993); and *Fact Sheets on the Federal Food Assistance Programs* (Washington, D.C.: Food Research and Action Center, May 1993).

74. Select Panel for the Promotion of Child Health, *Better Health for Our Children: A National Strategy,* vols. 1 and 2 (Washington, D.C.: U.S. Department of Health and Human Services, DHHS Pub. No. 79–55071, 1981).

75. Ibid., vol. 2, pp. 69–72.

76. ADA Reports, Nutrition services for children with special health care needs.

77. M. T. Baer and coauthors, Children with special health care needs, in *Call to Action: Better Nutrition for Mothers, Children, and Families,* ed. C. O. Sharbaugh (Washington, D.C.: National Center for Education in Maternal and Child Health, 1991), pp. 191–208.

78. S. Farnan, Role of nutrition in Crippled Children's Service agencies, *Topics in Clinical Nutrition* 3 (1988): 33–42, and Final Report, *Nutrition Programming for the Chronically Ill/Handicapped Child* (Birmingham, Ala.: Sparks Center for Developmental and Learning Disorders, University of Alabama, and Child Development Center, University of Tennessee Center for the Health Sciences, 1986).

79. ADA Reports, Nutrition services for children with special health care needs.

80. ADA Reports, Position of The American Dietetic Association: Nutrition in comprehensive program planning for persons with developmental disabilities, *Journal of the American Dietetic Association* 92 (1992): 613–15.

81. American Heart Association Schoolsite Program (Dallas: National Center, American Heart Association).

82. American Cancer Society "Changing the Course" Program (Minneapolis: Minnesota Division, American Cancer Society).

83. A description of the "Heart-Healthy Lessons for Children" program can be found in the *Journal of the American Dietetic Association* 92 (1992): 1558.

84. The American Dietetic Association and McDonald's Corporation, Partnership Kit (St. Charles, IL: McDonald's Educational Resource Center, 1993).

85. Behrens and Longe, *Hospital-Based Health Promotion Programs*.

86. Select Panel for the Promotion of Child Health, vol. 1, p. 2.

Growing Older: Nutrition Assessment, Services, and Programs

Something to Think About . . .

How far you go in life depends on your being tender with the young, compassionate with the aged, sympathetic with the striving, and tolerant of the weak and the strong. Because someday in life you will have been all of these.

—George Washington Carver

Introduction

It is easy to get the impression from mortality statistics that people are living longer and longer lives, but this is not the case. Certainly, the *average* age at death (life expectancy) has changed dramatically. Life expectancy at birth is now 74.8 years—most men die at a little past 71, and most women die at a little past 78.[1] On the other hand, the *maximum* age at which people die—that is, the *maximum life span*—has changed very little. It seems that the aging phenomenon cuts off life at a rather fixed point in time.

To what extent is aging inevitable? Apparently, aging is an inevitable, natural process programmed into our genes at conception. Nevertheless, we can adopt lifestyle habits, such as consuming a healthful diet, exercising, and paying attention to our work and recreational environments, that will slow the process within the natural limits set by heredity. Clearly, good nutrition can retard and ease the aging process in many significant ways. However, no potions, foods, or pills will prolong youth. People who claim to have found the fountain of youth have been selling its waters for centuries, but products purporting to prevent aging profit only the sellers, not the buyers.

One approach to the prevention of aging has been to study other cultures in the hope of finding an extremely long-lived people and then learning their secrets of long life. The views of the experts can best be summed up by saying that disease can *shorten* people's lives and that poor nutrition practices make diseases more likely to occur. Thus, by postponing and slowing disease processes, optimal nutrition can help to prolong life up to the maximum life span—but cannot extend it further.[2] This chapter focuses on the nutrient requirements of older adults, the diseases that seem to come with age, their risk factors, and the relevance of nutrition to them; it also examines the programs and services that target older adults for health promotion and disease prevention. We begin with a look at the demographic trends characteristic of this segment of the population and the national nutrition and health goals for improving the quality of life of Americans as they age.

Technically, the life span is the oldest documented age to which a member of a given species is known to have survived. For humans, this is about 113 years.

454

Demographic Trends and Aging

The number of elderly (aged 65 years and older) in the United States will double by 2030 to more than 65 million people. In 1988, the elderly accounted for 12.4 percent of the population, and this proportion is expected to rise to approximately 14 percent in 2010 and to nearly 22 percent by 2030. Nearly 12 percent of the population will be over age 74 by 2030. As Figure 14-1 shows, all age groups among elderly men and women in the United States are growing.[3]

Both the baby boom that took place between 1946 and 1964 and improved life expectancy are important contributors to the growing elderly population in the United States. Baby boomers will increase the numbers of the older middle-

Researchers and marketing analysts have struggled to find a useful way to segment—and, therefore, target—the elderly market. One frequently used segmentation divides the elderly into the "mature," aged 55–64; the "young-old," aged 65–74; and the "old-old," over age 74.

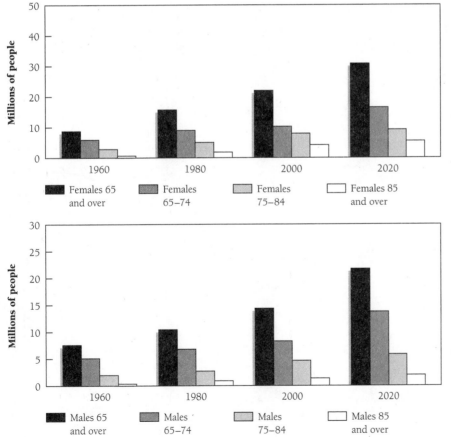

FIGURE

14-1

The Growing Population of Elderly Men and Women in the United States by Age Group (Projected)

Source: Reprinted from *Geriatric Nutrition: The Health Professional's Handbook* by R. Chernoff, p. 4, with permission of Aspen Publishers, Inc., © 1991.

aged (ages 46 through 63) until 2010, when they will begin to swell the ranks of the retired population.[4]

Life expectancy has risen as a result of better prenatal and postnatal care and improved means of combating disease in older adults. For example, the death rate from heart disease began to decline in the 1960s and continues to fall today. Over half of the drop is attributed to a decline in smoking and fewer people with high blood pressure or high blood cholesterol. As Figure 14-2 illustrates, life expectancy at birth has increased dramatically for both men and women and for both whites and nonwhites since 1900. The longer a person lives, too, the longer he or she is expected to live (see Table 14-1).

Policymakers and others concerned with meeting the health needs of older adults are alert to the implications of these demographic changes because the elderly tend to consume a large amount of total health care and long-term care resources. Consider that persons aged 65 years and over are just over 12 percent of the total population today—some 30 million men and women—yet they account for more than:[5]

◆ 30 percent of the country's health care costs,

◆ 25 percent of the prescription drugs used,

◆ 15 percent of all visits to doctors' offices, and

◆ 40 percent of all days in acute-care hospitals.

FIGURE

14-2

Life Expectancies at Birth, by Race and Sex, for the United States, 1900–1990

Source: National Center for Health Statistics, *Health United States and Prevention Profile, 1991* (Washington, D.C.: U.S. Department of Health and Human Services, 1991).

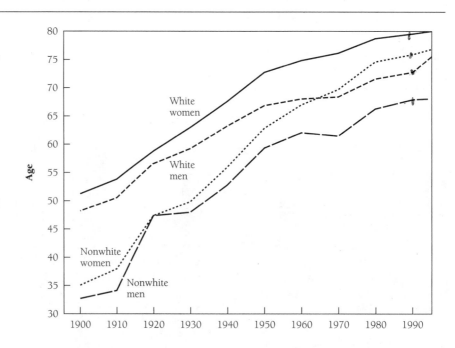

AGE, SEX, AND RACE	REMAINING LIFE EXPECTANCY IN YEARS[a]			
	1960[b]	1970	1980	1989
White male:				
At 65 years	12.9	13.1	14.2	15.2
At 85 years	4.4	5.2	5.0	5.3
Black male:				
At 65 years	12.7	12.5	13.0	13.6
At 85 years	5.7	5.9	4.5	5.6
White female:				
At 65 years	15.9	17.1	18.4	19.0
At 85 years	4.9	5.9	6.3	6.5
Black female:				
At 65 years	15.1	15.7	16.8	17.0
At 85 years	6.2	7.0	6.1	6.7

[a]From 1960 to 1989, life expectancy at age 65 was highest for white females, followed by black females, white males, and black males. In 1989, life expectancy at age 85 showed a crossover in that for each sex, life expectancy was higher for black than for white persons. This crossover also occurred in 1960 and 1970.
[b]Includes deaths of nonresidents of the United States.

TABLE

14-1

Life Expectancy at Specified Ages, by Race and Sex
Source: National Center for Health Statistics. *Vital Statistics of the United States,* Vol. 2 (Washington, D.C.: U.S. Department of Health and Human Services, 1992).

With the "graying of America," these health care demands can only increase. As Joseph A. Califano, a former secretary of health and human services, testified before the Committee on a National Research Agenda on Aging:

> The aging of America will challenge all our political, retirement, and social service systems. As never before, it will test our commitment to decent human values. Nowhere is the aging of America freighted with more risk and opportunity than in the area of health care.[6]

National Goals for Health Promotion

An individual's current health profile is substantially determined by behavioral risk factors. The leading causes of death for adults aged 25 through 64 are cancer, heart disease, stroke, injuries, chronic lung disease, and liver disease; all have been associated with behavioral risk factors. Thus, many adults today would benefit from changes in their lifestyle behaviors. For example, incorporating exercise and a balanced, low-fat diet into one's lifestyle can contribute to weight loss and to controlling three important risk factors for heart disease—high fat intake, overweight, and a sedentary lifestyle.

The most important goal of health promotion and disease prevention for adults as they age is maintaining health and functional independence. Many of the health problems associated with the later years are preventable or can be controlled.[7] For example, changing certain risk behaviors into healthy ones can improve the quality of life for older persons and lessen their risk of disability. Improvements in diet and nutrition status and weight control can enhance the health of older adults as well as help control risk factors for disease in middle-aged and younger adults. The *Surgeon General's Report on Nutrition and Health* demonstrates how the same set of dietary recommendations can both promote general health and help prevent a broad spectrum of chronic diseases.[8] As Figure 14-3 shows, these basic dietary recommendations reduce the risk of a variety of chronic diseases or their complications. The accompanying box presents the key national health objectives for the year 2000 that focus on improving the health of adults as they age.[9]

The first major effort to develop national policies to reduce chronic disease risk factors in older adults took place during the Surgeon General's Workshop on Health Promotion and Aging in 1988. The workshop issued several major nutrition policy recommendations for promoting the health of older adults that are related to dietary guidance and nutrition services (see Table 14-2 on page 461).[10]

Efforts at health promotion and disease prevention are conducted at several levels. *Primary* prevention efforts seek to prevent the occurrence of a disease in susceptible people by decreasing their risks for the disease, typically through behavior modification. Examples include the promotion of healthful behaviors such as stopping smoking, improved dietary behaviors, and regular physical activity. The goal of *secondary* prevention is to detect and treat a disease in its early stages. Health fairs offering blood pressure and cholesterol screening are an example of this type of prevention. *Tertiary* prevention seeks to minimize the disabling effects of a disease once it occurs. Rehabilitative services such as physical and occupational therapies are an example of this level of prevention. Thus,

---

FIGURE

14-3

Consistency of Recommendations for Reducing the Risk of Chronic Diseases or Their Complications
Source: J. M. McGinnis and M. Nestle, The Surgeon General's Report on nutrition and health: Policy implications and implementation strategies, *American Journal of Clinical Nutrition* 49 (1989): 26. © American Society for Clinical Nutrition.

Change diet → / Reduce risk ↓	Reduce fats	Control calories	Increase starch & fiber	Reduce sodium	Control alcohol
Heart disease	🍎	🍎		🍎	
Cancer	🍎	🍎	🍎		🍎
Stroke	🍎	🍎		🍎	🍎
Diabetes	🍎	🍎	🍎		
Gastrointestinal diseases	🍎	🍎	🍎		🍎

Starch refers to complex carbohydrates provided by fruits, vegetables, and whole-grain products. Gastrointestinal diseases affected by dietary factors are primarily gallbladder disease (fat and energy), diverticular disease (fiber), and cirrhosis of the liver (alcohol).

Healthy People 2000 Objectives

◆ **Health status objectives:**

◆ Reduce coronary heart disease deaths to no more than 100/100,000 people. (Baseline: 135/100,000 in 1987.)

◆ Reverse the rise in cancer deaths to achieve a rate of no more than 130/100,000. (Baseline: 133/100,000 in 1987.)

◆ Reduce overweight to a prevalence of no more than 20 percent among people aged 20 and older. (Baseline: 26 percent for people aged 20 through 74 in 1976–1980; for men, 24 percent; for women, 27 percent.)

◆ Reduce to no more than 90/1000 people the proportion of all people aged 65 and older who have difficulty performing two or more personal care activities, thereby preserving independence.* (Baseline: 111/1000 in 1984–1985.)

◆ **Risk-reduction objectives:**

◆ Increase to at least 30 percent the proportion of people aged 6 and older who engage regularly, preferably daily, in light to moderate physical activity for at least 30 minutes per day. (Baseline: 22 percent of people over 18 years were active for at least 30 minutes five or more times per week in 1985.)

◆ Reduce dietary fat intake to an average of 30 percent of calories or less and average saturated fat intake to less than 10 percent of calories among people aged 2 years and older. (Baseline: 36 percent of calories from total fat and 13 percent from saturated fat for people aged 20 through 74 in 1976–1980.)

◆ Increase complex-carbohydrate and fiber-containing foods in the diets of adults to 5 or more daily servings for vegetables (including legumes) and fruits, and to 6 or more daily servings for grain products. (Baseline: $2^1/_2$ servings of vegetables and fruits and 3 servings of grain products for women aged 19 through 50 in 1985.)

◆ Increase to at least 50 percent the proportion of overweight people aged 12 and older who have adopted sound dietary practices combined with regular physical activity to attain an appropriate body weight. (Baseline: 30 percent of overweight women and 25 percent of overweight men for people aged 18 and older in 1985.)

◆ Increase to at least 85 percent the proportion of people 18 years of age or older who use food labels to make nutritious food selections. (Baseline: 74 percent used labels in 1988.)

◆ **Services and protection objectives:**

◆ Increase to at least 90 percent the proportion of restaurants and institutional foodservice operations that offer identifiable low-fat, low-calorie food choices, consistent with the *Dietary Guidelines for Americans*. (Baseline: About 70 percent of fast-food and family restaurant chains with 350 or more units had at least one low-fat, low-calorie item on their menu in 1989.)

Continued

—Continued

- ◆ Increase to at least 80 percent the receipt of home foodservices by people aged 65 and older who have difficulty in preparing their own meals or are otherwise in need of home-delivered meals.
- ◆ Increase to at least 50 percent the proportion of worksites with 50 or more employees that offer nutrition education and/or weight-management programs for employees. (Baseline: 17 percent offered nutrition education activities, and 15 percent offered weight-control activities in 1985.)

*Personal care activities are bathing, dressing, using the toilet, getting in or out of bed or chair, and eating.

Source: Adapted from *Healthy People 2000: National Health Promotion and Disease Prevention* (Washington, D.C.: U.S. Department of Health and Human Services, Public Health Service, 1990), pp. 588–89, 611–13.

---

health promotion activities are designed to help adults of all ages change their eating patterns and other behaviors to reduce the risk of chronic disease.

Aging and Nutrition Status

Growing old is often associated with frailty, sickness, and a loss of vitality. Although the aging in our society do experience chronic illness and associated disabilities, this population is very heterogeneous: older people vary greatly in their social, economic, and lifestyle situations, functional capacity, and physical conditions.[11] Each person ages at a different rate, sometimes making chronologic age different from biologic age. Most older persons live at home (see Figure 14-4 on page 462), are fully independent, and have lives of good quality.[12] Only 5 to 6 percent of older adults live in nursing homes.[13] Older persons who have problems with the **activities of daily living (ADLs)** are known as the frail elderly. Because they depend on others to perform these essential activities, they are likely to be at risk for malnutrition.[14]

ADLs Activities of daily living include bathing, dressing, grooming, transferring from bed to chair, going to the bathroom, being continent, and feeding oneself.

◆ NUTRITIONAL NEEDS AND INTAKES

Many of the nutrient needs of older adults are the same as for younger persons, but some special considerations deserve emphasis. Energy needs decline with age because of a decrease in basal metabolism related to loss of lean tissue and a decrease in physical activity. The RDA for energy intake is lower for adults, beginning at age 51. Given their limited energy allowances, older adults are advised to select mostly nutrient-dense foods.

Water recommendation for adults: 1 to 1 1/2 oz/kg actual body weight.

Perhaps the most important nutrient of all is *water.* Older adults need to be reminded to take in fluids because they are likely to be somewhat insensitive to their own thirst signals. They should take in six to eight glasses of fluid a day.

Dietary guidance for older adults should:

◆ Target messages to the special concerns of this population.
◆ Emphasize the need for food intake and physical activity sufficient to meet nutrient requirements and maintain appropriate body weight.
◆ Promote general dietary guidelines to consume more fruits, vegetables, and grains, but to choose lean meats and low-fat dairy products.
◆ Address drug-nutrient interactions.
◆ Become integrated into the training of physicians, dietitians, and other health professionals.

Nutrition services should be:

◆ Structured to include nutrition assessment and guidance.
◆ Incorporated into institutional-, community-, or home-based health care programs for older adults.
◆ Tailored to the needs of older people who are homebound, live in isolation, or are chronically ill.
◆ Provided by credentialed nutrition professionals.

Food manufacturers should:

◆ Develop easy-to-prepare, tasty food products that have a high proportion of nutrients to calories.
◆ Use food labels set in larger type that provide sufficient information to guide older consumers.

The federal government should:

◆ Disseminate information about model programs that have successfully delivered nutrition education and services to older adults.
◆ Require its sponsored programs to address the caloric and nutrient needs of older participants.
◆ Promote research and surveillance programs to improve nutrition status.
◆ Develop a system for appropriate funding for nutrition services delivered to older people.

TABLE

14-2

Surgeon General's Nutrition Policy Recommendations for Health Promotion in Older Adults

Source: M. Nestle and J. A. Gilbride, Nutrition policies for health promotion in older adults: Education priorities for the 1990s. Reprinted with permission, *Journal of Nutrition Education* 22 (1990): 316, Society for Nutrition Education.

At present, the Committee on Dietary Allowances does not provide separate RDAs for the various categories of older adults (e.g., mature, young-old, old-old). Rather, all people over 50 are grouped together. Some nutritionists think the recommended intakes of some of the vitamins—vitamins D, B_6, and B_{12}—are too low for the over-65 group.[15] The elderly absorb vitamins B_6 and B_{12} less efficiently and therefore may need to increase their intake. People's needs for these and other nutrients may change as aging progresses. Some practitioners recommend supplements, particularly for the water-soluble vitamins. Other nutritionists, however, say that until more appropriate age-specific RDAs are established, the current RDAs should continue to be used as standards for healthy older persons.[16]

These nutritionists argue that recommending supplements often makes the elderly vulnerable to exploitation by quacks and that their money is better spent on nutrient-dense foods. Surveys designed to find out what kinds of nutrient supplements older people are using tend to support the view that, in many cases,

The RDA for older adults are shown inside the front cover.

The Canadian RNI divide older people into two age groups—50 to 74, and 75 and older.

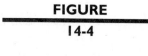

FIGURE

14-4

Living Arrangements of Older Adults by Age and Sex

Source: Adapted from E. L. Schneider and J. M. Guralank, The aging of America: Impact of health-care costs, *Journal of the American Medical Association* 263 (1990): 2335–40.

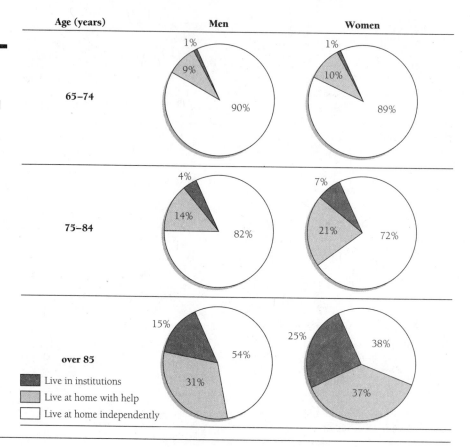

older people are wasting their money. A study in a Southern California retirement community showed that 72 percent of the subjects were taking nutrient supplements—mostly of vitamins C and E—but that these choices were not related to the users' dietary intakes; that is, they were not appropriate.[17] The older person would probably be wise to follow the rule of thumb that if food energy intake is below about 1500 calories, a vitamin-mineral supplement is recommended—just a once-daily type of supplement, not the megavitamin kind.

Table 14-3 shows a recommended eating pattern that would supply the amounts of food energy recommended by the RDA tables. Because overweight is recognized as a shortener of the life span, these seem to be life-sustaining recommendations. Clearly, an adequate intake of nutrients and fiber from a variety of foods throughout life, together with moderate intakes of food energy and fat, helps immensely to promote good health in the later years.

◆ PRIMARY NUTRITION-RELATED PROBLEMS

Although aging is not completely understood, we know that it involves progressive changes in every body tissue and organ: the brain, heart, lungs, digestive tract, and bones (see Table 14-4). After age 35, functional capacity declines in

FOOD GROUP/ SERVINGS PER DAY	EQUIVALENT SERVING SIZES
Milk 2–3+*	1 c milk, yogurt, custard, pudding, soft-serve ice cream, or frozen yogurt; $1\frac{1}{2}$ oz cheese; $1\frac{1}{2}$ c cream soup made with milk; 2 c cottage cheese, regular ice cream, or ice milk
Meat/substitute 2–3*	2–3 oz lean meat or fish (a piece the size of a deck of cards) or 2 eggs; 1 chicken breast or leg and thigh; 2–3 oz cheese; $\frac{1}{2}$–$\frac{3}{4}$ c cottage cheese, tuna, other flaked meat or fish; 1–$1\frac{1}{2}$ c dried beans or peas; 4–6 tbsp peanut butter; 2–3 slices low-fat cold cuts
Fruit 2+	$\frac{1}{2}$–$\frac{3}{4}$ c (1 piece) citrus or other vitamin C–source fruit
Vegetables 3–5+	$\frac{1}{2}$–1 c dark green/deep yellow vegetables
Bread/cereals 6+	1 slice whole-grain or enriched bread; $\frac{1}{2}$ bun, bagel, English muffin; $\frac{1}{2}$ c rice, pasta, cooked cereal; 1 c cold cereal; 3–6 crackers*
Fats/sweets As needed for calories	not applicable
Alcohol In moderation	not applicable

*Lower-fat, lower-calorie items are recommended.

TABLE

14-3

Recommended Eating Pattern for Older People
Source: Reprinted with permission by the Nutrition Screening Initiative, a project of the American Academy of Family Physicians, The American Dietetic Association, and the National Council on Aging, Inc. and funded in part by a grant from Ross Laboratories, a division of Abbott Laboratories.

almost every organ system. Such changes affect nutrition status: some, including oral problems, interfere with nutrient intake; others affect absorption, storage, and utilization of nutrients; and still others increase the excretion of, and need for, specific nutrients.[18] Examples of various conditions associated with aging that can affect nutrition status include sensory impairments, altered endocrine, gastrointestinal, and cardiovascular functions, and changes in the renal and musculoskeletal systems. Both genetic and environmental factors contribute to these declines.[19] Many of the changes are inevitable, but a healthful lifestyle that combines moderation with adequate intakes of all essential nutrients can forestall degeneration and improve the quality of life into the later years.

As a person gets older, the chances of suffering a chronic illness or functional impairment are greater. Among the diseases that befall some people in later life are heart disease, hypertension, cancer, diverticulosis, osteoporosis, dementia, diabetes, and gum disease. More than 60 percent of people over age 65 have high blood pressure, and approximately 30 percent have heart disease. Chronic conditions contributing to **disability** include arthritis, heart disease, strokes, disorders of vision and hearing, nutritional deficiencies, and oral-dental problems (see Figure 14-5). Dementia (especially Alzheimer's disease) is a major contributor to disability and placement in nursing homes for those over age 75.[20] Malnutrition can occur secondary to these conditions, as noted in Table 14-5 on page 466.[21] Many of these conditions require special diets that can further compromise nutrition status in the older adult.

Disability Any restriction on or impairment in performing an activity in the manner or within the range considered normal for a human being.

TABLE

14-4

Changes in Biologic Function between the Ages of 30 and 70

Source: E. L. Smith and coauthors, Physical activity prescription for the older adult, *The Physician and Sportsmedicine* 11 (1983): 92. Reprinted by permission of McGraw-Hill, Inc.

BIOLOGIC FUNCTION	CHANGE
Work capacity (%)	↓25–30
Cardiac output (%)	↓30
Maximum heart rate (beats min^{-1})	↓24
Blood pressure (mm Hg)	
Systolic	↑10–40
Diastolic	↑ 5–10
Respiration (%)	
Vital capacity	↓40–50
Residual volume	↑30–50
Basal metabolic rate (%)	↓ 8–12
Musculature (%)	
Muscle mass	↓25–30
Hand grip strength	↓25–30
Nerve conduction velocity (%)	↓10–15
Flexibility (%)	↓20–30
Bone (%)	
Women	↓25–30
Men	↓15–20
Renal function (%)	↓30–50

Polypharmacy The taking of three or more medications regularly; occurs in one-third of those over 65 years.

Polypharmacy, or the use of multiple drugs, is problematic for many older adults. Table 14-6 lists the drugs most commonly used by the elderly and their nutritional side effects.[22] The average older person receives more than 13 prescriptions a year and may take as many as six drugs at a time. Cardiac drugs are most widely used by the elderly, followed by drugs to treat arthritis, psychic disorders, and respiratory and gastrointestinal conditions. Long-term use of a variety of drugs increases the risk of drug-nutrient interactions. Individuals with impaired nutrition status and poor dietary intakes are at the highest risk.[23]

Individually or in combination, the social, economic, psychological, cultural, and environmental factors associated with aging may interact with the physiological changes and further affect nutrition status in older adults. These interactions are illustrated in Figure 14-6 on page 468.[24]

Evaluation of Nutrition Status

Up to one-quarter of all elderly patients and one-half of all hospitalized elderly may be suffering from malnutrition.[25] In addition, a national survey in 1990 found that one-third of noninstitutionalized Americans over the age of 65 live alone, 45 percent take multiple prescription drugs that can interfere with appetite and nutrient absorption, 30 percent skip meals almost daily, and 25 percent have annual incomes under $10,000—all factors placing elderly people at potential for nutritional risk.[26] Identifying older adults at nutritional risk is an important first step in maintaining quality of life and functional status.[27] The

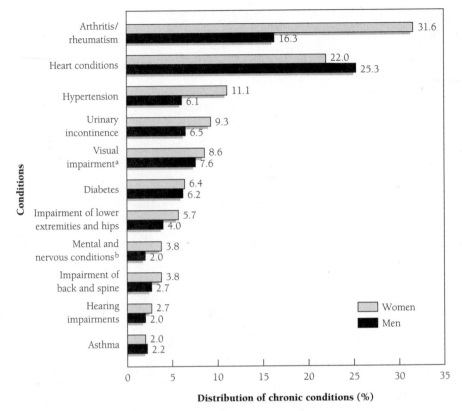

FIGURE

14-5

Distribution of Chronic Conditions That Cause Disability in People over Age 65 Years

Source: Reprinted from *Geriatric Nutrition: The Health Professional's Handbook* by R. Chernoff, p. 457, with permission of Aspen Publishers, Inc., © 1991.

a Cataracts.
b Rate for depression 147/1000. Rate for Alzheimer's disease 112/1000 (5% to 10% > age 65 years; 35% > age 85 years).

1988 Surgeon General's Workshop on Health Promotion and Aging recommended that a nutrition assessment be completed on all older adults admitted to health care institutions or community-based health services.[28] This recommendation is similar to those proposed by the American Dietetic Association (ADA) in its position paper on nutrition and aging. The ADA recommends that nutrition services including nutrition assessment and monitoring, therapeutic interventions as needed, and nutrition counseling and education be included throughout the continuum of health care services for older adults.[29] A discussion of the guidelines and tools for nutrition screening and assessment of older adults follows in the next two sections.

◆ NUTRITION SCREENING

The American Dietetic Association, the American Academy of Family Physicians, and the National Council on Aging collaborated in 1990 on a five-year effort to promote nutrition screening and early intervention as part of routine health care.

TABLE

14-5

Malnutrition That Is Secondary to Disease, Physiologic State, or Medication Use

Source: Adapted from Institute of Medicine, *The Second Fifty Years: Promoting Health and Preventing Disability* (Washington, D.C.: National Academy Press, 1992), pp. 168–69.

DISEASE OR CONDITION	EFFECTS ON NUTRITION STATUS
Atherosclerosis	May increase difficulties in regulating fluid balances if caused by congestive heart failure. If the individual is incapacitated, energy needs decrease.
Cancer	Weight loss, lack of appetite, and secondary malnutrition are common.
Dental and oral disease	May alter the ability to chew and thus reduce dietary intake. Increased likelihood of choking and aspiration.
Depression and dementia	Increased or decreased food intakes are common. A person with dementia may have decreased ability to get food, or the appetite may be very small or very great. Judgment and balance in meal planning are generally absent.
Diabetes mellitus (insulin-dependent)	If untreated, increased risk of undernutrition results; increased risk of other diet-related diseases, such as hyperlipidemia, and decreased resistance to infections.
Diabetes mellitus (non-insulin-dependent)	Increased risk of other diet-related diseases such as hyperlipidemia; weight loss is needed if obesity is present.
End-stage kidney disease	Alters fluid and electrolyte needs; uremia may alter appetite and increase risk of malnutrition. Infections and low-grade fever may increase energy output and weight loss.
Gastrointestinal disorders	Increased risk of malabsorption of nutrients and consequent undernutrition.
High blood pressure	Hyper- or hypokalemia can be increased by dietary means; weight gain may exacerbate high blood pressure.
Osteoarthritis	Makes motion difficult, including those activities related to purchasing, serving, eating, and cleaning up after meals. Predisposes people to a sedentary lifestyle and may give rise to obesity. Drug-nutrient relationships are common.
Osteoporosis	Limits the ability to purchase and prepare food if mobility is affected. If severe scoliosis is present, the appetite may be altered.
Smoking	Smoking may alter weight status. Alters serum levels of some nutrients such as ascorbic acid and carotenes. Chronic smoking gives rise to emphysema and chronic obstructive pulmonary diseases (COPD), which makes it difficult to eat owing to breathing problems.
Stroke	May alter abilities in the cognitive and motor realms related to food and eating. If the individual is incapacitated, his or her energy needs decrease.

Its initial focus is on the elderly, one of the largest population groups in the United States at risk of poor nutrition.

The Nutrition Screening Initiative has identified a number of specific risk factors and indicators of poor nutrition status in older adults (see Tables 14-7 and 14-8 on pages 469–470). Some of the risk factors shown in Table 14-7 increase the risks for dietary inadequacy, excess, or imbalance and involve social, economic, and lifestyle factors rather than physical health problems. Others indicate risks

DRUG	NUTRITIONAL SIDE EFFECTS
◆ **Drugs influencing appetite and food intake:**	
Antipsychotics and sedatives	Somnolence; disinterest in food
Digoxin	Marked anorexia; nausea; vomiting; weakness
Cancer chemotherapies	Nausea; vomiting; aversion to food
◆ **Drugs affecting absorption of nutrients:**	
Laxatives and cathartics	Malabsorption of fat-soluble vitamins; fluid and electrolyte loss
Corticosteroids	Decreased vitamin D activity
Anticonvulsants	Decreased vitamin D activity
H_2 receptor blockers	Vitamin B_{12} malabsorption
Aluminum or magnesium antacids	Phosphate depletion
Cholestyramine	Decreased absorption of lipids, folate, iron, vitamin B_{12}, and fat-soluble vitamins; gastro-intestinal side effects
◆ **Drugs affecting metabolism of nutrients:**	
Isoniazid, hydralazine, L-dopa	Vitamin B_6 antagonists
Salicylates	Iron loss secondary to gastrointestinal bleeding
Anticoagulants	Vitamin K antagonists
◆ **Drugs affecting excretion of nutrients:**	
Thiazides	Loss of potassium, sodium, magnesium, and zinc
Furosemide	Loss of potassium, magnesium, chloride, sodium, and water
Spironolactone	Potassium sparing; hyperkalemia; fluid and electrolyte changes

TABLE

14-6

Nutritional Side Effects of Drugs Commonly Used by the Elderly
Source: J. E. Kerstetter, B. A. Holthausen, and P. A. Fitz, Malnutrition in the institutionalized older adult. Copyright The American Dietetic Association. Reprinted by permission from *Journal of the American Dietetic Association* 92 (1992): 1113.

of malnutrition secondary to disease and/or treatment modalities rather than those caused primarily by lack of food.[30]

A key premise of the Nutrition Screening Initiative is that nutrition status is a "vital sign"—as vital to health assessment as blood pressure and pulse rate.[31] The Nutrition Screening Initiative has developed a ten-question self-assessment "checklist" that can be distributed at any office or agency for the elderly (see Figure 14-7 on page 471). Individuals identify factors placing them at nutritional risk to arrive at their score. This checklist addresses disease, eating status, tooth loss or mouth pain, economic hardship, reduced social contact, multiple medications, involuntary weight loss or gain, and need for assistance with self-care. The word DETERMINE is used as a mnemonic device with the checklist and helps to provide basic nutrition information (see Figure 14-8 on page 472). Each initial letter in DETERMINE stands for a risk factor.[32] As Figure 14-9 (on page 473) shows, people identified as being at risk should be followed up with more in-depth screening of risk factors and assessment of nutrition status (Level I or Level II screens) by a health professional (see Table 14-9 on page 474).

The Level I screen is a basic nutrition screen designed for social service and health professionals to use to identify older adults who may need medical attention or nutrition services. This screen includes determinations of height and weight and charts to convert these measures to body mass index (BMI). The

BMI = wt (kg)/ht (m)²

FIGURE
14-6

Factors Influencing the Nutrition Status of Older Adults

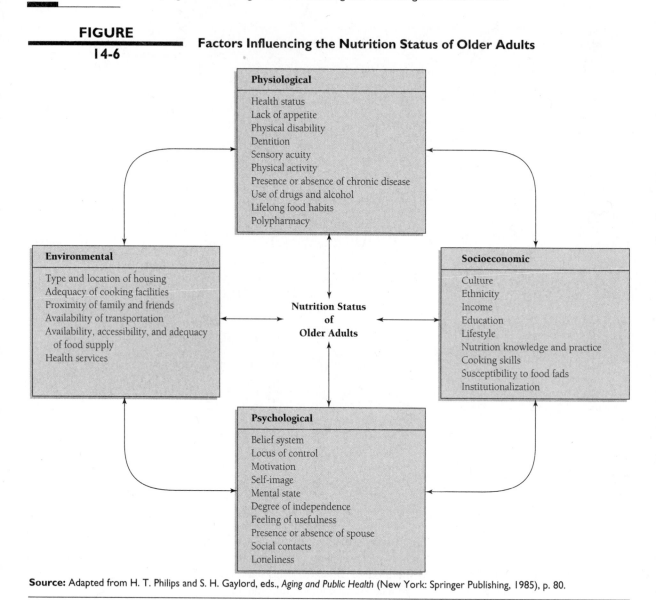

Source: Adapted from H. T. Philips and S. H. Gaylord, eds., *Aging and Public Health* (New York: Springer Publishing, 1985), p. 80.

Examples of the Nutrition Screening Initiative's in-depth assessments are provided in Appendix E.

Level I screen also evaluates eating habits and provides a brief review of socioeconomic and functional status.

The Level II screen provides more specific diagnostic information on nutrition status. It is designed for health and medical professionals to use with older adults who have a potentially serious medical or nutritional problem. This in-depth screening tool focuses on the components of nutrition assessment: anthropometric indicators (e.g., weight, height, body composition); clinical indicators (e.g., oral health and general physical exam); biochemical indicators (e.g., serum albumin, serum cholesterol, hemoglobin, plasma glucose); and dietary indicators

Inappropriate food intake
- Meal/snack frequency
- Quantity/quality:
  Milk/milk products
  Meat/meat substitutes
  Fruit/vegetables
  Bread/cereals
  Fats
  Sweets
- Dietary modifications:
  Self-imposed
  Prescribed
  Compliance
  Impact
- Alcohol abuse

Chronic medication use
- Prescribed/self-administered
- Self-prescribed over-the-counter
- Polypharmacy
- Nutritional supplements
- Quackery

Social isolation
- Support systems:
  Availability
  Utilization
- Living arrangements:
  Cooking/food storage
  Transportation
  Other

Dependency/disability
- Functional status
  Activities of daily living
  Instrumental activities of daily living*
- Disabling conditions:
  Lack of manual dexterity
  Use of assistive devices
- Inactivity/immobility

Acute/chronic diseases or conditions
- Abnormalities of body weight
- Alcohol abuse
- Cognitive or emotional impairment:
  Depression
  Dementias
- Oral health problems
- Pressure sores
- Sensory impairment
- Others

Poverty
- Income:
  Source
  Adequacy
- Food expenditures/resources
- Reliance on economic assistance
  programs:
  Food
  Housing
  Medical
  Other
  Adequacy

Advanced Age

*Instrumental activities of daily living include activities such as meal preparation, financial management, and housekeeping.

TABLE

14-7

Risk Factors Associated with Poor Nutrition Status in Aging Adults, including Elements by Which Risk Is Assessed

Source: Adapted from J. V. White and coauthors, Consensus of the Nutrition Screening Initiative: Risk factors and indicators of poor nutritional status in older Americans. Copyright The American Dietetic Association. Reprinted by permission from *Journal of the American Dietetic Association* 91 (1991): 784.

(e.g., dietary history). The Level II screen also assesses chronic medication use and the living environment of the individual (assistance, facilities, support systems, safety), cognitive status using the Mini Mental Test Exam, emotional status, and functional status.[33] These tools are presented in Tables 14-10 to 14-12 on pages 475–477.

◆ NUTRITION ASSESSMENT

Periodic nutrition assessment is useful for identifying and tracking elderly persons at nutritional risk.[34] The components of nutrition assessment for the elderly are listed in Table 14-13 (see page 478) along with indicators to determine risk. A geriatric nutrition assessment includes the elements discussed in the bullet list that follows.[35]

TABLE
14-8

Major Indicators of Poor Nutrition Status in Older Adults

Source: Reprinted with permission by the Nutrition Screening Initiative, a project of the American Academy of Family Physicians, The American Dietetic Association, and the National Council on Aging, Inc. and funded in part by a grant from Ross Laboratories, a division of Abbott Laboratories.

◆ **Significant weight loss over time:**
  ◆ 5.0% or more of prior body weight in 1 month.
  ◆ 7.5% or more of body weight in 3 months.
  ◆ 10.0% or more of body weight in 6 months or involuntary weight loss.
◆ **Significantly low or high weight for height:** 20% below or above desirable weight for height at a given age.
◆ **Significant reduction in serum albumin:** Serum albumin of less than 3.5 g/dL.
◆ **Significant change in functional status:** Change from "independent" to "dependent" in two of the ADLs or one of the nutrition-related IADLs.[a]
◆ **Significant and sustained inappropriate food intake:**
  ◆ Failure to consume the recommended minimum from one or more of the food groups suggested in the Dietary Guidelines for Americans, or a sufficient variety of foods for a period of 3 months or more.
  ◆ Excessive consumption of fat, saturated fat, and/or alcohol (alcohol: >1 oz/day, women; >2 oz/day, men).
◆ **Significant reduction in mid-arm circumference:** To less than 10th percentile (NHANES standards).
◆ **Significant increase or decrease in triceps skinfolds:** To less than 10th percentile or more than 95th percentile (NHANES standards).
◆ **Significant obesity:** More than 120% of desirable weight or body mass index over 27 or triceps skinfolds above 95th percentile (NHANES standards).
◆ **Other nutrition-related disorders:** Presence of osteoporosis, osteomalacia, folate deficiency, or vitamin B_{12} deficiency.

[a]IADLs are instrumental activities of daily living (e.g., meal preparation and financial management).

A nomogram for determining stature using knee-to-heel height is provided in Appendix E.

◆ **Anthropometric measures**. Height, weight, and skinfold measures are affected by aging. Height decreases over time due to changes in the integrity of the skeletal system as a result of bone loss. Measurements of height are sometimes difficult to obtain because of poor posture or the inability to stand erect unassisted. In such cases, a recumbent anthropometric measure such as knee-to-heel height can be used as an alternative measure of stature.[36]

Current weight using a calibrated balance beam scale and a weight history are important to obtain. Wheelchair and bed balance beam scales can be used for the nonambulatory client. The individual's hydration status should be noted because edema or dehydration can distort anthropometric measures.

Skinfold measurements (triceps skinfold and mid-arm muscle area) are affected by alterations in skin elasticity, compressibility, and distribution of body fat, which are all common in normal aging. For example, the centralization of body fat can cause the triceps skinfold measure to underestimate total body fat.

Standards for evaluating anthropometric measurements for the elderly are limited by the number of subjects included in the reference data. Currently, standards for people aged 55 to 74 years are taken from the NHANES I and NHANES II survey data. The NHANES III study is expect-

FIGURE

14-7

Checklist to Determine your Nutritional Health
Source: Reprinted with permission by the Nutrition Screening Initiative, a project of the American Academy of Family Physicians, The American Dietetic Association, and the National Council on Aging, Inc. and funded in part by a grant from Ross Laboratories, a division of Abbott Laboratories.

The warning signs of poor nutritional health are often overlooked. To see whether you (or people you know) are at nutritional risk, take this simple quiz. Read the statements below. Circle the number in the "yes" column for those that apply. To find your total nutritional score, add up all of the numbers you circled.

	Yes
I have an illness or condition that made me change the kind and/or amount of food I eat.	2
I eat fewer than two meals per day.	3
I eat few fruits, vegetables or milk products.	2
I have three or more drinks of beer, liquor, or wine almost every day.	2
I have tooth or mouth problems that make it hard for me to eat.	2
I don't always have enough money to buy the food I need.	4
I eat alone most of the time.	1
I take three or more different prescribed or over-the-counter drugs a day.	1
Without wanting to, I have lost or gained 10 pounds in the past six months.	2
I am not always physically able to shop, cook, and/or feed myself.	2
Total nutritional score:	

If your total nutritional score is:
0–2—Good! Recheck your nutritional score in six months.
3–5—You are at a moderate nutritional risk. See what can be done to improve your eating habits and lifestyle. A local office on aging, senior nutrition program, senior citizens center, or health department can help. Recheck your nutritional score in three months.
6 or more—You are at a high nutritional risk. Bring this checklist next time you see your doctor, dietitian, or other qualified health or social service professional. Talk with them about any problems you have experienced. Ask for nutrition counseling.

ed to provide improved standards for comparison, including data on people older than 74 years.

◆ **Clinical assessment.** The clinical assessment should evaluate the condition of hair, skin, nails, musculature, eyes, mucosa, and other physical attributes. An oral examination is useful for determining the condition of the mouth and teeth, the need for dentures or condition of existing dentures, and oral lesions. An assessment of the client's ability to chew, swallow, and self-feed is recommended.[37]

Refer to Appendix E for clinical signs of nutritional deficiencies.

◆ **Biochemical assessment.** Biochemical parameters are affected by the aging process, as well as by polypharmacy, chronic disease, and hydration status. However, serial measures of blood parameters can be useful in evaluating nutritional risk. Serum albumin is generally used to assess visceral protein status in the elderly. Low serum albumin levels are associated with increased morbidity and mortality in the elderly. Measurements of serum cholesterol, hemoglobin, and blood glucose and antigen-recall skin tests are also included.

◆ **Dietary assessment.** A detailed record of current food consumption and a history of changes in eating habits over time are needed to assess diet adequacy. The evaluation should detect persons who avoid certain food

FIGURE

14-8

The Nutrition Checklist Warning Signs

Source: Reprinted with permission by the Nutrition Screening Initiative, a project of the American Academy of Family Physicians, The American Dietetic Association, and the National Council on Aging, Inc. and funded in part by a grant from Ross Laboratories, a division of Abbott Laboratories.

Use the word DETERMINE to remind you of the warning signs.

DISEASE

Any disease, illness, or chronic condition that causes you to change the way you eat, or makes it hard for you to eat, puts your nutritional health at risk. Four out of five adults have chronic diseases that are affected by diet. Confusion or memory loss that keeps getting worse is estimated to affect one out of five or more of older adults. This can make it hard to remember what, when, or if you've eaten. Feeling sad or depressed, which happens to about one in eight older adults, can cause big changes in appetite, digestion, energy level, weight, and well-being.

EATING POORLY

Eating too little and eating too much both lead to poor health. Eating the same foods day after day or not eating fruit, vegetables, and milk products daily will also cause poor nutritional health. One in five adults skip meals daily. Only 13% of adults eat the minimum amount of fruit and vegetables needed. One in four older adults drink too much alcohol. Many health problems become worse if you drink more than one or two alcoholic beverages per day.

TOOTH LOSS/MOUTH PAIN

A healthy mouth, teeth, and gums are needed to eat. Missing, loose, or rotten teeth or dentures that don't fit well or cause mouth sores make it hard to eat.

ECONOMIC HARDSHIP

As many as 40% of older Americans have incomes of less than $6,000 per year. Having less—or choosing to spend less—than $25–30 per week for food makes it very hard to get the foods you need to stay healthy.

REDUCED SOCIAL CONTACT

One-third of all older people live alone. Being with people daily has a positive effect on morale, well-being, and eating.

MULTIPLE MEDICINES

Many older Americans must take medicines for health problems. Almost half of older Americans take multiple medicines daily. Growing old may change the way we respond to drugs. The more medicines you take, the greater chance for side effects such as increased or decreased appetite, change in taste, constipation, weakness, drowsiness, diarrhea, nausea, and others. Vitamins or minerals when taken in large doses act like drugs and can cause harm. Alert your doctor to everything you take.

INVOLUNTARY WEIGHT LOSS/GAIN

Losing or gaining a lot of weight when you are not trying to do so is an important warning sign that must not be ignored. Being overweight or underweight also increases your chance of poor health.

NEEDS ASSISTANCE IN SELF-CARE

Although most older people are able to eat, one of every five has trouble walking, shopping, buying and cooking food, especially as they get older.

ELDER YEARS ABOVE AGE 80

Most older people lead full and productive lives. But as age increases, risk of frailty and health problems increase. Checking your nutritional health regularly makes good sense.

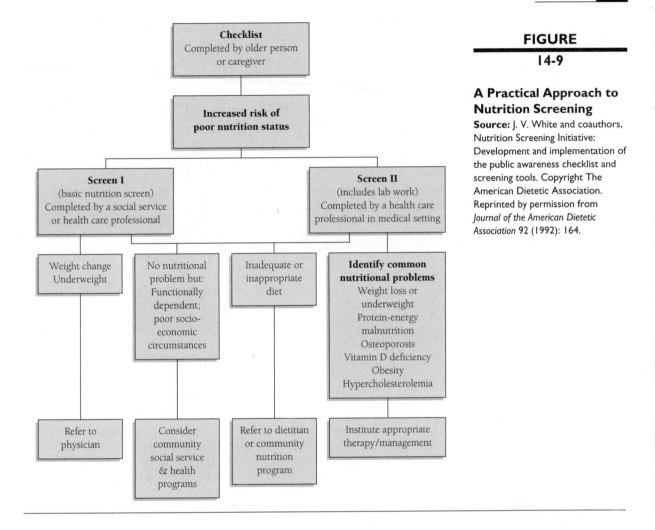

FIGURE

14-9

A Practical Approach to Nutrition Screening
Source: J. V. White and coauthors, Nutrition Screening Initiative: Development and implementation of the public awareness checklist and screening tools. Copyright The American Dietetic Association. Reprinted by permission from *Journal of the American Dietetic Association* 92 (1992): 164.

groups, adhere to unusual dietary practices, or consume excessive or insufficient amounts of essential nutrients. The adequacy of fluid intake should be assessed as well.

◆ **Functional assessment.** Functional assessment measures changes in the basic functions necessary to maintain independent living (refer to Table 14-12 on page 477). ADLs refer to self-care activities (e.g., bathing, dressing, feeding). Instrumental ADLs, or IADLs, which require a higher level of functioning, include activities such as meal preparation, financial management, and housekeeping. Many of these activities (e.g., shopping, cooking, self-feeding) are closely related to adequate nutrition status.

◆ **Medication assessment.** Note the types and doses of various prescription and over-the-counter drugs. Evaluate the individual's drug intake for possible nutrient-drug interactions that could affect the absorption, metabo-

	LEVEL I SCREEN	LEVEL II SCREEN
Primary User	Social workers and health care professionals	Physicians and other qualified health care professionals
Data Evaluation	Height	Height
	Weight	Weight
	Dietary data	Dietary data
	Daily food intake	Daily food intake
	Living environment	Living environment
	Functional status	Functional status
		Laboratory and anthropometric data
		Clinical features
		Mental/cognitive status
		Medication use

TABLE

14-9

Nutrition Screening Initiative: Level I and Level II Screens
Source: Adapted from Nutrition Screening Initiative, *Nutrition Screening Manual for Professionals Caring for Older Americans* (Washington, D.C.: The Nutrition Screening Initiative, 1991).

lism, and requirements for specific nutrients. Also identify any drugs that may depress the appetite or alter the perception of taste.

◆ **Social assessment.** Financial resources, living arrangements, and social support network, including availability of caregivers, should be evaluated as part of the nutrition assessment since these factors can directly impact a person's nutrition status. Poverty (e.g., annual income of less than $6000 per person) and social isolation particularly impair the nutrition status of many older adults as noted perceptively by a professor of psychiatry:

> It is not what the older person eats but with whom that will be the deciding factor in proper care for him. The oft-repeated complaint of the older patient that he has little incentive to prepare food for only himself is not merely a statement of fact but also a rebuke to the questioner for failing to perceive his isolation and aloneness and to realize that food . . . for one's self lacks the condiment of another's presence which can transform the simplest fare to the ceremonial act with all its shared meaning.[38]

Community-Based Programs and Services

Until the early 1970s, nutrition services for older adults, with the exception of food stamps, were found primarily in hospitals and long-term care facilities. Efforts were then made to expand nutrition services from the hospitals to include communities and homes.[39]

In response to the socioeconomic problems that trouble many older adults and may lead to malnutrition—low income, inadequate facilities for preparing food, lack of transportation, and inability to afford dental care, among others—federal, state, and local agencies have mandated nutrition programs for the elderly. Older adults' need for nutrition services depends on their level of independence, which can be depicted as a continuum, as in Figure 14-10 on page 479.[40]

Orientation:

♦ Ask for the date (What is the year/season/date/day/month?). (1 point each)
♦ Where are we (state) (county) (town) (hospital) (floor)? (1 point each)

Registration:

♦ Name 3 unrelated objects, (e.g., ball, tree, flag) clearly and slowly. Then ask the patient to say all 3 after you have said them. (Give 1 point for each correct answer. Then repeat them until the patient learns all 3. Count trials and record.)

Attention and calculation trial:

♦ Serial 7s: Ask patient to begin with 100 and count backward by 7. (1 point for each correct answer. Stop after 5 answers.) Alternatively, spell "world" backwards. (The score is the number of letters in the correct order.)

Recall trial:

♦ Ask the patient to recall the 3 objects repeated above. (Give 1 point for each correct answer.)

Language trial:

♦ Show the patient a wristwatch and ask him what it is. Repeat for a pencil. (Score 0–2.)
♦ Repeat the following "No ifs, ands, or buts." (1 point)
♦ Follow a 3-stage command: "Take a paper in your right hand, fold it in half, and put it on the floor." (3 points)
♦ On a blank piece of paper, print the sentence "Close your eyes." Ask patient to read it and do what it says. (1 point)
♦ Write a sentence. (1 point)
♦ Copy design: draw intersecting pentagons; ask the patient to copy it exactly as it is. All 10 angles must be present and two must intersect. (1 point)

ASSESS level of consciousness along a continuum.

Alert	Drowsy	Stupor	Coma

TABLE

14-10

Mini Mental Status Exam

Source: Reprinted from M. F. Folstein, S. E. Folstein, and P. McHugh. Mini-mental state: A practical method for grading the cognitive state of patients for the clinician, *Journal of Psychiatric Research* 12, Copyright 1975, with kind permission from Elsevier Science Ltd, The Boulevard, Langford Lane, Kidlington, OX5 1GB, UK. Some professional education and training are needed to administer and interpret this instrument.

Currently, community nutrition programs support the functional independence of older individuals in ambulatory care centers, adult day care centers, hospices, and home settings. Community nutritionists need to be familiar with organizations and programs providing nutrition and other health-related services to older adults.[41] A summary of the nutrition programs for older adults is provided in Table 14-14 on page 480.

♦ GENERAL ASSISTANCE PROGRAMS

The Supplemental Security Income (SSI) Program improves the financial plight of the very poor directly by increasing a person's or family's income to the defined poverty level. This sometimes helps older people retain their independence.

Another system of financial support to older Americans is the third-party reimbursement system, discussed earlier in Chapter 4. Third-party payers (e.g.,

TABLE

14-11

Geriatric Depression Scale

Source: Reprinted from T. Yesavage, T. Brink, and coauthors. Development and validation of a geriatric screening scale: A preliminary report, *Journal of Psychiatric Research* 17, Copyright 1983, with kind permission from Elsevier Science Ltd, The Boulevard, Langford Lane, Kidlington OX5 1GB UK.

Choose the best answer ("yes" or "no") for how you felt this past week.[a]

* 1. Are you basically satisfied with your life?
  2. Have you dropped many of your activities and interests?
  3. Do you feel that your life is empty?
  4. Do you often get bored?
* 5. Are you hopeful about the future?
  6. Are you bothered by thoughts you can't get out of your head?
* 7. Are you in good spirits most of the time?
  8. Are you afraid that something bad is going to happen to you?
* 9. Do you feel happy most of the time?
  10. Do you often feel helpless?
  11. Do you often get restless and fidgety?
  12. Do you prefer to stay at home, rather than going out and doing new things?
  13. Do you frequently worry about the future?
  14. Do you feel you have more problems with memory than most?
*15. Do you think it is wonderful to be alive now?
  16. Do you often feel downhearted and blue?
  17. Do you feel pretty worthless the way you are now?
  18. Do you worry a lot about the past?
*19. Do you find life very exciting?
  20. Is it hard for you to get started on new projects?
*21. Do you feel full of energy?
  22. Do you feel that your situation is hopeless?
  23. Do you think that most people are better off than you are?
  24. Do you frequently get upset over little things?
  25. Do you frequently feel like crying?
  26. Do you have trouble concentrating?
*27. Do you enjoy getting up in the morning?
  28. Do you prefer to avoid social gatherings?
*29. Is it easy for you to make decisions?
*30. Is your mind as clear as it used to be?

Norms:	Normal	5±4
	Mildly depressed	15±6
	Very depressed	23±5

*Appropriate (nondepressed) answers = yes, all others = no.

[a]This instrument is intended for professional administration and interpretation. Any significant score (depressed range) indicates probable need for professional advice.

Medicare, Medicaid, Blue Cross/Blue Shield) sometimes reimburse the costs of receiving health-related services, including such nutrition services as nutrition screening, assessment, and counseling and enteral or parenteral nutrition support.[42] Generally, the nutrition service must be deemed "medically necessary." Whether a service is reimbursable and the extent of reimbursement varies from state to state and from case to case.

Social work agencies can provide older adults with information about appropriate nutrition resources in the community, such as congregate meal sites or

ADLs[a]
  Bathing—May receive help with one body part
  Dressing—May receive help with tying shoes
  Toileting—May use bedpan/urinal at night
  Transferring—May use assistive devices
  Continence—Complete control at all times
  Feeding–May receive help with cutting meat, buttering bread
IADLs (nutrition-related)[a]
  Shopping—Takes care of all needs
  Food preparation—Plans, prepares, and serves adequate meals
  Transportation—Drives own car or uses public transportation or taxi alone or accompanied
  Other IADLs include use of the telephone and management of housekeeping, laundry, medications, and finances.
 	
[a]Change from "performing without assistance" (independence) to "needs assistance most of the time" (dependence) with 2 ADLs or 1 nutrition-related IADL indicates likelihood of poor nutrition status.
	TABLE
	14-12
	
	Functional Status Assessment Using Activities of Daily Living (ADLs) and Nutrition-Related Instrumental Activities of Daily Living (IADLs)

Source: J. V. White and coauthors, Consensus of the Nutrition Screening Initiative: Risk factors and indicators of poor nutritional status in older Americans. Copyright The American Dietetic Association. Reprinted by permission from *Journal of the American Dietetic Association* 91 (1991): 784.

Meals-on-Wheels programs.* On physician referral, Home Health Services, offered through local private and public organizations, provide home health aides to assist older people with shopping, housekeeping, and food preparation.

◆ NUTRITION PROGRAMS OF THE U.S. DEPARTMENT OF AGRICULTURE

The Food Stamp Program was not designed specifically for older people, but it can nevertheless help older adults in need of financial assistance. The Food Stamp Program, which is administered by the U.S. Department of Agriculture (USDA), enables qualifying people to obtain coupons that they can use to buy food at grocery stores or to pay for meals at "Dining Out Programs" sometimes offered by restaurants. Currently, the program reaches between 40 percent and 80 percent of eligible elders—some 2 million households. Reasons for nonparticipation by the elderly include the "stigma" of receiving assistance, confusing paperwork, and a lack of public information about eligibility requirements. In an effort to reach more eligible older adults, California and Wisconsin provide those over 65 years of age with a cash equivalent to their entitled food stamp benefit as part of their SSI check.

The Food Stamp Program is discussed in Chapter 11's Program Spotlight.

The USDA also contributes to the elderly nutrition programs through its Nutrition Program for the Elderly (NPE). The NPE provides cash and commodity foods to local senior citizen centers for use in the Congregate and Home-Delivered Meals Programs of the U.S. Department of Health and Human Services (DHHS). The USDA also sponsors meal programs for the Adult Day Care Centers operating in many communities through its Child and Adult Day Care Program. Adult day care facilities care for seniors while their care providers are away from

*The *Eldercare Locator* (800/677-1116) is a new service available nationwide that provides the name and telephone number for information resources on aging in local areas.

TABLE

14-13

Nutrition Assessment for Older Adults

Source: Adapted with permission by the Nutrition Screening Initiative, a project of the American Academy of Family Physicians, The American Dietetic Association, and the National Council on Aging, Inc. and funded in part by a grant from Ross Laboratories, a division of Abbott Laboratories.

NUTRITION ASSESSMENT COMPONENT	INDICATOR OF RISK
Anthropometric Measurements	
Weight	Measured weight-for-height 80% or below or 120% or
Height	above midpoint of medium frame (Metropolitan Life Tables)
	Reported usual body weight more than 5% less than actual weight
	Involuntary weight loss or gain of more than 10 lb
Body mass index (BMI)	Underweight: BMI <16
	Overweight: BMI >25
Body composition	Mid-arm muscle circumference 20% or more below NHANES standards
	Triceps skinfolds 40% or less, or 190% or more above NHANES standards
	Waist-to-hip ratio:
	>1.0 for men
	>0.8 for women
Clinical assessment	
Individual/family medical history	Use of tobacco, alcohol, drugs
	Chronic illness or disability
	Blood pressure >140/90 mm Hg
Oral cavity exam	Lesions in mouth, bleeding gums, mobile teeth, ill-fitting dentures, need for dentures
Physical examination	Signs and symptoms of possible diet-related problems
Biochemical assessment	
Total blood cholesterol	Elevated:
	>240 mg/dL on 2 occasions
	>200 mg/dL plus risk factors
LDL-C	Elevated: >130 mg/dL
HDL-C	Low: <35 mg/dL
Hemoglobin	Risk of anemia:
	Males: 45–64 yr: 13.2 g/dL; 65+ yr: 13.6 g/dL
	Females: 45–64 yr: 11.8 g/dL; 65+ yr: 11.9 g/dL
Serum albumin	Low: <3.5 g/dL
Blood glucose	Outside normal range of 70–110 mg/100 ml
Dietary assessment	
3-day food diary	Deficient or excessive intakes of calories and/or nutrients
Food frequency	
24-hour recall	
Functional assessment	
Activities of daily living (ADLs)	A change from independence to dependence (needs
Instrumental activities of daily living (IADLs)	assistance most of the time) with 2 ADLs or 1 nutrition-related IADL
Medication Assessment	Use of 3 or more prescribed medications; daily use of over-the-counter medications (e.g., aspirin, antacids); nutrition quackery

the home. USDA's Commodity Supplemental Food Program is also available in a limited number of states and can provide monthly food packages to persons 60 years of age and older.

| FIGURE 14-10 | Overview of Community Nutrition Programs for Older Adults |

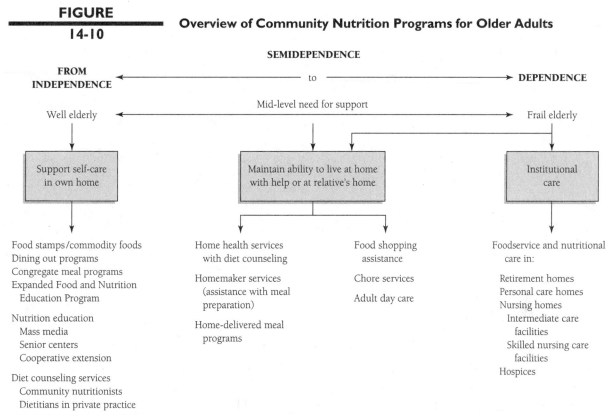

SEMIDEPENDENCE

FROM INDEPENDENCE ←———————— to ————————→ DEPENDENCE

Well elderly ←———— Mid-level need for support ————→ Frail elderly

| Support self-care in own home | Maintain ability to live at home with help or at relative's home | Institutional care |

Food stamps/commodity foods
Dining out programs
Congregate meal programs
Expanded Food and Nutrition
　Education Program

Nutrition education
　Mass media
　Senior centers
　Cooperative extension

Diet counseling services
　Community nutritionists
　Dietitians in private practice

Home health services
　with diet counseling

Homemaker services
　(assistance with meal
　preparation)

Home-delivered meal
　programs

Food shopping
　assistance

Chore services

Adult day care

Foodservice and nutritional
　care in:

Retirement homes
Personal care homes
Nursing homes
　Intermediate care
　　facilities
　Skilled nursing care
　　facilities
Hospices

Source: Adapted from H. T. Philips and S. H. Gaylord, eds., *Aging and Public Health.* Copyright Springer Publishing Company, Inc., New York 10012. Used by permission.

◆ NUTRITION PROGRAMS OF THE U.S. DEPARTMENT OF HEALTH AND HUMAN SERVICES

The Older Americans Act (OAA) of 1965 was amended in 1972 (P.L. 92-258) to establish the federal Nutrition Program for Older Americans (NPOA). This formula-grant program distributes funds under Title IIIc (formerly known as Title VII) of the OAA. NPOA funds are given to state agencies on aging, which coordinate community services for the elderly based on the number of elderly residing in each state. This chapter's Program Spotlight provides an overview of the congregate and home-delivered meals programs.

◆ PRIVATE SECTOR NUTRITION ASSISTANCE PROGRAMS

In some communities, food banks enable older people on limited incomes to buy good food for less money. A food bank project buys industry "irregulars"—products that have been mislabeled, underweighted, redesigned, or mispackaged and would therefore ordinarily be thrown away. Nothing is wrong with this food; the industry can credit it as a donation, and the buyer (often a food-preparing site)

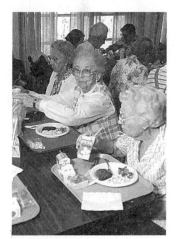

The social atmosphere can be as valuable as the foods served at congregate meal sites.

TABLE	Nutrition Programs for Older Adults
14-14	

PROGRAM	TYPE OF INTERVENTION	FUNDING SOURCE	ELIGIBLE/AVAILABLE SERVICES	PERCENT OF OLDER POPULATION SERVED
Nutrition Program for Older Americans	Congregate and home-delivered meals, therapeutic diets	DHHS OHDS AoA	Meals; transportation; shopping assistance; limited nutrition education, information, and referral	10% to 13% of population aged 60+ years
Food Stamps	Income subsidy	USDA Social Security	Coupons for food purchases or cash equivalent	50% to 80% of the eligible low-income elderly
Meals-on-Wheels America	Direct food delivery	Private	Home meals that complement weekday congregate programs; attention to needs of home-bound elderly	<1%
Child and Adult Day Care	Meal program, supervised day care	USDA	Day care programs for older Americans	Figures unknown
Medicare/Medicaid	Third-party payment system	DHHS HCFA SSA	Covers medical and related services provided by participating hospitals, HMOs, private medical practices, ambulatory centers, rehabilitation and skilled nursing facilities, home health agencies, and hospice programs. Eligible nutrition services vary depending on the setting of care and the deemed medical necessity. Home meals, enteral/parenteral nutrition, and weight reduction are particularly limited.	Virtually all people over age 65 years are eligible (but many eligible people reportedly lack coverage by either program).

AoA = U.S. Department of Health and Human Services, Administration on Aging.
DHHS = U.S. Department of Health and Human Services.
HCFA = U.S. Department of Health and Human Services, Health Care Financing Administration.
OHDS = U.S. Department of Health and Human Services, Office of Human Development Services.
SSA = Social Security Administration.
USDA = U.S. Department of Agriculture

Source: Adapted from *Geriatric Nutrition: The Health Professional's Handbook* by R. Chernoff, pp. 428–29, with permission of Aspen Publishers, Inc., © 1991.

can obtain the food for a small handling fee and make it available at a greatly reduced price.

The Meals-on-Wheels America program is a similar but separate program to the federal home-delivered meals program. Meals-on-Wheels is a national project operated under the auspices of local volunteer groups. Its purpose is to help fill gaps in services provided by the federal meals programs by reaching older adults in communities not fully serviced by the NPOA.[43] The preparation and delivery of the meals provided by Meals-on-Wheels is usually integrated into existing NPOA programs. In some communities, the Meals-on-Wheels program provides weekend and holiday meals in addition to the standard five luncheon meals.

◆ *The Nutrition Program for Older Americans*

The Federal Nutrition Program for Older Americans is intended to improve older people's nutrition status and enable them to avoid medical problems, continue living in communities of their own choice, and stay out of institutions. Its specific goals are to provide:

◆ Low-cost, nutritious meals.

◆ Opportunities for social interaction.

◆ Nutrition education and shopping assistance.

◆ Counseling and referral to other social and rehabilitation services.

◆ Transportation services.

The current Title IIIc legislation makes a hot noon meal available five days a week, supplying a third of the RDA (see Table 14-15). There is no cost for meals, but participants sometimes make voluntary contributions.

One aspect of Title IIIc is the Congregate Meals Program. Administrators try to select sites for congregate meals that will be accessible to as many of the eligible elderly as possible. The congregate meal sites are often community centers, senior citizen centers, religious facilities, schools, extended care facilities, or elderly housing complexes. Through the Home-Delivered Meals Program, meals are delivered to those who are homebound either permanently or temporarily. This program ensures nutrition, but its recipients miss out on the social benefit of the congregate meal sites; every effort is made to persuade them to come to the shared meals, if they can. The Administration on Aging of the DHHS administers these programs, while the states, usually in conjunction with local county and city agencies, are responsible for their daily operation and administration.

All persons over 60 years of age and their spouses (regardless of age) are eligible to receive meals from these programs, regardless of their income level. However, priority is given to minorities, those with low incomes, and extremely old individuals. Since 1972, these programs have grown significantly; currently,

FOOD TYPE	RECOMMENDED PORTION SIZE
Meat or meat alternate	3 oz, cooked portion
Vegetables and fruits	Two $\frac{1}{2}$ c portions*
Enriched white or whole-grain bread or alternate	1 serving (one slice bread or equivalent)
Butter or margarine	1 tsp
Milk	8 oz milk or calcium equivalent
Dessert	1 serving

*A Vitamin C–rich fruit or vegetable is to be served each day; a vitamin A–rich fruit or vegetable is to be served at least three times per week.

TABLE

14-15

Title IIIc Meal Pattern
Source: U.S. Department of Health and Human Services.

Continued

—Continued

they account for annual expenditures of about $1 billion, representing some 244 million meals served each year—144 million congregate meals and 100 million home-delivered meals. Funding assists with food purchasing and preparation, facilities, and transportation for persons otherwise unable to participate.

By the early 1980s, it was apparent that Title IIIc funds were insufficient to provide meals to the increasing numbers of frail elderly in need of home-delivered meals, which are usually more costly than congregate site meals. Some of this increased demand was due to the initiation of the prospective payment system for hospitals, which caused more of the elderly to be discharged early from hospitals. Certain states then initiated state-funded home-delivered meals programs for those who could not be served by the federal meals program. One such program is the Supplemental Nutrition Assistance Program (SNAP) initiated in New York State in 1984.[1]

Current evaluations of home-delivered meals programs ask whether the most needy elderly are going unserved, and who should be given priority for receiving assistance—those who do not have access to food because of social or economic disabilities or those with medical disabilities. Criteria for nutritional risk are needed in order to assign priority among the elderly experiencing food insecurity. The British have developed one such assessment tool to help social workers identify nutritional risk factors related to poverty, frailty, and loss of coping skills among the homebound elderly (see Table 14-16).[2] In the United States, eligibility for home-delivered meals varies according to whether the program is federal, state, or locally operated.

In an effort to reduce the cost of providing home-delivered meals, some states have initiated "luncheon clubs." In these clubs, several seniors who live near each other and receive home-delivered meals gather in a neighbor's home. Only one meal delivery stop is therefore required, and the seniors benefit from the social interaction.[3]

TABLE	1. Consumption of fewer than 8 main meals (hot or cold) per week.

14-16

Ten Nutritional Risk Factors Diagnostic for the Need for Assistance among the Elderly

1. Consumption of fewer than 8 main meals (hot or cold) per week.
2. Drinking of very little milk (less than half a pint per day).
3. Little or no intake of fruits or vegetables.
4. Wastage of food, even if supplied hot and ready to eat.
5. Long periods of the day without food or beverages.
6. Depression or loneliness.
7. Unexpected weight change (gain or loss).
8. Shopping difficulties.
9. Low income.
10. Presence of disabilities (including alcoholism).

Source: L. Davies, Nutrition and the elderly: Identifying those at risk, *Proceedings of the Nutrition Society* 43 (1984): 299. © 1984, reprinted with the permission of Cambridge University Press.

Continued

—Continued

Evaluations of the congregate and home-delivered meals programs generally show that they improve the dietary intake and nutrition status of their clients.[4] Participants generally have greater diversity in their diets, higher intakes of essential nutrients, and are less likely to report problems with food insecurity than nonparticipants.[5] Other benefits come as a result of the screening and referrals offered by the programs. The activities associated with the congregate meals provide additional advantages: diet counseling, exercise, adult education, and other classes and activities. Participants benefit, too, from the opportunity for improved socialization.[6]

Despite these positive outcomes, the meals programs also have several deficiencies. Weekend or evening meals are not available for those who cannot get food or cannot cook. Persons with special dietary needs (e.g., diabetes) cannot obtain special diets. Furthermore, the meals supplied are often too high in fat or lack nutrients that the participants are unlikely to obtain from the food they get for themselves (e.g., folate).[7]

The special needs of the homebound elderly should be given greater priority. The dietary intake of the homebound elderly might improve if meals were provided more than once a day and were supplied seven days a week rather than five. The meals should also furnish larger percentages of the RDA.[8]

Although Title IIIc nutrition programs are required to provide nutrition education to their clients, these efforts are usually limited to the congregate meal sites.[9] Except for a limited amount of printed material, those who purchase and prepare these meals receive virtually no education.[10] Thus, greater emphasis on nutrition education for both helpers and clients is warranted.

The OAA was amended most recently in 1992. This legislation reauthorizes the OAA until 1995 and permits the Administration on Aging to make significant changes in the OAA programs. Highlights of these changes include the following:[11]

◆ Nutrition education will be provided to nutrition program participants at least semiannually.

◆ Each state must establish and administer the nutrition programs under the advice of dietitians.

◆ Criteria for nonfinancial eligibility to receive nutrition services will be developed.

◆ States must ensure that meals comply with the Dietary Guidelines for Americans and provide one-third of the RDA for one meal, two-thirds of the RDA for two meals, and 100 percent of the RDA if three meals are served.

In addition, this legislation added a new part to Title III, known as Title IIIf, which authorizes the provision of services related to health promotion and disease prevention, as listed at the top of the next page.[12]

Continued

PROGRAM
SPOTLIGHT

—Continued

◆ Health Risk Appraisals.

◆ Routine health screening.

◆ Health promotion programs (e.g., substance abuse, weight loss, smoking cessation).

◆ Programs that focus on physical fitness, group exercise, music, art, and dance movement therapy.

◆ Home injury control services, including screening of high-risk home environments and injury prevention programs.

◆ Screening for the prevention of depression, coordination of community mental health services, provision of educational activities, and referral to psychiatric and psychological services.

◆ Educational programs about preventive health services covered under Medicare.

◆ Medication management programs and screening.

◆ Information about the diagnosis, prevention, treatment, and rehabilitation of age-related diseases like osteoporosis and cardiovascular disease.

Some states are using the new Title IIIf funds to incorporate the Nutrition Screening Initiative into the services that they already provide to elders.

1. D. A. Roe, Development and current status of home-delivered meals programs in the United States: Who is served? *Nutrition Reviews* 48 (1990): 181–85.
2. Ibid, p. 183.
3. S. Riggs, Serving the seventies: Meal programs for the elderly, together or at home, *Restaurants and Institutions* 95 (1984): 193–96.
4. D. M. Czajka-Narins and coauthors, Nutritional and biochemical effects of nutrition programs in the elderly, *Clinics in Geriatric Medicine* 3 (1987): 275–88; and M. Nestle and J. A. Gilbride, Nutrition policies for health promotion in older adults: Education Priorities for the 1990s, Journal of Nutrition Education 22 (1990): 314–17.
5. D. L. Edwards and coauthors, Home-delivered meals benefit the diabetic elderly, *Journal of the American Dietetic Association* 93 (1993): 585–87.
6. Institute of Medicine, *The Second Fifty Years: Promoting Health and Preventing Disability* (Washington, D.C.: National Academy Press, 1992), p. 182.
7. Roe, Development and current status of home-delivered meals programs, p. 185.
8. D. A. Stevens, L. E. Grivetti, and R. B. McDonald, Nutrient intake of urban and rural elderly receiving home-delivered meals, *Journal of the American Dietetic Association* 92 (1992): 714–18; and O. Walden and coauthors, The provision of weekend home-delivered meals by state and a pilot study indicating the need for weekend home-delivered meals, *Journal of Nutrition for the Elderly* 8 (1988): 31–43.
9. *Nutrition Services for the Elderly* (Washington, D.C.: U.S. House of Representatives Committee on Aging, Hearing Pub. No. Y4. Ag 4/2 N 95, June 10, 1988).
10. Stevens, Grivetti, and McDonald, Nutrient intake of urban and rural elderly.
11. Legislative highlights: Older Americans Act passes, *Journal of the American Dietetic Association* 92 (1992): 1458.
12. *Gerontological Nutritionists Newsletter,* Winter 1994, p. 7.

◆ NUTRITION EDUCATION PROGRAMS

Nutrition education strategies aimed at adults are found in both the public and the private sector. They strive to increase nutrition knowledge and skills and improve eating patterns among adults of all ages. Nutrition education for health promotion is generally based on the *Dietary Guidelines for Americans* and the Food Guide Pyramid.[44] The nutritional goals of these educational tools are to help consumers select diets that provide an appropriate amount of energy to maintain a healthful weight, meet the RDA for all nutrients without depending on supplements, are varied in types of fat and moderate in total fat, caloric sweeteners, sodium, cholesterol, and alcohol, and are adequate in complex carbohydrate and fiber.

Public nutrition education programs include the Expanded Food and Nutrition Education Program (EFNEP), described in Chapter 12, and the FDA and USDA public education campaign on the new food label in cooperation with other federal, state, and local agencies (e.g., state Cooperative Extension). For example, in Florida, the Area Agency on Aging of Central Florida has teamed with Florida Cooperative Extension to provide food labeling educational materials for the elderly and training programs for volunteers working with the elderly. The Michigan State University Cooperative extension offers a workbook for culturally diverse low-income consumers on how to use the food label to manage fat intake.

A primary challenge facing nutrition educators is to improve nutrition education strategies to reduce the major risk factors for coronary heart disease and cancer, the leading causes of death among older Americans.[45] Public efforts are now underway. The National Heart, Lung, and Blood Institute initiated the guidelines of the National Cholesterol Education Program (NCEP) to help prevent heart disease by reducing saturated fat and cholesterol in the American diet.[46] The National Cancer Institute (NCI) designed its *National 5 A Day for Better Health* program to increase per capita fruit and vegetable consumption. The NCI's 5 A Day program promotes a simple nutrition message that physicians, nurses, community nutritionists, and other health care professionals can reinforce to their clients: *Eat five or more servings of fruits and vegetables every day for better health.*[47]

A number of trade and professional organizations are likewise directing some of their nutrition education strategies to help consumers understand the role of nutrition in health promotion and disease prevention. Brochures, booklets, and videos that offer simple ways to trim dietary fat, interpret nutrition labels, implement the Dietary Guidelines, or improve shopping skills are available from the American Dietetic Association, American Association for Retired Persons, the National Dairy Council, General Mills, and the Produce Marketing Association, among others. For example, Kraft General Food's *A Matter of Balance: Using the New Food Labels* is a consumer brochure which uses the themes of balance and moderation to explain how to use the new food label to plan a healthful diet.

In many communities, food retailers and foodservice establishments provide point-of-purchase information and literature to their customers.[48] Other communities offer seminars and grocery store tours to help consumers understand the new food label.

Nationwide, about one-third of all seniors live in rural areas—communities with populations of 2500 or less.[49] Few nutrition education efforts for these seniors are available, although some new programs have been designed to target this large audience. The Harvest Health at Home—Eating for the Second Fifty

Years (HHH) project in North Dakota, which was designed using social learning theory, reaches rural communities through a series of newsletters.[50] The focus is on improving eating behaviors with emphasis on preventive nutrition messages such as decreasing fat intake and increasing fiber in the diet. Part of the intervention's success is due to the practical suggestions included in the newsletters (e.g., lists comparing the nutrient contents of brand name products); such measures are generally valuable and effective when working with elders. The HHH intervention has also been successful in collaborating with other health professionals; for example, the newsletter publicizes the schedule of routine screenings sponsored by local health departments and clinics.

Focus group interviews with older adults show that seniors are interested in changing their eating behavior.[51] Including practical activities in nutrition education programs can help motivate these changes. For example, at the White Crane Senior Health Center in Chicago, a combination health care and wellness center founded by seniors, monthly cooking classes provide an opportunity to modify and taste new recipes and try new foods.

◆ HEALTH PROMOTION PROGRAMS

Evidence continues to indicate that adults of all ages need to modify their current eating patterns and other behaviors to reduce the risk of chronic diseases. However, as mentioned in the discussion of social marketing in Chapter 9, behavior changes can be very difficult to make. An important characteristic of community nutrition interventions is that they can reach people in many different contexts of their daily lives. Supportive social environments can help individuals change their behavior.[52] For this reason, community- and employer-based programs for health promotion are expanding and are facilitating lifestyle changes. For example, many employers now provide worksite health promotion programs offering classes and activities for smoking cessation, weight loss, and stress management. These programs vary widely—some are simple and inexpensive (distribution of health information pamphlets), while others are more complex (comprehensive risk factor screening and intensive follow-up counseling).[53] In general, worksite health promotion efforts can be classified under four main areas:[54]

The national health promotion and disease prevention objectives for the nation include the target that by the year 2000, at least 85 percent of all workplaces with 50 or more employees will offer employee health promotion programs.

- ◆ **Policies.** Smoking, alcohol and other drugs, and AIDS/HIV infection.
- ◆ **Screenings.** Health risk/health status, cancer, high blood pressure, and cholesterol.
- ◆ **Information or activities.** Individual counseling, group classes, workshops, lectures, special events, and resource materials such as posters, brochures, pamphlets, and videos. Topics typically covered include cancer, high blood pressure, cholesterol, smoking, exercise and fitness, nutrition, weight control, prenatal care, medical self-care, mental health, stress management, alcohol and other drugs, AIDS/HIV infection, sexually transmitted diseases (STDs), job hazards and injury prevention, back care, and off-the-job accidents.
- ◆ **Facilities or services.** Nutrition, physical fitness, alcohol and other drugs, and stress management.

Figure 14-11 shows the prevalence of worksites with 50 or more employees offering information or activities in 17 subject areas. According to the DHHS, two out of three worksites with at least 50 employees offer some form of health promotion program.[55] Successful nutrition promotion programs range from introducing heart healthy menus into company cafeterias to reducing blood cholesterol levels through screening and intervention.[56] As described in Chapter 8, the Treatwell intervention project promoted dietary changes to reduce fat and increase dietary fiber consumption among employees at 8 worksites.[57]

Current efforts to help young adults identify their familial risk factors for chronic disease conditions and programs that tout the benefits of lifelong healthful eating and regular physical activity should enable the older adults of tomorrow to enjoy a productive and satisfying life well into advanced age. For older adults (those over 50), health promotion efforts seek to preserve independence, productivity, and personal fulfillment.[58] The premise of health promotion is that individuals can enjoy benefits from healthful behaviors at any age. To this end,

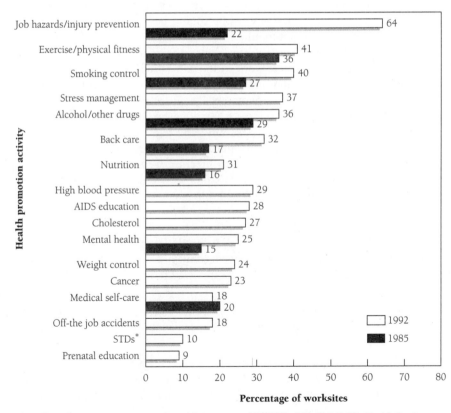

FIGURE

14-11

Worksites Offering Health Promotion Information or Activities, 1985 and 1992

Source: Reprinted with permission from U.S. Department of Health and Human Services, 1992 National Survey of Worksite Health Promotion Activities: Summary, *American Journal of Health Promotion* 7 (1993): 454.

The Office of Disease Prevention and Health Promotion (ODPHP) of the U.S. Public Health Service conducted a 1992 survey to measure the growth of worksite health promotion activities since its first survey in 1985. This figure shows the prevalence of worksites with information or activities in 17 subject areas in 1992 and comparisons with 1985 in eight areas.

*STDs = sexually transmitted diseases

most states now offer community wellness centers for seniors that include services at all levels of prevention.[59] Resource people for these efforts at the local level include public health nutritionists employed by county health departments, consultant registered dietitians working with local nursing homes and community hospitals, and county extension service home economists.[60] Community groups and churches also offer support and self-help groups.

Looking Ahead: And Then *We* Were Old

As a nation, we tend to value the future more than the present, putting off enjoying today so that we will have money, prestige, or time to have fun tomorrow. The elderly feel this loss of future. The present is their time for leisure and enjoyment, but often they have no experience in using leisure time.

The solution is to begin to prepare for old age early in life, both psychologically and nutritionally. Preparation for this period should, of course, include financial planning, but other lifelong habits should be developed as well. Each adult needs to learn to reach out to others to forestall the loneliness that will otherwise ensue. Adults need to develop some skills or activities that they can continue into their later years—volunteer work with organizations, reading, games, hobbies, or intellectual pursuits—and that will give meaning to their lives. Each adult needs to develop the habit of adjusting to change, especially when it comes without consent, so that it will not be seen as a loss of control over one's life. The goal is to arrive at maturity with as healthy a mind and body as possible; this means cultivating good nutrition status and maintaining a program of daily exercise.

In general, the ability of the elderly to function well varies from person to person and depends on several factors. The following "life advantages" seem to contribute to good physical and mental health in later years:[61]

◆ Genetic potential for extended longevity. Some persons seem to have inherited a reduced susceptibility to degenerative diseases.

◆ A continued desire for new knowledge and new experiences. Some studies suggest that "active" minds, ever involved in learning new things, may be more resistant to decline.

◆ Socialization, intimacy, and family integrity. Older persons thrive in situations where love, understanding, shared responsibility, and mutual respect are nurtured.

◆ Adherence to a prudent diet while avoiding excesses of food energy, fat, cholesterol, and sodium. A prudent diet with adequate intakes of all essential nutrients has a positive impact on health and weight management.

◆ Avoidance of substance abuse.

◆ Acceptable living arrangements.

◆ Financial independence.

Growing Seasoned

- ◆ Choose nutrient-dense foods.
- ◆ Maintain appropriate body weight.
- ◆ Reduce stress.
- ◆ For women, see a physician about estrogen replacement against osteoporosis.
- ◆ For people who smoke, quit.
- ◆ Expect to enjoy sex, and learn new ways of enhancing it.
- ◆ Use alcohol only moderately, if at all; use drugs only as prescribed.
- ◆ Take care to prevent accidents.
- ◆ Expect good vision and hearing throughout life; obtain glasses and hearing aids if necessary.
- ◆ Be alert to confusion as a disease symptom, and seek diagnosis.
- ◆ Control depression through activities and friendships.
- ◆ Drink 8 glasses of water every day.
- ◆ Practice mental skills. Keep on solving math problems and crossword puzzles, playing cards or other games, reading, writing, imagining, and creating.
- ◆ Make financial plans early to ensure security.
- ◆ Accept change. Work at recovering from losses; make new friends.
- ◆ Cultivate spiritual health. Cherish personal values. Make life meaningful.
- ◆ Go outside for sunshine and fresh air as often as possible.
- ◆ Be physically active. Walk, run, dance, swim, bike, row, or climb for aerobic activity. Lift weights, do calisthenics, or pursue some other activity to tone, firm, and strengthen muscles.
- ◆ Be socially active—play bridge, join an exercise group, take a class, teach a class, eat with friends, or volunteer time to help others.
- ◆ Stay interested in life—pursue a hobby, spend time with grandchildren, take a trip, read, grow a garden, or go to the movies.
- ◆ Enjoy life.

Source: Adapted by permission from *Understanding Nutrition,* 6th ed. by E. N. Whitney and S. R. Rolfes. Copyright © 1993 by West Publishing Company. All rights reserved.

◆ Access to health care, including a family physician, health clinic, public health nursing service providing home health care, dentist, podiatrist, physical therapist, pharmacist, and community nutritionist.

Everyone knows older people who have maintained many contacts—through relatives, church, synagogue, or fraternal orders—and have not allowed themselves to drift into isolation. Upon analysis, you will find that their favorable environment came through a lifetime of effort. These people spent their entire lives reaching out to others and practicing the art of weaving others into their own lives. Likewise, a lifetime of effort is required for good nutrition status in the later years. A person who has eaten a wide variety of foods, stayed trim, and remained physically active will be best able to withstand the assaults of change.

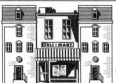 **COMMUNITY LEARNING ACTIVITY**

In this activity, we ask that you become familiar with an older adult's circumstances and needs. The older adult you choose to interview can be a relative, neighbor, associate, or other individual over the age of 65. Ask your interviewee to complete the checklist developed by the Nutrition Screening Initiative (see Figure 14-7). Next, depending on the results you obtain, refer to the schematic in Figure 14-8 and determine your appropriate next step. Use the Level I screen to further evaluate risk factors for poor nutrition status in this individual (see Appendix E). Finally, what nutrition interventions and referrals, if any, would you recommend to this person (e.g., nutrition education, food stamps, congregate or home-delivered meals programs, dental care, physical activity and exercise programs, homemaker or home health aide assistance, and socialization activities)?

Getting Where You Want to Go

Imagine for a minute that circumstances require you to travel from Kansas City to Chicago. Spreading a map across your lap, you plot your course. You could take an interstate highway all the way, starting with I-35 traveling north to Des Moines and then turning east toward Chicago on I-80. Or you might take I-70 to St. Louis and turn due north onto I-55, a course that would take you right into the Chicago Loop. Or you might decide to bypass the interstate highways altogether and stick to the so-called blue highways, those tiny threads on the map that snake along from town to town. Your decision about which route to take depends on many factors, including the purpose and urgency of your trip and how much time you can allocate for traveling.

In many respects, your decision about what you do in life is much like plotting a journey by car to a distant city. Many choices confront you, and the possibility always exists that circumstances may compel or entice you to change your route along the way. Right now, you might be asking yourself the following questions: How can I get where I want to go? More importantly, how do I determine where I want to go in the first place? The answers to these questions are unique to each of you, because each of you is unique. As you read through this discussion, write down your thoughts to help clarify your vision.

◆ SQUARE ONE: KNOW YOURSELF

The first step in determining where you want to go is to know yourself. Hold yourself up to the light, so to speak, so that you can see yourself from every angle. Evaluate your strong points and the areas marked for improvement. (The "To Be Improved" areas are sometimes called weaknesses. Weaknesses are not personality defects or deficits. They are areas of personal development that you have not had the time or inclination to explore and strengthen.) Consider your personality, your view of the world, and what you want out of life. Do you like working with people? Do you enjoy tinkering with gadgets and gizmos? Do you value public service? Are you an optimist or a cynic? Would you describe yourself as impulsive, dependable, funny, unfocused, inquisitive, theatrical, or lazy? Write down the words that describe all aspects of your personality and character. Remember, there are no right or wrong answers.

◆ SQUARE TWO: DEFINE YOUR DREAMS

Knowing who you are (and who you are not) will help you move to the next tier—defining your dreams. Your vision of your future lies in your dreams, for what you *imagine* yourself doing is what you are ultimately going to do. So, what do you see yourself doing? To help you define your dreams, answer the following questions:[1]

- ◆ What would you ideally most like to *be?*
- ◆ What would you ideally most like to *do?*
- ◆ What kind of experiences help you feel complete?
- ◆ In what kind of situations do you most want and tend to share yourself?

Continued

Let yourself dream freely and without constraints. Do not be concerned at this point about finances or family obligations. Give your dreams room to grow.

◆ SQUARE THREE: SET GOALS

Having dreams won't get you very far if you don't put some structure to them. As Thoreau stated so eloquently, "If you have built castles in the air, your work need not be lost; that is where they should be. Now put the foundations under them."[2]

Setting specific goals for your future is one of the most challenging tasks you will undertake. There are many areas in which goal setting is desirable: economic, spiritual, social, physical, mental, emotional, educational, personal, and vocational.

For this exercise, set at least one goal for your personal life. The goal should be achievable but broad enough to accommodate your dreams. Joe D. Batten, author of the book *Tough-Minded Leadership*, wrote his personal goal as follows: "I will make the lives of others richer by the richness of my own."[3] Your personal goal might be entirely different.

Another way to approach this exercise is to write your personal mission statement. A personal mission statement is much like a nation's constitution; it is a set of principles to live by. In his bestselling book *The 7 Habits of Highly Effective People,* Stephen R. Covey cites the personal mission statement developed by a friend, a portion of which is shown in the accompanying box.

◆ SQUARE FOUR: DEVELOP AN ACTION PLAN

To paraphrase a Chinese proverb, if you don't know where you are going, then any road will take you there. To get where you want to go, you *must* develop an action plan. Action

---

An Example of a Personal Mission Statement

◆ Succeed at home first.

◆ Never compromise with honesty.

◆ Be sincere yet decisive.

◆ Develop one new proficiency a year.

◆ Plan tomorrow's work today.

◆ Maintain a positive attitude.

◆ Keep a sense of humor.

◆ Do not fear mistakes—fear only the absence of creative, constructive, and corrective responses to those mistakes.

◆ Help subordinates achieve success.

◆ Concentrate all abilities and efforts on the task at hand; do not worry about the next job or promotion.

Source: Adapted from S. R. Covey, *The 7 Habits of Highly Effective People* (New York: Simon & Schuster, 1989), p. 106.

Continued

◆ PROFESSIONAL FOCUS—*Continued*

is the essence of achievement. Stephen Covey calls this "beginning with the end in mind." You must begin your journey with a clear picture of your destination; that is, you must mentally create the image of who you want to be and where you want to go before you physically create the image. Use the following steps to develop an action plan for your personal life:

1. Develop a picture in your mind's eye of what you want to do with your life. You may see yourself having a family and a career position with a major food company, or helping an isolated community in a developing country improve its standard of living, or starting your own business. The technique of mental imaging allows you to fine-tune your picture, so that when opportunities present themselves, you can determine whether they fit your action plan.

2. Pretest your mental picture. If your mental picture shows you working with small animals as part of a research project, then find a way to test your decision before you commit yourself to this path. You may discover that you don't like working with rats or hamsters! Pretesting your decisions saves time and allows you to discard opportunities that are not useful or don't fit your action plan.

3. Predetermine your alternatives. Have a backup plan to help you maximize your opportunities and forestall any crises. Explore your alternatives by talking to people who have pursued a similar dream.

◆ LEARN TO MANAGE YOURSELF

Shirley Hufstedler, a lawyer who became the secretary of education, remarked: "When I was very young, the things I wanted to do were not permitted by social dictates. I wanted to do a lot of things that girls weren't supposed to do. So I had to figure out ways to do what I wanted to do and still show up in a pinafore for a piano recital, so as not to blow my cover. You could call it manipulation, but I see it as observation and picking one's way around obstacles. If you think of what you want and examine the possibilities, you can usually figure out a way to accomplish it."[4]

Getting where you want to go is nearly impossible if you don't learn to manage yourself—your goals, your time, your work. Aristotle observed that the hardest victory is the victory over self. Successful people have mastered themselves through discipline. For some people, discipline is a dirty word. In truth, discipline means *training*. Any athlete will attest to the power of training, which builds, molds, and strengthens the body and mind for a strong performance. Discipline is as important to life as it is to athletic competition. Without it, little can be accomplished. Acquiring discipline, the mastery of self, is a lifelong process for most of us, and there is no simple pattern by which it can be attained. The process involves developing a vision, setting goals, and following through on an action plan to reach those goals. The first step in acquiring discipline begins at square one: Know yourself.

1. J. D. Batten, *Tough-Minded Leadership* (New York: American Management Association, 1989), p. 177.
2. As cited in R. N. Bolles, *The Three Boxes of Life* (Berkeley, Calif.: Ten Speed Press, 1981), p. 34.
3. As cited in Batten, *Tough-Minded Leadership*, p. 179.
4. As cited in W. Bennis, *On Becoming a Leader* (Reading, Mass.: Addison-Wesley, 1989), pp. 53–54.

NOTES

1. National Center for Health Statistics, *Health United States, 1988* (Washington, D.C.: U.S. Department of Health and Human Services, December 1988).

2. A. E. Harper, Nutrition, aging, and longevity, *American Journal of Clinical Nutrition* (Supplement) 36 (October 1982): 737–49.

3. The discussion of demographic trends was adapted from B. Senauer, E. Asp, and J. Kinsey, *Food Trends and the Changing Consumer* (St. Paul, Minn.: Eagan Press, 1991), pp. 199–213.

4. Ibid., p. 199.

5. C. W. Lecos, Diet and the elderly, *FDA Consumer*, January 1985, pp. 1–4; and C. C. Pegels, *Health Care and the Older Citizen* (Gaithersburg, Md.: Aspen Publishers, 1988).

6. Institute of Medicine, *Extending Life, Enhancing Life: A National Research Agenda on Aging* (Washington, D.C.: National Academy Press, 1991), p. 1.

7. *Healthy People 2000: National Health Promotion and Disease Prevention* (Washington, D.C.: U.S. Department of Health and Human Services, Public Health Service, 1990), pp. 579–92.

8. J. M. McGinnis and M. Nestle, The Surgeon General's report on nutrition and health: Policy implications and implementation strategies, *American Journal of Clinical Nutrition* 49 (1989): 23–28.

9. *Healthy People 2000,* pp. 588-89, 611–13.

10. M. Nestle and J. A. Gilbride, Nutrition policies for health promotion in older adults: Education priorities for the 1990s, *Journal of Nutrition Education* 22 (1990): 316.

11. Institute of Medicine, *The Second Fifty Years: Promoting Health and Preventing Disability* (Washington, D.C.: National Academy Press, 1992), pp. 1–21.

12. Institute of Medicine, *Extending Life.*

13. J. E. Kerstetter, B. A. Holthausen, and P. A. Fitz, Malnutrition in the institutionalized older adult, *Journal of the American Dietetic Association* 92 (1992): 1109–16.

14. J. T. Dwyer, J. J. Gallo, and W. Reichel, Assessing nutritional status in elderly patients, *American Family Physician* 47 (1993): 613–20.

15. J. B. Blumberg, Changing nutrient requirements in older adults, *Nutrition Today*, September/October 1992, pp. 15–20.

16. U.S. Department of Health and Human Services, *The Surgeon General's Report on Nutrition and Health* (Washington, D.C.: DHHS, 1988), pp. 595–617.

17. G. E. Gray, A. Paganini-Hill, and R. K. Ross, Vitamin supplement use in a Southern California retirement community, *Journal of the American Dietetic Association* 86 (1986): 800–802.

18. Nutrition of the elderly, *Dairy Council Digest* 48 (1977): 1–2.

19. E. L. Smith, P. E. Smith, and C. Gilligan, Diet, exercise, and chronic disease patterns in older adults, *Nutrition Reviews* 46 (1988): 52–61.

20. Institute of Medicine, *Extending Life,* pp. 1–39.

21. Institute of Medicine, *The Second Fifty Years,* pp. 168–69.

22. Kerstetter, Holthausen, and Fitz, Malnutrition, p. 1113.

23. F. G. Abdellah and S. R. Moore, eds., *Surgeon General's Workshop on Health Promotion and Aging: Proceedings* (Washington, D.C.: Office of the Surgeon General, 1988), pp. G1–G19.

24. M. T. Fanelli and M. Kaufman, Nutrition and older adults, in *Aging and Public Health*, ed. H. T. Philips and S. H. Gaylord (New York: Springer Publishing, 1985), pp. 70–100.

25. Community Nutrition Institute, *Nutrition Week,* April 30, 1993, p. 3.

26. *Nutrition Screening Initiative Survey* (Washington, D.C.: Peter D. Hart Research Associates, February, 1990); and President's page: The Nutrition Screening Initiative—An emerging force in public policy, *Journal of the American Dietetic Association* 93 (1993): 822.

27. Kerstetter, Holthausen, and Fitz, Malnutrition, p. 1114.

28. *Surgeon General's Workshop: Health Promotion and Aging* (Washington, D.C.: U.S. Department of Health and Human Services, 1988).

29. Position of the American Dietetic Association: Nutrition, aging, and the continuum of health care, *Journal of the American Dietetic Association* 93 (1993): 80–82.

30. J. T. Dwyer, *Screening Older Americans' Nutritional Health: Current Practices and Possibilities* (Washington, D.C.: Nutrition Screening Initiative, 1991), pp. 1–23.

31. M. A. Hess, President's page: ADA as an advocate for older Americans, *Journal of the American Dietetic Association* 91 (1991): 847–49.

32. J. V. White and coauthors, Nutrition Screening Initiative: Development and implementation of the public awareness checklist and screening tools, *Journal of the American Dietetic Association* 92 (1992): 163–67.

33. The discussion of tools used by the Nutrition Screening Initiative was adapted from White and coauthors, Nutrition Screening Initiative, pp. 163–67; J. V. White and coauthors, Consensus of the Nutrition Screening Initiative: Risk factors and indicators of poor nutritional status in older Americans, *Journal of the American*

Dietetic Association 91 (1991): 783–87; and J. V. White, Risk factors for poor nutritional status in older Americans, *American Family Physician* 44 (1991): 2087–97.

34. S. Mobarhan and L. S. Trumbore, Nutritional problems of the elderly, *Clinics in Geriatric Medicine* 7 (1991): 191–214.

35. The discussion of assessment in the elderly was adapted from P. P. Barry and M. Ibarra, Multidimensional assessment of the elderly, *Hospital Practice* 25 (1990): 117–28; Mobarhan and Trumbore, Nutritional problems of the elderly; C. O. Mitchell, Nutritional assessment of the elderly, *Clinics in Applied Nutrition* 1 (1991): 76–88; and R. Chernoff, Physiological aging and nutrition status, *Nutrition in Clinical Practice* 5 (1990): 8–13.

36. W. C. Chumlea, A. F. Roche, and M. L. Steinbaugh, Estimating stature from knee height for persons 60 to 90 years of age, *Journal of the American Geriatric Society* 33 (1985): 116–20.

37. Mitchell, Nutritional assessment of the elderly.

38. J. Weinberg, Psychologic implications of the nutritional needs of the elderly, *Journal of the American Dietetic Association* 60 (1972): 293–96.

39. U.S. Department of Health and Human Services, *The Surgeon General's Report,* pp. 598–99.

40. Fanelli and Kaufman, Nutrition and older adults, pp. 88–89.

41. S. Saffel-Shrier and B. M. Athas, Effective provision of comprehensive nutrition case management for the elderly, *Journal of the American Dietetic Association* 93 (1993): 439–444.

42. R. Chernoff, *Geriatric Nutrition: The Health Professional's Handbook* (Gaithersburg, Md.: Aspen, 1991), pp. 436–42.

43. *Meals-on-Wheels America: More Meals for the Homebound Through Public/Private Partnerships—A Technical Assistant Guide* (New York: New York City Department for the Aging, 1989).

44. J. V. White and coauthors, Beyond nutrition screening: A systems approach to nutrition intervention, *Journal of the American Dietetic Association* 93 (1993): 405–407.

45. B. G. Janas, C. A. Bisogni, and C. C. Campbell, Conceptual model for dietary change to lower serum cholesterol, *Journal of Nutrition Education* 25 (1993): 186–92; and T. Byers, Dietary trends in the United States: Relevance to cancer prevention, *Cancer* 72 (1993): 1015–18.

46. Report of the National Cholesterol Education Program Expert Panel on Detection, Evaluation, and Treatment of High Blood Cholesterol in Adults, *Archives of Internal Medicine* 148 (1988): 36–69.

47. J. Dwyer, Diet and nutritional strategies for cancer risk reduction: Focus on the 21st century, *Cancer* 72 (1993): 1024–31.

48. P. R. Thomas, Improving America's diet and health: From recommendations to action, *Journal of Nutrition Education* 23 (1991): 128–31.

49. E. D'urso-Fischer and coauthors, Reaching out to the elderly, *Nutrition Today* 25 (1990): 20–25.

50. Ibid, pp. 20–21.

51. Ibid.

52. A. Worick and M. Petersons, Weight-loss contests at the worksite: Results of repeat participation, *Journal of the American Dietetic Association* 93 (1993): 680–81.

53. R. W. Jeffery, The healthy worker project, *American Journal of Public Health* 83 (1993): 395–401; J. C. Erfurt, A. Foote, and M. A. Heirich, Worksite wellness programs: Incremental comparisons of screening and referral alone, health education, follow-up counseling, and plant organization, *American Journal of Health Promotion* 5 (1991): 438–48; and C. S. Wilbur, Live for life: The Johnson & Johnson program, *Preventive Medicine* 12 (1983): 672–81.

54. The list of classes of health promotion activities is from U.S. Department of Health and Human Services, 1992 National Survey of Worksite Health Promotion Activities: Summary, *American Journal of Health Promotion* 7 (1993): 452–64.

55. Jeffery, The healthy worker project, p. 395.

56. K. Richmond, Introducing heart healthy foods in a company cafeteria, *Journal of Nutrition Education* 18 (1986): S63; G. S. Peterson and coauthors, Strategies for lowering cholesterol at the worksite, *Journal of Nutrition Education* 18 (1986): S54; and H. Quigley, L. L. Bean cholesterol reduction program, *Journal of Nutrition Education* 18 (1986): S58.

57. J. R. Hebert and coauthors, A work-site nutrition intervention: Its effects on the consumption of cancer-related nutrients, *American Journal of Public Health* 83 (1993): 391–94.

58. M. G. Ory, Considerations in the development of age-sensitive indicators for assessing health promotion, *Health Promotion* 3 (1988): 139–49.

59. S. Maloney, Healthy older people, in *Surgeon General's Workshop on Health Promotion and Aging* (Washington, D.C.: U.S. Department of Health and Human Services, 1988).

60. Fanelli and Kaufman, Nutrition and older adults, p. 95.

61. The list of advantages was adapted from D. A. Roe, *Geriatric Nutrition,* 3rd ed. (Englewood Cliffs, N.J.: Prentice Hall, 1992), pp. 1–9.

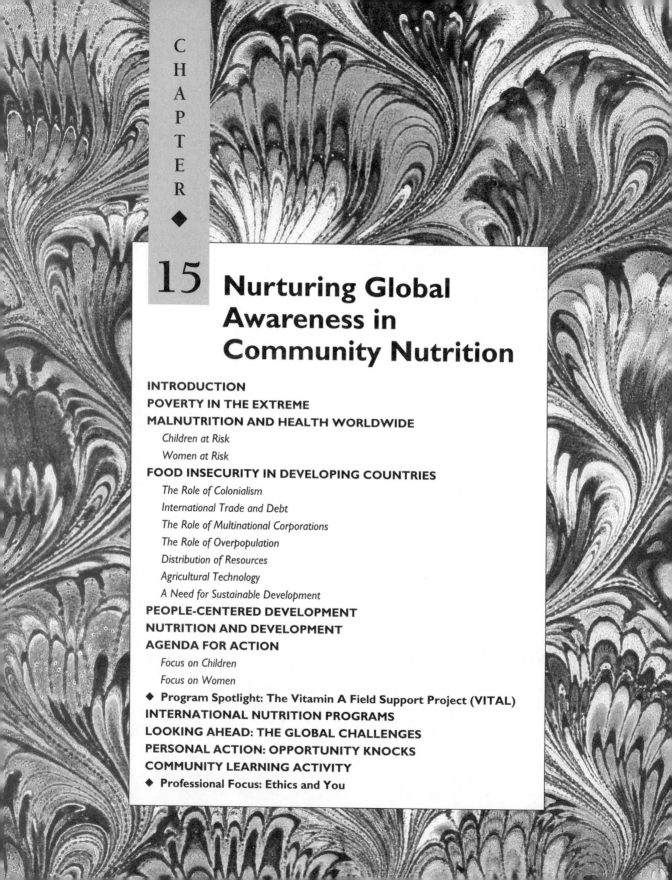

15 Nurturing Global Awareness in Community Nutrition

Something to Think About . . .

The world does not exist in a series of separately functioning compartments. The last lines from the chapter on poverty in the State of the World Report sum this up succinctly: "Sheets of rain washing off denuded watersheds flood exclusive neighborhoods as surely as slums. Potentially valuable medicines lost with the extinction of rain forest species are as unavailable to the rich in their private hospitals as they are to the poor in rural clinics. And the carbon dioxide released as landless migrants burn plots in the Amazon or the Congo warms the globe as surely as do the fumes from automobiles and factory smoke-stacks in Los Angeles or Milan."

Poverty, food security, environment, nutrition—they are all inescapably interlinked. Those of you who have the knowledge to embrace issues of nutrition education also have the power to ameliorate the human predicament. And there is no objective in this world more worth pursuing than improving the human condition.

—Stephen Lewis

Introduction

All people need food. Regardless of race, religion, sex, or nationality, our bodies experience similarly the effects of food insecurity and its companion malnutrition—listlessness, weakness, failure to thrive, stunted growth, mental retardation, muscle wastage, scurvy, anemia, rickets, osteoporosis, goiter, tooth decay, blindness, and a host of other effects, including death.[1] Apathy and shortened attention span are two of a number of behavioral symptoms that are often mistaken for laziness, lack of intelligence, or mental illness in undernourished people.

The Food and Agriculture Organization (FAO) estimates that of the more than 5 billion people in the world, at least half a billion—one in ten humans—suffer from chronic, severe undernutrition, consuming too little food each day to meet even minimum energy requirements.[2] About 190 million or more are children of preschool age, and 10 million of these weigh less than 60 percent of the standard weight for their age. Some 2 billion people, mostly women and children, are deficient in one or more of three major micronutrients: iron, iodine, and vitamin A.[3]

To qualify as chronically and severely undernourished by FAO standards, a person must consume fewer than the calories required to meet minimal energy needs as expressed by 1.4 × resting energy expenditure (REE).

Poverty in the Extreme

Food insecurity was once viewed as a problem of overpopulation and inadequate food production, but now many people recognize it as a problem of poverty (see

Food security is defined as access by all people at all times to enough food for an active and healthy life. Food security has two aspects: ensuring that adequate food supplies are available and ensuring that households whose members suffer from undernutrition have the ability to acquire food, either by producing it themselves or by being able to purchase it.

Figure 15-1).[4] Food is *available* but not *accessible* to the poor who have neither land nor money. In 1978, Robert McNamara, then-president of the World Bank, gave what stands as the classic description of *absolute* poverty: "A condition of life so limited by malnutrition, illiteracy, disease, squalid surroundings, high infant mortality, and low life expectancy as to be beneath any reasonable definition of human decency."[5]

The total numbers of people estimated to be living in poverty are given in Table 15-1. The present estimate of 1.2 billion people living in poverty translates to 23 percent of the world's population (200 million more people than in 1980). The 1980s have been called "the lost decade" for the poor of Africa, Latin America, and parts of Asia. Living standards declined due in part to accelerated rates of population growth and environmental decline, but also as a result of lower export earnings, rising inflation, and higher interest rates on foreign debts.[6] In other words, the poor earned less and paid more.

Those who live with chronic poverty must constantly face unsafe drinking water, intestinal parasites, insufficient food, a low-protein diet, stunted growth,

FIGURE

15-1

The Gap between Developed and Developing Countries

Source: U.S. Presidential Commission on World Hunger, *Overcoming World Hunger: The Challenge Ahead*, abridged ed. (Washington, D.C.: U.S. Government Printing Office, June 1980), p. 4.

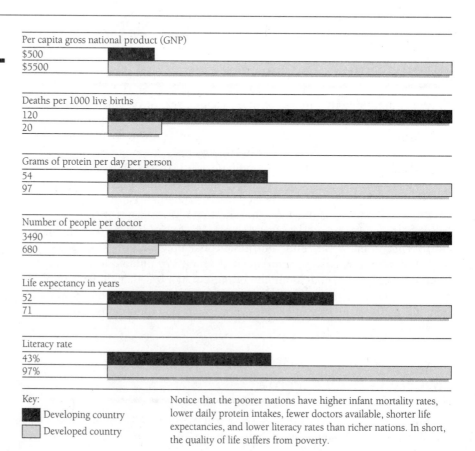

Per capita gross national product (GNP)
$500
$5500

Deaths per 1000 live births
120
20

Grams of protein per day per person
54
97

Number of people per doctor
3490
680

Life expectancy in years
52
71

Literacy rate
43%
97%

Key:
▓ Developing country
☐ Developed country

Notice that the poorer nations have higher infant mortality rates, lower daily protein intakes, fewer doctors available, shorter life expectancies, and lower literacy rates than richer nations. In short, the quality of life suffers from poverty.

REGION	NUMBER OF PEOPLE* (MILLIONS)	PERCENTAGE OF TOTAL POPULATION
Asia	675	25
Sub-Saharan Africa	325	62
Latin America	150	35
North Africa and Middle East	75	28
World	1225	23

*Estimates are best thought of as mid-points of ranges that extend 10% above and 10% below listed figures.

TABLE

15-1

People Estimated to be Living in Absolute Poverty, 1989
Source: Worldwatch Institute.

low birth weights, illiteracy, disease, shortened life spans, and death. In *Quiet Violence: View from a Bangladesh Village*, Hartman and Boyce provide a good introduction to life in the villages of the developing world. The lives of these villagers are more difficult than anything we have ever known, and yet their hopes and dreams are not unlike our own. They exhibit resourcefulness, hard work, and dignity in the midst of circumstances that require a persistence and personal strength that most of us will never need to call upon in our lifetimes. Hari, one of the landless laborers in the village, reflects on his life just days before his death: "Between the mortar and the pestle, the chili cannot last. We poor are like chilies—each year we are ground down, and soon there will be nothing left."[7]

Poverty is much more than an economic condition and exists for many reasons, including overpopulation, the greed of others, unemployment, and the lack of productive resources such as land, tools, and credit. Consequently, if we are to provide adequate nutrition for all the earth's hungry people, we must transform the economic, political, and social structures that both limit food production, distribution, and consumption and create a gap between rich and poor.

Malnutrition and Health Worldwide

Worldwide, about 40,000 to 50,000 people die each day as a result of undernutrition. Millions of children die each year from the parasitic and infectious diseases associated with poverty: dysentery, whooping cough, measles, tuberculosis, cholera, and malaria (see Table 15-2). These diseases interact with poor nutrition to form a vicious cycle in which the outcome for many is death, as shown in Figure 15-2.[8] UNICEF estimates that malnutrition and disease claim the lives of 250,000 children *every week*.[9]

UNICEF estimates that most child malnutrition in the developing world could be eliminated with the expenditure of an additional $25 billion a year (see Figure 15-3 on page 502 to put this sum of money in perspective). This amount would cover the cost of the resources needed to control the major childhood diseases, halve the rate of child malnutrition, bring clean water and safe sanitation to all communities, make family planning services universally available, and provide almost every child with at least a basic education.[10]

No famine, no flood, no earthquake, no war has ever claimed the lives of 250,000 children in a single week. Yet malnutrition and disease claim that number of child victims every week.

UNICEF The United Nations International Children's Emergency Fund, now referred to as the United Nations Children's Fund.

TABLE

15-2

The Five Leading Diseases That Kill Children, Late 1980s
Source: UNICEF 1990.

CONDITION	PERCENTAGE OF CHILD DEATHS	ANNUAL NUMBER OF CHILD DEATHS	READILY PREVENTABLE?
Diarrhea	34.6	5,000,000	Yes, with clean water and medication
Acute respiratory diseases	27.7	4,000,000	Yes, with immunization and medication
Measles	13.8	2,000,000	Yes, with immunization
Tetanus	12.4	1,800,000	Yes, with immunization
Malaria	6.9	1,000,000	Yes, with medication

Protein-energy malnutrition (PEM) The world's most widespread malnutrition problem, includes **kwashiorkor** (a deficiency disease caused by inadequate protein intake), **marasmus** (a deficiency disease caused by inadequate food intake—starvation), and the states in which they overlap.

Hungry people receive such small quantities of food that they develop multiple nutrient deficiencies. Their undernutrition may result from lack of food energy or from a lack of both food energy and protein—protein-energy malnutrition (PEM). Such distinctions can easily be made on paper, and the extremes are evident in individuals; but for the most part, the differences blur.

Protein-energy malnutrition (PEM) is the most widespread form of malnutrition in the world today, affecting over 500 million children. Children who are thin for their height may be suffering from acute PEM (recent severe food restriction), whereas children who are short for their age may be suffering from chronic PEM (long-term food deprivation). PEM includes the classifications of **kwashiorkor**, a protein deficiency disease, **marasmus**, a deficiency disease caused by inadequate food intake, and the states in which these two extremes overlap.* Children suffering from PEM are likely to develop infections, nutrient deficiencies, and diarrhea.

Worldwide, three micronutrient deficiencies are of particular concern: vitamin A deficiency, the world's most common cause of preventable child blindness and vision impairment; iron-deficiency anemia; and iodine deficiency, which causes high levels of goiter and child retardation.[11]

This chapter's Program Spotlight highlights the international activities of the Vitamin A Field Support Project (VITAL).

◆ Vitamin A deficiency. Some 13 million children below six years of age have xerophthalmia. Of these, an estimated 500,000 children become partially or totally blind as a result of insufficient vitamin A in the diet. Vitamin A deficiency is also associated with other forms of malnutrition, infection, diarrhea, and a high rate of mortality.

◆ Iron deficiency. Iron-deficiency anemia is estimated to affect some 1.3 billion people, or one-fourth of all people living. Iron deficiency in infancy

* The exact cause of kwashiorkor remains uncertain. Some research suggests that kwashiorkor may involve more than protein deficiency and develops when malnourished children eat moldy grains or peanuts. The mold *Aspergillus flavus*, commonly found in hot, humid areas, produces a potent aflatoxin that inhibits protein synthesis. (R. G. Hendickse, Kwashiorkor: The hypothesis that incriminates aflatoxins, *Pediatrics* 88 [1991]: 376–79.)

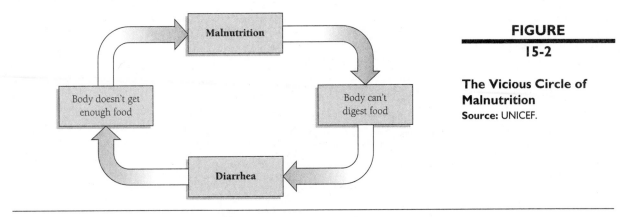

FIGURE

15-2

The Vicious Circle of Malnutrition
Source: UNICEF.

and early childhood is associated with decreased cognitive abilities and resistance to disease.

◆ Iodine deficiency. Iodine deficiency, the major preventable cause of mental retardation worldwide, is a risk factor for both physical and mental retardation in about 1 billion people. About 200 million people worldwide—especially in mountainous regions—are estimated to have goiter, and over 3 million suffer overt cretinism.

The malnutrition that comes from living with food insecurity is one of the major factors influencing life expectancy. According to the *1990 World Population Data Sheet*, life expectancy at birth in the United States and Canada is now about 77 years.[12] In Japan, Switzerland, and Sweden, it is about 78 years. Worldwide, life expectancy averages about 62 years, but in Africa it is approximately 50, and in the small African country of Sierra Leone it is only 43.

Hunger and malnutrition can be found in people of all ages, sexes, and nationalities. Even so, these problems hit some groups harder than others.

◆ CHILDREN AT RISK

When nutrient needs are high (as in times of rapid growth), the risk of undernutrition increases. If family food is limited, pregnant and lactating women, infants, and children are the first to show the signs of undernutrition. Effects of food insecurity can be devastating to this group of the population.

As Chapter 12 pointed out, to support normal fetal growth and development, women must gain adequate weight during pregnancy. Healthy women in developed countries gain an average of about 27 pounds. Studies among poor women show a weight gain of only 11 to 15 pounds.[13] As a consequence, they give birth to babies with low birth weights.

Birth weight is a potent indicator of an infant's future health status. A low–birth weight baby (less than $5\frac{1}{2}$ pounds or 2500 grams) is more likely to experience complications during delivery than a normal baby and has a statistically greater-than-normal chance of having physical and mental birth defects,

FIGURE

15-3

Affording the Cost
Source: UNICEF, derived from various sources.

It is no longer possible to say that the task of meeting basic human needs is too vast or expensive. With present knowledge, the task could be accomplished within a decade and at a cost of an extra $25 billion per year. Some comparisons:

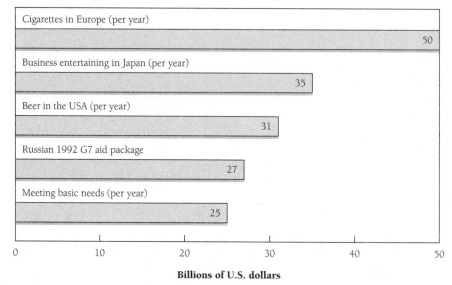

Billions of U.S. dollars

This $25 billion is UNICEF's estimate of the extra resources required to control the major childhood diseases, halve child malnutrition, reduce child deaths by 4 million a year, bring safe water and sanitation to all communities, provide basic education for children, and make family planning universally available.

Developing countries
Countries with low per capita incomes and low standards of living. Such countries make up most of Africa, Latin America, and Asia.

contracting diseases, and dying early in life. Worldwide, low birth weight contributes to more than half of the deaths of children under five years of age. Low–birth weight infants suffering undernutrition after their births incur even greater risks. They are more likely to get sick, to fail to obtain nourishment by sucking, and to be unable to win their mothers' attention by energetic, vigorous cries and other healthy behavior. They can become apathetic, neglected babies, and this compounds the original malnutrition problems.

Until the middle of the twentieth century, in most **developing countries,** babies were breastfed for their first year of life—with supplements of other milk and cereal gruel added to their diets after the first several months. Today, the percentage of infants who are exclusively breastfed to the age of four months has dropped to below 10 percent.[14] A number of factors contributed to this unfortunate decline including the aggressive promotion and sale of infant formula to new mothers; the encouragement of bottlefeeding by health care practitioners, who send mothers home from the hospital with free samples of formula after delivery of the newborn; and the global pattern of urbanization and accompanying loss of cultural ties supporting breastfeeding combined with more women working outside the home.[15] Overall, the World Health Organization (WHO) estimates that more than a million children's lives could be saved each year if all mothers gave their babies nothing but breast milk for the first four to six months of life.[16]

Breastfeeding permits infants in many developing countries to achieve weight and height gains equal to those of children in developed countries until about six months of age, but then the majority of these children fall behind in growth and development because inadequate supplementary foods are added to their diets. Visitors to developing countries may underestimate childhood undernutrition because they do not realize that the children they think are three or four years old are actually eight or nine years old. Failure of children to grow is a warning of the extreme malnutrition that may soon follow.

Replacing breast milk with infant formula in environments and economic circumstances that make it impossible to feed formula safely may lead to infant undernutrition. Breast milk, the recommended food for infants, is sterile and contains antibodies that enhance an infant's resistance to disease. In the absence of sterilization and refrigeration, formula in bottles is an ideal breeding ground for bacteria. More than 1.9 billion people in developing countries do not have access to safe drinking water.[17] Thus, feeding infants formula prepared with contaminated water often causes infections leading to diarrhea, dehydration, and failure to absorb nutrients. In countries where poor sanitation is prevalent, breastfeeding should take priority over feeding formula. Failure to breastfeed an infant who lives in a house without indoor plumbing incurs twice the risk of perinatal mortality as breastfeeding an infant who lives in a house with good sanitation.[18]

Even if infants are protected by breastfeeding at first, they must be weaned. The **weaning period** is one of the most dangerous times for children in developing countries for a number of reasons. For one, newly weaned infants often receive nutrient-poor diluted cereals or starchy root crops. For another, infants' foods are often prepared with contaminated water, making infection almost inevitable. Attitudes toward food may also affect nutrition. In some areas of India, for example, a child may be forbidden to eat curds and fruit because they are "cold" or bananas because they "cause convulsions."[19]

Weaning period The time during which an infant's diet is changed from breast milk to other nourishment.

Mortality statistics reflect the hazards to infants and children. The infant mortality rate ranges from about 17 (Costa Rica) to over 162 (Afghanistan) in the poorest of the developing countries (see Table 15-3). The death rate for children from one to four years of age is no more favorable; it ranges from 20 to 30 times higher in developing countries than in developed countries.[20] Maternal mortality rates are equally shocking (see Figure 15-4).

UNICEF regards the **under-5 mortality rate** (U5MR) as the single best indicator of children's overall health and well-being.[21] UNICEF argues that this rate reflects the overall resources a country directs at children:

Under-five mortality rate (U5MR) The number of children who die before the age of five for every 1000 live births.

> . . . the U5MR reflects the nutritional health and the health knowledge of mothers; the level of immunization and ORT (oral rehydration therapy) use; the availability of maternal and health services (including prenatal care); income and food availability in the family; the availability of clean water and safe sanitation; and the overall safety of the child's environment.[22]

◆ WOMEN AT RISK

Women are more susceptible than men to food insecurity and undernutrition for a number of reasons. In addition to their increased nutrient needs during child-

DEVELOPING COUNTRIES WITH IMR OVER 120[b]		DEVELOPING COUNTRIES WITH IMR UNDER 25	
Asia and Middle East			
Afghanistan	162	Fiji	24
		North Korea	24
		Sri Lanka	24
		Thailand	24
		United Arab E.	22
		South Korea	21
		Malaysia	20
		Kuwait	15
		Singapore	8
Africa			
Mali	159	Mauritius	20
Sierra Leone	143		
Guinea-Bissau	140		
Malawi	138		
Guinea	134		
Gambia	132		
Mozambique	130		
Angola	127		
Burkina Faso	127		
Liberia	126		
Niger	124		
Chad	122		
Ethiopia	122		
Somalia	122		
Latin America			
-----		Panama	21
		Uruguay	20
		Chile	19
		Costa Rica	17
		Jamaica	14
		Trinidad	14
		Cuba	13

[a]This table provides the countries with the highest and lowest infant mortality rates (IMRs) found among developing nations. For countries at war, the IMR is likely to be appreciably higher than these United Nations' estimates. Table 12-1 on page 370 lists IMRs for selected developed countries.
[b]IMR = infant deaths under one year of age, expressed as a rate per thousand live births.
----- = No countries reported at this level of IMR.

bearing years, many women in developing countries are responsible, even during their pregnancies, for most of the physical labor required to procure food for their families. The poor nutrition of some women results from both their family's lack of access to food and unequal distribution of food within the family itself. A woman will feed her husband, children, and other family members first, eating only whatever is left. Furthermore, each time she becomes pregnant, her body's nutrient reserves are drained.

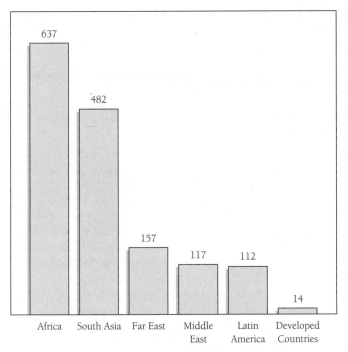

FIGURE

15-4

Maternal Mortality in Developing Regions Compared with Average for Developed Countries, 1985
Source: Reproduced with permission from *World Military and Social Expenditures,* 13th ed. by R. L. Sivard. Copyright 1989 by World Priorities, Inc., Washington, D.C., p. 31.

Death rate per 100,000 live births

Social beliefs may also limit women's food intakes. In the Indian Punjab, the director of a program aimed at relieving undernutrition in local villages found that an undernutrition rate of 10 to 15 percent persisted even after a major effort to provide supplementary foods to families. The majority of those affected were young girls, who were unable to demand their share and were regarded by other family members as not deserving a fair share.[23]

Food Insecurity in Developing Countries

World hunger is more extreme than domestic hunger. In fact, most people would find it hard to imagine the severity of poverty in the developing world:

> Many hundreds of millions of people in the poorest countries are preoccupied solely with survival and elementary needs. For them, work is frequently not available or pay is low, and conditions barely tolerable. Homes are constructed of impermanent materials and have neither piped water nor sanitation. Electricity is a luxury. Health services are thinly spread, and in rural areas only rarely within walking distance. Permanent insecurity is the condition of the poor. . . . In the wealthy countries, ordinary men and women face genuine economic problems. . . . But they rarely face anything resembling the total deprivation found in the poor countries.[24]

Table 15-4 reveals the human dimensions of the world hunger problem; Table 15-5 shows some of its many causes. World hunger is a problem of supply and demand, inappropriate technology, environmental abuse, demographic distribution, unequal access to resources, extremes in dietary patterns, and unjust economic systems. Two generalizations and an important question are suggested by these tables:

◆ The underlying causes of global hunger and poverty are complex and interrelated.

◆ Hunger is a product of poverty resulting from the ways in which governments and businesses manage national and international economies.

◆ The question then is, Why are people poor?

Poverty contributes to hunger in many important ways.[25] Oftentimes, people who are poor are powerless to change their situation because they have little access to vital resources such as education, training, food, health services, and other vehicles of change. The roots of hunger and poverty, like those of many other current problems, can be found in numerous historical and natural developments, including colonialism, economic institutions, corporate systems, population pressure, resource distribution, and agricultural technology.

TABLE

15-4

The Realities of Hunger

Source: Adapted from *World Hunger: Facts,* available from Oxfam America, 26 West St., Boston, MA 02111; Office on Global Education, Church World Service, 2115 N. Charles St., Baltimore, MD 21218.

◆ The United Nations reports that there are 520 million malnourished people in the world.

◆ Each year, 15 to 20 million people die of hunger-related causes, including diseases brought on by lowered resistance due to malnutrition. Of every four of these, three are children.

◆ Over 40% of all deaths in poor countries occur among children under five years old.

◆ The United Nations (UNICEF) states that 17 million children died last year from preventable diseases—one every two seconds, 40,000 a day. (A vaccination immunizing one child against a major disease costs 7 cents.) At least 500,000 children are partially or totally blinded each year simply through lack of vitamin A.

◆ More than 1 billion people in poor countries suffer from chronic anemia.

◆ Every day, the world produces 2 lb of grain for every man, woman, and child on earth. This is enough to provide everyone with 3000 kcal/day, well above the average need of 2300 kcal.

◆ A person born in the rich world will consume 30 times as much food as a person born in the poor world.

◆ The poor countries have nearly 75% of the world's population, but consume only about 15% of the world's available energy.

◆ One-eighth of the world's population lives on an income of less than $300 a year—many use 80 to 90% of that income to obtain food.

◆ Of the 5 billion people on earth, more than 1 billion drink contaminated water. Water-related disease claims 25 million lives a year. Of these, 15 million are under five years of age.

◆ An estimated 1 billion adults can't read or write. In many countries, half of the population over 15 is illiterate. Two-thirds of these are women.

TABLE

15-5

Causes of the World Food Problem

Source: Adapted from C. G. Knight and R. P. Wilcox, *Triumph or Triage? The World Food Problem in Geographical Perspective,* Resource Paper no. 75–3 (Washington, D.C.: Association of American Geographers, 1976), p. 4.

WORLDWIDE PROBLEMS

- Natural catastrophes—drought, heavy rains and flooding, crop failures.
- Environmental degradation—soil erosion and inadequate water resources.
- Food supply-and-demand imbalances.
- Inadequate food reserves.
- Warfare and civil disturbances.
- Migration—refugees.
- Culturally based food prejudices.
- Declining ecological conditions in agricultural regions.

PROBLEMS OF THE DEVELOPING WORLD	PROBLEMS OF THE INDUSTRIALIZED WORLD
<ul><li>Underdevelopment.</li><li>Excessive population growth.</li><li>Lack of economic incentives—farmers using inappropriate methods and laboring on land they may lose or can never hope to own.</li><li>Parents lacking knowledge of basic nutrition for their children</li><li>Insufficient government attention to the rural sector.</li></ul>	<ul><li>Excessive use of natural resources.</li><li>Pollution.</li><li>Inefficient animal protein diets.</li><li>Inadequate research in science and technology to meet basic human needs.</li><li>Excessive government bureaucracy.</li><li>Loss of farmland to competing uses.</li></ul>

PROBLEMS LINKING THE INDUSTRIALIZED AND DEVELOPING WORLDS

- Unequal access to resources.
- Inadequate transfer of research and technology.
- Lack of development planning.
- Insufficient food aid.
- Excessive food aid that undermines local initiatives for food production.
- Politics of food aid and nutrition education.
- Inappropriate technological research.
- Inappropriate role of multinational corporations.
- Insufficient emphasis on agricultural development for self-sufficiency.

◆ THE ROLE OF COLONIALISM

The colonial era led to hunger and malnutrition for millions of people in developing countries. Although no longer called colonialism, much of this same activity still continues today. The African experience provides a good example of the colonial process.

Britain, the Netherlands, Germany, France, and other nations originally colonized the African continent largely to gain a source of raw materials for industrial use. Accordingly, the colonial powers created a governing infrastructure designed merely to move Africa's minerals, metals, cash crops, and wealth to Europe. They provided few opportunities for education, disrupted traditional family structures and community organization, and greatly diminished the ability of the African people to produce their own food.

Before the Europeans arrived, small landowners throughout much of Africa had cleared forests to grow beans, grains, or vegetables for their own use. With colonialism, wealthy Africans and foreign investors took over the fertile farmland and forced the rural poor onto marginal lands that could produce adequate food only with irrigation and fertilizer, which were beyond the means of the poor. The fertile lands were used to grow cotton, sesame, sugar, cocoa, coffee, tea, tobacco, and livestock for export. As more raw materials were exported, more food and manufactured products had to be imported. Imported goods cost money—also beyond the reach of the poor.

Per capita production of grains for food use has declined for the last 20 years in Africa, while sugar cane production has doubled and tea production has quadrupled. The country of Chad recently harvested a record cotton crop in the same year that it experienced an epidemic of famine. Sixty percent of the gross national product of Ghana, Sudan, Somalia, Ethiopia, Zambia, and Malawi is derived from cash crops that finance both luxury imported goods for the minority and international debts. Huge amounts of soybeans and grains are fed to livestock to produce protein foods the poor cannot afford to purchase.

◆ INTERNATIONAL TRADE AND DEBT

Over the years, developing countries have seen the prices of imported fuels and manufactured items rise much faster than the prices they receive for their export goods, such as bananas, coffee, and various raw materials, on the international market. The combination of high import costs and low export profits often pushes a developing country into accelerating international debt that sometimes leads to bankruptcy.

Debt and trade are closely related to the progress a country can make toward achieving adequate diets for its people. As import prices increase relative to export prices, a country's money moves abroad to pay for the imports. With more and more of its money abroad, the country is forced to borrow money, usually at high interest rates, to continue functioning at home. Many of its financial resources must then go to pay the interest on the borrowed money, thus draining the economy further. Creditor nations may not demand much, or any, capital back, but they do require that interest be paid each year, and the interest can consume most of a country's gross national product. Large and growing debts can slow or halt a nation's attempt to deal effectively with its problems of local food insecurity. As more and more of its financial resources are used to pay off interest on the country's trade debts, less and less money is available to deal with food insecurity at home.[26] Each year, the debt crisis worsens and leads to further problems with hunger.

Currently, the developed and developing countries in the United Nations are discussing ways to lighten this burden of international debt. These discussions are known as the **North-South Dialogue** and represent what is referred to as a **New International Economic Order (NIEO)**. The NIEO proposals include rescheduling interest payments or even totally forgiving the debts of developing

North-South Dialogue Discussions between the developed countries and the developing countries aimed at achieving global economic change and addressing the economic imbalance in international trade experienced by the developing countries. (The more developed countries, with the exceptions of New Zealand and Australia, are located geographically to the north of most of the developing countries.)

New International Economic Order (NIEO) Proposals made by the developing countries, requesting structural changes in the international economic system.

countries. As Stephen Lewis, formerly Canada's ambassador and permanent representative to the United Nations, noted: "It would scarcely be felt if we [the North] forgave the entire African debt. Industrial capitalism lost on the stock exchange, in one day in October 1987, 10 times the African debt."[27]

Little consensus has been reached on the merits of these proposals. Some fear the loss of profits that the lender nations and multinational banks will sustain. Others believe that the loans were ill-advised to begin with and that the lenders have collected sufficient interest already, often many times the original value of the loans. In any case, the NIEO may have identified one of the key steps in solving debtor countries' hunger problems. Once the tremendous financial drain caused by their international debt is eliminated, the countries can allocate more financial resources to economic development that will lead to less hunger. Undoubtedly, the debate between the developing and developed world will continue. These North-South discussions are likely to be as crucial to the future of both sides as the arms control negotiations between the East and West were during the Cold War.

◆ THE ROLE OF MULTINATIONAL CORPORATIONS

National economic policies based on the export of cash crops, such as coffee, often have a negative effect on household food security. The competition between cash crops and food crops for farmland provides a classic example of the plight of the poor. Typically, the fertile farmlands are controlled by large landowners and **multinational corporations** who hire indigenous people for below-subsistence wages to grow crops to be exported for profit, leaving little fertile land for the local farmers to use to grow food. The local people work hard cultivating cash crops for others, not food crops for themselves. The money they earn is not even enough to buy the products they help produce. As a result, imported foods—bananas, beef, cocoa, coconuts, coffee, pineapples, sugar, tea, winter tomatoes, and the like—fill the grocery stores of developed countries, while the poor who labored to grow these foods have less food and fewer resources than when they farmed the land for their own use. Additional cropland is diverted for nonfood, cash crops such as tobacco, rubber, and cotton. These practices have also had an adverse effect on many U.S. farmers. The foreign cash crops often undersell the same U.S.-grown produce. The U.S. farmers cannot compete against these lower-priced imported foods and may be forced out of business.

Export-oriented agriculture thus uses the labor, land, capital, and technology that is needed to help local families produce their own food. For example, the resources used to produce bananas for export could be reallocated to provide food for the local people. Some have suggested that the developed countries could help alleviate the world food problem not by *giving* more food aid to the poor countries, but by *taking* less food away from them.[28]

Countless examples can be cited to illustrate how natural resources are diverted from producing food for domestic consumption to producing luxury crops for those who can afford them:

◆ Africa is a net *exporter* of barley, beans, peanuts, fresh vegetables, and cattle (not to mention luxury crops such as coffee and cocoa), yet it has a

Multinational corporations
International companies with direct investments and/or operative facilities in more than one country. U.S. oil and food companies are examples.

higher incidence of protein-energy malnutrition among young children than any other continent.

◆ Over half of the U.S. supply of several winter and early spring vegetables comes from Mexico where infant deaths associated with poor nutrition are common.

◆ Half of the agricultural land in Central America produces food for export, while in several Central American countries the poorest 50 percent of the population eat only half the protein they need.[29]

Besides diverting acreage away from the traditional staples of the local diet, some multinational corporations may also contribute to hunger through their marketing techniques. Their advertisements lead many consumers with limited incomes to associate products like cola beverages, cigarettes, infant formulas, and snack foods with Western culture and prosperity. A poor family's nutrition status suffers when its tight budget is pinched further by the purchase of such goods. Even worse is the inappropriate use of infant formula. Use of formula leads a mother to wean her infant. Then, when her money runs out and she cannot afford to buy more formula, her breast milk has ceased to flow, and she cannot resume breastfeeding. All too often, the result is malnutrition, sickness, and death of the infant.[30]

The United Nations has commissioned several studies in the hopes of establishing an international code of conduct for multinational corporations.[31] These corporations could increase the credit and capital available to the developing world; and these resources, if properly used, could help to eliminate food insecurity. The multinational corporations also possess the scientific knowledge and organizational skills needed to help develop improved food and agricultural systems. Experience shows, however, that sustained outside pressure may have to be applied to some of these corporations to help ensure that human needs do not become subordinate to political and financial gains. U.S. consumers can often influence these multinational corporations because they are shareholders in them.

◆ THE ROLE OF OVERPOPULATION

The current world population is approximately 5 billion, and the United Nations projects 6 billion by the year 2000. The earth may not be able to support this many people adequately. The world's present population is certainly of concern as is the projected increase in that population. Nevertheless, population is only one aspect of the world food problem. Poverty seems to be at the root of both problems—hunger and overpopulation.

Three major factors affect population growth: birth rates, death rates, and standards of living. Low-income countries have high birth rates, high death rates, and low standards of living.

When people's standard of living rises, giving them better access to health care, family planning, and education, the death rate falls. In time, the birth rate also falls. As the standard of living continues to improve, the family earns sufficient income to risk having smaller numbers of children. A family depends on its children to cultivate the land, secure food and water, and provide for the adults in their old age. Under conditions of ongoing poverty, parents will choose to have many children to ensure that some will survive to adulthood. Children represent the "social security" of the poor. Improvements in economic status help relieve the need for this "insurance" and so help reduce the birth rate. Table 15-6 shows the relationships between the infant mortality rate and the population growth rate and reveals that hunger and poverty reflect both the level of national development and the people's sense of security.[32]

In many countries where economic growth has occurred and all groups share resources relatively equally, the rate of population growth has decreased. Examples include Costa Rica, Sri Lanka, Taiwan, and Malaysia. In countries where economic growth has occurred but the resources are unevenly distributed, population growth has remained high. Examples include Brazil, Mexico, the Philippines, and Thailand, where a large family continues to be a major economic asset for the poor.[33]

As the world's population continues to grow, it threatens the world's capacity to produce adequate food in the future. The activity of billions of human beings on the earth's limited surface is seriously and adversely affecting our planet: wiping out many varieties of plant life, using up our freshwater supplies, and destroying the protective ozone layer that shields life from the sun's damaging rays—in short, overstraining the earth's ability to support life. Population control is one of the most pressing needs of this time in history. Until the nations of the world resolve the population problem, they must all deal with its effects and make efforts to support the life of the populations that currently exist.

The transition of population growth rates from a slow-growth stage (high birth rates and high death rates) through a rapid-growth stage (high birth rates and low death rates) to a low-growth stage (low birth rates and low death rates) is known as the **demographic transition.**

◆ DISTRIBUTION OF RESOURCES

Land reform—giving people a meaningful opportunity to produce food for local consumption, for example—can combine with population control to increase everyone's assets. Some background information is important to understanding this relationship:

◆ Much of the world's agriculture is primitive. More than 50 percent of all food consumed in the world is still produced by hand.

◆ In many countries, up to 90 percent of the population live on rural land.

◆ Most governments dictate the day-to-day lives of their people, and their policies may not be equitable.

	HUNGRY COUNTRIES	NONHUNGRY COUNTRIES
Average infant mortality rate	113 per 1000	35 per 1000
Total infant deaths per year	10.6 million	1.4 million
Size of population	2.6 billion	2.4 billion
Average rate of population increase	2.4% per year	1.0% per year
Total births per year	86.4 million	38.6 million

TABLE

15-6

Effect of Hunger on the Population Growth Rate
Source: Adapted from *The Ending Hunger Briefing Workbook* (1982), pp. 26, 30.

◆ Securing enough food on a day-to-day basis is a problem for as many as a billion human beings.

◆ Even the best land in many parts of the world does not support the growing of food, even by those who can afford fertilizer and irrigation.[34]

Resources are distributed unequally not only between the rich and the poor within nations, but also between rich and poor nations. But if the wealthy nations simply give aid to the poor nations, the poor nations will be weakened further. Instead, the wealthy nations must foster self-reliance in the poor nations. Doing so will initially require some economic sacrifices by the wealthy nations, but will ultimately benefit large numbers of hungry people.

Poor nations must be allowed to increase their agricultural productivity. Much is involved, but to put it simply, poor nations must gain greater access to five things simultaneously: land, capital, water, technology, and knowledge.[35] Equally important, each nation must make improving the condition of all its people a political priority. International food aid may be required temporarily during the development period, but eventually this aid will be less and less necessary.

If you give a man a fish, he will eat for a day. If you teach him to fish, he will eat for a lifetime.

◆ AGRICULTURAL TECHNOLOGY

Governments can learn from recent history the importance of developing local agricultural technology. A major effort made in the 1960s and 1970s—the **green revolution**—demonstrated both the potential for increased grain production in Asia and the necessity of considering local conditions. The industrial world made an effort to bring its agricultural technology to the developing countries, but the high-yielding strains of wheat and rice that were selected required irrigation, chemical fertilizers, and pesticides—all costly and beyond the economic means of many of the farmers in the developing world.

Green revolution The development and widespread adoption of high-yielding strains of wheat and rice in developing countries. The term *green revolution* is also used to describe almost any package of modern agricultural technology delivered to developing countries.

International research centers need to examine the conditions of developing countries and orient their research toward **appropriate technology**—labor-intensive rather than energy-intensive agricultural methods. Instead of transplanting industrial technology into the developing countries, small, efficient farms and local structures for marketing, credit, transportation, food storage, and agricultural education should be developed.

Appropriate technology A technology that utilizes locally abundant resources in preference to locally scarce resources. Developing countries usually have a large labor force and little capital; the appropriate technology would therefore be labor-intensive.

For example, labor-intensive technology, such as the use of manual grinders for grains, is appropriate in some places because it makes the best use of human, financial, and natural resources. A manual grinder can process 20 pounds of grain per hour, replacing the mortar and pestle, which can grind a maximum of only 3 pounds in the same time.[36] The specific technology that is appropriate for use varies from situation to situation.

◆ A NEED FOR SUSTAINABLE DEVELOPMENT

Environmental concerns must be taken more seriously as well. The amount of land available for crop production is as important as the condition of the soil and the availability of water. Soil erosion is now accelerating on every continent at a

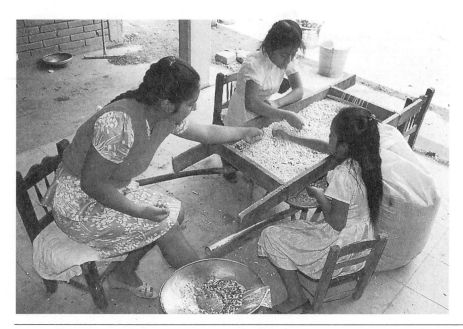

Most often, the appropriate technology in developing countries is labor-intensive.

rate that threatens the world's ability to continue feeding itself. Erosion of soil has always occurred; it is a natural process. But in the past, processes that build up the soil—such as the growth of trees—have compensated for erosion.

Where forests have already been converted to farmland and there are no trees, farmers can practice crop rotation, alternating soil-devouring crops with soil-building crops. An acre of soil planted one year in corn, the next in wheat, and the next in clover loses 2.7 tons of topsoil each year, but if it is planted only in corn three years in a row, it will lose 19.7 tons a year.[37] When farmers must choose whether to make three times as much money planting corn year after year or to rotate crops and go bankrupt, many choose the short-term profits. Ruin may not follow immediately, but it will follow.[38]

As the 1990 State of the World Report puts it:

> Poverty drives ecological deterioration when desperate people overexploit their resource space, sacrificing the future to salvage the present. The cruel logic of short-term needs forces landless families to raise plots in the rain forest, plow steep slopes, and shorten fallow periods. Ecological decline, in turn, perpetuates poverty as degraded ecosystems offer diminishing yields to their poor inhabitants. A self-defeating spiral of economic deprivation and ecological degradation takes hold.

There is a growing recognition that governments need to encourage and support efforts at sustainable development. **Sustainable development** is defined as the successful management of agricultural resources to satisfy changing human needs while maintaining or enhancing the natural resource base and avoiding environmental degradation.[39]

Sustainable development
Development that meets the needs of the present without compromising the ability of future generations to meet their own needs.

People-Centered Development

We have used the word "developing" in this chapter to classify certain countries, but what is development? According to Oxfam America, a nonprofit international agency that funds self-help development and disaster relief projects worldwide, development enables people to meet their essential needs, extends beyond food aid and emergency relief, reverses the process of impoverishment, enhances democracy, and makes possible a balance between populations and resources. It also improves the well-being and status of women, respects local cultures, sustains the natural environment, measures progress in human, not just monetary terms, and involves change, not just charity. Finally, development requires the empowerment of the poor and promotes the interests of the majority of people worldwide, in the global North as well as the South.[40]

Consider, for example, the history of development in Sri Lanka.[41] This island nation off the southeastern coast of India is the size of Ireland with a population of 14 million people. Sri Lanka, which achieved independence in 1948 and developed welfare and education programs in the 1960s and 1970s, now boasts a literacy rate of 85 percent and an infant mortality rate that has dropped from 141 to 37 deaths per 1000 live births. Despite these improvements, the national average income of $270 remains one of the lowest in the world.

Many of the villagers live in mud huts with little more than 100 square feet of space; light enters only from the open doorway. Several children, parents, and grandparents live in each home. Food procurement and preparation head the list of endless chores each day. Children must be cared for, rice must be dried and pounded into flour, chilies must be dried and ground for curry, water must be collected from the well when it's working, the animals must be grazed, the garden needs to be cultivated, and laundry must be carried to the reservoir. Parents often spend time working away from the home as well. In the poorer villages, less time is needed for meal preparation—there are fewer meals.

In an effort to improve these conditions by increasing average income, the current government has shifted its emphasis away from human welfare programs. To stimulate the economy, it has created free trade zones and maintains a cheap labor force to attract multinational corporations whose products are chiefly for export. Tourism is being widely developed on the tropical island to generate national income. These monies are largely spent to provide imported food and luxury goods for those who can afford them. Thus, the *average* income of Sri Lanka is rising, but only because the rich are becoming richer; the poor remain poor.

Contrast this consumer-oriented, high-technology, import-oriented, plantation-crop form of development with an alternative grass roots development movement called the *Sarvodaya Shramadana*, which is active in about 30 percent of the 23,000 villages on the island. Believing national development should begin with the villages, Sarvodaya helps people organize themselves to deal directly with their own problems and sponsors programs in health, education, agriculture, and local industry. Villagers have identified 10 basic needs: fuel, housing, basic health care, minimum requirements of clothing, a balanced and adequate diet, communication facili-

Sarvodaya *means awakening, or the well-being of all; Shramadana is the sharing of one's time, thought, and labor for the welfare of all.*

ties (including roads), an adequate supply of clean water, education relevant to their lives, a clean beautiful environment, and a spiritual and cultural life. Villagers are asked to describe projects that would fulfill their basic needs, and then set priorities. They are expected to furnish the maximum amount of their own human and material resources. The remaining input is supplied by other able Sarvodaya villages and district and national Sarvodaya headquarters. Training is provided as necessary in community organization, health and preschool education, and practical income-generating skills. Resources from the national headquarters include savings and loan programs, health and nutrition monitoring programs, community and marketing cooperatives, and appropriate agricultural technology.

Sarvodaya demonstrates that development cannot be measured by gross national product or the quantity of the community harvest. Instead, development should serve the people. A preschool may be struck by lightning and burn the day after it is built, but what matters most is that the people saw the need for a school and labored together to build it. Harsha Navarante, a Sarvodaya district director, summarizes the movement: "When the politician goes into a village plagued by poor roads he announces, 'The roads are terrible! Change the government! Vote for me!' Sarvodaya's message is that the roads are terrible, therefore the villagers must join together to fix them. We build the road and the road builds us."

The Sri Lankan experience highlights the need for ongoing community involvement and participation in project development and implementation. In Tanzania, the Iringa Nutrition Program involves community members in the assessment and analysis of problems and decisions about appropriate actions.[42] The program is designed to increase people's awareness of malnutrition and thus improve their capacity to take action. Fundamental to the program are the United Nations' child survival activities; these include the regular quarterly weighing of children under five years of age in the villages with discussion of the results by the village health committees. From this analysis, a set of appropriate interventions for solving problems can be identified. Recent evaluations indicate that this process has contributed to significant decreases in infant and child malnutrition and mortality.[43]

The cornerstone of true development was best expressed decades ago by Mahatma Gandhi: "Whenever you are in doubt . . . apply the following test. Recall the face of the poorest and the weakest man whom you may have seen, and ask yourself if the step you contemplate is going to be of any use to him. Will he gain anything by it? Will it restore him to a control over his own life and destiny?"[44]

Nutrition and Development

The first global International Conference on Nutrition (ICN), held in December 1992 in Rome, Italy, was organized by the food and health agencies of the United Nations (FAO and WHO). The intergovernmental conference focused world attention on nutritional and diet-related problems, especially among the poor and other vulnerable groups, in hopes of mobilizing governments, United Nations

Organizations and groups working to end world hunger are listed in Appendix B.

organizations, nongovernmental organizations, local communities, the private sector, and individuals in the fight against hunger and malnutrition.[45]

The ICN reflects not only the recognition of the problems surrounding food insecurity but also the realization that solutions are possible, especially for children. The United Nations views a healthy nutritious diet as a basic human right—one that the FAO and WHO are pledged to secure. However, achieving improved nutritional well-being worldwide requires broad action on many issues, including the following, which were explored at the ICN:

◆ Ensuring that the poor and malnourished have adequate access to food.

◆ Preventing and controlling infectious diseases by providing clean water, basic sanitation, and effective health care.

◆ Promoting healthy diets and lifestyles.

◆ Protecting consumers through improved food quality and safety.

◆ Preventing micronutrient deficiencies.

◆ Assessing, analyzing, and global monitoring of nutrition status of populations at risk.

◆ Incorporating nutrition objectives into development policies and programs.

The ICN helped focus world attention for the first time on the role of nutrition in achieving sustainable development. Nutrition and health are now seen as instruments or tools of economic development as well as goals. The inclusion of nutrition objectives in growth and development policies holds the promise of increasing the productivity and earning power of people worldwide. Well-nourished people are more productive, are sick less often, and earn higher incomes.[46] For this reason, spending on World Bank–assisted nutrition programs grew from $50 million in 1985 to $600 million in 1991.[47]

The World Bank is a group of international financial institutions owned by the governments of more than 150 nations. The bank provides loans for economic development.

Agenda for Action

Although the problem of world hunger may seem overwhelming, it can be broken down into many small, local problems. Significant strides can then be made toward solving them at the local level. Even if the problem of poverty itself is not immediately or fully solved, progress is possible. For example, infants and children need not be raised in middle-class homes to be protected from malnutrition. Slight modifications of the children's diets can be immensely beneficial.

◆ FOCUS ON CHILDREN

GOBI An acronym formed from the elements of UNICEF's Child Survival campaign— Growth charts, Oral rehydration therapy, Breast milk, and Immunization.

Children are the group most strongly affected by poverty, malnutrition, and food insecurity and its related effects on the environment.[48] However, there is hopeful news for children in developing countries. GOBI, a child survival plan set forth by UNICEF in 1983, has made outstanding progress in cutting the number of hunger-related child deaths. GOBI is an acronym formed from four simple, but profoundly important, elements of UNICEF's "Child Survival" campaign: growth charts, oral rehydration therapy (ORT), breast milk, and immunization.

The use of growth monitoring to determine the adequacy of child feeding requires a worldwide education campaign. A mother can learn to weigh her child every month and chart the child's growth on specially designed paper. She can learn to detect the early stages of hidden malnutrition that can leave a child irreparably retarded in mind and body. Then at least she will know she needs to take steps to remedy the malnutrition—if she can.

Most children who die of malnutrition do not starve to death—they die because their health has been compromised by dehydration from infections causing diarrhea. Until recently, there was no easy way of stopping the infection-diarrhea cycle and saving their lives; now, the spread of **oral rehydration therapy (ORT)** is preventing an estimated 1 million dehydration deaths each year.[49] ORT involves the administration of a simple solution that mothers can make themselves, using locally available ingredients; the solution increases a body's ability to absorb fluids 25-fold.[50] International development groups also provide mothers with packets of premeasured salt and sugar to be mixed with *boiled* water in rural and urban areas.* A safe, sanitary supply of drinking water is a prerequisite for the success of the ORT program. Contaminated water perpetuates the infection-diarrhea cycle.

Oral rehydration therapy (ORT) The treatment of dehydration (usually due to diarrhea caused by infectious disease) with an oral solution; as developed by UNICEF, ORT is intended to enable a mother to mix a simple solution for her child from substances that she has at home.

The promotion of breastfeeding among mothers in developing countries has many benefits. Breast milk is hygienic, readily available, and nutritionally sound, and it provides infants with immunologic protection specific for their environment. In the developing world, its advantages over formula feeding can mean the difference between life and death.

An important contributor to children's malnutrition in developing countries is the high bulk and low energy content of the available foods. The diet may be based on grains, such as wheat, rice, millet, sorghum, and corn, as well as starchy root crops, such as the cassava, sweet potato, plantain, and banana. These may be supplemented with legumes (peas or beans), but rarely with animal proteins. Infants have small stomachs, and most cannot eat enough of these staples (grains or root crops) to meet their daily energy and protein requirements. They need to be fed more nutrient-dense foods during the weaning period. The most promising weaning foods are usually concentrated mixtures of grain and locally available **pulses**— that is, peas or beans—which are both nourishing and inexpensive.[51] Mothers are advised to continue breastfeeding while they introduce weaning foods.

Pulses A term used for legumes, especially those that serve as staples in the diet of developing countries.

As for immunizations (the *I* of GOBI), they could prevent most of the 5 million deaths each year from measles, diphtheria, tetanus, whooping cough, poliomyelitis, and tuberculosis. However, adequate protein nutrition is necessary for vaccinations to be effective; otherwise the body may use the vaccine itself as a source of protein. It used to be difficult to keep vaccines stable in their long journeys from laboratory to remote villages. Now, however, the discovery of a new measles vaccine that does not require refrigeration has made universal measles immunization for young children possible, and many countries are reporting cov-

*Oral rehydration solutions are easily prepared from common ingredients including: $\frac{1}{3}$ to $\frac{2}{3}$ tsp table salt, $\frac{3}{4}$ tsp sodium bicarbonate, $\frac{1}{3}$ tsp potassium chloride, and $3\frac{1}{3}$ tbsp sugar in one liter of boiled water. Several commercial preparations are also available. (F. J. Zeman, *Clinical Nutrition and Dietetics,* 2nd ed. [New York: MacMillan Publishing Co., 1991], p. 241.)

erage rates of 80 to 90 percent. The immunization achievements of the 1980s are credited with preventing approximately 3 million deaths a year and the protection of many millions more from disease, malnutrition, blindness, deafness, and polio.[52]

The first World Summit for Children in history was convened by UNICEF in September of 1990, bringing together representatives of 159 nations for the purpose of making a renewed commitment to ending child deaths and child malnutrition on today's scale by the year 2000. Significantly, *nutrition* was mentioned for the first time in world history as an internationally recognized human right.[53] The overall goal of ending child deaths and malnutrition was broken down into 24 specific targets in a Plan of Action agreed upon by the countries in attendance (see the box). An immediate result of this summit has been an increase in the number of governments actively adopting the child survival strategies of UNICEF and WHO.

UNICEF's goals for nutrition and food security to be reached by the year 2000 include the following:

◆ A 50 percent reduction in the 1990 levels of moderate to severe malnutrition among children under five years old; this in itself would save the lives of 100 million children by the year 2000.

◆ A 50 percent reduction in the 1990 levels of low–birth weight infants.

◆ The virtual elimination of blindness and other consequences of vitamin A deficiency.

Strategies devised to achieve these goals by the year 2000 include universal immunization; oral rehydration therapy; a massive effort to promote breastfeeding as the ideal food for at least the first four to six months of an infant's life; an attack on malnutrition involving nutrition surveillance that focuses on growth monitoring and weighing of infants at least once every month for the first 18 months of life; and nutrition and literacy education that will empower women in developing countries and lead to a reduction in nutrition-related diseases among vulnerable children.[54]

◆ FOCUS ON WOMEN

Women make up 50 percent of the world's population. With their children, they represent the majority of those living in poverty. Thus, any solution to the problems of poverty and hunger is incomplete and even hopeless if it fails to address the role of women in developing countries (see Table 15-7 on page 524).

In many countries, over 90 percent of the population live in rural areas. Women living in rural poverty endure oppressive conditions. They are often overworked and underfed, yet they are expected to carry most of the burden of their family's survival. In many cultures, they are the last to get food, although they spend long hours each day procuring water and firewood and pounding grain by hand (see Figure 15-5 on page 525). In many countries, women in rural areas not only are the primary food producers, but also are responsible for child

[This discussion continues on page 522.]

Plan of Action from the World Summit for Children

The following is a partial list of goals, to be attained by the year 2000, which were adopted by the World Summit for Children on September 30, 1990.

Overall Goals, 1990–2000

◆ A one-third reduction in under-five death rates (or a reduction to below 70 per 1000 live births—whichever is lower).

◆ A halving of maternal mortality rates.

◆ A halving of severe and moderate malnutrition among the under fives.

◆ Safe water and sanitation for all families.

◆ Basic education for all children and completion of primary education by at least 80 percent.

◆ A halving of the adult illiteracy rate and the achievement of equal educational opportunity for males and females.

Protection for Girls and Women

◆ Family planning education and services to be made available to all couples to empower them to prevent unwanted pregnancies and births. Such services should be adapted to each country's cultural, religious, and social traditions.

◆ All women to have access to prenatal care, a trained attendant during childbirth, and facilities for high-risk pregnancies and emergencies.

◆ Universal recognition of the special health and nutritional needs of females during early childhood, adolescence, pregnancy, and lactation.

Nutrition

◆ A reduction in the incidence of low birth weight to less than 10 percent.

◆ A one-third reduction in iron-deficiency anemia among women, and virtual elimination of vitamin A deficiency and iodine deficiency disorders.

◆ All families to know the importance of supporting women in the task of exclusive breastfeeding for the first four to six months of a child's life.

◆ Growth monitoring and promotion to be institutionalized in all countries.

◆ Dissemination of knowledge to enable all families to ensure food security.

Child Health

◆ The eradication of polio, a 90 percent reduction in measles cases, and a 95 percent reduction in measles deaths, compared to pre-immunization levels.

◆ Achievement and maintenance of at least 90 percent immunization coverage of one-year-old children and universal tetanus immunization for women in the childbearing years.

◆ A halving of child deaths caused by diarrhea and a 25 percent reduction in the incidence of diarrheal diseases.

◆ A one-third reduction in child deaths caused by acute respiratory infections.

Source: Adapted from UNICEF, *The State of the World's Children 1993* (London: Oxford University Press, 1993), p. 32.

◆ *The Vitamin A Field Support Project (VITAL)*

Eye damage caused by vitamin A deficiency (VAD) affects an estimated 13 million preschool children worldwide.[1] Millions more children consume inadequate amounts of vitamin A–rich foods and are thus at risk for VAD. Manifestations of VAD range from mild xerophthalmia (night blindness and/or Bitot's spots) to dryness of the conjunctiva and cornea and, in severe cases, to melting of the cornea and blindness. In Asia alone, 200,000 children are blinded each year, with two-thirds of these children dying soon afterward. Recent epidemiological research has identified a relationship between marginal VAD, documented by reduced levels of circulating serum retinol, and higher mortality and morbidity rates from infectious diseases in children.[2] Researchers meeting at the International Conference on Nutrition in 1992 confirmed that even mild VAD significantly increases the death rate among children aged six months to six years. In particular, VAD significantly increases the severity and risk for diarrheal disease, measles, and pneumonia—the three main health threats facing children in the developing world.[3] Evidence from Africa suggests that vitamin A supplements can substantially reduce mortality and complications among children with measles, presumably by protecting epithelial tissue and ensuring the proper maintenance and functioning of the immune system.[4]

The most common factor contributing to the magnitude of VAD worldwide is the chronic inadequate dietary intake of vitamin A. Other contributors include poor nutrition status of mothers during pregnancy and lactation, low prevalence of breastfeeding, delayed or inappropriate introduction of supplementary foods, high incidence of infection (e.g., diarrhea, acute respiratory infection, measles), low levels of maternal education, drought, civil strife, poverty, and ecologic deprivation in some regions resulting in limited availability of vitamin A–rich foods.[5] For example, the production and consumption of vitamin A–rich foods in Africa (dark green, leafy vegetables, orange-colored fruits and tubers, and red palm oil) are influenced strongly by seasonal trends and cultural practices.[6]

VITAL is a VAD program administered by the U.S. Agency for International Development (USAID). Like other programs designed to eradicate and prevent VAD in developing countries, VITAL focuses on three approaches:

◆ **Dietary diversification**. VITAL strategies include stimulating the production and consumption of vitamin A–rich foods through agricultural production, home gardening, food preservation, nutrition education, and social marketing. For example, VITAL promotes the consumption of papayas, an excellent source of vitamin A, by pregnant women in the South Pacific. In some regions, foods containing vitamin A—especially vegetables and fruits—are readily available but underutilized by vulnerable groups, particularly weaning-age children and pregnant and lactating women, due to traditional customs and beliefs. Consequently, dietary

Continued

—Continued

diversification programs in these areas focus on intensive nutrition education and social marketing campaigns to foster necessary community understanding, motivation, and participation.

Home gardens play a critical role in alleviating VAD in many communities. They provide a regular and secure supply of household food.

VITAL also sponsors several projects aimed at increasing vitamin A consumption by improving food processing techniques. Solar drying has been introduced as the appropriate technology for the preservation of mangoes, papayas, sweet potatoes, pumpkins, green leaves, and other vitamin A–rich foods in several countries. When solar dried, these foods retain both flavor and carotene content and can alleviate seasonal variation in the availability of food. For example, the MANGOCOM Project in Senegal attempts to improve the vitamin A intake of weaning-age children by promoting dried mangoes, produced by women's cottage industries, as finger foods and fruit purees for toddlers.[7]

◆ **Food fortification**. Fortifying food is generally a large-scale undertaking and will only be effective if the target groups can buy and will consume the fortified product. In several developed countries, commonly consumed foods (e.g., margarine and milk) have been successfully fortified with vitamin A. Sugar is fortified with the vitamin in several regions of Central America, notably through VITAL projects in Guatemala, El Salvador, and Honduras.[8] Pilot trials with vitamin A–fortified rice are underway in Brazil. In both Indonesia and the Philippines, monosodium glutamate (MSG) was fortified with vitamin A. Program evaluations in both countries showed improvements in vitamin A status in the target populations. However, MSG fortification programs have since been halted due to unresolved technological problems, the questionable safety of MSG, and the lack of political will to support the fortification efforts. A pilot program in the Philippines is currently testing vitamin A–fortified margarine as an alternative means of improving the vitamin A status of children.

◆ **Distribution of vitamin A supplements**. Most commonly, VAD intervention programs periodically distribute vitamin A supplements in the form of high-dose capsules or oral dispensers. UNICEF typically donates the vitamin A capsules and helps organize the distribution efforts.* Often, supplements are delivered in conjunction with ongoing local health ser-

---

*The recommended dosing schedule for a vitamin A capsule distribution program is 200,000 IU given twice a year. The dose for children less than one year of age or those who are significantly underweight is 100,000 IU twice a year. (A. Gadomski and C. Kjolhede, *Vitamin A Deficiency and Childhood Morbidity and Mortality* [Baltimore, Md.: Johns Hopkins University Publications, 1988].)

Continued

—Continued

vices, primary health care programs (e.g., maternal-child health projects), or national vaccination campaigns.

Vitamin A supplementation programs to date have reported a number of operational obstacles: low priority given to the distribution of the supplements by primary health care workers, a lack of community demand for vitamin A, and a lack of awareness among policymakers of the critical nature of vitamin A nutrition status. However, similar obstacles have been overcome by immunization programs, which now reach 80 percent of targeted children worldwide.[9] For this reason, WHO and UNICEF have suggested that vitamin A supplementation be integrated into existing immunization programs: "The provision of vitamin A supplementation through immunization services could dramatically expand the coverage of children in late infancy, giving a boost to vitamin A status before the critical period of weaning." Since immunization programs primarily target infants under 12 months of age, similar coverage would need to be provided by other means to children from one to six years of age.

Supplementation is considered a temporary measure for the control and prevention of VAD. More permanent solutions include cultivating vitamin A–rich foods, fortifying foods with vitamin A, promoting improved food habits, eliminating poverty, and improving sanitation worldwide.[10] Therefore, countries pursuing the high coverage achieved by integrating vitamin A supplement distribution into immunization programs are encouraged to also allocate resources to these alternative efforts.

Continued

care and food preparation. Often they have to work as harvesters on other people's lands as well. Husbands are frequently absent from their homes—not by choice, but because the changing global economy has forced many men to leave home to find paying jobs. They have gone to look for work in the cities or to find employment growing export crops on distant commercial farms.

Development projects are often large in scale and highly technological, but they frequently overlook women's needs. Typically, only men have access to education and training programs (see Figure 15-5). Yet women play a vital role in the nutrition of their nation's people. Their nutrition during pregnancy and lactation determines the future health of their children. If women are weakened by malnutrition themselves or ignorant about how to feed their families, the consequences ripple outward to affect many other individuals. The importance of women in these countries is increasingly being appreciated, and many countries now offer development programs with women in mind.

Seven basic strategies are at the heart of women's programs:

—Continued

Fortunately, the problem of VAD is not insurmountable. The numerous VITAL projects worldwide have demonstrated three principles critical to successful VAD intervention efforts. First, successful interventions include preliminary formative research (e.g., focus group interviews), target audience segmentation, pretesting, and evaluation in program planning. Secondly, support by policymakers and participation by local community members is critical to sustaining the program. Lastly, multiple channels of communication are recommended (e.g., mass media, traditional forms of media, and personal communications).

In the final analysis, individual countries will need to choose the most practical and cost-effective mix of VAD interventions based on local customs, resources, and needs. Numerous international agencies, including WHO, UNICEF, FAO, the World Bank, and USAID have made the commitment to support country efforts to meet the 1990 World Summit for Children's goal of virtually eliminating VAD by the year 2000.

1. Vitamin A deficiency in Asia, *VITAL NEWS* 3 (1992): 1–11.
2. K. P. West and coauthors, Efficacy of vitamin A in reducing preschool child mortality in Nepal, *Lancet* 338 (1991): 67–71.
3. UNICEF, *The State of the World's Children, 1993*, p. 12.
4. Vitamin A deficiency in Africa, *VITAL NEWS* 3 (1992): 1–10.
5. Vitamin A deficiency in Asia, p. 2.
6. Vitamin A deficiency in Africa, p. 4.
7. J. Rankins, MANGOCOM: A nutrition social marketing module for field use, *Journal of Nutrition Education* 24 (1992): 192–94.
8. Vitamin A deficiency in Latin America and the Caribbean, VITAL NEWS 3 (1992): 8.
9. The discussion of vitamin A supplementation and immunization programs was adapted from Linking vitamin A activities to primary health care programs, *VITAL NEWS* 2 (1991): 1–7.
10. M. G. Herrera and coauthors, Vitamin A supplementation and child survival, *Lancet* 340 (1992): 267–71.

◆ Removing barriers to financial credit so women can obtain loans for raw materials and equipment to enhance their role in food production.

◆ Providing access to time-saving technologies—seed grinders, for example.

◆ Providing appropriate training to make women self-reliant.

◆ Teaching management and marketing skills to help women avoid exploitation.

◆ Making health and day care services available to provide a healthy environment for the women's children.

◆ Forming women's support groups to foster strength through cooperative efforts.[55]

◆ Providing information and technology to promote planned pregnancies.

The recognition of women's needs by some development organizations is an encouraging trend in the efforts to contend with the world hunger crisis. The fol-

TABLE

15-7

Women and Development: Fiction and Fact

Source: Reproduced with permission from *Women . . . A World Survey* by R. L. Sivard. Copyright © 1985 by World Priorities, Inc., Washington, D.C.

◆ **Men produce the world's food; women prepare it for the table.** In developing countries, where three-fourths of the world's people live, rural women account for more than half the food produced.

◆ **Women work to supplement the family's income.** Women are the sole breadwinners in one-fourth to one-third of the families in the world. The number of female-headed families is rapidly increasing.

◆ **When women receive the same education and training as men, they will receive equal pay.** So far, earning differentials persist even at equivalent levels of training. In professional fields, for example, comparisons of men's and women's salaries show a large gap between them even when samples are matched for training and experience.

◆ **Men are the heavy workers, and where food is short, they should have first priority.** As a rule, women work longer hours than men. Many carry triple work loads—in their household, labor force, and reproductive roles. Rural women often average an 18-hour day. Anemia resulting from a primary or secondary nutrient deficiency is a serious health problem for women in developing countries.

◆ **In modern societies, women have moved into all fields of work.** Relatively few women have entered occupations traditionally dominated by men. Most women remain highly segregated in low-paid jobs.

◆ **Women contribute a minor share of the world's economic product.** Women are a minority in the conventional measures of economic activity because these measures undercount women's paid labor and do not cover their unpaid labor. The value of women's work in the household alone, if given economic value, would add an estimated one-third to the world's gross national product.

lowing examples from Sierra Leone and Ghana illustrate how women's development programs work:[56]

Balu Kamara is a farmer in Sierra Leone in West Africa, where farming is difficult, particularly for women. There women have little money and must take out loans to buy seed rice and to pay for the use of oxen. The price of rice is so low, though, that at the end of the growing season the women do not earn enough money to repay their loans. Yet, as the economy worsens, it is up to the women to carry the burdens; it is up to the women to stretch what resources are available to feed their families regardless of hardships.

Balu is the leader of the Farm Women's Club, a basket cooperative the women formed to make and sell baskets so they could pay their debts and continue farming. Finding time to weave baskets is difficult. Yet the women and their cooperative are succeeding. On the value of the Farm Women's Club, Balu says, "We have access to credit and a cash income. We have the opportunity to learn improved methods of agriculture and marketing and to increase our belief in ourselves and ease our families through the hungry season."

Gari, or processed cassava, is a bland tasting food served in a form like porridge.

Gari (processed cassava) is becoming increasingly popular in Ghana because of the shortage of many other food items and because, once prepared, it is easy to cook. But it is very time-consuming to prepare gari—peeling and grating the fresh cassava, fermenting it over several days, squeezing the water from the fermented cassava, and, finally roasting it over a wood fire.

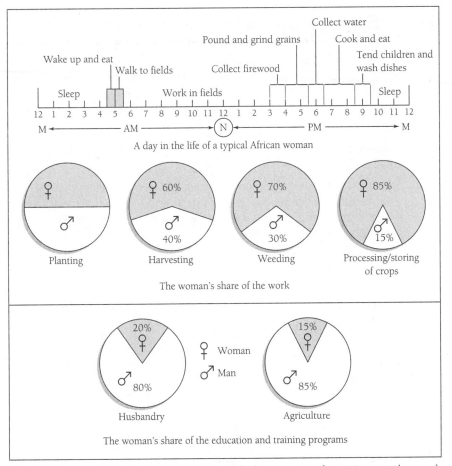

A day in the life of a typical African woman

The woman's share of the work

The woman's share of the education and training programs

FIGURE

15-5

Women and Development
Source: Adapted from T. Flynn, Women in development, *Seeds* (Sprouts edition), May 1988.

Note that the women do the work for their families, while the men receive the training to produce goods and crops for export.

To help village women in the Volta Region increase their income through gari processing, an improved technology was introduced with the help of the National Council on Women and Development. The process involves a special mechanical grater, a pressing machine to squeeze the water from the grated cassava and a large enamel pan for roasting. This pan holds ten times the volume of the traditional cassava pot. The system was developed locally, with advice from the women themselves contributing to the success of the project.

Before, the women produced 50 gari bags every week. Now they are able to produce 5000 to 6000 bags a week. However, this increased output of gari can only be maintained with a higher yield of cassava in the area. Therefore, a male cassava growers' association has been formed to step up cassava production, and a tractor has been acquired by the women's cooperative so as to put more land under cassava cultivation.

International Nutrition Programs

Nutrition programs in developing countries vary considerably. They include both large-scale and small-scale operations, may be supported with private or public funds, and may focus on emergency relief or long-term development.[57] In developing countries, emphasis has generally been placed on four types of nutrition interventions:

1. Breastfeeding promotion programs with guidance on preparing appropriate weaning foods.

2. Nutrition education programs typically focusing either on infant and child feeding guidelines and practices and child survival activities or on the incorporation of nutrition education into primary school curriculums and teacher training programs.

3. Food fortification and/or the distribution of nutrient supplements (e.g., vitamin A capsules) and the identification of local food sources of problem nutrients.

4. Special feeding programs designed to provide particularly vulnerable groups with nutritious supplemental foods.[58]

In many countries, there is mounting evidence of grass roots progress in improving agricultural, water, education, and health services, especially for children.[59] Experiences in Sierra Leone and Nepal are encouraging examples.

In Sierra Leone, a food product was developed from rice, sesame (benniseed), and peanuts that were hand pounded and cooked to make a flour meal. The local children not only found it tasty, but whereas they had been malnourished before, they thrived when this product supplemented their diets. The village women formed a cooperative to reduce the drudgery of preparing the food and rotated the work on a weekly or monthly basis.[60] The government also established a manufacturing plan to produce and market the mixture at subsidized prices. The success of the venture lies in the involvement of the local people in identifying the problem and devising a solution that meets their needs.

A similar success story is told in Nepal. A supplementary food made from soybeans, corn, and wheat, mixed in a 2:1:1 proportion, yielded a concentrated "superflour" of high biological value suitable for infants and children. A nutrition rehabilitation center tested this superflour by giving undernourished children and their mothers two cereal-based meals a day, and giving the children three additional small meals of superflour porridge daily. Within 10 days, the undernourished children had gained weight, lost their edema, and recovered their appetites and social alertness. The mothers, who saw the remarkable recoveries of their children, were motivated to learn how to make the tasty supplementary food and incorporate it into their local foodstuffs and customs.

These two examples offer hope, but the real issue of poverty remains to be addressed. One-shot intervention programs offering nutrition education, food distribution, food fortification, and the like are not enough. It is difficult to describe the misery a mother feels when she has received education about nutrition but cannot grow or purchase the foods her family needs. She now knows *why* her child is sick and dying but is unable to *apply* her new knowledge.

Looking Ahead: The Global Challenges

In 1977, the thirtieth annual World Health Assembly, convened in Alma Ata, decided unanimously that the main social target of member governments and WHO itself should be "the attainment by all citizens of the world by the year 2000 of a level of health that will permit them to lead a socially and economically productive life." This goal is now referred to simply as "Health for All by the Year 2000."[61] The assembly hoped to make primary health care services accessible and affordable for all people in every country of the world. Today, however, over a billion and a half of the world's people continue to live without access to basic health care, and some 40,000 children die each day from the effects of malnutrition and related diseases—an estimated 100 million deaths in the 1990s.

In the developing world, the health care crisis revolves around the daily struggle for survival and the growing disparity between the haves and the have-nots. For the poor, the struggle for safe water, adequate nutrition, and access to basic health care leaves no energy or resources for other concerns—and most have little hope of winning the battle. For most of us, living in the developed world, health care reform means we are assured of meeting our own and our family's ongoing health care needs, including access to the latest miracle drug or the availability of a bone marrow transplant. But as one physician from the hospital ship *M/V Anastasis* remarked on visiting Ghana in West Africa: "We are foolhardy to believe that we can be a healthy society when the world around us is languishing with diseases and poverty that we could alleviate."[62]

In addition, we face many new challenges not even thought of in 1977 when the goal of "Health for All by the Year 2000" was set.[63] Before we can attain this goal, we must deal with these issues, among others:

◆ The HIV/AIDS pandemic. In late 1991, WHO estimated that there were 10 million AIDS cases throughout the world, 6 million in Africa.

◆ The recent upsurge in cases of tuberculosis in the United States among the urban poor, homeless persons, migrant workers, immigrants and refugees from countries with high tuberculosis rates, intravenous drug users, residents of correctional facilities, nursing home residents, and those infected with HIV.[64]

◆ The trend toward urbanization. Urbanization has been a factor in the worldwide decline in breastfeeding, the increased consumption of empty-calorie foods, and the outbreak of cholera in several Latin American countries since 1990 due to contamination of the urban water supply. As nations continue the rural-to-urban transition, the incidence of chronic diarrhea from polluted water and foodborne contamination remains a major public health problem in urban slums.

◆ The growing number of elderly persons in the developed world. This demographic change requires fundamental health care reform, as discussed earlier in Chapter 14, to ensure the maintenance of quality living and functional ability in the later years.

◆ The upward surge in global poverty. The proportion of the world's population that is poor, approximately 1.2 billion people, has increased over the last decade, halting a 40-year downward trend.[65]

◆ Rapid population growth. The earth's population will nearly double within the next 40 years—most of these people will be born into poor families in developing countries. Agricultural production will need to increase to feed these people. The number of nonagricultural jobs must also increase to support those not working in agriculture.

◆ Destruction of the global environment. The earth's capacity to sustain life is being impaired by many complex interrelated developments, including overconsumption, industrial pollution, overgrazing, and deforestation. This destruction of natural resources threatens the health and well-being of both today's people and future generations as well.

Personal Action: Opportunity Knocks

The problems addressed in this chapter may appear to be so great that they can be approached only through worldwide political decisions. Indeed, the members of the International Conference on Nutrition stressed that intensive worldwide efforts were needed to overcome hunger and malnutrition and to foster self-reliant development. To this end, many individuals and groups are working to improve the future well-being of the world and its people through a number of national and international organizations.*

Individuals can help change the world through their personal choices.[66] Our choices have an impact on the way the rest of the world's people live and die. As mentioned in Chapter 11, our nation, with 6 percent of the world's population, consumes about 40 percent of the world's food and energy resources. The world food problem depends partly on the demands we place on the world's finite natural resources. In a sense, we contribute to the world food problem. People in affluent nations have the freedom and means to choose their lifestyles; people in poor nations do not. We can find ways to reduce our consumption of the world's resources by using only what is required.

It is ironic that whereas other societies cannot secure enough clean water for people to drink, our society produces bottles of soda that contain one calorie of artificial sweetener in 12 ounces of water that cost 800 calories to produce. In the United States, $5 billion is spent annually to lower calorie consumption, while

*For information, contact Bread for the World Institute or Oxfam America; or request a copy of *Who's Involved with Hunger: An Organization Guide for Education and Advocacy* from World Hunger Education Service (See Appendix B for addresses).

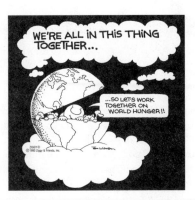

500 million people in the rest of the world can rarely find an adequate number of calories to consume.[67] Thus, choosing a diet at the level of necessity, rather than excess, would reduce the resource demands made by our industrial agriculture. In fact, those who study the future are convinced that the hope of the world lies in everyone's adopting a simple lifestyle. As one such person put it, "the widespread simplification of life is vital to the well-being of the entire human family."[68] Personal lifestyles do matter, for a society is nothing more than the sum of its individuals. As we go, so goes our world.

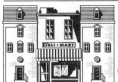

COMMUNITY LEARNING ACTIVITY

You probably cannot solve the world food problem single-handedly, but the place to start is with yourself and your community. Phrases such as "think globally, act locally" reinforce this message—start where you are.

1. This activity asks you to consider what changes you could make in your personal life that might affect the problem of world hunger and the issues associated with it that were discussed in this chapter. We ask that you consider the following list of suggestions and then identify other strategies to add to this list:

   ◆ Examine your diet to become more conscious of your dependence on others.

   ◆ Consider your lifestyle and make intentional choices as you use resources.

   ◆ Grow some of your own food. (Try community gardens in the city.)

   ◆ As you buy, think about who benefits.[69]

2. Contact one or more of the organizations working to end world hunger (see Appendix B). Learn more about their activities and share a profile of an organization with your class.

Ethics and You

Life is full of paradoxes. Chapter 4 demonstrated that although health promotion and disease prevention are paramount to halting the escalating cost of health care in this country, the United States spends only 4 percent of its health care dollars on disease prevention. Chapter 11 presented the goal of nutrition as applying scientific knowledge to feed all people adequately, yet every fifth child in the United States is vulnerable to hunger. Although the United States spends more on health care than other nations, Chapters 11 through 14 revealed certain health disparities between racial and ethnic groups, particularly in pregnancy outcome, infant mortality rate, nutrition status, life expectancy, and food insecurity. And finally, Chapter 15 described the issues confronting developing countries and asked: Is it fundamentally wrong that so much preventable sickness and death occur in the world?

As a community nutritionist, how do you address such issues? This Professional Focus reviews some of the ethical questions in the field of health promotion that relate specifically to community nutritionists. Its intent is not to arrive at a conclusion or present solutions to ethical dilemmas; rather, it seeks to present the issues for your consideration and stresses the need for moral sensitivity in the planning and implementation of community nutrition programs. As Aristotle once said, "We are what we repeatedly do." Moral sensitivity and characteristics such as honesty, integrity, loyalty, and candor are developed by practice.[1]

◆ WHAT IS ETHICS?

Philosophers throughout history have struggled with questions of how to live and work ethically. Ethics is a philosophical discipline dealing with what is morally good and bad, right and wrong. Ethics helps decision makers search for criteria to evaluate different moral stances.[2]

As a community nutritionist, you may wonder what ethics has to do with your professional activities. Certainly, as a community nutritionist, you will not often confront such media issues as euthanasia, abortion, capital punishment, insider trading, maternal surrogacy, infanticide, the withdrawal of nutrition support for terminally ill patients, or the right to die. Nevertheless, situations arise in community settings that will force you to make ethical decisions.

Community nutritionists working with the media or food industry must consider the accuracy of product descriptions and claims as well as words and images that can mislead the public.[3] As a manager, the community nutritionist may face ethical dilemmas in allocating resources. In setting priorities, she may have to make some decisions that call upon her ethics. If she believes that all eligible clients have the right to receive optimal nutrition care, then how should she decide which clients will actually receive the care? (In this case optimal nutrition care may mean the receipt of home-delivered meals by a homebound elderly person.) The community nutritionist involved in research emphasizes honesty, accuracy, and integrity in conducting studies and publishing the results. Consider the impact of using falsified data in determining nutrition policy for funding a new or existing nutrition program.

Continued

◆ PROFESSIONAL FOCUS—*Continued*

◆ CODES OF ETHICS

Simple answers to ethical questions are elusive, but many health care organizations and professional associations have established codes of ethics to provide guidance in resolving ethical dilemmas.[4] Codes of ethics are written to guide decision making in areas of moral conflict; outline the obligations of the practitioner to self, clients, society, and the profession; and "assist in protecting the nutritional health, safety, and welfare of the public."[5] The American Dietetic Association (ADA) published its first Code of Ethics in 1942.[6] The most recent code (see the box) became effective in 1989 and applies to all ADA members and credentialed practitioners.

A code of ethics for nutritionists and other professionals working in international situations is likewise critical, as C. E. Taylor notes: "Needs are so obvious that the temptation is great to rush in with programs that seem reasonable; but international work is full of surprises. Each new activity needs to be carefully tested."[7] Consider the story of the monkey and the fish:

> After a dam burst, a flood raged through an African countryside. A monkey, standing in safety on the riverbank, watched a fish swim into view. "I will save this poor fish from drowning," thought the monkey. And, swinging from a tree branch, he scooped up the fish and carried it, gasping, to land. "Throw me back," pleaded the fish. Reluctantly, the monkey agreed, scratching his head in bewilderment at the fish's lack of appreciation for the aid he had so selflessly offered.[8]

◆ GUIDING PRINCIPLES

Three basic principles are used in ethical decision making and in developing guidelines for professional practice:[9] (1) autonomy—respecting the individual's rights of self-determination, independence, and privacy; (2) beneficence—protecting clients from harm and maximizing possible benefits; and (3) justice—striving for fairness in one's actions and equality in the allocation of resources.

To determine whether an issue in the community setting raises an ethical question, consider these ethical principles expressed as questions:[10]

1. Does the nutrition program, message, product, or service foster or deter the individual's ability to act freely? (The ADA Code of Ethics items 6, 10, and 15 address this principle of autonomy.)

2. Does the nutrition program, message, product, or service help people or harm them? (Items 7, 8, 9, 17, and 18 in the ADA Code of Ethics address this principle of beneficence.)

3. Does the nutrition program, message, product, or service unfairly or arbitrarily discriminate among persons or groups? (Items 1, 2, and 16 in the ADA Code of Ethics address this principle of justice.)

Consumers are eager to know about nutrition. As nutrition educators, the principle of beneficence moves us to provide consumers with truthful and convincing information based on current scientific knowledge. In this way, we protect them from fraudulent mis-

Continued

Code of Ethics for the Profession of Dietetics

The dietetic practitioner:

1. Provides professional services with objectivity and with respect for the unique needs and values of individuals.
2. Avoids discrimination against other individuals on the basis of race, creed, religion, sex, age, and national origin.
3. Fulfills professional commitments in good faith.
4. Conducts himself/herself with honesty, integrity, and fairness.
5. Remains free of conflict of interest while fulfilling the objectives and maintaining the integrity of the dietetic profession.
6. Maintains confidentiality of information.
7. Practices dietetics based on scientific principles and current information.
8. Assumes responsibility and accountability for personal competence in practice.
9. Recognizes and exercises professional judgment within the limits of his or her qualifications and seeks counsel or makes referrals as appropriate.
10. Provides sufficient information to enable clients to make their own informed decisions.
11. Who wishes to inform the public and colleagues of his or her services does so by using factual information; does not advertise in a false or misleading manner.
12. Promotes or endorses products in a manner that is neither false nor misleading.
13. Permits use of his or her name for the purpose of certifying that dietetic services have been rendered only if he or she has provided or supervised the provision of those services.
14. Accurately presents professional qualifications and credentials:
    - ◆ Uses "RD" or "registered dietitian" and "DTR" or "dietetic technician registered" only when registration is current and authorized by the Commission on Dietetic Registration.
    - ◆ Provides accurate information and complies with all requirements of the Commission on Dietetic Registration program in which he or she is seeking initial or continued credentials from the Commission on Dietetic Registration.
    - ◆ Is subject to disciplinary action for aiding another person in violating any Commission on Dietetic Registration requirements or aiding another person in representing himself/herself as an RD or DTR when he or she is not.

Continued

◆ **PROFESSIONAL FOCUS**—*Continued*

Code of Ethics for the Profession of Dietetics

15. Presents substantiated information and interprets controversial information without personal bias, recognizing that legitimate differences of opinion exist.

16. Makes all reasonable effort to avoid bias in any kind of professional evaluation; provides objective evaluation of candidates for professional association memberships, awards, scholarships, or job advancements.

17. Voluntarily withdraws from professional practice under the following circumstances:

    ◆ Has engaged in any substance abuse that could affect his or her practice;

    ◆ Has been adjudged by a court to be mentally incompetent;

    ◆ Has an emotional or mental disability that affects his or her practice in a manner that could harm the client.

18. Complies with all applicable laws and regulations concerning the profession; is subject to disciplinary action under the following circumstances:

    ◆ Has been convicted of a crime under the laws of the United States which is a felony or a misdemeanor, an essential element of which is dishonesty and which is related to the practice of the profession.

    ◆ Has been disciplined by a state and at least one of the grounds for the discipline is the same or substantially equivalent to these principles.

    ◆ Has committed an act of misfeasance or malfeasance that is directly related to the practice of the profession as determined by a court of competent jurisdiction, a licensing board, or an agency of a governmental body.

19. Accepts the obligation to protect society and the profession by upholding the Code of Ethics for the Profession of Dietetics and by reporting alleged violations of the Code through the defined review process of The American Dietetic Association and its credentialing agency, the Commission on Dietetic Registration.

Source: From the American Dietetic Association, Code of Ethics for the Profession of Dietetics, *Journal of the American Dietetic Association* 88 (1988): 1592–93. Copyright © 1988 The American Dietetic Association, Chicago, Illinois. Reprinted by permission.

information and also motivate them to change their diet accordingly.[11] The principle of autonomy motivates us to provide the consumer with factual information that includes both the weaknesses and the strengths of the scientific data supporting a given behavior, service, or product; with this information, the individual can exercise his right to make an informed choice or decision.

Continued

◆ PROFESSIONAL FOCUS—*Continued*

◆ HEALTH PROMOTION AND ETHICS

The purpose of health promotion is to motivate people to adopt and maintain healthful practices in order to prevent illness and functional impairment. Many hold that by investing in health promotion and disease prevention activities, we can avoid the much greater economic and social costs of disease and disability. The challenge today is to provide the public with the opportunity to benefit from appropriate nutrition knowledge and services. However, this challenge raises a hidden moral issue worthy of consideration. At what point is scientific knowledge sufficiently documented to warrant translating it into dietary messages to the public? What responsibilities and rights do we have to alter individual lifestyles in our effort to promote public health? As health promoters, we are sometimes criticized for taking a paternalistic approach with a "We know better than you" attitude. Moral sensitivity demands that we respect the dignity of persons—their right to make their own choices. We may carefully and creatively design messages for older women at risk of osteoporosis, encouraging them to use dairy products in their daily diet, but our target audience has the right to resist our efforts and choose not to do so. An adequate calcium intake is a good thing, but life offers many other good things as well.

Health promotion for a number of issues (e.g., cigarette smoking and drinking and driving) necessitates a paternalistic approach that both restricts private liberties and promotes group virtues like beneficence and concern for the common good. Such paternalism is for the most part considered legitimate and reflects the view that the good of each of us is not the same thing as the good of all of us together.[12]

Community nutritionists, as health promoters, call attention to other health risks—a diet high in saturated fat or low in fiber, commercial advertising of empty-calorie foods to children, and nutrition fraud in the marketplace, among others. Should governments, therefore, move from taxing cigarettes and alcohol to taxing companies that manufacture high-fat confections or cereals high in sugar? Since obesity and a sedentary lifestyle are associated with a number of chronic diseases (e.g., hypertension, coronary artery disease, diabetes) and increased health care costs, should persons who eat too many calories or too much fat or those who fail to exercise regularly be taxed to discourage these lifestyles and raise revenues for health costs? Should we fine pregnant women who smoke or drink? In other words, to what extent should society tolerate and bear the burden for the health risks that individuals choose to take? Such are the ethical dilemmas facing those working in health promotion. The ethical conflict is how to achieve the goal of protecting and promoting public health while ensuring an individual's freedom of choice.

◆ ETHICAL DECISION MAKING

Analytical skills are necessary to resolve ethical dilemmas. One must objectively evaluate the individual circumstances of each situation, gather relevant data, consider possible alternatives, consult with experts as necessary, and take appropriate actions to accomplish the greatest good for the greatest number. The particular action chosen must adhere to the general ethical principles of autonomy, beneficence, and justice.

As community nutritionists, you are certain to face ethical dilemmas in both your professional and personal lives. In closing this book, we leave you with a set of questions.[13] In the months to come, consider your responses to these questions based on your

Continued

moral sensitivity regarding these situations, your understanding of ethical principles, and your discussions with other professionals experienced in making ethical decisions:

◆ Is it right to save lives by immunization, nutrition, ORT, or chemotherapy when those who are saved may face a life of despair?

◆ Do the United States and Canada and other developed countries have a moral obligation toward the less-developed countries?

◆ When setting priorities in program planning in the face of limited resources, who should receive benefits—infants? Children? Pregnant women? Working people? Elderly persons?

◆ What are the ethical limits to promotional activities of multinational corporations? Is it acceptable to market infant formula or soft drinks in developing countries? Should we ban television advertising of empty-calorie foods to children?

◆ In setting program priorities, are there situations in which one ethnic group should be favored over another?

◆ Do we have the right to ask individuals to adjust and, in some cases, to abandon their ethnic and cultural customs, traditions, or cuisines for the goal of improved health?

1. S. L. Anderson, Dietitians' practices and attitudes regarding the Code of Ethics for the Profession of Dietetics, *Journal of the American Dietetic Association* 93 (1993): 88–91.
2. S. Tamborini-Martin and K. V. Hanley, The importance of being ethical, *Health Progress* 70 (1989): 24.
3. J. N. Neville and R. Chernoff, Professional ethics: Everyone's issue, *Journal of the American Dietetic Association* 88 (1988): 1286.
4. J. Sobal, Research ethics in nutrition education, *Journal of Nutrition Education* 24 (1992): 234–38.
5. American Dietetic Association and Commission on Dietetic Registration, *Code of Ethics for the Profession of Dietetics* (Chicago: American Dietetic Association, 1988).
6. Neville and Chernoff, Professional ethics, p. 1287.
7. C. E. Taylor, Ethics for an international health profession, *Science* 153 (1966): 716–20, as cited by P. F. Basch, *Textbook of International Health* (New York: Oxford University Press, 1990), pp. 407–8.
8. C. Levine, Ethics, justice, and international health, *Hasting Center Report* 4 (1977): 5–6.
9. M. Barry, Ethical considerations of human investigations in developing countries: The AIDS dilemma, *New England Journal of Medicine* 319 (1988): 1083–85.
10. M. W. Kreuter, M. J. Parsons, and M. P. McMurry, Moral sensitivity in health promotion, *Health Education*, November/December 1982, pp. 11–13.
11. K. McNutt, Ethics: A cop or a counselor? *Nutrition Today* 26 (1991): 36–39.
12. D. Beauchamp, Lifestyle, public health and paternalism, in *Ethical Dilemmas in Health Promotion,* ed. S. Doxiadis (New York: John Wiley & Sons, 1987), pp. 69–81.
13. Adapted from Basch, *Textbook of International Health*.

NOTES

1. G. G. Graham, Starvation in the modern world, *New England Journal of Medicine* 328 (1993): 1058–61.

2. World food supplies and prevalence of chronic under-nutrition in developing regions as assessed in 1992 (Rome: FAO Statistical Analysis Service, 1992).

3. United Nations International Conference on Nutrition, *World Declaration and Plan of Action for Nutrition* (Rome: U.N. Food and Agriculture Organization, 1992), p. 1.

4. The description of food security in the margin is from World Bank, *The Challenge of Hunger in Africa: A Call to Action* (Washington, D.C.: World Bank, 1988), p. 1.

5. A. Durning, Life on the brink, *World Watch* 3 (1990): 22–30.

6. Ibid., p. 25.

7. B. Hartman and J. Boyce, *Quiet Violence: View from a Bangladesh Village* (San Francisco: Institute for Food and Development Policy, 1983).

8. D. R. Gwatkin, How many die? A set of demographic estimates of the annual number of infant and child deaths in the world, *American Journal of Public Health* 70 (1980): 1286–89.

9. This estimate and the margin comment are from UNICEF, *The State of the World's Children 1993* (London: Oxford University Press, 1993), p. 57.

10. Ibid., pp. 1–3.

11. B. A. Carlson and T. M. Wardlaw, A global, regional, and country assessment of child malnutrition, *UNICEF Staff Working Papers*, no. 7 (New York: UNICEF, 1990), pp. 1–30.

12. Population Reference Bureau, *1990 World Population Data Sheet* (Washington, D.C.: Population Reference Bureau, 1990).

13. M. Cameron and Y. Hofvander, *Manual on Feeding Infants and Young Children*, 3rd ed. (New York: Protein Advisory Board of the United Nations, 1989), pp. 11–13.

14. UNICEF, *The State of the World's Children 1993*, p. 44.

15. L. Robertson, Breastfeeding practices in maternity wards in Swaziland, *Journal of Nutrition Education* 23 (1991): 284–87.

16. UNICEF, *The State of the World's Children 1992* (London: Oxford University Press, 1992).

17. Bread for the World Institute on Hunger and Development, *Hunger 1992* (Washington, D.C.: Bread for the World Institute, 1992), p. 83.

18. J. P. Habicht, J. DaVanzo, and W. P. Butz, Mother's milk and sewage: Their interactive effects on infant mortality, *Pediatrics* 81 (1988): 456–61.

19. Dr. Carol Dyer's findings related to social and cultural beliefs about food in India are from A. Berg, *The Nutrition Factor* (Washington, D.C.: Brookings Institute, 1973), p. 46.

20. World Bank, *World Development Report 1991* (New York: Oxford University Press, 1991), Table 21.

21. Y. W. Bradshaw and coauthors, Borrowing against the future: Children and third world indebtedness, *Social Forces* 71 (1993): 629–56.

22. UNICEF, *The State of the World's Children 1989* (London: Oxford University Press, 1989), p. 82.

23. Berg, *The Nutrition Factor*, p. 46.

24. Independent Commission on International Issues, *North–South: A Program for Survival* (Cambridge, Mass.: MIT Press, 1980), pp. 49–50.

25. The following discussions were adapted from E. N. Whitney, E. M. N. Hamilton, and S. Rolfes, *Understanding Nutrition*, 5th ed. (St. Paul, Minn.: West Publishing, 1990), pp. 575–87.

26. The Hunger Project, *Ending Hunger: An Idea Whose Time Has Come* (New York: Praeger, 1985), pp. 314–15.

27. S. Lewis, Realism and vision in Africa, *Development: A Journal of the Society for International Development* 1 (1988): 46.

28. G. Kent, Food Trade: The poor feed the rich, *Food and Nutrition Bulletin* 4 (1982): 25–33.

29. F. M. Lappe and J. Collins, *Food First: Beyond the Myth of Scarcity* (Boston: Houghton Mifflin, 1978), p. 15.

30. G. M. Guthrie, Six to eighteen—the perilous months, *Nutrition Today* 23 (1988): 4–11.

31. Interreligious Taskforce on U.S. Food Policy, *Identifying a Food Policy Agenda for the 1990s: A Working Paper* (Washington, D.C.: Interreligious Taskforce on U.S. Food Policy, 1989), pp. 1–30.

32. J. Kocher, Not too many but too little, in J. D. Gussow, *The Feeding Web: Issues in Nutritional Ecology* (Palo Alto, Calif.: Bull Publishing, 1978), pp. 81–83.

33. M. R. Langham, L. Polopolus, and M. L. Upchurch, *World Food Issues* (Gainesville, Fla.: University of Florida Press, 1982), pp. 18–20.

34. R. R. Spitzer, *No Need for Hunger* (Danville, Ill.: Interstate Printers and Publishers, 1981), pp. 20–23.

35. E. O'Kelly, Appropriate technology for women, *Development Forum*, June 1984, p. 2.

36. National Agricultural Lands Study, *Soil Degradation: Effects on Agricultural Productivity*, Interim Report no. 4 (Washington, D.C.: U.S. Department of Agriculture, November 1980), as cited by L. R. Brown, World Population growth, soil erosion, and food security, *Science* 214 (1981): 995–1002.

37. Brown, World population growth.

38. T. Peterson, Hunger and the environment, *Seeds,* October 1987, pp. 6–13.

39. B. Stutz, The landscape of hunger, *Audobon,* March/April 1993, pp. 54–57; Newsbreaks: Effects of environmental degradation on nutrition, *Nutrition Today,* March/April, 1992, p. 4.

40. *Oxfam America News,* Fall 1992, p. 8.

41. The discussion of Sri Lankan development was adapted from M. Boyle, New heartbeat for an ancient people, *Seeds,* December 1984, pp. 14–18.

42. Mobilization for nutrition: Results from Iringa, *Mothers and Children: Bulletin on Infant Feeding and Maternal Nutrition* 8 (1989): 1–3; and Improving child survival and nutrition, *Evaluation Report: Joint WHO/UNICEF Nutrition Support Program in Iringa, Tanzania* (United Republic of Tanzania: WHO/UNICEF, 1989).

43. *Evaluation Report: Joint WHO/UNICEF Nutrition Support Program.*

44. Durning, Life on the brink, p. 29.

45. World Declaration on Nutrition, *Nutrition Reviews* 51 (1993): 41–43.

46. L. Miring'U and C. R. Mumaw, Needs assessment for in-service training for community nutrition educators in the Kiambu district in Kenya, *Journal of Nutrition Education* 25 (1993): 70–73.

47. *Nutrition: Linking Food, Health, and Development* (Washington, D.C.: U.S. National Committee for World Food Day, 1992), pp. 1–18.

48. S. Lewis, Food security, environment, poverty, and the world's children, *Journal of Nutrition Education* 24 (1992): 3S–5S.

49. UNICEF, *The State of the World's Children 1993,* p. 1.

50. Oral rehydration therapy, *World Health* (Geneva: World Health Organization, June 1985).

51. P. Pellet, The role of food mixtures in combating childhood malnutrition, in *Nutrition in the Community,* ed. D. McLaren (New York: John Wiley & Sons, 1978), pp. 185–202; and Graham, Starvation in the modern world, p. 1060.

52. UNICEF, *The State of the World's Children 1993,* p. 1.

53. Lewis, Food security, 1992.

54. Ibid., p. 5S.

55. Oxfam America, *Facts for Action: Women Creating a New World,* no. 3 (Boston: Oxfam America, 1991), pp. 2–3.

56. Trade and Development Program, *Exploring the Linkages: Trade Policies, Third World Development, and U.S. Agriculture* (Washington, D.C.: Bread for the World Institute, 1989), p. 23 as adapted from M. Carr, *Blacksmith, Baker, Roofing Sheet Maker* (London: Intermediate Technology Publications, 1984); and Bread for the World, *Women in Development* (Washington,

57. K. R. Nelson, R. M. Jenkins, and S. K. Nelson, A third world supplemental feeding project: Expectations and realities—A dichotomy, *Nutrition Today* 24 (1989): 19–26.

58. The list of types of programs was adapted from G. M. Wardlaw, Hunger and undernutrition in the world, *Nutri-News* (St. Louis: Mosby–Year Book, Inc., 1990), p. 14.

59. S. Pauling, Overcoming post–cold war challenges in Africa, *Bread for the World Background Paper* 130 (1993): 1–4.

60. *National Conference on Primary Health Care* (Kathmandu: Ministry of Health, Health Services Coordination Committee, World Health Organization, and UNICEF, 1977), pp. 9, 25, as cited by M. E. Frantz, Nutrition problems and programs in Nepal, *Hunger Notes* 2 (1980): 5–8.

61. L. C. Chen, Primary health care in developing countries: Overcoming operational, technical, and social barriers, *Lancet* 2 (1986): 1260–65; and P. F. Basch, *Textbook of International Health* (New York: Oxford University Press, 1990), pp. 200–205.

62. C. Aroney-Sine, Health care crisis: The global challenge, *Seeds* 15 (1993): 9–11.

63. L. R. Brown, *Vital Signs 1993: The Trends That Are Shaping Our Future* (New York: Norton, 1993); and L. R. Brown, A decade of discontinuity, *World Watch,* July/August 1993, pp. 19–26.

64. Report of the Special Initiative on AIDS of the American Public Health Association, *Tuberculosis and HIV Disease* (Washington, D.C.: American Public Health Association, 1992), pp. 1–5; and R. Bayer, N. Neveloff, and S. Landesman, The dual epidemics of tuberculosis and AIDS: Ethical and policy issues in screening and treatment, *American Journal of Public Health* 83 (1993): 649–54.

65. K. Selvaggio and N. Alexander, *Foreign aid at the crossroads* (Washington, D.C.: Bread for the World Institute, 1992), pp. 2–3.

66. The case for optimism, in E. Cornish, *The Study of the Future: An Introduction to the Art and Science of Understanding and Shaping Tomorrow's World* (Washington, D.C.: World Future Society, 1977), pp. 34–37.

67. 1990 State of the World Report.

68. D. Elgin, *Voluntary Simplicity: Toward a Way of Life That Is Outwardly Simple, Inwardly Rich* (New York: Morrow, 1981), p. 25.

69. Trade and Development Program, *Exploring the Linkages,* p. 25.

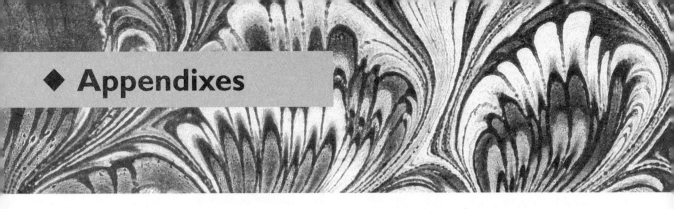

◆ Appendixes

F

Tips for Successful Grantwriting

G

The SMOG Readability Formula

H

Healthy Communities 2000: Model Standards—Guidelines for Community Attainment of the Year 2000 National Health Objectives

Appendix A

ORGANIZATION CHARTS

APPENDIX A-1   THE ORGANIZATION CHART FOR A HYPOTHETICAL STATE HEALTH AGENCY

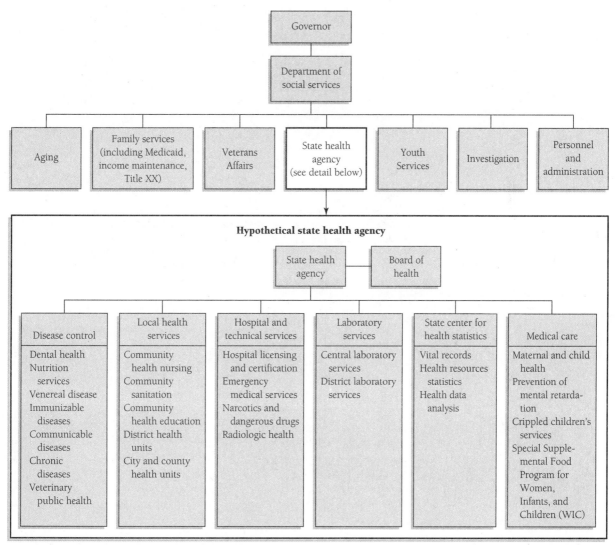

Source: G. Pickett and J. J. Hanlon, *Public Health: Administration and Practice* (St. Louis: Times Mirror/Mosby College Publishing, 1990), p. 109. (From National Public Health Program Reporting System.) Used with permission.

APPENDIX A-2   THE ORGANIZATION CHART FOR A HYPOTHETICAL LOCAL HEALTH DEPARTMENT

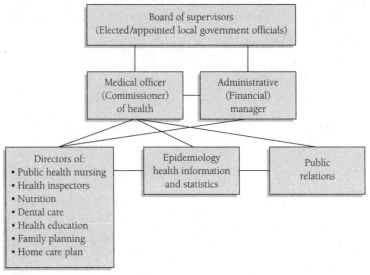

Source: Adapted, with permission, from J. M. Last, *Public Health and Human Ecology* (East Norwalk, Conn.: Appleton & Lange, 1987), p. 290.

Appendix B

COMMUNITY NUTRITION RESOURCES

APPENDIX B-1 A NUTRITIONIST'S GUIDE TO WASHINGTON, D.C.

Congress and Federal Legislation Resources

The *Congressional Handbook,* an annual directory of members of Congress, is available from:

- ◆ U.S. Chamber of Commerce
  Legislative Action Department
  1615 H Street, NW
  Washington, D.C. 20062

The *Congressional Insight Handbook: An Information Guide to the U.S. House of Representatives* is available from:

- ◆ Public Affairs Department
  National Association of Manufacturers
  Washington, D.C. 20004–1703

The *Congressional Record Scanner,* which provides a synopsis of the *Congressional Record;* the *Congressional Monitor,* a newsletter summarizing weekly activities of Congress and the Supreme Court; and the *CQ Quarterly,* which summarizes current issues and documents related to government activities, are available from:

- ◆ Congressional Quarterly, Inc.
  1414 22nd Street, NW
  Washington, D.C. 20037

The *Congressional Yellowbook,* which provides a directory of congressional staff and federal agencies, is available from:

- ◆ The Washington Monitor
  1301 Pennsylvania Avenue, NW
  Washington, D.C. 20004

House and Senate bills and committee reports are available from individual offices of members of Congress or from:

- ◆ House Document Room
  U.S. Capitol
  226 House Annex I
  Washington, D.C. 20515

- ◆ Senate Document Room
  Hart Senate Office Building
  Room B-04
  Washington, D.C. 20515

The *Federal Register* and the *Congressional Record,* which contains congressional and agency reports, and the *Congressional Directory,* which lists government offices and congressional committees, are available from:

◆ U.S. Government Printing Office
The Superintendent of Documents
Washington, D.C. 20402
(202) 783-3238

Reports of congressional audits of federal programs (e.g., Food Stamps, WIC) are available from:

◆ U.S. General Accounting Office
Reports and Publications
P.O. Box 6015
Gaithersburg, MD 20884–6015
(202) 512-6000

U.S. Government Agencies

The U.S. Department of Agriculture (USDA) has several divisions. The USDA's Food Safety and Inspection Service (FSIS) inspects and analyzes domestic and imported meat, poultry, and meat and poultry food products; establishes standards and approves recipes and labels of processed meat and poultry products; and monitors the meat and poultry industries for violations of inspection laws. To obtain publications or ask questions, write or call:

◆ FSIS, USDA
Public Awareness
14th Street SW and Independence Avenue
Room 1165 S
Washington, D.C. 20250
(202) 690-0351
USDA also maintains a meat and poultry hotline:
(800) 535-4555

The USDA's Agricultural Research Service (ARS) conducts research to fulfill the diverse needs of agricultural users—from farmers to consumers—in the areas of crop and animal production, protection, processing, and distribution; food safety and quality; and natural resources conservation. Write or call the information staff:

◆ ARS, USDA
Information Staff
Room 307, Building 005
BARC—West
Beltsville, MD 20705
(301) 504-6264

The USDA's Human Nutrition Information Service (HNIS) maintains the USDA's Nutrient Data Bank, conducts the Nationwide Food Consumption Survey, monitors the nutrient content of the U.S. food supply, provides nutrition guidelines for education and action programs, collects and disseminates food and nutrition materials, and conducts nutrition education research. Write or call:

◆ HNIS, USDA
5505 Belcrest Road
Hyattsville, MD 20782
(301) 436-8498

The USDA's Food and Nutrition Service (FNS) administers the Food Stamp
Program; the National School Lunch and School Breakfast programs; the Special
Supplemental Food Program for Women, Infants, and Children (WIC); and the
food distribution, child and adult care food, summer food service, and special
milk programs. Write or call:

◆ FNS, USDA
3101 Park Center Drive
Alexandria, VA 22302
(703) 756-3284

The USDA's Agricultural Marketing Service (AMS) operates a variety of marketing programs and services—several of interest to consumers. Its activities include
developing grades and standards for the trading of food and other farm products
and carrying out grading services on request from packers and processors;
inspecting egg products for wholesomeness; administering marketing orders that
aid in the marketing of milk, fruits, vegetables, and related specialty crops like
nuts; and administering truth-in-seed labeling and other regulatory programs.
Write or call:

◆ AMS, USDA
P.O. Box 96456
Washington, D.C. 20090–6456
(202) 447-8998

The USDA's *Food News for Consumers,* a quarterly newsletter, is available from
the U.S. Government Printing Office. Other government addresses and telephone
numbers follow:

◆ Food and Drug Administration
Office of Consumer Affairs
5600 Fishers Lane
Rockville, MD 20852
(301) 443-1544

◆ The Food and Nutrition Information
Center
National Agriculture Library
10301 Baltimore Boulevard, Room 304
Beltsville, MD 20705–2351
(301) 344-3719

◆ Administration on Aging
330 Independence Avenue, SW
Washington, D.C. 20201
(202) 619-0724

◆ Centers for Disease Control and
Prevention Information Hotline:
(404) 332-4555

◆ Centers for Disease Control
and Prevention
Division of Chronic Disease
Control and Community
Intervention

◆ Centers for Disease Control and
Prevention
Office on Smoking and Health
National Center for Chronic Disease
Prevention and Health Promotion

National Center for Chronic
Disease Prevention and
Health Promotion
Community Health
Promotion Branch
4770 Buford Highway, NE
Mailstop K-46
Atlanta, GA 30341
(404) 488-5426

Mail Stop K-50
1600 Clifton Road, NE
Atlanta, GA 30333
(404) 488-5705

◆ Centers for Disease Control
and Prevention
Public Health Program
Practice Office
Division of Public
Health Systems
1600 Clifton Road
Mailstop E-20
Atlanta, GA 30333
(404) 639-1967

◆ Environmental Protection Agency
401 M Street, NW
Washington, D.C. 20460
(202) 382-3535
EPA Safe Drinking Water Hotline:
(800) 426-4791

◆ Federal Trade Commission
Public Reference Branch
Washington, D.C. 20418
(202) 326-2222

◆ Food and Drug Administration
Office of Consumer Affairs
5600 Fishers Lane
Rockville, MD 20852
(301) 443-1544

◆ FDA Consumer Information
Line:
(800) 535-4555

◆ FDA Office of Nutrition and Food
Sciences
200 C Street, SW
Washington, D.C. 20204
(202) 205-4561

◆ The Food and Nutrition
Information Center
National Agriculture Library
10301 Baltimore Boulevard,
Room 304
Beltsville, MD 20705–2351
(301) 344-3719

◆ National Academy of Sciences/
National Research Council
(NAS/NRC)
2101 Constitution Avenue, NW
Washington, D.C. 20418
(202) 334-2000

◆ National Cancer Institute
9000 Rockville Pike
Building 31, Room 10A-24
Bethesda, MD 20892
(800) 4-CANCER

◆ National Center for Health Statistics
Public Health Service
U.S. Department of Health and
Human Services
6525 Belcrest Road
Hyattsville, MD 20782
(301) 436-8500

◆ National Health Information
Center

◆ National Heart, Lung, and Blood
Institute Information Center

P.O. Box 1133
Washington, D.C. 20013–1133
(301) 565-4167
(800) 336-4797

◆ National Institutes of Health
9000 Rockville Pike
Bethesda, MD 20892
(301) 496-4000

4733 Bethesda Avenue, Suite 530
Bethesda, MD 20814-4820
(301) 951-3260

◆ Office of Disease Prevention and
Health Promotion
Public Health Service
U.S. Department of Health and
Human Services
333 C Street, SW
Room 2132
Washington, D.C. 20201
(202) 205-8611

◆ U.S. Public Health Service Public Affairs Office
Hubert H. Humphrey Building
Room 725-H
200 Independence Avenue, SW
Washington, D.C. 20201
(202) 245-6867

APPENDIX B-2 GENERAL COMMUNITY NUTRITION RESOURCES

Consumer and Advocacy Groups

◆ American Dietetic Association
Office of Government Affairs
1225 Eye Street, NW
Suite 1250
Washington, D.C. 20005
(202) 371-0500

◆ Center for Science in the Public
Interest
1875 Connecticut Avenue, NW
Suite 300
Washington, D.C. 20009–5728
(202) 332-9110

◆ Center on Budget and Policy
Priorities
777 N. Capitol Street, NE
Room 705
Washington, D.C. 20002
(202) 408-1080

◆ Children's Defense Fund
122 C Street, NW
Washington, D.C. 20001
(202) 628-8787

◆ Children's Foundation
725 Fifteenth Street, NW
Suite 505
Washington, D.C. 20005
(202) 347-3300

◆ Community Nutrition Institute
2001 S Street, NW
Suite 530
Washington, D.C. 20009
(202) 462-4700

◆ Consumer Association of
Canada
307 Gilmour Street

◆ The Consumer Information Center
Pueblo, CO 81009
(719) 948-3334

Ottawa, Ontario K2P 0P7
Canada

◆ Consumer's Union
101 Truman Avenue
Yonkers, N.Y. 10703
(914) 378-2000

◆ Food Research and Action Center
1875 Connecticut Avenue, NW
Suite 540
Washington, D.C. 20009
(202) 986-2200

◆ Interfaith Impact for Justice
and Peace
110 Maryland Avenue, NE
Washington, D.C. 20002
(202) 543-2800

◆ National Council Against Health
Fraud, Inc.
P.O. Box 1276
Loma Linda, CA 92354
(714) 824-4690

◆ National Council of Senior
Citizens
1331 F Street, NW
Washington, D.C. 20004
(202) 347-8800

◆ Nutrition Legislative News
P.O. Box 75035
Washington, D.C. 20013
(202) 488-8879

◆ Public Voice for Food and
Health Policy
1001 Connecticut
Avenue, NW
Room 522
Washington, D.C. 20036
(202) 659-5930

◆ Urban Institute
2100 M Street, NW, 5th floor
Washington, D.C. 20037
(202) 833-7200

Professional and Service Organizations

◆ AIDS Referral
1620 Eye Street, NW
Washington, D.C. 20006
(202) 293-7330
National AIDS Hotline (CDC):
(800) 342-AIDS (English)
(800) 344-SIDA (Spanish)
(800) 2437-TTY (Deaf)
(900) 820-2437

◆ Al-Anon Family Group Headquarters
826 Midtown Station
New York, NY 10018
(212) 302-7240
(800) 356-9996

◆ Alateen
1372 Broadway
New York, NY 10018

◆ Alcohol and Drug Abuse
Information Line:
(800) 252-6465

◆ Alcoholics Anonymous (AA)
General Service Office
475 Riverside Drive
New York, NY 10015
(212) 870-3400

◆ Alliance for Food and Fiber
Food Safety Hotline:
(800) 266-0200

◆ Alzheimer's Disease
Information and Referral
Service
919 North Michigan Avenue
Chicago, IL 60611
(800) 272-3900

◆ American Anorexia/Bulimia
Association, Inc.
418 East 76 Street
New York, NY 10021
(212) 734-1114

◆ American Cancer Society
Cancer Information Center
1701 Rickenbacker Drive
Suite 5B
Sun City Center, FL
33573–5361
(800) ACS-2345

◆ American Council of the
Blind Information Line:
(800) 424-8666

◆ American Dental Association
211 East Chicago Avenue
Chicago, IL 60611
(312) 440-2500

◆ American Dietetic Association
216 West Jackson Boulevard
Suite 800
Chicago, IL 60606–6995
(312) 899-0040

◆ American Academy of Pediatrics
P.O. Box 927
141 Northwest Point Boulevard
Elk Grove Village, IL 60009–0927
(708) 228-5005

◆ American Association of Retired
Persons
601 E Street, NW
Washington, D.C. 20049
(202) 434-2277

◆ American College of Sports Medicine
P.O. Box 1440
Indianapolis, IN 46204
(317) 637-9200

◆ American Council on Science and
Health
1995 Broadway
New York, NY 10023
(212) 362-7044

◆ American Diabetes Association
1660 Duke Street
Alexandria, VA 22314
(703) 549-1500
(800) 232-3472

◆ American Health Foundation
320 E. 43rd Street
New York, NY 10017
(212) 953-1900

The American Dietetic Association's National Center on Nutrition and
Dietetics operates a toll-free nutrition hotline for consumers:
(800) 366-1655

◆ American Heart Association
7320 Greenville Avenue
Dallas, TX 75231
(214) 373-6300
(800) 242-8721

◆ American Institute for
Cancer Research

◆ American Home Economics
Association
1555 King Street
Alexandria, VA 22314
(703) 706-4600

◆ American Institute of Nutrition
9650 Rockville Pike

1759 R Street, NW
Washington, D.C. 20009
(202) 328-7744
(800) 843-8114

Bethesda, MD 20014
(301) 530-7050

◆ American Medical Association
515 North State Street
Chicago, IL 60610
(312) 464-5000

◆ American Public Health Association
1015 Fifteenth Street, NW
Washington, D.C. 20005
(202) 789-5600

◆ American Public Welfare
Association
(Food Stamp Program
Administrators)
810 First Street, NE
Room 500
Washington, D.C. 20002
(202) 682-0100

◆ American Red Cross
National Headquarters
431 Eighteenth Street, NW
Washington, D.C. 20006
(202) 737-8300

◆ American School Food
Service Association
(Child Nutrition Program
Personnel)
1600 Duke Street, 7th floor
Alexandria, VA 22314
(703) 739-3900

◆ American School Health Association
7263 State Route 43
Kent, OH 44240
(216) 678-4526

◆ American SIDS (Sudden
Infant Death) Institute
Information Line:
(800) 232-SIDS;
in Georgia: (800) 847-7437

◆ American Society for Clinical
Nutrition
9650 Rockville Pike
Bethesda, MD 20814
(301) 530-7110

◆ Anorexia Nervosa and
Related Eating Disorders, Inc.
P.O. Box 5102
Eugene, Oregon 97405
(503) 344-1144

◆ Arthritis Foundation
Information Line:
(800) 283-7800

◆ Asthma and Allergy
Foundation of America
Information Line:
(800) 7-ASTHMA

◆ Bulimia Anorexia Self-Help
Crisis Line:
(800) 227-4785
(800) 762-3347

◆ Canadian Diabetes Association
78 Bond Street
Toronto, Ontario M5B 2J8
Canada
(416) 362-4440

◆ Canadian Dietetic Association
480 University Avenue
Suite 601
Toronto, Ontario M5G 1V2, Canada
(416) 596-0857

◆ Canadian Public Health
Association

◆ Canadian Sport Medicine and Science
Council of Canada

Publications, Suite 400
1565 Carling Avenue
Ottawa, Ontario K1Z 8R1
Canada

◆ Courage Stroke Network
Information Line:
(800) 553-6921

◆ Healthy Kids Resource Center
California Comprehensive
Health Education Resource
Center
321 Wallace Avenue
Vallejo, CA 94590
(707) 557-0680

◆ International Life Sciences
Institute—Nutrition
Foundation
1126 Sixteenth Street, NW
Suite 111
Washington, D.C. 20036
(202) 659-0074

◆ March of Dimes Birth
Defects Foundation
National Headquarters
1275 Mamaroneck Avenue
White Plains, NY 10605
(914) 428-7100

◆ National Association for
Sickle Cell Disease
Information Line:
(800) 421-8453

◆ National Child Abuse Hotline:
(800) 422-4453

◆ National Eating Disorder
Information Centre of Canada
200 Elizabeth Street,
College Wing 1-328
Toronto, Ontario M5G 2C4
Canada

1600 James Naismith Drive
Suite 502
Gloucester, Ontario K1B 5N4
Canada

◆ Dial a Hearing Screening Test:
(800) 222-EARS

◆ Institute of Food Technologists
221 North LaSalle Street
Chicago, IL 60601
(312) 782-8424

◆ La Leche League International, Inc.
9616 Minneapolis Avenue
Franklin Park, IL 60131
(708) 455-7730

◆ Narcotics Anonymous (NA)
P.O. Box 9999
Van Nuys, CA 91409
(818) 780-3951

◆ National Association of WIC
Directors
P.O. Box 53405
Washington, D.C. 20009
(202) 232-5492

◆ National Council on Alcoholism
12 West 21st Street
New York, NY 10010
(212) 206-6770
(800) 527-5344

◆ National Institute of Nutrition
302-265 Carling Avenue
Ottawa, Ontario K1S 2E1, Canada

◆ National Osteoporosis
Foundation
2100 M Street, NW
Suite 602
Washington, D.C. 20037
(202) 223-2226

◆ National Safety Council Lead
Poisoning Hotline:
(800) 532-3394

◆ Nutrition Screening Initiative
1010 Wisconsin Avenue, NW
Suite 800
Washington, D.C. 20007
(202) 625-1662

◆ Pennsylvania State Nutrition
Center
The Pennsylvania State
University
Ruth Building
417 East Calder Way
University Park, PA
16802-5663
(814) 865-6323

◆ Sexually Transmitted Diseases
Hotline:
(800) 227-8922

◆ *Tufts University Diet &*
Nutrition Letter
203 Harrison Avenue
Boston, MA 02111
(800) 274-7581

◆ Williams & Wilkins
(Publisher of *Nutrition Today*)
428 East Preston Street
Baltimore, MD 21202
(410) 528-4000

◆ National Pesticide
Telecommunications Network
Texas Tech University
Thompson Hall, Room S129
Lubbock, TX 79430
NPTN Hotline: (800) 858-PEST

◆ Nutrition Information Service
University of Alabama at Birmingham
Room 447 Webb Building
UAB Station
Birmingham, AL 35294–3360
(800) 231-DIET

◆ Overeaters Anonymous (OA)
P.O. Box 92870
Los Angeles, CA 90009
(213) 618-8835

◆ PM, Inc. (Publisher of *Nutrition*
and the MD)
P.O. Box 10172
Van Nuys, CA 91410
(818) 997-8011

◆ Society for Nutrition Education
2001 Killebrew Drive
Suite 340
Minneapolis, MN 55425–1882
(612) 854-0035

◆ Weight Watchers
Consumer Affairs Department A
500 North Broadway
Jericho, NY 11753–2196
(800) 874-4170

Trade Organizations

◆ American Egg Board
1460 Renaissance Drive
Park Ridge, IL 60068
(708) 296-7043

◆ Beech-Nut
Checkerboard Square, 1B
St. Louis, MO 63164
(800) 523-6633

◆ Borden Farm Products
Borden Company
Consumer Affairs
180 East Broad Street
Columbus, OH 43215
(614) 225-4000

◆ General Mills
Nutrition Department
P.O. Box 1113
Minneapolis, MN 55440
(612) 540-7206

◆ H. J. Heinz
Consumer Relations
P.O. Box 57
Pittsburgh, PA 15230
(412) 456-5700

◆ Kellogg Company
Battle Creek, MI 49016–1986
(616) 961-2000

◆ Mead Johnson Nutritionals
2400 West Lloyd Expressway
Evansville, IN 47721
(812) 429-5000

◆ National Dairy Council
O'Hare International Center

◆ American Meat Institute
1700 North Moore Street
Suite 1600
Arlington, VA 22209
(703) 841-2400

◆ Best Foods
Consumer Service Department
Division of CPC International
International Plaza
P.O. Box 8000
Englewood Cliffs, NJ 07632
(201) 894-4000

◆ Campbell Soup Company
Campbell Place
Camden, NJ 08103–1799
(609) 342-4800

◆ Gerber Products Company
445 State Street
Fremont, MI 49413
(616) 928-2000

◆ Hunt-Wesson Foods
1645 West Valencia Drive
Fullerton, CA 92633
(714) 680-1000

◆ Kraft General Foods Consumer
Center
250 North Street
White Plains, NY 10625
(914) 335-2500

◆ Nabisco Consumer Affairs
100 DeForest Avenue
East Hanover, NJ 07936
(800) 932-7800
(800) NABISCO

◆ National Live Stock & Meat Board
444 North Michigan Avenue

10255 West Higgins Road
Suite 900
Rosemont, IL 60018–5616
(708) 803-2000

Chicago, IL 60611
(312) 467-5520

◆ Nestlé Company
100 Manhattanville Road
Purchase, NY 10577
(914) 251-3000

◆ NutraSweet Simplesse Company
P.O. Box 830
Deerfield, IL 60015
(800) 321-7254

◆ Oscar Mayer Company
P.O. Box 7188
Madison, WI 53707
(608) 241-3311

◆ Pillsbury Company
200 South Sixth Street
Minneapolis, MN 55402–1464
(612) 330-4966

◆ The Potato Board
1385 South Colorado
Boulevard
Suite 512
Denver, CO 80222
(303) 758-7783

◆ Procter and Gamble Company
One Procter and Gamble Plaza
Cincinnati, OH 45202
(513) 983-1100

◆ Rice Council
P.O. Box 740123
Houston, TX 77274
(713) 270-6699

◆ Ross Laboratories
Abbott Laboratory
625 Cleveland Avenue
Columbus, OH 43215
(614) 624-7900
(800) 227-5767

◆ Soy Protein Council
1255 23rd Street, NW
Washington, D.C. 20037
(202) 467-6610

◆ Sunkist Growers
Consumer Service, Division BB
Box 7888
Valley Annex
Van Nuys, CA 91409
(818) 986-4800

◆ United Fresh Fruit and
Vegetable Association
727 N. Washington Street
Alexandria, VA 22314
(703) 836-3410

◆ Vitamin Nutrition Information
Service (VNIS)
Hoffman-LaRoche, Inc.
340 Kingsland Street
Nutley, NJ 07110
(201) 235-1194

Organizations Concerned with Hunger and Poverty

◆ Bread for the World Institute
1100 Wayne Avenue
Suite 1000
Silver Spring, MD 20910
(301) 608-2400

◆ CARE
Office of Education
660 First Avenue
New York, NY 10016
(212) 686-3110

For legislative updates:
(301) 588-7439

◆ Catholic Relief Services
209 West Fayette Street
Baltimore, MD 21201–3443
(410) 625-2220
(800) 647-4788

◆ Center on Hunger, Poverty,
and Nutrition Policy
Tufts University School
of Nutrition
126 Curtis Street
Medford, MA 02155
(617) 381-3223

◆ End Hunger Network
365 Sycamore Road
Santa Monica, CA 90402
(310) 454-3716

◆ Foodchain
970 Jefferson Street
Atlanta, GA 30318
(800) 845-3008

◆ The Hunger Project
One Madison Avenue
New York, NY 10010
(212) 532-4255

◆ Oxfam America
26 West Street
Boston, MA 02111
(617) 482-1211

◆ Seeds
P.O. Box 6170
Waco, TX 76706
(817) 755-7745

◆ U.S. Committee for UNICEF
333 East 38th Street

◆ Center for Global Education
Augsburg College
731 21st Avenue South
Minneapolis, MN 55454
(612) 330-1159

◆ Church World Service/CROP
P.O. Box 968
Elkhart, IN 46515
(219) 264-3102
(800) 456-1310

◆ Food and Agriculture
Organization (FAO)
North American Regional Office
1001 22nd Street, NW
Washington, D.C. 20437
(202) 653-2402

◆ Freedom from Hunger
P.O. Box 2000
1644 DaVinci Court
Davis, CA 95617
(916) 758-6200

◆ Institute for Food and Development
Policy
398 60th Street
Oakland, CA 94618
(510) 654-4400
(800) 888-3314

◆ Second Harvest
116 Michigan Avenue
Room 4
Chicago, IL 60603
(312) 263-2303

◆ UNICEF
Information Division
866 UN Plaza
New York, NY 10017
(212) 326-7000

◆ U.S. Agency for International
Development

New York, NY 10016
(212) 686-5522

Office of Nutrition
Department of State
Washington, D.C. 20523
(202) 647-4000

◆ U.S. Conference of Mayors
1620 Eye Street, NW,
4th Floor
Washington, D.C. 20009
(202) 293-7330

◆ U.S. National Committee for World
Food Day
1001 22nd Street, NW
Washington, D.C. 20437
(202) 653-2404

◆ VITAL
1616 North Fort Meyer Drive
Suite 1240
Arlington, VA 22209
(703) 841-0652

◆ World Bank
Publications Department
1818 H Street, NW
Washington, D.C. 20433
(202) 477-8350

◆ World Health
Organization (WHO)
1211 Geneva 27
Switzerland

◆ World Health Organization
Regional Office
525 23rd Street, NW
Washington, D.C. 20037
(202) 861-3200

◆ World Health Organization
Publications
49 Sheridan Avenue
Albany, NY 12210
(518) 436-9686

◆ World Hunger Education Service
P.O. Box 29056
Washington, D.C. 20017
(202) 298-9503

◆ World Hunger Year
261 West 35th Street
Room 1402
New York, NY 10001
(212) 629-8850

◆ World Vision
919 W. Huntington Drive
Monrovia, CA 91016
(818) 357-7979

◆ Worldwatch Institute
1776 Massachusetts Avenue, NW
Washington, D.C. 20036
(202) 452-1999

Canadian Government
Federal

◆ Bureau of Nutritional Sciences
Food Directorate
Health Protection Branch
Health Canada
Banting Building
Tunney's Pasture
Ottawa, Ontario K1A 0L2

◆ Nutrition Programs Unit
Health Promotion Directorate
Health Canada
Room 456, Jeanne Mance Building
Tunney's Pasture
Ottawa, Ontario K1A 1B4, Canada
(613) 957-8328

Canada
(613) 957-0911

◆ Nutrition Consultant
Epidemiology and Community
Health, Indian and Northern
Health Services
Health Canada
Room 1116, Jeanne Mance Building
Tunney's Pasture
Ottawa, Ontario K1A 0L3, Canada
(613) 954-7757

Provincial and Territorial

◆ Nutrition Coordinator
Special Services
Department of Health
and Social Services
16 Fitzroy St.
P.O. Box 2000
Charlottetown, Prince Edward
Island C1A 7J9, Canada
(902) 368-5004

◆ Senior Nutrition Consultant
Public Health Services
Department of Health and
Community Services
P.O. Box 5100
Fredericton, New Brunswick
E3B 5G8, Canada

◆ Responsable des programmes
de nutrition
Direction de la Santé
Ministère de la Santé et
des Services sociaux
10e étage, 1075 chemin
Saint-Foy
Québec, Québec G1S 2M1
Canada

◆ Program Specialist Nutrition
Health and Wellness Branch
Healthy Public Policy
Program Division
Manitoba Health
303–800 Portage Avenue

◆ Provincial Nutrition Consultant
Health Promotion and Nutrition
Division
Department of Health
Box 4750
St. John's, Newfoundland A1C 5T7
Canada

◆ Nutrition Coordinator
Department of Health and Fitness
P.O. Box 488
Halifax, Nova Scotia B3J 2R8, Canada

◆ Senior Nutrition Consultant
Public Health Branch
Ministry of Health, 5th Floor
15 Overlea Boulevard,
Toronto, Ontario M4H 1A9, Canada

◆ Provincial Nutritionist
Community Services
Saskatchewan Health
3475 Albert Street
Regina, Saskatchewan
S4S 6X6, Canada

Winnipeg, Manitoba
R3G 0N4, Canada

◆ Community Nutrition
Program
Family Health Services
Public Health Division
Alberta Health
Seventh Street Plaza,
South Tower
10030–107 Avenue
Edmonton, Alberta T5J 3E4
Canada

◆ Director Nutrition
Family Health Division
Ministry of Health
5th Floor, 1515 Blanshard Street
Victoria, British Columbia V8W 3C8
Canada

◆ A/Director Dietetics
Department of Health and
Human Resources
#5 Hospital Road
Whitehorse, Yukon Y1A 2C6
Canada

◆ Nutritionist, Community Health
Department of Health
7th Floor, Lahm Ridge Tower,
Box 1320
Yellowknife, Northwest Territories
X1A 2L9, Canada

APPENDIX B-3 CLEARINGHOUSES, INFORMATION CENTERS, AND DATA ARCHIVES

Clearinghouses and Information Centers

◆ National Clearinghouse on Bilingual Education
1118 22nd Street NW
Washington, D.C. 20037
(202) 467-0867

◆ National Clearinghouse for Alcohol and Drug
Information (NCADI)
P.O. Box 2345
Rockville, MD 20847–2345
(301) 468-2600

◆ Office of Cancer Communications
National Cancer Institute
Information Resources Branch
Bethesda, MD 20892

(800) 4-CANCER
(800) 638-6070 (in Alaska)
(808) 524-1234 (in Oahu, Hawaii)

◆ National Heart, Lung, and Blood Institute (NHLBI)
NHLBI Information Center
P.O. Box 30105
Bethesda, MD 20824–0105
(301) 951-3260

◆ Superintendent of Documents
U.S. Government Printing Office
Washington, D.C. 20402
(202) 783-3238

Data Archives

Information about population survey data, including data related to nutrition, can be obtained from both the government and private sectors. Several organizations publish catalogs of the data they collect and/or store. Each organization sets its own priorities, terms for accessing the data, and charge for obtaining the data and supporting documentation. A few of these organizations are listed below.

- ◆ National Center for Health Statistics
  Scientific and Technical Information Branch
  Room 1064, Presidential Building
  6525 Belcrest Road
  Hyattsville, MD 20782
  (301) 436-8500

- ◆ Louis Harris Data Center
  Contact: David Sheaves
  CB #3355, Manning Hall
  University of North Carolina
  Chapel Hill, NC 27599–3355
  (919) 966-3346

- ◆ Institute for Research in Social Science
  Demographic Data Services
  CB #3355, Manning Hall

University of North Carolina
Chapel Hill, NC 27599–3355
(919) 962-0512

- ◆ National Technical Information Service (NTIS)
  Contact: Document Library
  5285 Port Royal Rd.
  Springfield, VA 22161
  (703) 487-4650

- ◆ National Archive of Computerized Data on Aging
  Inter-university Consortium for Political and Social Research
  University of Michigan
  P.O. Box 1248
  Ann Arbor, MI 48106–1248
  (313) 764-2570

APPENDIX B-4 ELECTRONIC RESOURCES FOR THE COMMUNITY NUTRITIONIST

Compiled by Edward H. Weiss, PhD, RD
D'Youville College
Buffalo, New York
1994

Electronic bulletin boards and remote access databases are becoming important resources for the community nutritionist. These resources have on-line help and user guides. Access can be made by modem through a telephone or an Internet connection. An excellent introduction to Internet (electronic highway) is found in *Navigating the Internet* by Mark Gibbs and Richard Smith (published by Sams Publishing, Carmel, IN, 1993) and *The Whole Internet* by Ed Krol (published by O'Reilly & Associates, Inc., Sebastopol, CA, 1992). These texts were written for the newcomer and provide an introduction to the "tools" and terms needed to navigate around the Internet. The amount of information and variety of methods of accessing and searching databases can be confusing to the novice. Seeking out someone who has already been successful will speed the process.

You can begin to search out and access electronic resources using the free resources listed below. Information on both telephone and Internet access is included when available.

Name:	PENpages—The Pennsylvania State University
Service:	Searchable databases containing information and reports on agriculture, human nutrition, food safety, gerontology, and family issues.
Information:	(814) 863-3449 (voice) or 865-1229 (voice)
Internet:	Telnet to PSUPEN.PSU.EDU
	At prompt username: type PENPAGES (press return).
Modem:	(814) 863-4820 (VT100 or VT102) 8-N-1*
	At prompt Local > type CONNECT PEN (press return).
	At prompt username: type PENPAGES (press return).

*All telephone settings are Data bit: 8, Parity: None, Stop bit: 1, Duplex: full (8-N-1), unless otherwise noted.

Name:	FDA Bulletin Board System
Service:	News releases, congressional testimony, *FDA Consumer Magazine*, speeches, AIDS information, recall lists, and more.
Information:	(301) 443-3285 (voice): general information
	(301) 443-7318 (voice): technical support
Internet:	Telnet to FDABBS.FDA.GOV
	At prompt type: bbs (all lowercase).
Modem:	1 (800) 222-0185 (VT100, VT102, ANSI) 7-E-1
	At prompt type: bbs (all lowercase).

Name: WONDER P/C—Centers for Disease Control and Prevention (CDC)

Service: MMWR articles (searchable), data sets and/or documentation on topics that include NHANES I, II; diabetes, AIDS, U.S. Census, National Hospital Discharge Survey, CDC Prevention Guidelines, resource contacts, data analysis, and E-mail to CDC users and staff.

Information: (404) 332-4569 (voice)
CDC Wonder Customer Support
1600 Clifton Rd., NE Mailstop F-51
Atlanta, GA 30333

Modem: Via CDC-supplied software and a toll-free 800 number. Software and access codes are mailed free of charge but preregistration is required.

Name: Fed World BBS

Service: Bulletin board run by the National Technical Information Service, provides information and access to over 80 bulletin boards (BBS) run by federal government agencies (e.g., National Agricultural Library, Human Nutrition Information Service, Indian Health Service, Library of Congress, and NIH Information Center). Once identified, these BBS can be contacted directly via the telephone or Internet.

Information: (703) 487-4608 (voice)

Internet: Telnet to FEDWORLD.DOC.GOV
Follow directions at prompt.

Modem: (703) 321-8020 (VT100, VT102) 8-N-1
Follow directions at prompt.

Name: CENET—Cornell Extension Network

Service: Information on human nutrition, food safety, agriculture, community development, and many non-nutrition-related topics. (Access is free to guests after 5:00 P.M. and weekends.)

Information: (607) 255-8127 (voice)

Internet: Telnet to EMPIRE.CCE.CORNELL.EDU
At prompt type: guest (lowercase only).

Modem: (607) 255-6196 (VT100) 8-N-1
Connect to EMPIRE.CCE.CORNELL.EDU
At prompt type: guest (lowercase only).

Name: CUFAN—Clemson University Food and Agriculture Network

Service: Full-text documents on agricultural and customer topics and cooperative extension.

Information: (803) 656-5080 (voice)

Internet: Telnet to PRISM.CLEMSON.EDU
At prompt type: PUBLIC.

Modem: Telephone access not available.

Name: QUERRI—Questions on University Extension Regional Resource Information

Service: Bibliographic database of a variety of educational resources about agriculture, food, and nutrition (see family and consumer science), and related consumer issues. Listed materials can be ordered. Basically, an on-line catalog of resources.

Information: (515) 294-8802 (voice)

Internet: Telnet to ISN.RDNS.IASTATE.EDU
At prompt type: QUERRI.

Modem: (515) 294-2400 (VT100) 8-N-1
Press return after connection is made.
At prompt (Dial:) type: QUERRI.

Name: UnCover

Service: Searchable periodical index database and fax delivery service. Individuals may search the database for free, the cost for faxing is $8.50 (plus a copyright fee, approximately $3.00–$5.00). The UnCover database can be searched by topic, journal title, or author. You may also browse the table of contents of individual journal issues.

Info: (800) 787-7979

Internet: Telnet to DATABASE.CARL.ORG. At prompt, select UnCover from the menu, and connect to the free open access version.

Modem: (303) 756-3600 (VT100) 8-N-1

Appendix C

NATIONAL NUTRITION MONITORING SYSTEM

APPENDIX C-I   Dietary and Nutrition Status Surveys and Surveillance Activities of the National Nutrition Monitoring System

DATE	AGENCY[a]	SURVEY	TARGET U.S. POPULATION	SAMPLE SELECTED	NUMBER INTERVIEWED (RESPONSE RATE)	NUMBER EXAMINED (RESPONSE RATE)
1909–annual	USDA	U.S. Food Supply Series	NA[b]	~350 foods currently	NA	NA
1936–37	USDA	Household Food Consumption Survey—Household Food Use	Housekeeping households, with husband and wife, native born, nonrelief	NR[c]	20,466 households	NA
1942	USDA	Household Food Consumption Survey—Household Food Use	Housekeeping households	3060 households	2748 households	NA
1948	USDA	Household Food Consumption Survey—Household Food Use	Urban housekeeping households	5681 households	4489 households	NA
1955	USDA	Household Food Consumption Survey—Household Food Use	Civilian, housekeeping households	6792 households	6060 households	NA
1965–66	USDA	Household Food Consumption Survey—Household Food Use	Civilian, housekeeping households	18,890 households	15,112 households	NA
1965	USDA	Nationwide Food Consumption Survey—Individual Intakes	Eligible individuals residing in eligible households (all except half of persons 20–64 yr)	NR	14,519 persons	NA
1968–70	DHEW	Ten State Nutrition Survey	Low-income families in 10 states	29,935 families	23,846 (80%) families 86,352 persons	40,847 (47%)
1971–74	NCHS	First National Health and Nutrition Examination Survey	Civilian, noninstitutionalized individuals, 1–74 yr	28,043 persons	27,753 (99%)	20,749 (74%)
1974–75	NCHS	NHANES I Augmentation Sample	Civilian, noninstitutionalized persons, 25–74 yr	4300 persons	4288 (94%)	3053 (71%)

Continued

Dietary and Nutrition Status Surveys and Surveillance Activities of the National Nutrition Monitoring System—*Continued*

DATE	AGENCY[a]	SURVEY	TARGET U.S. POPULATION	SAMPLE SELECTED	NUMBER INTERVIEWED (RESPONSE RATE)	NUMBER EXAMINED (RESPONSE RATE)
1973–continuous	CDC	Pediatric Nutrition Surveillance System	Low-income, high-risk children, 0–17 yr	5 states (in 1987, 36 states plus District of Columbia and Puerto Rico)	NA	NA
1976–80	NCHS	Second National Health and Nutrition Examination Survey	Civilian, noninstitutionalized individuals, 0.5–74 yr	27,801 persons	25,286 (91%)	20,322(73%)
1977–78	USDA	Nationwide Food Consumption Survey—Household Food Use	Civilian households	24,408 households	14,964 households	NA
1977–78	USDA	Nationwide Food Consumption Survey—Individual Intakes	Eligible individuals residing in eligible households (All except half of persons over 18 yr in summer, fall, and winter)	44,169 persons	30,770 persons	NA
1977–78	USDA	Supplemental Nationwide Food Consumption Survey–Household Food Use	Civilian households in Puerto Rico, Alaska, Hawaii. Elderly adults in 48 states.	18,162 households	10,341 households	NA
1977–78	USDA	Supplemental Nationwide Food Consumption Survey—Individual Intakes	Individuals residing in eligible households	28,984 persons	21,465 persons	NA
1977–78	USDA	Low-income Nationwide Food Consumption Survey—Household Food Use	Low-income civilian households in 48 states.	NR	4623 households	NA
1977–78	USDA	Low-Income Nationwide Consumption Survey—Individual Intakes	Individuals residing in eligible households	16,208 persons	12,847 persons	NA

Continued

APPENDIX			**Dietary and Nutrition Status Surveys and Surveillance Activities of the National Nutrition Monitoring System—***Continued*				
C-1							

DATE	AGENCY[a]	SURVEY	TARGET U.S. POPULATION	SAMPLE SELECTED	NUMBER INTERVIEWED (RESPONSE RATE)	NUMBER EXAMINED (RESPONSE RATE)
1979–continuous	CDC	Pregnancy Nutrition Surveillance System	Low-income, high-risk pregnant women	13 states (in 1986, 12 states plus District of Columbia)	NA	NA
1979–80	USDA	Low-Income Nationwide Food Consumption Survey—Household Food Use	Low-income civilian households	NR	3002 households	NA
1979–80	USDA	Low-Income Nationwide Food Consumption Survey—Individual Intakes	Individuals in eligible households	NR	8492 persons	NA
1982–84	NCHS	Hispanic Health and Nutrition Examination Survey	Civilian, noninstitutionalized individuals, 0.5–74 yr			
			Mexican-American (AZ, CA, CO, NM, TX)	9894 persons	8554 (87%)	7462 (75%)
			Cuban (FL)	2244 persons	1766 (79%)	1357 (61%)
			Puerto Rican (CT, NJ, NY)	3786 persons	3369 (89%)	2834 (75%)
1985–86	USDA	Continuing Survey of Food Intakes by Individuals	Women and men, 19–50 yr, children, 1–5 yr	4359 households	3224 households 4618 persons	NA
1985–86	USDA	Continuing Survey of Food Intakes by Individuals in Low-Income Households	Low-income, women and men, 19–50 yr, children 1–5 yr	3711 households	3239 households 5619 persons	NA
1987	CDC	Surveillance of Severe Pediatric Undernutrition	Low-income, high-risk children, 0–5 yr	4 states	NA	
1987–88	USDA	Nationwide Food Consumption Survey–Household Food Use	Civilian households	NR		NA
1987–88	USDA	Nationwide Food Consumption Survey—Individual Intakes	Individuals residing in eligible households	NR		NA

Continued

APPENDIX C-1   Dietary and Nutrition Status Surveys and Surveillance Activities of the National Nutrition Monitoring System—*Continued*

DATE	AGENCY[a]	SURVEY	TARGET U.S. POPULATION	SAMPLE SELECTED	NUMBER INTERVIEWED (RESPONSE RATE)	NUMBER EXAMINED (RESPONSE RATE)
1988–94	NCHS	Third National Health and Nutrition Examination Survey	Civilian, noninstitutionalized individuals, 2 mo+	~40,000 persons		
1989–96	USDA	Continuing Survey of Food Intakes by Individuals	Individuals of all ages residing in eligible households			
			All income	1500 each year		
			Low income	750 each year		

[a]USDA, U.S. Department of Agriculture; DHEW, Department of Health, Education and Welfare; NCHS, National Center for Health Statistics; CDC, Centers for Disease Control and Prevention.
[b]Not applicable.
[c]Not reported.

Source: Reprinted with permission from *Present Knowledge in Nutrition,* 6th ed., International Life Sciences Institute.

APPENDIX
C-2

Specialized Activities Contributing to the National Nutrition Monitoring System

DATE	AGENCY[a]	SURVEY	TARGET U.S. POPULATION	SAMPLE INTERVIEWED	OBJECTIVE
1957–annual	NCHS	National Health Interview Survey	Civilian, noninstitutionalized individuals	~50,000 households	To collect data on personal and demographic features, incidence of acute illness and injuries, prevalence of chronic conditions and impairments, and utilization of health resources and other current health issues
1984	NCHS	Supplemental topics: Aging	Persons, 55+ yr	16,148 persons	To assess health status and care of elderly people
1985	NCHS	Health Promotion/Disease Prevention	Persons, 18+ yr	33,630 persons	To measure progress toward 1990 Health Objectives for the Nation
1986	NCHS	Vitamin/Mineral Supplements	Children, 2–6 yr Persons, 18+ yr	1877 children 1775 persons	To determine supplement usage and intake levels
1987	NCHS	Cancer Epidemiology and Control	Persons 18+ yr	~45,000 persons	To assess cancer risk factors
1961–annual	FDA	Total Diet Study	Specific age-sex groups	NA[b]	To assess levels of a variety of nutritional components and contaminants in food supply and representative diets of target population
1980	FDA	Vitamin/Mineral Supplement Intake Survey	Civilian, noninstitutionalized persons, 16+ yr	2991 persons	To assess nutrient intakes from supplements and to examine characteristics of supplement users
1981–83, 1984–continuous	CDC	Behavioral Risk Factor Surveillance System	Persons, 18+ yr, residing in participation states in households with telephones	23,113 persons (30,730 persons in 1986)	To assess prevalence of personal health practices related to leading causes of death
1982–84, 1986	NCHS	NHANES I Epidemiologic Followup Study	Persons examined in NHANES I, 25–75 yr at baseline	12,220 persons (1982)	To examine relationship of baseline clinical, nutritional, and behavioral factors assessed in NHANES I to subsequent morbidity and mortality
1982, 1984, 1986, 1988	FDA	Health and Diet Study	Civilian, noninstitutionalized persons, 18+ yr	4000 persons response rate of 70–75%	To assess public knowledge, attitudes, and practices about diet and health and public's use of information on food labels
1988–90	NCHS	National Maternal and Infant Health Survey	Reproductive-age women	20,000 vital records, 60,000 persons linked with sampled vital records	To examine factors associated with low birth weight and fetal and infant deaths

[a]NCHS, National Center for Health Statistics; CDC, Centers for Disease Control and Prevention; FDA, Food and Drug Administration.
[b]Not applicable.

Source: Reprinted with permission from *Present Knowledge in Nutrition*, 6th ed., International Life Sciences Institute.

APPENDIX
C-3

Data Elements of the 1987 Nationwide Food Consumption Survey

Household Component: In this part of the survey, questions appear on the screen of a laptop computer, the interviewer asks the question, and enters the response directly into the computer.

Household composition and meals
Sex, age of each member
Pregnancy/lactation status
For each person, number of morning, noon and evening meals last week:
◆ From home food supplies
◆ Bought and eaten away from home
◆ Free as guest or in payment
Expense for food bought and eaten away from home by members
Number of meals and snacks served to guests and employees last week

Household food use during past week (Food is reported in the form as it is purchased or brought into household from garden, restaurant, or other place, with the quantity used during the week. Food used includes food that gets eaten or is carried in packed lunches, picnics, etc.; leftovers fed to pets, and food thrown away for any reason.):
◆ Quantity of each food used by household
◆ Source of food—purchased, home-produced, or received as gift or pay
◆ Unit of purchase and price of each purchased food
◆ Source of drinking water

Food assistance program participation
WIC
School lunch and breakfast
Food stamps
Direct distribution of cheese and butter

Household characteristics
Race
Ethnicity
Income last month
Income last year
Cash assets
Size of household

Food shopping practices
Education of male and female heads
Age of male and female heads
Employment of male and female heads
Description of dwelling
Presence of selected kitchen equipment

Continued

APPENDIX
C-3

Data Elements of the 1987 Nationwide Food Consumption Survey—
Continued

Individual Component: Interviewer asks for each individual to recall the kinds and quantities of each food eaten at home and away on the full day before the interview and enters the information on the form. Then each individual is asked to record food eaten on the day of and following the interview on forms left by the interviewer. Interviewer returns after 2 days to review and collect records.

Food intake: For each food eaten on each of 3 days
Time eaten
Name of eating occasion—breakfast, lunch, snack, etc.
With whom eaten—alone, other household members, nonhousehold members, both member and nonmembers
Description of food—descriptors as indicated in easy-to-use instruction book
Quantity consumed. Measuring utensils are provided to help estimate quantities
Food sources—home supplies, carried out in packed lunch, picnic, etc., obtained and eaten away
If eaten away, type of place—restaurant, cafeteria, fast food, school, someone's house, etc.
Identify any food eaten at home that was from fast-food place or meals on wheels.
For food preparer only, was salt or fat used in preparation? If fat was used, what type?
Quantity of water

Related elements

About diet—
Was intake typical?
If not, why?
Healthfulness of diet (self-evaluation)
Was salt added at table?
On special diet?
Vegetarian?
Supplement use: How often and type?
Frequency of consumption of calcium-rich foods
Was alcoholic beverage consumption typical?

About individual—
Height and weight (self-reported)
Health status (self-evaluation)
Disability, handicap
Diagnosed disease
Problem chewing food. Why?
Leisure physical activity
Smoking

Source: Reprinted with permission from B. B. Peterkin, R. L. Rizek, and K. S. Tippett, Nationwide Food Consumption Survey, 1987, *Nutrition Today* (January/February 1988): 22. © Williams & Wilkins.

APPENDIX C-4

Sources of Data on Nutrients and Other Food Constituents in Food Consumption Surveys

NUTRIENT OR FOOD CONSTITUENT[a]	NATIONAL FOOD SUPPLY	NATIONWIDE FOOD CONSUMPTION SURVEY			NHANES		TOTAL DIET STUDY	FOOD COMPOSI- TION
		Household	Individual	CSFII[b]	I	II		
Water . . .	—	—	—	Yes	—	—	—	Yes
Energy (kcal) . . .	Yes	Yes	Yes	Yes	Yes	Yes	—	Yes
Protein:								
Total . . .	Yes	Yes	Yes	Yes	Yes	Yes	—	Yes
Amino acids . . .	—	—	—	—	—	—	—	([c])
Carbohydrate:								
Total . . .	Yes	Yes	Yes	Yes	—	Yes	—	Yes
Sugars . . .	Yes	—	([d])	—	—	—	—	—
Lipids:								
Total fat . . .	Yes	Yes	Yes	Yes	Yes	Yes	—	Yes
Saturated fat . . .	Yes	—	—	Yes	Yes	Yes	—	([c])
Oleic acid . . .	Yes	—	—	—	Yes	Yes	—	([c])
Total monounsaturated . . .	—	—	—	Yes	—	—	—	([c])
Linoleic acid . . .	Yes	—	—	—	Yes	Yes	—	([c])
Total polyunsaturated . . .	—	—	—	Yes	—	—	—	([c])
Cholesterol . . .	Yes	—	([d])	Yes	Yes	Yes	—	([c])
Vitamins:								
A (IU)[e] . . .	Yes	Yes	Yes	Yes	Yes	Yes	—	Yes
A (RE)[e] . . .	—	—	—	Yes	—	—	—	([c])
Carotene . . .	—	—	—	Yes	—	—	—	—
E . . .	—	—	—	Yes	—	—	—	([c])
Thiamin (B_1) . . .	Yes	Yes	Yes	Yes	Yes	Yes	—	Yes
Riboflavin (B_2) . . .	Yes	Yes	Yes	Yes	Yes	Yes	—	Yes
Niacin (preformed) . . .	Yes	Yes	Yes	Yes	Yes	Yes	—	Yes
Pantothenic acid . . .	([d])	—	—	—	—	—	—	([c])
B_6 . . .	Yes	Yes	Yes	Yes	—	—	—	Yes

Continued

APPENDIX C-4

Sources of Data on Nutrients and Other Food Constituents in Food Consumption Surveys—Continued

NUTRIENT OR FOOD CONSTITUENT[a]	NATIONAL FOOD SUPPLY	NATIONWIDE FOOD CONSUMPTION SURVEY			NHANES		TOTAL DIET STUDY	FOOD COMPOSI-TION
		Household	Individual	CSFII[b]	I	II		
Folate . . .	(d) ·	—	—	Yes	—	—	—	(c)
B$_{12}$ . . .	Yes	Yes	Yes	Yes	—	—	—	Yes
C . . .	Yes	Yes	Yes	Yes	Yes	Yes	—	Yes
Minerals:								
Calcium . . .	Yes	Yes	Yes	Yes	Yes	Yes	Yes	Yes
Phosphorus . . .	Yes	Yes	Yes	Yes	—	Yes	Yes	Yes
Magnesium . . .	Yes	Yes	Yes	Yes	Yes	Yes	Yes	Yes
Iron . . .	—	—	—	—	—	—	Yes	—
Iodine . . .	—	—	—	—	—	—	Yes	—
Sodium . . .	Yes	—	Yes	Yes	—	Yes	Yes	Yes
Potassium . . .	Yes	—	—	Yes	—	Yes	Yes	Yes
Copper . . .	—	—	—	Yes	—	—	Yes	(c)
Zinc . . .	Yes	—	—	Yes	—	—	Yes	(c)
Manganese . . .	—	—	—	—	—	—	Yes	(c)
Selenium . . .	—	—	—	—	—	—	Yes	—
Chromium . . .	—	—	—	—	—	—	Yes	—
Fiber:								
Crude . . .	Yes	—	—	—	—	—	—	Yes
Dietary . . .	—	—	—	Yes	—	—	—	Yes
Alcoholic beverages . . .	—	Yes	Yes	Yes	—	Yes	Yes	Yes

[a]Alcoholic beverages are included.

[b]Continuing Survey of Food Intakes by Individuals.

[c]Nutrient data available at the completion of revision of U.S. Department of Agriculture's Handbook No. 8.

[d]From Food Supply and Nationwide Food Consumption Survey data supplied by Dr. Susan Welsh, Human Nutrition Information Service, U.S. Department of Agriculture.

[e]IU = International Units, RE = Retinol Equivalents

Source: C. E. Woteki, Appendix VIII: Measuring dietary patterns in surveys, in U.S. Department of Health and Human Services, *Vital and Health Statistics: Dietary Methodology for the Third National Health and Nutrition Examination Survey* (Washington, D.C.: U.S. Government Printing Office, 1992), p. 103.

Appendix D

CANADIAN DIETARY GUIDELINES AND RECOMMENDATIONS
APPENDIX D-1 CANADA'S GUIDELINES FOR HEALTHY EATING

Canada's Guidelines for Healthy Eating were developed by the Communications/Implementation Committee as the key nutrition messages to be communicated to healthy Canadians over two years of age. The guidelines encourage people to:

- Enjoy a variety of foods.
- Emphasize cereals, breads, other grain products, vegetables, and fruits.
- Choose lower-fat dairy products, leaner meats, and foods prepared with little or no fat.
- Achieve and maintain a healthy body weight by enjoying regular physical activity and healthy eating.
- Limit salt, alcohol, and caffeine.

APPENDIX D-2 CANADA'S RECOMMENDED NUTRIENT INTAKES (RNI)

Like the RDA on the inside front cover pages, the Recommended Nutrient Intakes (RNI) for Canadians make recommendations for intakes of vitamins, minerals, protein, and energy. The RNI are presented in Tables D2-1 and D2-2.

TABLE D2-1

Recommended Nutrient Intakes for Canadians, 1990

AGE	SEX	WEIGHT (kg)	PROTEIN (g/day)[a]	FAT-SOLUBLE VITAMINS Vitamin A (RE/day)[b]	Vitamin D (µg/day)[c]	Vitamin E (mg/day)[d]
Infants (months)						
0–4	Both	6	12[f]	400	10	3
5–12	Both	9	12	400	10	3
Children and adults (years)						
1	Both	11	13	400	10	3
2–3	Both	14	16	400	5	4
4–6	Both	18	19	500	5	5
7–9	M	25	26	700	2.5	7
	F	25	26	700	2.5	6
10–12	M	34	34	800	2.5	8
	F	36	36	800	5	7
13–15	M	50	49	900	5	9
	F	48	46	800	5	7
16–18	M	62	58	1000	5	10
	F	53	47	800	2.5	7
19–24	M	71	61	1000	2.5	10
	F	58	50	800	2.5	7
25–49	M	74	64	1000	2.5	9
	F	59	51	800	2.5	6
50–74	M	73	63	1000	5	7
	F	63	54	800	5	6
75+	M	69	59	1000	5	6
	F	64	55	800	5	5
Pregnancy (additional amount needed)						
1st trimester			5	0	2.5	2
2nd trimester			20	0	2.5	2
3rd trimester			24	0	2.5	2
Lactation (additional amount needed)			22	400	2.5	3

Note: Recommended intakes of energy and certain nutrients are not listed in this table because of the nature of the variables upon which they are based. The figures for energy are estimates of average requirements for expected patterns of activity. For nutrients not shown, the following amounts are recommended based on at least 2000 kcalories per day and body weights as given: thiamin, 0.4 milligrams per 1000 kcalories (0.48 milligrams/5000 kilojoules); riboflavin, 0.5 milligrams per 1000 kcalories (0.6 milligrams/5000 kilojoules); niacin, 7.2 niacin equivalents per 1000 kcalories (8.6 niacin equivalents/5000 kilojoules); vitamin B$_6$, 15 micrograms, as pyridoxine, per gram of protein. Recommended intakes during periods of growth are taken as appropriate for individuals representative of the midpoint in each age group. All recommended intakes are designed to cover individual variations in essentially all of a healthy population subsisting upon a variety of common foods available in Canada.

Continued

TABLE D2-1 — Recommended Nutrient Intakes for Canadians, 1990—*Continued*

WATER-SOLUBLE VITAMINS			MINERALS					
Vitamin C (mg/day)[e]	Folate (µg/day)	Vitamin B$_{12}$ (µg/day)	Calcium (mg/day)	Phosphorus (mg/day)	Magnesium (mg/day)	Iron (mg/day)	Iodine (µg/day)	Zinc (mg/day)
20	25	0.3	250	150	20	0.3[g]	30	2[h]
20	40	0.4	400	200	32	7	40	3
20	40	0.5	500	300	40	6	55	4
20	50	0.6	550	350	50	6	65	4
25	70	0.8	600	400	65	8	85	5
25	90	1.0	700	500	100	8	110	7
25	90	1.0	700	500	100	8	95	7
25	120	1.0	900	700	130	8	125	9
25	130	1.0	1100	800	135	8	110	9
30	175	1.0	1100	900	185	10	160	12
30	170	1.0	1000	850	180	13	160	9
40	220	1.0	900	1000	230	10	160	12
30	190	1.0	700	850	200	12	160	9
40	220	1.0	800	1000	240	9	160	12
30	180	1.0	700	850	200	13	160	9
40	230	1.0	800	1000	250	9	160	12
30	185	1.0	700	850	200	13[i]	160	9
40	230	1.0	800	1000	250	9	160	12
30	195	1.0	800	850	210	8	160	9
40	215	1.0	800	1000	230	9	160	12
30	200	1.0	800	850	210	8	160	9
0	200	0.2	500	200	15	0	25	6
10	200	0.2	500	200	45	5	25	6
10	200	0.2	500	200	45	10	25	6
25	100	0.2	500	200	65	0	50	6

[a]The primary units are expressed per kilogram of body weight. The figures shown here are examples.

[b]One retinol equivalent (RE) corresponds to the biological activity of 1 microgram of retinol, 6 micrograms of beta-carotene, or 12 micrograms of other carotenes.

[c]Expressed as cholecalciferol or ergocalciferol.

[d]Expressed as δ-α-tocopherol equivalents, relative to which β - and γ-tocopherol and α-tocotrienol have activities of 0.5, 0.1, and 0.3, respectively.

[e]Cigarette smokers should increase intake by 50 percent.

[f]The assumption is made that the protein is from breast milk or is of the same biological value as that of breast milk, and that between 3 and 9 months, adjustment for the quality of the protein is made.

[g]Based on the assumption that breast milk is the source of iron.

[h]Based on the assumption that breast milk is the source of zinc.

[i]After menopause, the recommended intake is 8 milligrams per day.

Source: Health and Welfare Canada, *Nutrition Recommendations: The Report of the Scientific Review Committee* (Ottawa: Canadian Government Publishing Centre, 1990), Table 20, p. 204. Used with permission.

TABLE D2-2   Average Energy Requirements for Canadians

Age	Sex	AVERAGE HEIGHT (cm)	AVERAGE WEIGHT (kg)	REQUIREMENTS[a] (kcal/kg)[b]	(MJ/kg)[b]	(kcal/day)	(MJ/day)	(kcal/cm)	(MJ/cm)
Infants (months)									
0–2	Both	55	4.5	120–100	0.50–0.42	500	2.0	9	0.04
3–5	Both	63	7.0	100–95	0.42–0.40	700	2.8	11	0.05
6–8	Both	69	8.5	95–97	0.40–0.41	800	3.4	11.5	0.05
9–11	Both	73	9.5	97–99	0.41	950	3.8	12.5	0.05
Children and adults (years)									
1	Both	82	11	101	0.42	1100	4.8	13.5	0.06
2–3	Both	95	14	94	0.39	1300	5.6	13.5	0.06
4–6	Both	107	18	100	0.42	1800	7.6	17	0.07
7–9	M	126	25	88	0.37	2200	9.2	17.5	0.07
	F	125	25	76	0.32	1900	8.0	15	0.06
10–12	M	141	34	73	0.30	2500	10.4	17.5	0.07
	F	143	36	61	0.25	2200	9.2	15.5	0.06
13–15	M	159	50	57	0.24	2800	12.0	17.5	0.07
	F	157	48	46	0.19	2200	9.2	14	0.06
16–18	M	172	62	51	0.21	3200	13.2	18.5	0.08
	F	160	53	40	0.17	2100	8.8	13	0.05
19–24	M	175	71	42	0.18	3000	12.6		
	F	160	58	36	0.15	2100	8.8		
25–49	M	172	74	36	0.15	2700	11.3		
	F	160	59	32	0.13	1900	8.0		
50–74	M	170	73	31	0.13	2300	9.7		
	F	158	63	29	0.12	1800	7.6		
75+	M	168	69	29	0.12	2000	8.4		
	F	155	64	23	0.10	1500	6.3		

[a]Requirements can be expected to vary within a range of ±30 percent.
[b]First and last figures are averages at the beginning and end of the three-month period.

Source: Health and Welfare Canada, *Nutrition Recommendations: The Report of the Scientific Review Committee* (Ottawa: Canadian Government Publishing Centre, 1990), Tables 5 and 6, pp. 25, 27. Used with permission.

APPENDIX D-3 CANADA'S FOOD GUIDE TO HEALTHY EATING

The 1992 *Canada's Food Guide to Healthy Eating* gives consumers detailed information for selecting foods to meet *Canada's Guidelines for Healthy Eating* (1990). The *Food Guide* was designed to meet the nutritional needs of all Canadians four years of age and older and takes a total diet approach, rather than emphasizing a single food, meal, or day's meals and snacks.

The rainbow side of the Food Guide shows the four food groups with their revised names and pictorial examples of foods in each group. Key statements direct consumers about selecting foods generally from all the groups, and more specifically within each group. The bar side shows the number of servings recommended for each group, using a range of servings instead of a single minimum number. Other notable changes include the number of servings for some food groups and the size of servings for some foods.

Healthy Canada

Health and Welfare Canada

Santé et Bien-être social Canada

CANADA'S

Food Guide

TO HEALTHY EATING

Enjoy a variety of foods from each group every day.

Choose lower-fat foods more often.

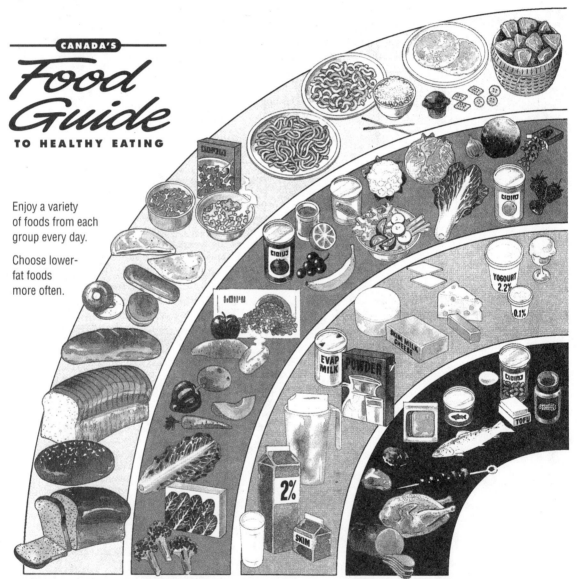

Grain Products
Choose whole grain and enriched products more often.

Vegetables & Fruit
Choose dark green and orange vegetables and orange fruit more often.

Milk Products
Choose lower-fat milk products more often.

Meat & Alternatives
Choose leaner meats, poultry and fish, as well as dried peas, beans and lentils more often.

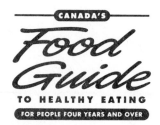

Different People Need Different Amounts of Food

The amount of food you need every day from the 4 food groups and other foods depends on your age, body size, activity level, whether you are male or female and if you are pregnant or breast-feeding. That's why the Food Guide gives a lower and higher number of servings for each food group. For example, young children can choose the lower number of servings, while male teenagers can go to the higher number. Most other people can choose servings somewhere in between.

Grain Products
5–12
SERVINGS PER DAY

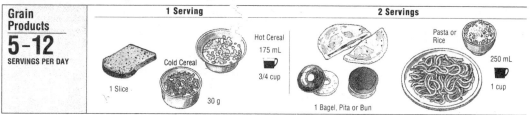

1 Serving

1 Slice
Cold Cereal
30 g
Hot Cereal
175 mL
3/4 cup

2 Servings

Pasta or Rice
250 mL
1 cup
1 Bagel, Pita or Bun

Vegetables & Fruit
5–10
SERVINGS PER DAY

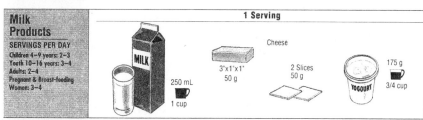

1 Serving

1 Medium Size Vegetable or Fruit

Fresh, Frozen or Canned Vegetables or Fruit
125 mL
1/2 cup

Salad
250 mL
1 cup

Juice
125 mL
1/2 cup

Milk Products
SERVINGS PER DAY
Children 4–9 years: 2–3
Youth 10–16 years: 3–4
Adults: 2–4
Pregnant & Breast-feeding Women: 3–4

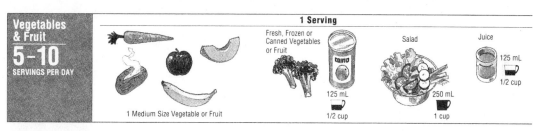

1 Serving

MILK
250 mL
1 cup

Cheese
3"x1"x1"
50 g
2 Slices
50 g

175 g
3/4 cup

Other Foods

Taste and enjoyment can also come from other foods and beverages that are not part of the 4 food groups. Some of these foods are higher in fat or Calories, so use these foods in moderation.

Meat & Alternatives
2–3
SERVINGS PER DAY

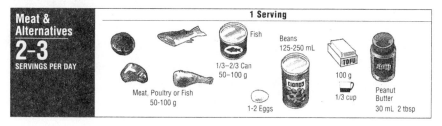

1 Serving

Meat, Poultry or Fish
50-100 g

Fish
1/3–2/3 Can
50–100 g

1-2 Eggs

Beans
125-250 mL

TOFU
100 g
1/3 cup

Peanut Butter
30 mL 2 tbsp

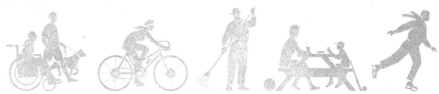

Enjoy eating well, being active and feeling good about yourself. That's VITALIT

Appendix E

NUTRITION ASSESSMENT AND SCREENING
APPENDIX E-I DIETARY ASSESSMENT

_____ **TABLE** _____ **Form for Collecting Historical Data**
EI-I

Name _____ Date _____
Address _____ Date of last medical checkup _____
_____ Age _____ Sex _____
_____ Height _____ Weight _____
Phone _____ Usual weight _____
Reason for admission _____ Ideal weight _____

Health History

1. Have you been told that you have (check any that apply):
   ____ Diabetes   ____ Heart disease   ____ Ulcers
   ____ GI disorders   ____ Lung disease   ____ Cancer
   ____ High blood pressure ____ Kidney disease   ____ Other
   ____ Hardening of arteries ____ Liver disease
2. Do you have complaints about any of the following:
   ____ Lack of appetite   ____ Diarrhea   ____ Nausea
   ____ Difficulty chewing or swallowing ____ Indigestion ____ Vomiting
   ____ Constipation   ____ Fever   ____ Other
3. For females:
   Are you pregnant? _____ How many months? _____
   How many pregnancies have you carried to term? _____
   When was your last child born? _____
   Are your menstrual periods normal? ____ If not, please explain: _____

Socioeconomic History

1. Last grade of school completed _____ Still in school? _____
2. Are you employed? _____ Occupation _____
3. Does someone else live with you? _____ Who? _____
4. Do you use tobacco in any way? _____ How much? _____
5. Where do you eat most of your meals? _____
6. Do you have a refrigerator? _____ Stove? _____
7. How often do you shop for food? _____

Drug History

1. Do you take medication, either prescribed by a doctor or over-the-counter?

Name of drug	Reason for taking	Dose	Frequency	Duration of intake
_____	_____	_____	_____	_____
_____	_____	_____	_____	_____
_____	_____	_____	_____	_____

2. Have you noticed any side effects from taking these medications? ____ If so, please explain: _____
3. Do you take vitamins or any kind of supplements? ____ Which ones? _____
   How often? _____ For what reason? _____

Continued

TABLE EI-I
Form for Collecting Historical Data—*Continued*

Diet History

1. Have you recently lost or gained more than 10 lb? _____ If yes, explain the surrounding circumstances (including associated illness, dietary changes, and time frame): _____
2. Do you eat at regular times each day? _____ How many times per day? _____
3. Do you usually eat snacks? _____ When? _____
4. What foods do you particularly like? _____
5. Are there foods you don't eat for other reasons? _____
6. Do you have difficulty eating? _____
7. How would you describe your feelings about food? _____
8. How do your eating habits change when you are emotionally upset? _____
9. Are you, or any member of your family, on a special diet? _____ If yes, who and what kind? _____
10. Do you drink alcohol? _____ How much? _____ How often? _____
11. How would you describe your exercise habits? _____ Type of exercise _____
    Intensity _____ Duration _____ Frequency _____
12. Are there any other facts about your lifestyle that you think might be related to your nutritional health? _____
    Explain _____

Note: Use the appropriate form to record food intake data.

Source: Reprinted by permission from *Understanding Nutrition,* 6th ed., by E. N. Whitney and S. R. Rolfes. Copyright © 1993 by West Publishing Company. All rights reserved.

TABLE EI-2
Food Intake Form for a 24-Hour Recall or Usual Intake Pattern

Source: Reprinted by permission from *Understanding Nutrition,* 6th ed., by E. N. Whitney and S. R. Rolfes. Copyright © 1993 by West Publishing Company. All rights reserved.

Name and address _____ Date _____

Did you take a vitamin mineral supplement? _____
If yes, what kind? _____ Dose _____
Please record the amount and type of foods and beverages consumed today.
[Or: Please record the amount and type of foods and beverages you typically consume each day.]

Food	Amount (c, tbsp, or piece)	Description (how cooked, how served)

| Name _____ Date _____ | | | | | |
Time	Place	With Whom	Emotional State	Hungry or Not Hungry	Food Eaten (Amount)

TABLE

E1-3

Food Diary Form

Source: Reprinted by permission from *Understanding Nutrition*, 6th ed., by E. N. Whitney and S. R. Rolfes. Copyright © 1993 by West Publishing Company. All rights reserved.

TABLE
EI-4

Food Frequency Checklist

The following information will help us to understand your regular eating habits so that we may offer you the best service possible. If you have any doubt about some items, be sure to underestimate the "goodness" of your habits rather than to overestimate.

1. How many times *per week* do you eat the following foods? Circle the appropriate number:

PER WEEK

Poultry	0	<1	1	2	3	4	5	6	7	8	9	>9 ____
Fish	0	<1	1	2	3	4	5	6	7	8	9	>9 ____
Hot dogs	0	<1	1	2	3	4	5	6	7	8	9	>9 ____
Bacon	0	<1	1	2	3	4	5	6	7	8	9	>9 ____
Lunch meat	0	<1	1	2	3	4	5	6	7	8	9	>9 ____
Sausage	0	<1	1	2	3	4	5	6	7	8	9	>9 ____
Pork or ham	0	<1	1	2	3	4	5	6	7	8	9	>9 ____
Salt pork	0	<1	1	2	3	4	5	6	7	8	9	>9 ____
Liver	0	<1	1	2	3	4	5	6	7	8	9	>9 ____
Beef or veal	0	<1	1	2	3	4	5	6	7	8	9	>9 ____
Other meats (which?) _____	0	<1	1	2	3	4	5	6	7	8	9	>9 ____
Cooked dry beans or peas	0	<1	1	2	3	4	5	6	7	8	9	>9 ____
Eggs	0	<1	1	2	3	4	5	6	7	8	9	>9 ____
Fast foods	0	<1	1	2	3	4	5	6	7	8	9	>9 ____

2. How many times *per day* do you eat the following foods? Circle the appropriate number:

PER DAY

Bread, toast, rolls, muffins	0	<1	1	2	3	4	5	6	7	8	9	>9 ____
Milk (including on cereal)	0	<1	1	2	3	4	5	6	7	8	9	>9 ____
Yogurt or tofu	0	<1	1	2	3	4	5	6	7	8	9	>9 ____
Cheese or cheese dishes	0	<1	1	2	3	4	5	6	7	8	9	>9 ____
Sugar, jam, jelly, syrup, honey	0	<1	1	2	3	4	5	6	7	8	9	>9 ____
Butter or margarine	0	<1	1	2	3	4	5	6	7	8	9	>9 ____

3. How many times *per week* do you eat the following foods? Circle the appropriate number:

PER WEEK

Fruits or fruit juices	0	<1	1	2	3	4	5	6	7	8	9	>9 ____
Vegetables other than potatoes	0	<1	1	2	3	4	5	6	7	8	9	>9 ____
Potatoes and other starchy vegetables	0	<1	1	2	3	4	5	6	7	8	9	>9 ____
Salads or raw vegetables	0	<1	1	2	3	4	5	6	7	8	9	>9 ____

Continued

Cereal (which kind?) _____ ....0 <1 1 2 3 4 5 6 7 8 9 >9 ____
Pancakes or waffles ....0 <1 1 2 3 4 5 6 7 8 9 >9 ____
Rice or other cooked grains ....0 <1 1 2 3 4 5 6 7 8 9 >9 ____
Noodles (macaroni, spaghetti) ....0 <1 1 2 3 4 5 6 7 8 9 >9 ____
Crackers or pretzels ....0 <1 1 2 3 4 5 6 7 8 9 >9 ____
Sweet rolls or doughnuts ....0 <1 1 2 3 4 5 6 7 8 9 >9 ____
Peanut butter or nuts ....0 <1 1 2 3 4 5 6 7 8 9 >9 ____
Milk or milk products ....0 <1 1 2 3 4 5 6 7 8 9 >9 ____
TV dinners, pot pies,
   other prepared meals ....0 <1 1 2 3 4 5 6 7 8 9 >9 ____
Sweet bakery goods (cake, cookies) ....0 <1 1 2 3 4 5 6 7 8 9 >9 ____
Snack foods (potato or corn chips) ....0 <1 1 2 3 4 5 6 7 8 9 >9 ____
Candy ....0 <1 1 2 3 4 5 6 7 8 9 >9 ____
Soft drinks (which?) _____ ....0 <1 1 2 3 4 5 6 7 8 9 >9 ____
Coffee or tea ....0 <1 1 2 3 4 5 6 7 8 9 >9 ____
Frozen sweets (which?) _____ ....0 <1 1 2 3 4 5 6 7 8 9 >9 ____
Instant meals such as breakfast bars or diet
   meal beverages (which?) _____ ....0 <1 1 2 3 4 5 6 7 8 9 >9 ____
Wine ....0 <1 1 2 3 4 5 6 7 8 9 >9 ____
Beer ....0 <1 1 2 3 4 5 6 7 8 9 >9 ____
Whiskey, vodka, rum, etc. ....0 <1 1 2 3 4 5 6 7 8 9 >9 ____

4. What specific kinds of the following foods do you eat the most often?
   Include the name of the food; whether it is fresh, canned, or frozen; and how it is
   prepared.

Fruits and fruit juices _____
Vegetables _____
Milk and milk products _____
Meats and meat alternates _____
Breads and cereals _____
Desserts _____
Snack foods _____

5. Please list the names of any liquid, powder, or pill forms of vitamin or mineral
   products you take, and state how often you take them. Please list also any diet supplement you use (such as protein milk shakes or brewer's yeast), how much you
   use, and how often you use it.

_____

6. Is there anything else we should know about your food/nutrient intake?

_____

TABLE

E1-4

**Food Frequency
Checklist—Continued**

APPENDIX E-2 ANTHROPOMETRIC ASSESSMENT

TABLE E2-1   1983 Metropolitan Height and Weight Tables

| MEN | | | | | WOMEN | | | | |
| Height | | Frame | | | Height | | Frame | | |
Feet	Inches	Small	Medium	Large	Feet	Inches	Small	Medium	Large
5	2	128–134	131–141	138–150	4	10	102–111	109–121	118–131
5	3	130–136	133–143	140–153	4	11	103–113	111–123	120–134
5	4	132–138	135–145	142–156	5	0	104–115	113–126	122–137
5	5	134–140	137–148	144–160	5	1	106–118	115–129	125–140
5	6	136–142	139–151	146–164	5	2	108–121	118–132	128–143
5	7	138–145	142–154	149–168	5	3	111–124	121–135	131–147
5	8	140–148	145–157	152–172	5	4	114–127	124–138	134–151
5	9	142–151	148–160	155–176	5	5	117–130	127–141	137–155
5	10	144–154	151–163	158–180	5	6	120–133	130–144	140–159
5	11	146–157	154–166	161–184	5	7	123–136	133–147	143–163
6	0	149–160	157–170	164–188	5	8	126–139	136–150	146–167
6	1	152–164	160–174	168–192	5	9	129–142	139–153	149–170
6	2	155–168	164–178	172–197	5	10	132–145	142–156	152–173
6	3	158–172	167–182	176–202	5	11	135–148	145–159	155–176
6	4	162–176	171–187	181–207	6	0	138–151	148–162	158–179

Note: To use the table, add an inch to your barefoot height (you are assumed to be wearing shoes with 1-inch heels), and adjust for clothing (the tables assume 5 pounds for clothes for men and 3 pounds for women). Weights are at age 25 to 29 based on lowest mortality, in pounds according to frame size.

Source: Reproduced courtesy of Metropolitan Life Insurance Company. Source of basic data: 1979 Build Study, Society of Actuaries and Association of Life Insurance Medical Directors of America, 1980.

TABLE E2-2   How to Determine Body Frame by Elbow Breadth

To make a simple approximation of frame size, do the following: Extend the arm, and bend the forearm upward at a 90° angle. Keep the fingers straight, and turn the inside of the wrist away from the body. Place the thumb and index finger on the two prominent bones on either side of the elbow. Measure the space between the fingers against a ruler or a tape measure.[a] Compare the measurements with the following standards.

These standards represent the elbow measurements for medium-framed men and women of various heights. Measurements smaller than those listed indicate a small frame, and larger measurements indicate a large frame.

| MEN | | WOMEN | |
Height in 1-Inch Heels	Elbow Breadth	Height in 1-Inch Heels	Elbow Breadth
5 ft 2 in to 5 ft 3 in	$2^1/_2$ to $2^7/_8$	4 ft 10 in to 4 ft 11 in	$2^1/_4$ to $2^1/_2$ in
5 ft 4 in to 5 ft 7 in	$2^5/_8$ to $2^7/_8$ in	5 ft 0 in to 5 ft 3 in	$2^1/_4$ to $2^1/_2$ in
5 ft 8 in to 5 ft 11 in	$2^3/_4$ to 3 in	5 ft 4 in to 5 ft 7 in	$2^3/_8$ to $2^5/_8$ in
6 ft 0 in to 6 ft 3 in	$2^3/_4$ to $3^1/_8$ in	5 ft 8 in to 5 ft 11 in	$2^3/_8$ to $2^5/_8$ in
6 ft 4 in and over	$2^7/_8$ to $3^1/_4$ in	6 ft 0 and over	$2^1/_2$ to $2^3/_4$ in

[a] For the most accurate measurement, measure elbow breadth with a caliper.

Source: Metropolitan Life Insurance Company.

FRAME SIZE	MALE r VALUES	FEMALE r VALUES
Small	> 10.4	> 11.0
Medium	9.6–10.4	10.1–11.0
Large	< 9.6	< 10.1

$^a r = \dfrac{\text{height (cm)}}{\text{wrist circumference (cm)}}$. The wrist is measured where it bends (distal to the styloid process), on the right arm (see the accompanying figure).

TABLE

E2-3

Frame Size from Height-Wrist Circumference Ratios (r)^a

Source: Reprinted by permission from *Understanding Nutrition*, 6th ed., by E. N. Whitney and S. R. Rolfes. Copyright © 1993 by West Publishing Company. All rights reserved.

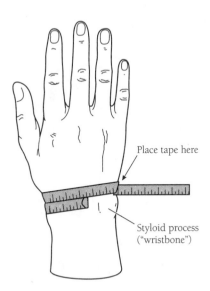

Place tape here

Styloid process ("wristbone")

Wrist Circumference

The wrist circumference is measured just above the wrist bone.

TABLE E2-4

Percentiles for Triceps Fatfold (in Millimeters) for Whites, United States

	MALE					FEMALE				
AGE	5th	25th	50th	75th	95th	5th	25th	50th	75th	95th
1–1.9	6	8	10	12	16	6	8	10	12	16
2–2.9	6	8	10	12	15	6	9	10	12	16
3–3.9	6	8	10	11	15	7	9	11	12	15
4–4.9	6	8	9	11	14	7	8	10	12	16
5–5.9	6	8	9	11	15	6	8	10	12	18
6–6.9	5	7	8	10	16	6	8	10	12	16
7–7.9	5	7	9	12	17	6	9	11	13	18
8–8.9	5	7	8	10	16	6	9	12	15	24
9–9.9	6	7	10	13	18	8	10	13	16	22
10–10.9	6	8	10	14	21	7	10	12	17	27
11–11.9	6	8	11	16	24	7	10	13	18	28
12–12.9	6	8	11	14	28	8	11	14	18	27
13–13.9	5	7	10	14	26	8	12	15	21	30
14–14.9	4	7	9	14	24	9	13	16	21	28
15–15.9	4	6	8	11	24	8	12	17	21	32
16–16.9	4	6	8	12	22	10	15	18	22	31
17–17.9	5	6	8	12	19	10	13	19	24	37
18–18.9	4	6	9	13	24	10	15	18	22	30
19–24.9	4	7	10	15	22	10	14	18	24	34
25–34.9	5	8	12	16	24	10	16	21	27	37
35–44.9	5	8	12	16	23	12	18	23	29	38
45–54.9	6	8	12	15	25	12	20	25	30	40
55–64.9	5	8	11	14	22	12	20	25	31	38
65–74.9	4	8	11	15	22	12	18	24	29	36

Note: If measurements fall between the percentiles shown here, the percentile can be estimated from the information in this table. For example, a measurement of 7 millimeters for a 27-year-old male would be about the 20th percentile.

Source: Adapted from A. R. Frisancho, New norms of upper limb fat and muscle areas for assessment of nutritional status, *American Journal of Clinical Nutrition* 34 (1981): 2541. © 1981 American Society for Clinical Nutrition.

TABLE E2-5   Percentiles of Mid-Arm Circumference (in Centimeters) for Whites, United States

AGE	MALE					FEMALE				
	5th	25th	50th	75th	95th	5th	25th	50th	75th	95th
<1	Reliable data unavailable					Reliable data unavailable				
1–1.9	14.2	15.0	15.9	17.0	18.3	13.8	14.8	15.6	16.4	17.7
2–2.9	14.1	15.3	16.2	17.0	18.5	14.2	15.2	16.0	16.7	18.4
3–3.9	15.0	16.0	16.7	17.5	19.0	14.3	15.8	16.7	17.5	18.9
4–4.9	14.9	16.2	17.1	18.0	19.2	14.9	16.0	16.9	17.7	19.1
5–5.9	15.3	16.7	17.5	18.5	20.4	15.3	16.5	17.5	18.5	21.1
6–6.9	15.5	16.7	17.9	18.8	22.8	15.6	17.0	17.6	18.7	21.1
7–7.9	16.2	17.7	18.7	20.1	23.0	16.4	17.4	18.3	19.9	23.1
8–8.9	16.2	17.7	19.0	20.2	24.5	16.8	18.3	19.5	21.4	26.1
9–9.9	17.5	18.7	20.0	21.7	25.7	17.8	19.4	21.1	22.4	26.0
10–10.9	18.1	19.6	21.0	23.1	27.4	17.4	19.3	21.0	22.8	26.5
11–11.9	18.6	20.2	22.3	24.4	28.0	18.5	20.8	22.4	24.8	30.3
12–12.9	19.3	21.4	23.2	25.4	30.3	19.4	21.6	23.7	25.6	29.4
13–13.9	19.4	22.8	24.7	26.3	30.1	20.2	22.3	24.3	27.1	33.8
14–14.9	22.0	23.7	25.3	28.3	32.3	21.4	23.7	25.2	27.2	32.2
15–15.9	22.2	24.4	26.4	28.4	32.0	20.8	23.9	25.4	27.9	32.2
16–16.9	24.4	26.2	27.8	30.3	34.3	21.8	24.1	25.8	28.3	33.4
17–17.9	24.6	26.7	28.5	30.8	34.7	22.0	24.1	26.4	29.5	35.0
18–18.9	24.5	27.6	29.7	32.1	37.9	22.2	24.1	25.8	28.1	32.5
19–24.9	26.2	28.8	30.8	33.1	37.2	21.1	24.7	26.5	29.0	34.5
25–34.9	27.1	30.0	31.9	34.2	37.5	23.3	25.6	27.7	30.4	36.8
35–44.9	27.8	30.5	32.6	34.5	37.4	24.1	26.7	29.0	31.7	37.8
45–54.9	26.7	30.1	32.2	34.2	37.6	24.2	27.4	29.9	32.8	38.4
55–64.9	25.8	29.6	31.7	33.6	36.9	24.3	28.0	30.3	33.5	38.5
65–74.9	24.8	28.5	30.7	32.5	35.5	24.0	27.4	29.9	32.6	37.3

Source: Adapted from A. R. Frisancho, New norms of upper limb fat and muscle areas for assessment of nutritional status, *American Journal of Clinical Nutrition* 34 (1981): 2542. © 1981 American Society for Clinical Nutrition.

TABLE E2-6	Percentiles of Mid-Arm Muscle Circumference (in Centimeters) for Whites, United States

	MALE					FEMALE				
AGE	5th	25th	50th	75th	95th	5th	25th	50th	75th	95th
1–1.9	11.0	11.9	12.7	13.5	14.7	10.5	11.7	12.4	13.9	14.3
2–2.9	11.1	12.2	13.0	14.0	15.0	11.1	11.9	12.6	13.3	14.7
3–3.9	11.7	13.1	13.7	14.3	15.3	11.3	12.4	13.2	14.0	15.2
4–4.9	12.3	13.3	14.1	14.8	15.9	11.5	12.8	13.6	14.4	15.7
5–5.9	12.8	14.0	14.7	15.4	16.9	12.5	13.4	14.2	15.1	16.5
6–6.9	13.1	14.2	15.1	16.1	17.7	13.0	13.8	14.5	15.4	17.1
7–7.9	13.7	15.1	16.0	16.8	19.0	12.9	14.2	15.1	16.0	17.6
8–8.9	14.0	15.4	16.2	17.0	18.7	13.8	15.1	16.0	17.1	19.4
9–9.9	15.1	16.1	17.0	18.3	20.2	14.7	15.8	16.7	18.0	19.8
10–10.9	15.6	16.6	18.0	19.1	22.1	14.8	15.9	17.0	18.0	19.7
11–11.9	15.9	17.3	18.3	19.5	23.0	15.0	17.1	18.1	19.6	22.3
12–12.9	16.7	18.2	19.5	21.0	24.1	16.2	18.0	19.1	20.1	22.0
13–13.9	17.2	19.6	21.1	22.6	24.5	16.9	18.3	19.8	21.1	24.0
14–14.9	18.9	21.2	22.3	24.0	26.4	17.4	19.0	20.1	21.6	24.7
15–15.9	19.9	21.8	23.7	25.4	27.2	17.5	18.9	20.2	21.5	24.4
16–16.9	21.3	23.4	24.9	26.9	29.6	17.0	19.0	20.2	21.6	24.9
17–17.9	22.4	24.5	25.8	27.3	31.2	17.5	19.4	20.5	22.1	25.7
18–18.9	22.6	25.2	26.4	28.3	32.4	17.4	19.1	20.2	21.5	24.5
19–24.9	23.8	25.7	27.3	28.9	32.1	17.9	19.5	20.7	22.1	24.9
25–34.9	24.3	26.4	27.9	29.8	32.6	18.3	19.9	21.2	22.8	26.4
35–44.9	24.7	26.9	28.6	30.2	32.7	18.6	20.5	21.8	23.6	27.2
45–54.9	23.9	26.5	28.1	30.0	32.6	18.7	20.6	22.0	23.8	27.4
55–64.9	23.6	26.0	27.8	29.5	32.0	18.7	20.9	22.5	24.4	28.0
65–74.9	22.3	25.1	26.8	28.4	30.6	18.5	20.8	22.5	24.4	27.9

Source: Adapted from A. R. Frisancho, New norms of upper limb fat and muscle areas for assessment of nutritional status, *American Journal of Clinical Nutrition* 34 (1981): 2542. © 1981 American Society for Clinical Nutrition.

TABLE E2-7	Selected Distribution Statistics for Weight (in Kilograms) in Mexican-American Children and Adolescents

			PERCENTILES						
AGE (YR)	MEAN	SEM	5th	10th	25th	50th	75th	90th	95th
Males									
1.00–1.99	11.37	0.22	8.90	9.55	10.35	11.30	12.20	12.90	13.65
2.00–2.99	13.86	0.14	11.25	11.65	12.85	14.05	14.90	15.85	16.25
3.00–3.99	15.71	0.22	11.95	12.80	14.35	15.40	16.70	18.65	20.15
4.00–4.99	17.39	0.14	14.35	14.85	15.85	17.15	18.60	20.15	21.65
5.00–5.99	19.87	0.25	15.55	16.25	17.95	19.35	21.05	23.65	25.20
6.00–6.99	22.18	0.48	16.30	17.70	19.30	21.55	24.20	27.05	29.10
7.00–7.99	25.40	0.56	18.55	19.30	22.15	24.25	28.15	31.95	35.60
8.00–8.99	28.21	0.51	22.75	23.20	24.25	27.15	30.00	34.65	39.70
9.00–9.99	32.34	0.66	23.90	24.90	27.00	30.00	36.40	41.95	47.75
10.00–10.99	36.18	1.04	—	26.00	28.15	34.15	42.70	50.70	—
11.00–11.99	43.11	0.79	29.30	31.20	35.05	40.45	49.70	58.00	62.25
12.00–12.99	45.33	0.80	32.25	33.90	37.95	44.20	49.80	54.70	69.40
13.00–13.99	52.25	1.24	38.60	40.35	44.45	50.20	58.00	68.40	73.10
14.00–14.99	58.66	1.30	—	43.75	49.00	56.60	65.15	72.60	—
15.00–15.99	59.25	0.90	—	47.55	53.05	57.35	64.50	71.15	—
16.00–16.99	64.47	1.38	—	47.70	56.90	61.75	70.60	81.10	—
17.00–17.99	63.65	1.19	—	52.40	55.95	60.85	68.05	79.45	—
18.00–18.99	67.51	1.33	—	53.10	58.95	67.50	74.05	81.90	—
Females									
1.00–1.99	10.88	0.22	8.80	9.10	9.75	10.65	11.75	13.20	13.55
2.00–2.99	12.96	0.16	10.80	11.10	11.85	12.85	13.70	15.20	15.65
3.00–3.99	15.12	0.19	—	12.50	13.30	14.90	16.65	17.65	—
4.00–4.99	17.36	0.26	—	14.80	15.65	16.80	18.75	20.40	—
5.00–5.99	19.66	0.24	15.10	16.15	17.25	18.65	20.60	24.25	26.50
6.00–6.99	22.15	0.45	17.10	18.05	19.15	20.85	23.15	28.25	32.60
7.00–7.99	24.80	0.41	—	19.65	21.15	23.75	27.30	32.25	—
8.00–8.99	28.24	0.64	20.75	21.65	23.95	27.05	30.90	36.25	41.70
9.00–9.99	33.55	0.40	21.90	23.25	27.20	32.65	38.40	44.85	48.65
10.00–10.99	38.17	0.94	—	27.70	31.15	36.15	43.20	52.35	—
11.00–11.99	40.72	0.78	27.15	29.15	33.20	39.10	46.70	53.40	60.00
12.00–12.99	47.51	0.70	34.40	36.75	40.70	46.70	52.75	58.55	66.35
13.00–13.99	52.56	0.84	—	41.45	45.45	51.80	56.95	65.15	—
14.00–14.99	54.39	1.12	—	44.00	47.85	53.05	59.15	69.45	—
15.00–15.99	56.98	1.13	—	44.85	49.00	55.30	62.40	74.90	—
16.00–16.99	56.76	1.52	—	43.30	48.30	53.10	58.25	77.65	—
17.00–17.99	55.90	1.22	—	44.55	49.35	52.95	60.55	72.30	—
18.00–18.99	57.17	1.00	—	46.20	50.90	56.40	62.95	69.25	—

Source: Adapted from A. F. Roche and coauthors, Reference data for weight, stature, and weight/stature^2 in Mexican Americans from the Hispanic Health and Nutrition Examination Survey (HHANES 1982–1984), *American Journal of Clinical Nutrition* 51 (1990): 918S. © 1990 American Society for Clinical Nutrition.

TABLE
E2-8

Selected Distribution Statistics for Stature (in Centimeters) in Mexican-American Children and Adolescents

AGE (YR)	MEAN	SEM	PERCENTILES						
			5th	10th	25th	50th	75th	90th	95th
Males									
1.00–1.99[a]	81.0	0.70	71.9	75.9	78.1	81.1	83.9	88.0	90.1
2.00–2.99[a]	91.3	0.50	84.2	85.3	87.9	91.4	93.9	96.8	99.0
3.00–3.99	98.0	0.59	89.5	91.2	95.2	98.4	100.8	103.7	105.4
4.00–4.99	104.7	0.29	96.6	98.5	101.2	104.3	108.3	111.6	112.6
5.00–5.99	111.4	0.30	102.7	104.5	108.1	111.0	115.3	118.4	120.7
6.00–6.99	117.6	0.45	108.2	109.7	114.4	118.2	121.2	124.1	125.2
7.00–7.99	123.1	0.68	112.8	115.3	118.8	123.4	127.5	130.9	131.8
8.00–8.99	129.0	0.37	122.0	122.6	125.7	128.3	132.5	135.6	137.3
9.00–9.99	133.8	0.37	124.4	126.4	129.1	133.0	137.4	142.8	145.0
10.00–10.99	139.5	0.46	128.4	130.7	133.1	138.9	145.5	148.8	151.4
11.00–11.99	146.1	0.64	135.5	137.9	141.3	145.6	150.9	155.2	156.8
12.00–12.99	152.1	0.71	140.4	141.9	146.8	151.3	157.2	162.6	164.5
13.00–13.99	159.9	0.85	148.0	150.3	154.9	159.7	165.5	170.3	171.1
14.00–14.99	165.5	0.79	—	156.9	160.3	166.2	170.4	174.1	—
15.00–15.99	168.1	0.73	—	158.5	163.2	169.0	173.5	177.2	—
16.00–16.99	169.8	0.66	—	162.1	165.0	170.9	174.1	177.7	—
17.00–17.99	171.2	1.00	—	163.0	166.4	171.0	175.6	179.3	—
18.00–18.99	170.3	0.88	—	163.5	166.1	169.2	173.8	181.4	—
Females									
1.00–1.99[a]	79.8	0.66	72.1	74.3	77.0	79.7	83.8	85.9	87.3
2.00–2.99[a]	89.4	0.45	83.5	84.2	86.9	89.4	92.2	94.2	96.4
3.00–3.99	97.0	0.44	—	89.7	93.4	97.1	101.1	102.9	—
4.00–4.99	104.6	0.53	—	98.2	101.8	104.9	108.2	110.2	—
5.00–5.99	110.8	0.48	102.9	104.4	107.4	110.7	114.4	116.3	118.9
6.00–6.99	117.6	0.40	109.1	111.8	114.8	117.4	120.6	124.3	126.1
7.00–7.99	122.0	0.47	—	116.1	117.8	121.9	125.6	128.4	—
8.00–8.99	127.8	0.74	118.5	119.9	123.4	127.9	132.0	135.7	139.6
9.00–9.99	135.5	0.43	123.4	126.5	130.5	136.1	140.5	144.7	145.6
10.00–10.99	141.4	0.64	—	132.5	137.2	140.3	146.6	150.2	—
11.00–11.99	146.3	0.73	133.4	135.4	141.4	146.2	151.8	156.7	158.2
12.00–12.99	152.8	0.79	142.8	144.7	149.1	153.3	158.1	158.7	163.5
13.00–13.99	156.4	0.49	—	149.5	152.1	157.3	160.2	163.6	—
14.00–14.99	157.0	0.41	—	150.5	153.0	157.8	160.4	164.0	—
15.00–15.99	160.2	0.65	—	152.9	156.5	160.4	164.4	168.0	—
16.00–16.99	157.6	1.06	—	149.3	153.2	157.7	162.2	165.7	—
17.00–17.99	159.1	1.18	—	151.9	155.4	159.0	161.8	165.0	—
18.00–18.99	157.9	0.80	—	149.5	154.6	158.3	161.9	164.6	—

[a]Recumbent length.

Source: Adapted from A. F. Roche and coauthors, Reference data for weight, stature, and weight/stature[2] in Mexican Americans from the Hispanic Health and Nutrition Examination Survey (HHANES 1982–1984), *American Journal of Clinical Nutrition* 51 (1990): 920S. © 1990 American Society for Clinical Nutrition.

TABLE E2-9	Selected Distribution Statistics for Weight/Stature^2 (in kg/m^2) in Mexican-American Children and Adolescents

			PERCENTILES						
AGE (YR)	MEAN	SEM	5th	10th	25th	50th	75th	90th	95th
Males									
1.00–1.99[a]	17.22	0.12	14.41	14.84	16.23	17.15	18.12	19.36	20.40
2.00–2.99[a]	16.60	0.16	14.33	14.74	15.52	16.65	17.46	18.39	19.01
3.00–3.99	16.29	0.08	14.38	14.57	15.22	16.09	16.95	17.96	19.03
4.00–4.99	15.81	0.10	13.93	14.56	15.15	15.69	16.51	17.10	17.56
5.00–5.99	15.95	0.18	13.70	14.09	14.80	15.57	16.60	17.98	18.97
6.00–6.99	16.13	0.22	13.92	14.08	14.60	15.72	16.68	18.56	20.24
7.00–7.99	16.55	0.27	14.12	14.52	15.10	15.82	17.20	19.49	21.12
8.00–8.99	16.94	0.24	14.04	14.40	15.35	16.22	17.98	20.29	21.43
9.00–9.99	17.93	0.32	14.29	14.65	15.56	16.78	19.24	22.53	23.83
10.00–10.99	18.35	0.43	14.45	15.02	15.55	17.42	20.96	23.90	25.13
11.00–11.99	20.04	0.38	15.20	15.70	16.90	19.08	22.14	25.35	27.05
12.00–12.99	19.46	0.29	15.95	16.09	17.07	18.44	21.08	23.52	27.41
13.00–13.99	20.31	0.40	16.64	17.40	18.06	19.53	21.57	24.47	27.82
14.00–14.99	21.35	0.44	16.32	16.82	18.25	20.24	22.95	27.13	31.28
15.00–15.99	20.90	0.28	17.50	17.65	18.71	20.54	22.47	24.78	25.76
16.00–16.99	22.28	0.44	17.03	17.93	19.67	20.98	24.26	29.64	31.15
17.00–17.99	21.73	0.50	17.18	18.30	19.41	20.73	23.71	26.68	28.83
18.00–18.99	23.27	0.42	17.98	19.22	20.60	22.21	25.19	28.85	31.17
Females									
1.00–1.99[a]	17.20	0.35	14.29	14.93	15.92	16.77	17.87	19.33	20.10
2.00–2.99[a]	16.15	0.11	14.22	14.63	15.21	15.97	16.82	17.60	18.16
3.00–3.99	16.07	0.18	13.58	14.34	15.18	16.03	16.79	17.93	18.38
4.00–4.99	15.80	0.14	14.03	14.31	14.76	15.47	16.40	18.24	18.79
5.00–5.99	15.92	0.20	13.54	13.96	14.80	15.38	16.78	18.51	20.19
6.00–6.99	15.74	0.25	13.28	13.70	14.35	15.27	16.70	18.20	20.54
7.00–7.99	16.36	0.14	13.70	14.07	14.89	15.82	17.69	19.70	21.73
8.00–8.99	17.16	0.25	13.83	14.30	15.28	16.57	18.38	21.42	23.80
9.00–9.99	18.07	0.23	13.72	14.49	15.63	17.77	20.13	22.40	23.84
10.00–10.99	18.90	0.41	14.28	14.96	16.42	17.93	21.33	24.21	26.24
11.00–11.99	18.79	0.27	14.43	14.99	16.22	17.94	21.37	24.24	26.47
12.00–12.99	20.29	0.24	15.08	16.24	17.40	19.43	22.29	25.35	28.75
13.00–13.99	21.44	0.34	16.96	17.61	18.56	20.54	23.14	27.80	30.43
14.00–14.99	22.02	0.38	17.00	17.75	19.69	21.41	23.45	28.04	28.81
15.00–15.99	22.20	0.38	17.25	18.10	19.04	21.42	24.52	27.69	29.43
16.00–16.99	22.89	0.32	17.44	18.49	19.54	21.17	25.11	30.06	33.22
17.00–17.99	22.22	0.32	17.72	18.32	19.63	21.67	24.52	28.00	29.97
18.00–18.99	22.99	0.28	18.38	19.65	20.71	22.37	24.78	27.02	31.19

[a]Weight/recumbent length^2.

Source: Adapted from A. F. Roche and coauthors, Reference data for weight, stature, and weight/stature^2 in Mexican Americans from the Hispanic Health and Nutrition Examination Survey (HHANES 1982–1984), *American Journal of Clinical Nutrition* 51 (1990): 922S. © 1990 American Society for Clinical Nutrition.

TABLE E2-10	Median Triceps Skinfold Thickness Values (in Millimeters) for Mexican-American, White, and Black Children and Adolescents

AGE (YR)	MEXICAN AMERICANS[a]	WHITES[a,b]	BLACKS[a,b]
Males			
1.00–1.99	10.0	10.0	10.0
2.00–2.99	10.0	10.0	9.5
3.00–3.99	9.5	9.5	9.0
4.00–4.99	9.0	9.0	8.0
5.00–5.99	8.0	8.5	7.5
6.00–6.99	8.0	8.5	6.0
7.00–7.99	9.0	9.0	6.0
8.00–8.99	10.0	9.5	7.0
9.00–9.99	10.0	9.5	7.5
10.00–10.99	12.0	11.5	9.0
11.00–11.99	14.5	11.5	8.0
12.00–12.99	11.0	12.0	8.5
13.00–13.99	10.5	9.5	8.0
14.00–14.99	9.5	9.5	6.5
15.00–15.99	9.0	7.5	7.0
16.00–16.99	10.0	8.5	7.0
17.00–17.99	9.0	7.0	6.0
18.00–18.99	10.5	9.5	7.0
Females			
1.00–1.99	9.5	10.5	10.5
2.00–2.99	10.5	10.5	10.0
3.00–3.99	10.5	10.5	8.5
4.00–4.99	10.0	10.0	9.5
5.00–5.99	10.0	10.5	9.0
6.00–6.99	10.0	11.0	8.5
7.00–7.99	11.5	10.0	9.0
8.00–8.99	12.5	11.5	9.0
9.00–9.99	14.5	13.0	11.5
10.00–10.99	15.0	13.5	12.0
11.00–11.99	13.5	14.5	14.5
12.00–12.99	15.5	13.0	12.5
13.00–13.99	17.0	15.0	13.0
14.00–14.99	19.5	17.0	14.0
15.00–15.99	19.0	16.5	12.5
16.00–16.99	18.0	19.0	17.5
17.00–17.99	18.5	20.0	16.5
18.00–18.99	20.5	18.0	18.0

[a]The sets of median triceps skinfold thickness values for Mexican-American boys and girls (ages 1–18 years) are significantly larger ($p < 0.05$) than the corresponding sets for white and black boys and girls.

[b]The sets of median triceps skinfold thickness values for white boys and girls (ages 1–18 years) are significantly larger ($p < 0.05$) than the corresponding sets for black boys and girls.

Source: Adapted from A. S. Ryan and coauthors, Median skinfold thickness distributions and fat-wave patterns in Mexican-American children from the Hispanic Health and Nutrition Examination Survey (HHANES 1982–1984), *American Journal of Clinical Nutrition* 51 (1990): 926S. © 1990 American Society for Clinical Nutrition.

GIRLS: BIRTH TO 36 MONTHS
PHYSICAL GROWTH
NCHS PERCENTILES*

NAME _____ RECORD # _____

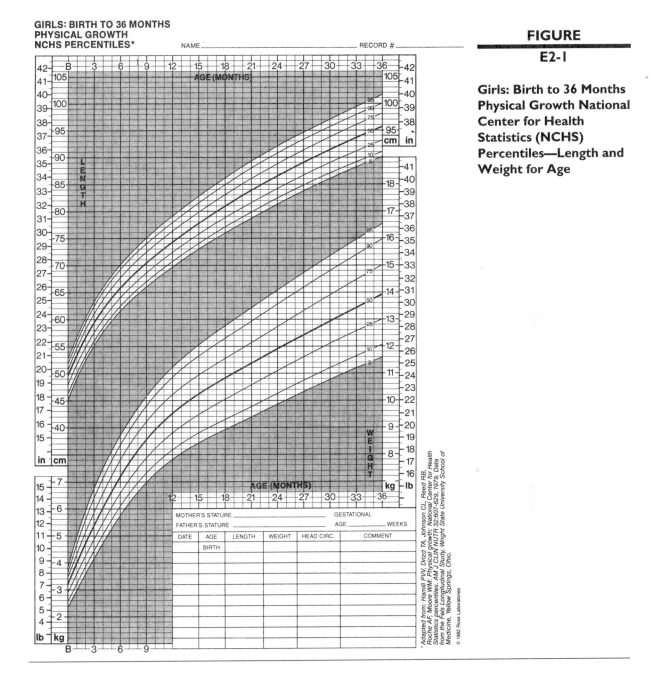

FIGURE

E2-1

Girls: Birth to 36 Months Physical Growth National Center for Health Statistics (NCHS) Percentiles—Length and Weight for Age

*Adapted from: Hamill PVV, Drizd TA, Johnson CL, Reed RB, Roche AF, Moore WM: Physical growth: National Center for Health Statistics percentiles. AM J CLIN NUTR 32:607-629, 1979. Data from the Fels Longitudinal Study, Wright State University School of Medicine, Yellow Springs, Ohio.

© 1982 Ross Laboratories

MOTHER'S STATURE _____ GESTATIONAL
FATHER'S STATURE _____ AGE _____ WEEKS

DATE	AGE	LENGTH	WEIGHT	HEAD CIRC.	COMMENT
	BIRTH				

FIGURE
E2-2

Boys: Birth to 36 Months Physical Growth NCHS Percentiles—Length and Weight for Age

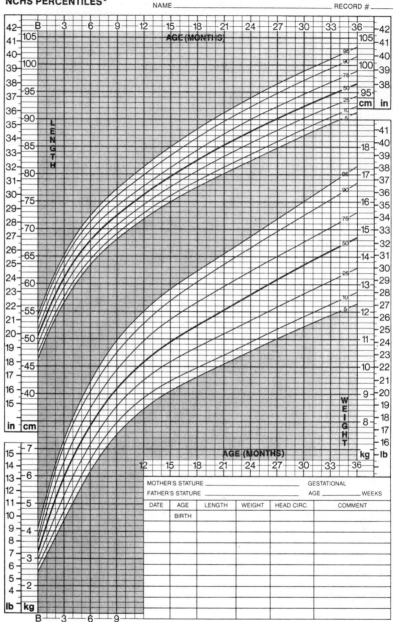

BOYS: BIRTH TO 36 MONTHS PHYSICAL GROWTH NCHS PERCENTILES*

NAME _____   RECORD # _____

*Adapted from: Hamill PVV, Drizd TA, Johnson CL, Reed RB, Roche AF, Moore WM: Physical growth: National Center for Health Statistics percentiles. AM J CLIN NUR 32:607-629, 1979. Data from the Fels Longitudinal Study, Wright State University School of Medicine, Yellow Springs, Ohio.

© 1982 Ross Laboratories

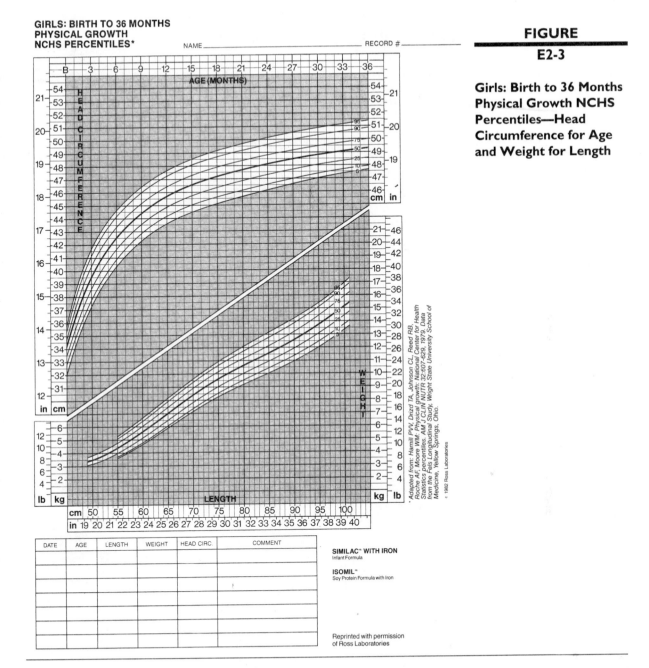

GIRLS: BIRTH TO 36 MONTHS
PHYSICAL GROWTH
NCHS PERCENTILES*

NAME_____   RECORD #_____

FIGURE

E2-3

**Girls: Birth to 36 Months
Physical Growth NCHS
Percentiles—Head
Circumference for Age
and Weight for Length**

* Adapted from: Hamill PVV, Drizd TA, Johnson CL, Reed RB, Roche AF, Moore WM. Physical growth: National Center for Health Statistics percentiles. AM J CLIN NUTR 32:607-629, 1979. Data from the Fels Longitudinal Study, Wright State University School of Medicine, Yellow Springs, Ohio.

© 1982 Ross Laboratories

DATE	AGE	LENGTH	WEIGHT	HEAD CIRC.	COMMENT

SIMILAC® WITH IRON
Infant Formula

ISOMIL®
Soy Protein Formula with Iron

Reprinted with permission
of Ross Laboratories

FIGURE
E2-4

Boys: Birth to 36 Months Physical Growth NCHS Percentiles—Head Circumference for Age and Weight for Length

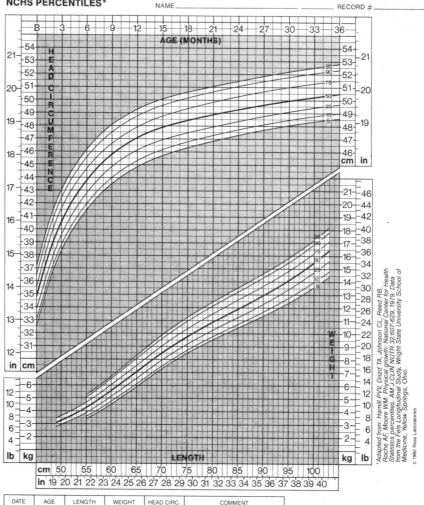

BOYS: BIRTH TO 36 MONTHS
PHYSICAL GROWTH
NCHS PERCENTILES*

NAME _____   RECORD # _____

*Adapted from: Hamill PVV, Drizd TA, Johnson CL, Reed RB, Roche AF, Moore WM: Physical growth: National Center for Health Statistics percentiles. AM J CLIN NUTR 32:607-629, 1979. Data from the Fels Longitudinal Study, Wright State University School of Medicine, Yellow Springs, Ohio.

© 1982 Ross Laboratories

DATE	AGE	LENGTH	WEIGHT	HEAD CIRC.	COMMENT

SIMILAC™ WITH IRON
Infant Formula

ISOMIL™
Soy Protein Formula with Iron

Reprinted with permission
of Ross Laboratories

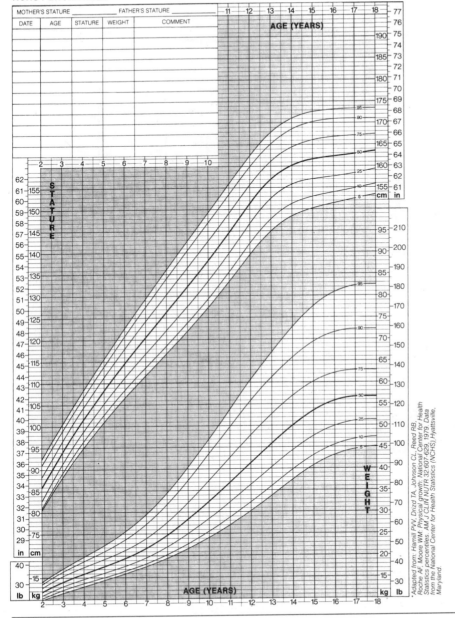

*Adapted from: Hamill PVV, Drizd TA, Johnson CL, Reed RB, Roche AF, Moore WM. Physical growth: National Center for Health Statistics percentiles. AM J CLIN NUTR 32:607-629, 1979. Data from the National Center for Health Statistics (NCHS), Hyattsville, Maryland.

FIGURE

E2-5

Girls: 2 to 18 Years Physical Growth NCHS Percentiles—Height and Weight for Age

FIGURE
E2-6

**Boys: 2 to 18 Years
Physical Growth NCHS
Percentiles—Height and
Weight for Age**

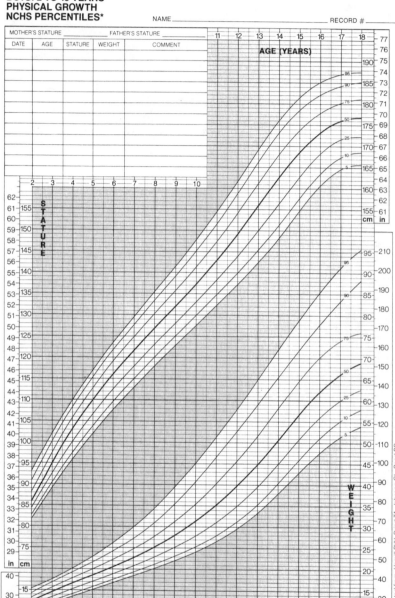

BOYS: 2 TO 18 YEARS
PHYSICAL GROWTH
NCHS PERCENTILES*

NAME_____   RECORD #_____

*Adapted from: Hamill PVV, Drizd TA, Johnson CL, Reed RB, Roche AF, Moore WM. Physical growth: National Center for Health Statistics percentiles. AM J CLIN NUTR 32:607-629, 1979. Data from the National Center for Health Statistics (NCHS), Hyattsville, Maryland

© 1982 Ross Laboratories

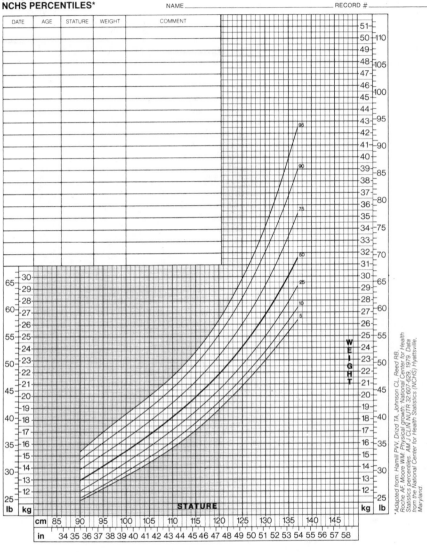

GIRLS: PREPUBESCENT PHYSICAL GROWTH NCHS PERCENTILES*

SIMILAC® WITH IRON
Infant Formula

ISOMIL®
Soy Protein Formula with Iron

Reprinted with permission
of Ross Laboratories

FIGURE
E2-7

Girls: Prepubescent Physical Growth NCHS Percentiles—Weight for Height

FIGURE
E2-8

**Boys: Prepubescent
Physical Growth NCHS
Percentiles—Weight for
Height**

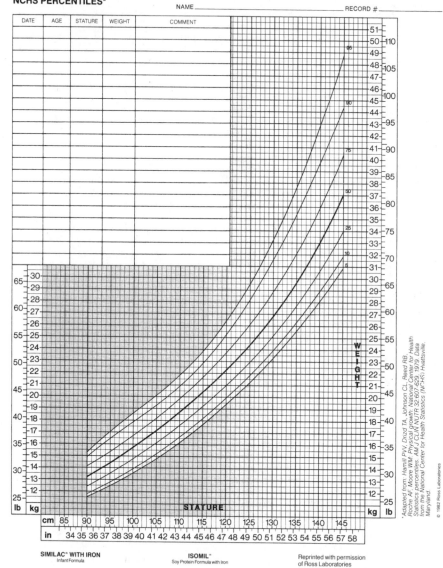

BOYS: PREPUBESCENT
PHYSICAL GROWTH
NCHS PERCENTILES*

FIGURE E2-9

Nomogram for Estimating Stature from Knee Height* in the Elderly

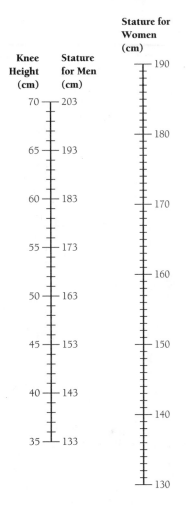

Directions

1. Locate the person's age on the column furthest to the left.
2. Locate the person's knee height on the next column.
3. Lay a ruler or straightedge so that it touches these two points—age and knee height.
4. Note where the straightedge crosses the stature column for the appropriate sex. The point where the ruler crosses the appropriate column is the person's estimated stature.

For example, a woman of 76.5 years has a knee height of 51.8 cm. Her estimated stature is 161.5 cm, the point where the line connecting the corresponding points on the age and knee-height scales crosses the scale for stature for women.

* Knee height estimate: Measure knee height (cm) from the bottom of the foot to the anterior of the knee with the ankle and the knee at a 90° angle.

Source: W. C. Chumlea, A. F. Roche, and D. Mukherjee, *Nutritional Assessment of the Elderly through Anthropometry*, p. 11. Reproduced with permission of Ross Products Division, Abbott Laboratories, Columbus, Ohio 43216, © 1987 Ross Products Division, Abbott Laboratories.

APPENDIX E-3 PHYSICAL ASSESSMENT

TABLE E3-1 Physical Signs Indicative or Suggestive of Malnutrition

	NORMAL APPEARANCE	SIGNS ASSOCIATED WITH MALNUTRITION
SKIN	No signs of rashes, swellings, dark or light spots	Dryness of skin (xerosis); sandpaper feel of skin (follicular hyperkeratosis); flakiness of skin; skin swollen and dark; red swollen pigmentation of exposed areas (pellagrous dermatosis); excessive lightness or darkness of skin (dyspigmentation); black and blue marks resulting from skin bleeding (petechiae); lack of fat under skin
NAILS	Firm, pink	Nails are spoon-shaped (Koilonychia); brittle & ridged
MUSCULAR & SKELETAL SYSTEM	Good muscle tone; some fat under skin; can walk and run without pain	Muscles have "wasted" appearance; baby's skull bones are thin and soft (craniotabes); round swelling of front and side of head (frontal and parietal bossing); swelling of ends of bones (epiphyseal enlargement); small bumps on both sides of chest wall (on ribs)—beading of ribs; baby's soft spot on head does not harden at proper time (persistently open anterior fontanelle); knock-knees or bowlegs; bleeding into muscle (musculo-skeletal hemorrhages); persons cannot get up or walk properly
CARDIOVASCULAR SYSTEM	Normal heart rate and rhythm; no murmurs or abnormal rhythms; normal blood pressure for age	Heart rate above 100 (tachycardia); enlarged heart; abnormal rhythm; elevated blood pressure
GASTROINTESTINAL SYSTEM	No palpable organs or masses (in children, however, liver edge may be palpable)	Liver enlargement; enlargement of spleen (usually indicates other associated diseases)
NERVOUS SYSTEM	Psychological stability; normal reflexes	Mental irritability and confusion; burning and tingling of hands and feet (paresthesia); loss of position and vibratory sense; weakness and tenderness of muscles (may result in inability to walk); decrease and loss of ankle and knee reflexes

Continued

TABLE
E3-1

Physical Signs Indicative or Suggestive of Malnutrition—Continued

	NORMAL APPEARANCE	SIGNS ASSOCIATED WITH MALNUTRITION
HAIR	Shiny; firm; not easily plucked	Lack of natural shine; hair dull and dry; thin and sparse; hair fine, silky, and straight; color changes; can be easily plucked
FACE	Skin color uniform with a smooth, pink, healthy appearance; not swollen	Skin color loss (depigmentation); skin dark over cheeks and under eyes (malar and supraorbital pigmentation); lumpiness or flakiness of skin of nose and mouth; swollen face; enlarged parotid glands; scaling of skin around nostrils (nasolabial seborrhea)
EYES	Bright, clear, shiny; no sores at corners of eyelids; membranes are a healthy pink and are moist. No prominent blood vessels or mound of tissues or sclera	Eye membranes are pale (pale conjunctivae); redness of membranes (conjunctival injection); Bitot's spots; redness and fissuring of eyelid corners (angular palpebritis); dryness of eye membranes (conjunctival xerosis); cornea has dull appearance (corneal xerosis); cornea is soft (keratomalacia); scar on cornea; ring of fine blood vessels around cornea (circumcorneal injection)
LIPS	Smooth, not chapped or swollen	Redness and swelling of mouth or lips (cheilosis); especially at corners of mouth (angular fissures and scars)
TONGUE	Deep red in appearance; not swollen or smooth	Swelling; scarlet and raw tongue; magenta (purplish) color of tongue; smooth tongue; swollen sores; hyperemic and hypertrophic papillae; atrophic papillae
TEETH	No cavities; no pain; bright	May be missing or erupting abnormally; gray or black spots (fluorosis); cavities (caries)
GUMS	Healthy; red; do not bleed; not swollen	"Spongy" and bleed easily; recession of gums
FACE/NECK	Face and neck not swollen	Thyroid enlargement (front of neck); parotid enlargement (cheeks become swollen)

Source: From G. Christakis, Nutritional assessment in health programs, *American Journal of Public Health* 63 (1973, supplement): 1–82. Copyright 1973 American Public Health Association. Used with permission.

TABLE
E3-2

Major Risk Factors for Malnutrition

Source: M. Nestle, *Nutrition in Clinical Practice* (Greenbrae, Calif.: Jones Medical Publications, 1985), pp. 64–65. Used with permission of R. Jones.

Nutritional History

◆ **Medical risk factors**
  Recent weight loss of 10% or more
  Surgery on gastrointestinal tract
  No food intake for 5 days or more
  Excessive nutrient losses (e.g., malabsorption, short-bowel syndrome, fistulas, abscesses, dialysis, wounds, vomiting, diarrhea)
  Increased metabolic requirements (e.g., pregnancy, lactation, fever, infections, burns, trauma)
  Chronic drug usage (e.g., alcohol, antacids, antibiotics, anticonvulsants, antitumor agents, diuretics, immunosuppressants, laxatives, corticosteroids)
  Associated disease conditions (e.g., anemia, cancer, eating disorders, heart disease, diabetes, renal disease, psychoses)

◆ **Dietary risk factors**
  Loss of appetite
  Inadequate food intake
  Lack of variety
  Fad, weight-loss diets
  Inadequate fiber, pica
  Excessive fat, sodium, sugar, alcohol

◆ **Social risk factors**
  Poverty
  Old age
  Immobility
  Social isolation
  Substance abuse

Physical Examination

◆ **Body weight**
  Low body weight: below 80% reference ranges

Continued

Excessive body weight: above 120–130% reference ranges

◆ **Anthropometric measurements**
Triceps (and other) skinfolds
Mid-arm muscle circumference

◆ **Clinical signs**
Nail: spooned, ridged
Hair: depigmented, easily plucked
Skin: dry, scaling, rough
Eyes: dull, dry
Lips: angular stomatitis, cheilosis
Tongue: fissured, magenta, glossitis
Gums: swollen, bleeding
Teeth: decayed
Muscles: wasted, weak, tender
Bones: painful, tender, swollen
Neurologic: apathy, lethargy, paresthesia, disoriented, memory loss

◆ **Laboratory Tests**
Hemoglobin
Hematocrit
Mean corpuscular volume
Serum glucose
Serum cholesterol
Serum albumin
Serum transferrin
Blood urea nitrogen
Total lymphocyte count
Prothrombin time
Alkaline phosphatase
Serum and urine nutrient levels

TABLE

E3-2

Major Risk Factors for Malnutrition—*Continued*

APPENDIX E-4 BIOCHEMICAL ASSESSMENT

TABLE E4-1 Selected Normal Values for Biochemical Tests Useful for Assessing Nutrition Status of Adults

NUTRIENT	ASSESSMENT TESTS	NORMAL RANGES
Protein	Blood urea nitrogen (BUN)	10 to 20 mg/100 ml
	Nitrogen	1 to 2 g/24 hr
	Retinol-binding protein (RBP)	2.6 to 7.6 mg/100 ml
	Serum albumin	3.5 to 5.0 g/dL
	Serum prealbumin (PA)	16.6 to 40.2 mg/dL
	Serum transferrin	250 to 300 mg/100 ml
	Total lymphocyte count (TLC)	1500 to 3000/mm^3
	Urinary creatinine excretion	15 to 25 mg/kg/day
Vitamins		
Vitamin A	Vitamin A	40 to 80 mcg/100 ml
	Carotene	25 to 50 mcg/100 ml
Vitamin D	Serum alkaline phosphatase	15 to 35 U/ml
	Serum cholecalciferol	24 to 40 ng/ml
Vitamin E	Serum tocopherol	0.89 to 1.07 mg/100 ml
	Erythrocyte hemolysis	<10%
Vitamin K	Prothrombin time	11 to 18 seconds
Thiamin	Urinary thiamin	≥66 mcg/g creatinine
Riboflavin	Urinary riboflavin	≥80 mcg/g creatinine
Niacin	Urinary N-methylnicotinamide	≥1.6 mg/g creatinine
	Urinary ratio of 2-pyridone: N-methylnicotinamide	≥1.0
Vitamin B$_6$	Urinary xanthurenic acid excretion	<25 mg/day
	Urinary vitamin B$_6$	≥20 mcg/g creatinine
Vitamin B$_{12}$	Serum vitamin B$_{12}$	150 to 900 pg/ml
	Erythrocyte vitamin B$_{12}$	155 to 195 pg/ml cells
	Methylmalonic acid excretion	<12 mg/day
Folate	Serum folate	≥6.0 ng/ml
	Erythrocyte folate	≥160 ng/ml
	Urinary formiminoglutamic acid (FIGLU) excretion	5 to 20 mg
Biotin	Serum biotin	120 to 240 mcg/100 ml
	Urinary biotin	30 to 60 mcg/day

Continued

TABLE E4-1	Selected Normal Values for Biochemical Tests Useful for Assessing Nutrition Status of Adults—*Continued*	

NUTRIENT	ASSESSMENT TESTS	NORMAL RANGES
Vitamin C	Serum or plasma ascorbic acid	≥13.0 mg/100 ml
	Leukocyte vitamin C	≥15 mg/100 ml
Minerals		
Calcium	Serum calcium	8.5 to 11 mg/100 ml
Chloride	Serum chloride	100 to 106 meq/L
Copper	Serum copper	75 to 150 mcg/100 ml
Iron	Hemoglobin	Women: 10 to 16 g/dL
		Men: 14 to 18 g/dL
	Hematocrit	Women: 34.5 to 43.9%
		Men: 38.6 to 48.0%
	Serum ferritin	Women: 20 to 120 µg/L
		Men: 20 to 300 µg/L
	Total iron-binding capacity (TIBC)	240 to 450 µg/dL
	Mean corpuscular volume (MCV)	82 to 92 mm^3
	Mean corpuscular hemoglobin concentration (MCHC)	32 to 36%
	Serum iron	Women: 65 to 165 µg/dL
		Men: 75 to 175 µg/dL
	Percent transferrin saturation	20 to 55%
Iodine	Serum protein-bound iodine (PBI)	4.0 to 8.0 mcg/100 ml
Magnesium	Serum magnesium	1.7 to 2.1 mg/dL
Potassium	Serum potassium	3.5 to 5.5 meq/L
Phosphorus	Serum phosphorus	2.0 to 4.5 mg/dL
Sodium	Serum sodium	135 to 145 meq/L
Zinc	Serum zinc	101 to 139 mcg/100 ml
Miscellaneous		
Glucose, fasting	Serum glucose	70 to 110 mg/dL
Glycosylated hemoglobin	Hemoglobin A$_{1c}$	4.0 to 7.0%
Lipids:		
Cholesterol	Serum cholesterol	Desirable: <200 mg/dL
		High risk: >240 mg/dL
HDL-c	Serum HDL-c	Desirable: >50 mg/dL
		High risk: <35 mg/dL
LDL-c	Serum LDL-c	Desirable: <130 mg/dL
		High risk: >160 mg/dL
Triglycerides	Serum triglycerides	Risk: >250 mg/dL
Ketones	Urinary acetone plus acetoacetate	0

Source: Adapted from A. Grant and S. DeHoog, *Nutritional Assessment and Support,* 3rd ed. (available from Anne Grant and Susan DeHoog, Box 75057, Northgate Station, Seattle, WA 98125).

APPENDIX E-5 NUTRITION SCREENING

Level 1 Screen

Body Weight

Measure height to the nearest inch and weight to the nearest pound. Record the values below and mark them on the Body Mass Index (BMI) scale to the right. Then use a straight edge (ruler) to connect the two points and circle the spot where this straight line crosses the center line (body mass index). Record the number below.

Healthy older adults should have a BMI between 24 and 27.

Height (in):_____
Weight (lbs):_____
Body Mass Index:_____
(number from center column)

Check any boxes that are true for the individual:

❑ Has lost or gained 10 pounds (or more) in the past 6 months.

❑ Body mass index <24

❑ Body mass index >27

For the remaining sections, please ask the individual which of the statements (if any) is true for him or her and place a check by each that applies.

NOMOGRAM FOR BODY MASS INDEX

WEIGHT — KG LB

BODY MASS INDEX $[WT/(HT)^2]$

WOMEN — OBESE / OVERWEIGHT / ACCEPTABLE

MEN — OBESE / OVERWEIGHT / ACCEPTABLE

HEIGHT — CM IN

© George A Bray 1978

Eating Habits

❑ Does not have enough food to eat each day

❑ Usually eats alone

❑ Does not eat anything on one or more days each month

❑ Has poor appetite

❑ Is on a special diet

❑ Eats vegetables two or fewer times daily

❑ Eats milk or milk products once or not at all daily

❑ Eats fruit or drinks fruit juice once or not at all daily

❑ Eats breads, cereals, pasta, rice, or other grains five or fewer times daily

❑ Has difficulty chewing or swallowing

❑ Has more than one alcoholic drink per day (if woman); more than two drinks per day (if man)

❑ Has pain in mouth, teeth, or gums

A physician should be contacted if the individual has gained or lost 10 pounds unexpectedly or without intending to during the past 6 months. A physician should also be notified if the individual's body mass index is above 27 or below 24.

Living Environment

☐ Lives on an income of less than $6000 per year (per individual in the household)

☐ Lives alone

☐ Is housebound

☐ Is concerned about home security

☐ Lives in a home with inadequate heating or cooling

☐ Does not have a stove and/or refrigerator

☐ Is unable or prefers not to spend money on food (<$25-30 per person spent on food each week)

Functional Status

Usually or always needs assistance with (check each that apply):

☐ Bathing

☐ Dressing

☐ Grooming

☐ Toileting

☐ Eating

☐ Walking or moving about

☐ Traveling (outside the home)

☐ Preparing food

☐ Shopping for food or other necessities

If you have checked one or more statements on this screen, the individual you have interviewed may be at risk for poor nutritional status. Please refer this individual to the appropriate health care or social service professional in your area. For example, a dietitian should be contacted for problems with selecting, preparing, or eating a healthy diet, or a dentist if the individual experiences pain or difficulty when chewing or swallowing. Those individuals whose income, lifestyle, or functional status may endanger their nutritional and overall health should be referred to available community services: home-delivered meals, congregate meal programs, transportation services, counseling services (alcohol abuse, depression, bereavement, etc.), home health care agencies, day care programs, etc.

Please repeat this screen at least once each year--sooner if the individual has a major change in his or her health, income, immediate family (e.g., spouse dies), or functional status.

These materials developed by the Nutrition Screening Initiative.

FIGURE
E5-2

Level II Screen

Complete the following screen by interviewing the patient directly and/or by referring to the patient chart. If you do not routinely perform all of the described tests or ask all of the listed questions, please consider including them but do not be concerned if the entire screen is not completed. Please try to conduct a minimal screen on as many older patients as possible, and please try to collect serial measurements, which are extremely valuable in monitoring nutritional status. Please refer to the manual for additional information.

Anthropometrics

Measure height to the nearest inch and weight to the nearest pound. Record the values below and mark them on the Body Mass Index (BMI) scale to the right. Then use a straight edge (paper, ruler) to connect the two points and circle the spot where this straight line crosses the center line (body mass index). Record the number below; healthy older adults should have a BMI between 24 and 27; check the appropriate box to flag an abnormally high or low value.

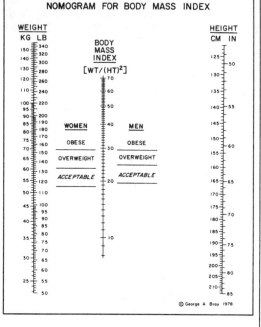

Height (in):_____
Weight (lbs):_____
Body Mass Index
(weight/height^2):_____

Please place a check by any statement regarding BMI and recent weight loss that is true for the patient.

❏ Body mass index <24

❏ Body mass index >27

❏ Has lost or gained 10 pounds (or more) of body weight in the past 6 months

Record the measurement of mid-arm circumference to the nearest 0.1 centimeter and of triceps skinfold to the nearest 2 millimeters.

Mid-Arm Circumference (cm):_____
Triceps Skinfold (mm):_____
Mid-Arm Muscle Circumference (cm):_____

Refer to the table and check any abnormal values:

❏ Mid-arm muscle circumference <10th percentile

❏ Triceps skinfold <10th percentile

❏ Triceps skinfold >95th percentile

Note: mid-arm circumference (cm) - [0.314 x triceps skinfold (mm)]= mid-arm *muscle* circumference (cm)

For the remaining sections, please place a check by any statements that are true for the patient.

Laboratory Data

❏ Serum albumin below 3.5 g/dl

❏ Serum cholesterol below 160 mg/dl

❏ Serum cholesterol above 240 mg/dl

Drug Use

❏ Three or more prescription drugs, OTC medications, and/or vitamin/mineral supplements daily

Clinical Features

Presence of (check each that apply):

❑ Problems with mouth, teeth, or gums

❑ Difficulty chewing

❑ Difficulty swallowing

❑ Angular stomatitis

❑ Glossitis

❑ History of bone pain

❑ History of bone fractures

❑ Skin changes (dry, loose, nonspecific lesions, edema)

Percentile	Men		Women	
	55-65 y	65-75 y	55-65 y	65-75 y
Arm circumference (cm)				
10th	27.3	26.3	25.7	25.2
50th	31.7	30.7	30.3	29.9
95th	36.9	35.5	38.5	37.3
Arm muscle circumference (cm)				
10th	24.5	23.5	19.6	19.5
50th	27.8	26.8	22.5	22.5
95th	32.0	30.6	28.0	27.9
Triceps skinfold (mm)				
10th	6	6	16	14
50th	11	11	25	24
95th	22	22	38	36

From: Frisancho AR. *New norms of upper limb fat and muscle areas for assessment of nutritional status.* Am J Clin Nutr 1981; 34:2540-2545. © 1981 American Society for Clinical Nutrition.

Eating Habits

❑ Does not have enough food to eat each day

❑ Usually eats alone

❑ Does not eat anything on one or more days each month

❑ Has poor appetite

❑ Is on a special diet

❑ Eats vegetables two or fewer times daily

❑ Eats milk or milk products once or not at all daily

❑ Eats fruit or drinks fruit juice once or not at all daily

❑ Eats breads, cereals, pasta, rice, or other grains five or fewer times daily

❑ Has more than one alcoholic drink per day (if woman); more than two drinks per day (if man)

Living Environment

❑ Lives on an income of less than $6000 per year (per individual in the household)

❑ Lives alone

❑ Is housebound

❑ Is concerned about home security

❑ Lives in a home with inadequate heating or cooling

❑ Does not have a stove and/or refrigerator

❑ Is unable or prefers not to spend money on food (<$25-30 per person spent on food each week)

Functional Status

Usually or always needs assistance with (check each that apply):

❑ Bathing

❑ Dressing

❑ Grooming

❑ Toileting

❑ Eating

❑ Walking or moving about

❑ Traveling (outside the home)

❑ Preparing food

❑ Shopping for food or other necessities

Mental/Cognitive Status

❑ Clinical evidence of impairment, e.g. Folstein<26

❑ Clinical evidence of depressive illness, e.g. Beck Depression Inventory>15, Geriatric Depression Scale>5

Patients in whom you have identified one or more major indicator (see pg 2) of poor nutritional status require immediate medical attention; if minor indicators are found, ensure that they are known to a health professional or to the patient's own physician. Patients who display risk factors (see pg 2) of poor nutritional status should be referred to the appropriate health care or social service professional (dietitian, nurse, dentist, case manager, etc.).

Appendix F

TIPS FOR SUCCESSFUL GRANTWRITING

Each year both the public and private sectors award billions of dollars in grants to individuals, agencies, organizations, and schools for a variety of activities and projects. According to some, "If you can find an effective solution to a pressing community problem, you can find funders to help you implement it."[1]

In the past, monies have been awarded to grantseekers for everything from training Good Humor peddlers to determining why children fall off tricycles and studying the biological rhythms of Indian catfish.[2] Today, competition for grant funding has increased while monies available from the public and private sectors have decreased. For this reason, learning the steps of successful grantwriting can help the novice grantseeker better compete for available funding. A glossary of grant-related terminology is provided at the end of this appendix.

How can you get a grant? The key to successful grantsmanship (the art of seeking and being awarded funds) lies in developing a clearly written proposal based on a good idea that complements the goals of the funding agency. The grant proposal should serve as a bridge between the grantee's vision and the grantor's funds and resources.[3] Experts advise that the task of writing a grant proposal be divided into a series of steps. Consider the following grant preparation steps:[4]

◆ **Develop the idea for your proposal.** Explore the problem and the available resources for dealing with the problem. Conduct a formal and informal needs assessment for your proposed project in the target or service area. Survey the related literature. Has this idea been considered in the past? How does your idea differ from or complement the existing resources or activities? Why is it likely to succeed? Be able to describe the problem clearly and concisely and explain the uniqueness of the proposed project or activity in two to three minutes. This will help you when contacting funders by phone or in person.

◆ **Identify a funding source.** Funding for grants in the United States is usually derived from one of three sources: (1) governmental agencies, (2) foundations and community trusts, and (3) business and industrial organizations (see Table F-1). A basic step in grantseeking is to identify funding agencies with similar interests, intentions, and needs regarding the proposed project or activity. Use personal and professional contacts in your funding search. Also, it is helpful to examine an organization's past pattern of giving. Table F-2 provides information on potential funding sources.

◆ **Obtain grant application materials from the chosen funding source.** Follow the application instructions exactly. Make special note of proposal deadlines. Contact the funding agency's grant contact person for assistance during proposal development when necessary to clarify details or answer

TABLE

F-1

Types of Funding Agencies
Source: Adapted from M. R. Schiller and J. C. Burge, How to write proposals and obtain funding, in *Research: Successful Approaches,* ed. E. R. Monsen (Chicago, Ill.: American Dietetic Association, 1992), pp. 49–69.

TYPE	EXAMPLES
Federal	National Institutes of Health, National Cancer Institute, National Institute on Aging, Department of Health and Human Services, U.S. Agency for International Development, National Heart, Lung, & Blood Institute
State and local	Department of education, department of human services, arts council, local school district
Foundations	Ford Foundation, Spencer Foundation, Rockefeller Foundation, International Life Sciences Institute—Nutrition Foundation
Nonprofit organizations	American Diabetes Association, American Heart Association, American Dietetic Association
Industry	IBM, Eli Lilly, Ross Laboratories, Mead Johnson, National Dairy Council, National Live Stock & Meat Board

questions about the application procedures. Identify all requested information. Remember that the basic requirements, application forms, information, and procedures will vary from one funding agency to another.

◆ **Plan the project.** Utilize local resources when addressing local problems. What is your purpose in developing the proposal? Who will be the beneficiaries and how will they benefit? Think through how you will execute the project from start to finish. What resources are needed? Seek the advice of colleagues.

◆ **Write the proposal.** Keep three principles in mind as you write: (1) be candid; (2) be brief; and (3) be on target (e.g., why is this project relevant to the funder's mission?). The components of a proposal will vary from one funding source to another, but they generally include:

   ◆ Title page.

   ◆ Table of contents.

   ◆ Abstract or summary. The proposal summary outlines the proposed project and appears at the beginning of the proposal. The summary is usually one page in length and should be written last to ensure that it contains all the key points necessary to present the objectives of the project. The abstract should also include a needs statement (why the project is important and needs to be done), the main goal of the project, the beginning and ending dates, and the amount of money requested. Many consider the abstract to be the most important page of the proposal. Grant reviewers form their initial impression of your project from the abstract, and it can be critical to the success of your venture.

   ◆ Introduction of the organization and grantseeker. This section establishes the credibility of the applicant or organization. What training and experience do you have? Why should the grant monies be awarded to your project or organization? What are your organization's goals,

Recommended Books on Grantwriting

◆ T. E. Ogden, *Research Proposals: A Guide to Success* (New York: Raven Press, 1991).
◆ L. Reif-Lehrer, *Writing a Successful Grant Application,* 2nd ed. (Boston, Mass.: Jones & Bartlett, 1989).

Funding Sourcebooks

General

◆ *DRG: Directory of Research Grants* is an international directory of programs sponsored by government agencies, private foundations, corporations, and professional organizations; available from Oryx Press, 4041 N. Central at Indian School Road, Phoenix, AZ 85012–3397.
◆ The *Grantseekers Guide,* by J. R. Shellow and N. C. Stella, includes a select group of funders with an understanding of, and commitment to, the social and economic justice projects of smaller organizations—often grass roots or community-based; available from Moyer Bell Publishing, New York.
◆ The *Grantsmanship Center Whole Nonprofit Catalog* advertises Grantsmanship Center workshops and contains useful articles, published quarterly; available from Grantsmanship Center, 650 S. Spring Street, Suite 507, P.O. Box 507, Los Angeles, CA 90014.
◆ The *Grassroots Fundraising Journal* is written for persons working in small to medium-sized organizations; available from Grassroots Fundraising Journal, 517 Union Avenue, Suite 206, Knoxville, TN 37902.

Corporations

◆ *Corporate 500: The Directory of Corporate Philanthropy* includes corporations that give support either directly or through foundations funded by them; available from Public Management Institute, 358 Brannan Street, San Francisco, CA 94107.
◆ *Taft Corporate Giving Directory* and the *Directory of International Corporate Giving* include profiles of over 500 major corporate foundations and corporate charitable giving programs; available from The Taft Group, 12300 Twinbrook Parkway, Suite 450, Rockville, MD 20895–9830.

Foundations

◆ *America's Newest Foundations* is available from The Taft Group, 12300 Twinbrook Parkway, Suite 450, Rockville, MD 20895–9830.
◆ *The Foundation Directory* provides descriptions of foundations including purpose, activities, financial data, and application information; *The Foundation Grants Index* lists grants of $5000 and over given by each foundation, with the recipient, amount, date, duration, and brief description of the grant; *Foundation Grants to Individuals* identifies 1233 foundations making ongoing grants to individuals; *National Directory of Corporate Giving* lists over 1500 companies making contributions to nonprofit organizations; available from The Foundation Center, 79 Fifth Avenue, New York, NY 10003.
◆ *Annual Register of Grant Support* includes profiles of foundations, arranged by subject field; available from National Register Publishing, 3004 Glenview Road, Wilmette, IL 60091.
◆ State and local foundation directories are also available from most local libraries.

Government

◆ *Catalog of Federal Domestic Assistance* is published annually and provides a listing of federal agencies with detailed information on each program funded by them; the

Continued

TABLE

F-2

Sources of Information on Funding Agencies and Grantwriting—*Continued*

Commerce Business Daily summarizes available grants, contracts, and applications; and the *Federal Register*, which is published weekdays except holidays, contains announcements of federal grants; available from U.S. Government Printing Office, Superintendent of Documents, Washington, D.C. 20402–9372.

Newsletters

◆ *Education Funding News* is a weekly newsletter; available from Education Funding Research Council, 4301 N. Fairfax Drive, Suite 875, Arlington, VA 22203, (703) 528-1000.

◆ *Foundation and Corporate Grants Alert* and *Health Grants & Contracts Weekly* are monthly/weekly newsletters giving information on "project opportunities in research, training, and services"; available from Capitol Publications, P.O. Box 1453, Alexandria, VA 22313–2053; (800) 327-7203.

◆ *Foundation Giving Watch* and *Corporate Giving Watch* are published monthly; available from The Taft Group, 835 Penobscot Building, Detroit, MI 48226.

◆ *NIH Guide for Grants and Contracts* is a weekly newsletter (also available electronically); available from NIH Guide, Printing and Reproduction Branch, National Institutes of Health, Room B4BN23, Building 31, Bethesda, MD 20892.

Online Funding Sources

◆ **Federal Information Exchange (FEDIX).** Information on 11 federal agencies, no charge for access. Via modem—800-232-4879; via Internet—fedix.fie.com or 192.111.228.1

◆ **Science and Technology Information System (STIS).** The National Science Foundation's electronic dissemination service; includes publications, grant announcements, newsletters, telephone listings, and awards; no charge for access; via modem—202-357-0359; via Internet—stis.nsf.gov or 128.150.195.40

◆ **DIALOG.** A commercial information service; includes hundreds of databases including the *Grants Database, The Foundation Directory and Index*, and *Federal Register*; charges for subscription, connection, searching, and printing vary with each database. Contact DIALOG Information Services, P.O. Box 10010, Palo Alto, CA 94303–0993; (800) 334-2564.

◆ **NIH Grant Line.** Includes the weekly *NIH Guide to Grants and Contracts*, full text of NIH Requests for Proposals, telephone directory, general NIH information; no charge for access; via modem—202-260-9950.

◆ **Federal Register Table of Contents.** Provides daily *Federal Register* table of contents, as well as public law numbers; via modem—202-275-1538.

◆ **Sponsored Programs Information Network.** Monitors federal and nonfederal programs; charges based on service and size of institution; demo available. Contact InfoEd, Inc., 453 Karner Road, Albany, NY 23305; (800) 727-6427.

◆ **Prospector's Choice.** Electronic source profiles of 8000 corporate and foundation grantors; $295 for smaller regional databases. Contact The Taft Group, 835 Penobscot Building, Detroit, MI 48226; (800) 877-TAFT.

philosophy, and track record with other grantors? What are your success stories?

◆ Project description. This includes a clear, concise, and well-supported problem statement (or needs assessment) with a review of the current literature related to the problem; a statement of the goals and measurable objectives; project methodology showing how you will achieve the stated objectives; a time line showing how the project will proceed, including activities that will occur and the resources and staff needed to operate the project (inputs). This section also identifies the kinds of facilities, transportation, and support services required (throughputs); explains what will be achieved in measurable terms (outputs); justifies your course of action (why did you select these activities?); highlights innovative or unique features of your project; and should convey a sense of urgency regarding the problem.

◆ Itemized project budget. The well-prepared budget is realistic, justifies all expenses of the project, and is consistent with the proposal narrative. Itemize overall project costs including such things as salaries, fringe benefits, consultant fees, equipment, computer costs, facilities, materials and supplies, travel, postage, telephone, and indirect costs.

◆ Project evaluation. The evaluation plan shows how you will measure and communicate outcomes or impact. How will you determine that objectives have been met? How do you plan to disseminate the results? Note any specific evaluation methods required by the grantor.

◆ Future funding needs. This section reflects long-term project needs and describes a plan for continuation of the project beyond the grant period and/or the availability of other resources necessary to implement the grant.

◆ Appendixes should be used to provide details about the project, supplementary data, sample data collection instruments, references of cited literature, and information requiring in-depth analysis. (Such materials might otherwise detract from the readability of the proposal, and are better placed in an appendix.) Appendixes also include personnel vitaes, time tables, letters of support and endorsements for the project, legal papers, and reprints of relevant articles written by the grantseeker.

◆ **Proofread your proposal.** Check grammar and spelling. Have you included all required information? Review your proposal with colleagues and seek their input and constructive criticism (e.g., have you used unsupported assumptions, jargon, or excessive language in the proposal?). Revise the proposal as necessary.

◆ **Submit the proposal to the funding source.** Keep in mind that several submissions may be necessary to one or more funding agencies. Be persistent and resilient. Learn from your rejections (see Table F-3 for the most frequently cited reasons for grant request rejections).

In summary, the grantseeker requires many qualities, but four are critical to successful grantsmanship: (1) diligence in researching funding sources; (2) creativity in matching your project's goals with those of a funding source; (3) attention to detail in proposal preparation; and (4) persistence in revising and resub-

TABLE
F-3

Common Reasons for Grant Proposal Rejections

Source: Adapted from D. Richards, Ten steps to successful grant writing, *Journal of Nursing Administration* 20 (1990): 20–23.

◆ Did not follow guidelines.
◆ Missed the deadline for submission of application.
◆ Topic falls outside the grantor's funding priorities.
◆ Proposal lacks a well thought-out plan of action.
◆ Personnel and resources are lacking to implement the proposal.
◆ The grantseeker lacks knowledge of the problem.
◆ The grant application was incompletely or incorrectly prepared.
◆ The proposal lacks a new or original idea.
◆ Errors in the budget or inconsistent budget estimates throughout the proposal.
◆ Inadequate evaluation criteria.

mitting proposals to potential funding sources. Remember that in grantwriting, "failure often precedes success."[5] Table F-4 lists several key tips for quality grantwriting.

1. A. Quinn, Writing a grant proposal that works, *Leader in Action,* Spring 1992, pp. 9–16.
2. V. P. White, *Grants: How to Find out about Them and What to Do Next* (New York: Plenum Press, 1985), p. vii.
3. Quinn, Writing a grant proposal that works, p. 11.
4. The steps for proposal writing were adapted from D. Richards, Ten steps to successful grant writing, *Journal*

of Nursing Administration 20 (1990): 20–23; C. Kemp, A practical approach to writing successful grant proposals, *Nurse Practitioner* 16 (1991): 51–56; and Appendix VI: Developing and Writing Grant Proposals, *1993 Catalog of Federal Domestic Assistance* (Washington, D.C.: U.S. Government Printing Office, 1993), pp. FF1–FF7.
5. Kemp, A practical approach, p. 53.

TABLE
F-4

Tips for Successful Grantwriting

Source: B. R. Ferrell and coauthors, Applying for Oncology Nursing Society and Oncology Nursing Foundation Grants, *Oncology Nursing Forum* 16 (1989): 728–30. Used by permission.

1. Grantwriting is not a solo activity; seek consultation and collaboration from others.
2. Have your proposal reviewed by peers before submitting it for funding.
3. Follow the directions in detail, including margins, page limits, and the use of references or appendixes.
4. State ideas clearly and succinctly; give attention to spelling and grammar.
5. Use letter-quality printing rather than dot matrix and use a good quality copier.
6. Plan ahead and develop a time frame for completing your grant. Avoid the last-minute rush that will compromise the quality of your proposal.
7. Use appendixes to include study instruments, procedures, or other supporting materials.
8. Include support letters from individuals who are important to the success of your study (e.g., medical staff, administrators, consultants, and co-investigators).

Glossary of Grants

Types of grants

block grant A grant from the federal government to states or local communities for broad purposes as authorized by legislation. Recipients have great flexibility in distributing such funds as long as the basic purposes are fulfilled.

capitation grant A grant made to an institution to provide a dependable support base, usually for training purposes. The amount of the grant is dependent on the size of enrollment or number of people served.

categorical grant A grant similar to a block grant, except funds must be expended within specific categories, such as maternal and child care.

conference grant A grant awarded to support the costs of meetings, symposia, or special seminars.

demonstration grant A grant, usually of limited duration, made to establish or demonstrate the feasibility of a theory or an approach.

formula grant A grant in which funds are provided to specified grantees on the basis of a specific formula, prescribed in legislation or regulation, rather than on the basis of an individual project review. The formula is usually based on such factors as population, enrollment, per capita income, morbidity and mortality, or a specific need. Capitation grants are one type of formula grant, and block grants are also usually awarded on the basis of a formula.

planning grant A grant made to support planning, developing, designing, and establishing the means for performing research or accomplishing other approved objectives.

project grant The most common form of grant, made to support a discrete, specified project to be performed by the named investigator(s) in an area representing his or her specific interest and competencies.

research grant A grant made to support investigation or experimentation aimed at the discovery and interpretation of facts, revision of accepted theories in light of new facts, or the application of such new or revised theories.

service grant A grant that supports costs of organizing, establishing, providing, or expanding the delivery of health or other essential services to a specified community or area. This may also be done through a block grant.

training grant A grant awarded to an organization to support costs of training students, personnel, or prospective employees in research, or in the techniques or practices pertinent to the delivery of health services in the particular area of concern.

Related terms

annual reports A summary of all research and training activities from all funding sources.

budget The itemized list of expenditures required for an activity.

consultant A person who is asked to participate in a grant because of expertise in a particular area.

Continued

—Continued

contract The legal agreement between the grantee and grantor establishing the work to be performed, products to be delivered, time schedules, financial arrangements, and other provisions or conditions governing the arrangement.

direct costs A budget item that reflects the direct expenditure of funds for salaries, fringe benefits, travel, equipment, supplies, communication, publications, and similar items.

grant A sum of money comprising an award of financial assistance to recipient individuals or organizations with assurances that a particular use will or will not be made of it.

grantee The institution, public or private nonprofit corporation, organization, agency, individual, or other legally accountable entity that receives a grant and assumes legal and financial responsibility and accountability both for the awarded funds and for the performance of the grant-supported activity.

grant-in-aid Another name for a project or formula grant.

grantor The agency (government, foundation, corporation, nonprofit organization, individual) awarding a grant to a recipient.

indirect costs Costs that are incurred for common or joint objectives and therefore cannot be identified specifically with a particular project or activity. They are costs involving operational support for mixed purposes (e.g., building maintenance, heating and cooling).

proposal A formal written document containing a descriptive narrative of an idea for a proposed program or project and a budget to be submitted to a funding agency.

request for proposal (RFP) If an agency has a particular area it wishes to fund, it will put out an RFP in that area. The RFP invites the submission of proposals and specifies the requirements that the proposal must meet.

Sources: Adapted from R. Lefferts, *Getting a Grant: How to Write Successful Grant Proposals* (Englewood Cliffs, N.J.: Prentice-Hall, 1982), pp. 156–62; and V. P. White, *Grants: How to Find out about Them and What to Do Next* (New York: Plenum Press, 1985), pp. 293–94.

Appendix G

THE SMOG READABILITY FORMULA

To calculate the SMOG reading grade level, begin with the entire written work that is being assessed, and follow these four steps:

1. Count off 10 consecutive sentences near the beginning, in the middle, and near the end of the text.

2. From this sample of 30 sentences, circle all of the words containing three or more syllables (polysyllabic), including repetitions of the same word, and total the number of words circled.

3. Estimate the square root of the total number of polysyllabic words counted. This is done by finding the nearest perfect square, and taking its square root.

4. Finally, add a constant of three to the square root. This number gives the SMOG grade, or the reading grade level that a person must have reached if he or she is to fully understand the text being assessed.

A few additional guidelines will help to clarify these directions:

- A sentence is defined as a string of words punctuated with a period (.), an exclamation point (!), or a question mark (?).

- Hyphenated words are considered as one word.

- Numbers that are written out should also be considered, and if in numeric form in the text, they should be pronounced to determine if they are polysyllabic.

- Proper nouns, if polysyllabic, should be counted, too.

- Abbreviations should be read as unabbreviated to determine if they are polysyllabic.

Not all pamphlets, fact sheets, or other printed materials contain 30 sentences. To test a text that has fewer than 30 sentences:

1. Count all of the polysyllabic words in the text.

2. Count the number of sentences.

3. Find the average number of polysyllabic words per sentence as follows:

$$\text{Average} = \frac{\text{Total number of polysyllabic words}}{\text{Total number of sentences}}$$

4. Multiply that average by the number of sentences *short of 30*.

5. Add that figure to the total number of polysyllabic words.

6. Find the square root and add the constant of 3.

Perhaps the quickest way to administer the SMOG grading test is by using the SMOG conversion table. Simply count the number of polysyllabic words in your chain of 30 sentences and look up the approximate grade level on the chart.

An example of how to use the SMOG Readability Formula and the SMOG Conversion Table is provided on the next page.

In Controlling Cancer—You Make A Difference

The key is ACTION. You can help protect yourself against cancer. Act promptly to:

Prevent some cancers through simple changes in lifestyle.

Find out about early detection tests in your home.

Gain peace of mind through regular medical checkups.

Cancers You Should Know About

Lung Cancer is the number one cancer among men, both in the number of new cases each year (79,000) and deaths (70,500). Rapidly increasing rates are due mainly to cigarette smoking. By not smoking, you can largely prevent lung cancer. The risk is reduced by smoking less, and by using lower tar and nicotine brands. But quitting altogether is by far the most effective safeguard. The American Cancer Society offers Quit Smoking Clinics and self-help materials.

Colorectal Cancer is second in cancer deaths (25,100) and third in new cases (49,000). When it is found early, chances of cure are good. A regular general physical usually includes a digital examination of the rectum and a guaiac slide test of a stool specimen to check for invisible blood. Now there are also Do-It-Yourself Guaiac Slides for home use. Ask your doctor about them. After you reach the age of 40, your regular check-up may include a "Procto," in which the rectum and part of the colon are inspected through a hollow, lighted tube.

Prostate Cancer is second in the number of new cases each year (57,000) and third in deaths (20,600). It occurs mainly in men over 60. A regular rectal exam of the prostate by your doctor is the best protection.

A Check-Up Pays Off

Be sure to have a regular, general physical including an oral exam. It is your best guarantee of good health.

How Cancer Works

If we know something about how cancer works, we can act more effectively to protect ourselves against the disease. Here are the basics:

1. Cancer spreads; time counts—Cancer is uncontrolled growth of abnormal cells. It begins small and if unchecked, spreads. If detected in an early, local stage, the chances for cure are best.
2. Risk increases with age—This is not a reason to worry, but a signal to have more regular thorough physical check-ups. Your doctor or clinic can advise you on what tests to get and how often they should be performed.
3. What you can do—Don't smoke and you will sharply reduce your chances of getting lung cancer. Avoid too much sun, a major cause of skin cancer. Learn cancer's Seven Warning Signals, listed on the back of this leaflet, and see your doctor promptly if they persist. Pain usually is a late symptom of cancer; don't wait for it.

Unproven Remedies

Beware of unproven cancer remedies. They may sound appealing, but they are usually worthless. Relying on them can delay good treatment until it is too late. Check with your doctor or the American Cancer Society.

More Information

For more information of any kind about cancer—free of cost—contact your local Unit of the American Cancer Society.

Know Cancer's Seven Warnings Signals

1. Change in bowel or bladder habits.
2. A sore that does not heal.
3. Unusual bleeding or discharge.
4. Thickening or lump in breast or elsewhere.
5. Indigestion or difficulty in swallowing.
6. Obvious change in wart or mole.
7. Nagging cough or hoarseness.

If you have a warning signal, see your doctor.

*This pamphlet is from the American Cancer Society.

We have calculated the reading grade level for this example. Compare your results to ours, then check both with the SMOG Conversion Table:

Readability Test Calculations

Total number of polysyllabic words	= 38
Nearest perfect square	= 36
Square root	= 6
Constant	= 3
SMOG reading grade level	= 9

SMOG Conversion Table*

TOTAL POLYSYLLABIC WORD COUNTS	APPROXIMATE GRADE LEVEL (+1.5 GRADES)
0–2	4
3–6	5
7–12	6
13–20	7
21–30	8
31–42	9
43–56	10
57–72	11
73–90	12
91–110	13
111–132	14
133–156	15
157–182	16
183–210	17
211–240	18

*Developed by: Harold C. McGraw, Office of Educational Research, Baltimore County Schools, Towson, Maryland.

Source: U.S. Department of Health and Human Services, Public Health Service, *Pretesting in Health Communications* (Bethesda, Md.: National Cancer Institute, NIH Pub.No. 84–1493, 1984), pp. 43–45.

Appendix H

HEALTHY COMMUNITIES 2000 MODEL STANDARDS: GUIDELINES FOR COMMUNITY ATTAINMENT OF THE YEAR 2000 NATIONAL HEALTH OBJECTIVES*

Healthy Communities 2000: Model Standards puts the objectives of *Healthy People 2000* into practice and encourages communities to establish achievable community health targets. It covers the priority areas and age groups used in *Healthy People 2000* and includes all of the national objectives. Community leaders can adapt the national targets according to local needs and can establish objectives based on their own situations using the fill-in-the-blank approach used in *Healthy Communities 2000: Model Standards* (see Table H-1). By its direct use of the *Healthy People 2000* goals and objectives, *Model Standards* provides a framework for communities to work toward their own priorities while pursuing national health objectives. *Model Standards* has been used successfully in large urban communities, in sparsely populated rural communities, and by city, county, district, and state health agencies.

MODEL STANDARDS PRINCIPLES

The *Healthy Communities 2000* document serves as a guidebook and a process for planning community public health services as the following principles for using *Model Standards* illustrate.

◆ **Emphasis on health outcomes.** Making progress in attacking major health problems depends on establishing an understandable set of health status objectives that are measurable and realistic and are accompanied by local process objectives for their achievement.

◆ **Flexibility.** *Model Standards* is a flexible planning tool using a "fill-in-the-blanks" approach that allows communities to establish and quantify objectives and develop strategies based on their own situations.

◆ **Focus upon the entire community.** Cooperation among major community groups and organizations creates the foundation for communities to establish and achieve the goals and objectives suggested by *Healthy Communities 2000: Model Standards.*

◆ **A government presence at the local level (AGPALL).** Every locale and population should be served by a unit of government that takes a leadership role in assuring the public's health. Assuring that vital services are provided in all communities is an indispensable role of government. Government assures services by encouraging actions by other entities, requiring such actions by regulation, or providing services directly.

*Adapted from *Healthy Communities 2000: Model Standards,* 3rd ed. (Washington, D.C.: American Public Health Association, 1991). Reprinted with permission.

◆ **The importance of negotiation.** Negotiation is the principal way to maintain local flexibility and promote agreement among agencies and individuals who have an interest in and responsibility to protect the public's health.

◆ **Standards and guidelines.** "Standards" implies uniform objectives to assure equity and social justice, and "guidelines" emphasizes local discretion for decision making.

◆ **Accessibility of services.** *Healthy Communities 2000* is designed to help communities tailor special population targets to assure services for those most in need.

◆ **Emphasis on programs.** *Model Standards* focuses on programs rather than professional practice because professional practice standards are usually set by the specialty practice organization.

STEPS FOR PUTTING *MODEL STANDARDS* TO USE

A series of 11 steps have been developed to assist local health agencies in implementing *Model Standards:**

1. **Assess and determine the role of one's health agency.** The local health department develops a mission statement and a long-range vision that provides employees and the community with a clear description of the agency's role and serves as a guide for the steps that follow.

2. **Assess the lead agency's organizational capacity.** The director and the staff of the agency should assess the organization's readiness to exercise leadership. Such an assessment can be accomplished by reviewing the department's structure to determine if it has the skills, community support, and staff capacity to lead the community.

3. **Develop an agency plan to build the necessary organizational capacity.** The agency should develop a plan to build on its internal strengths, overcome its weaknesses, and enhance its organizational effectiveness for carrying out community-wide efforts.

4. **Assess the community's organizational and power structures.** Each local health department should work with key community agencies, community leaders, interest groups, and community members. The agency should conduct an assessment of the community's organizational and power structures on either a formal or an informal basis.

5. **Organize the community to build a stronger constituency and establish a partnership for public health.** The local health agency should convene community groups to assess health needs, address health problems, and assist in the coordination of responsibilities.

---

*These steps were adapted from *The Guide to Implementing Model Standards: Eleven Steps toward a Healthy Community* (Washington, D.C.: American Public Health Association, 1993), pp. 1–22.

6. **Assess the health needs and available community resources.** A community assessment provides the information needed to identify a community's most critical health problems (see this textbook's Chapter 7).

7. **Determine local priorities.** Establishing priorities should involve major health agencies, community organizations, and key interest groups and individuals. The community assessment aids in determining local priorities.

8. **Select outcome and process objectives that are compatible with local priorities and the *Healthy People 2000* objectives.** *Healthy Communities 2000: Model Standards* provides an array of goals and objectives (see Table H-1) to establish measurable health status (outcome) objectives. After establishing these objectives, a community coalition can develop process objectives for achieving them.

9. **Develop community-wide intervention strategies.** Developing community-wide interventions provides the means to achieve selected community goals and objectives. Responsibilities should then be assigned so that activities can be distributed and coordinated among agencies and organizations.

10. **Develop and implement a plan of action.** Establishing goals, objectives, and community-wide intervention strategies is an important step, but success depends on developing and executing a plan of action that implements intervention activities and services.

11. **Monitor and evaluate the effort on a continuing basis.** The achievement of improved health status will attest to the effectiveness of community efforts. In the short term, achievement of local process objectives will show movement toward improved health status, if effective interventions have been selected.

Two planning tools have been developed to assist in the performance of these 11 steps. The *Assessment Protocol for Excellence in Public Health (APEXPH)* enhances the capacity of the public health agency to address assessment, policy development, and quality assurance functions. APEXPH is presented in a workbook that local health departments can use to:

◆ Assess and improve their organizational capacity.

◆ Assess the health status of the community.

◆ Involve the community in improving public health.

The *Planned Approach to Community Health (PATCH)* is a program designed to help communities plan, implement, and evaluate health promotion and education programs that are directed at preventing and controlling chronic diseases. PATCH is a community health promotion methodology that increases a community's capacity to organize and mobilize members, collect and use local area data, set health priorities, select and implement appropriate interventions, and perform process and impact evaluation.

Local health agencies and communities can use *Healthy Communities 2000: Model Standards* and the complementary planning processes such as APEXPH and

PATCH to translate national health objectives into community health action plans responsive to community needs.

MODEL STANDARDS NUTRITION GOALS AND OBJECTIVES

Model Standards has established the following goal for nutrition: Community residents will achieve optimal nutrition status that will reduce premature death and disability. The *Model Standards* health status objectives for the nutrition goal provide specific indicators focusing on nutrition-related disorders, deaths from coronary heart disease, cancer deaths, prevalence of overweight, low birth weight, weight gain during pregnancy, and growth retardation among low-income children. These are listed in Table H-1.

The *Model Standards* risk reduction objectives focus on dietary fat and saturated fat intake, consumption of complex carbohydrates and fiber-containing foods, practices to attain appropriate body weight, consumption of calcium-rich foods, salt and sodium intake, iron deficiency, breastfeeding, prevention of baby bottle tooth decay, and food labels. Specific objectives and indicators are provided in each category.

The *Model Standards* nutrition section also includes services and protection objectives. These focus on the development of a comprehensive nutrition plan, community nutrition education, nutrition services for at-risk populations, nutrition labeling, the availability of processed foods reduced in fat and saturated fat, the provision of nutrition information in grocery stores, healthful food choices in restaurants and foodservice operations, adequate delivery of home-delivered meals for older adults in need, nutrition education in schools and at worksites, nutrition assessment, counseling, and services as a provision of primary care services, breastfeeding promotion, and nutrition monitoring.

TABLE H-1   *Model Standards* **Goal for Nutrition**

Goal: Community residents will achieve optimal nutrition status that will reduce premature death and disability.

FOCUS	OBJECTIVE	INDICATOR
Health status objectives		
Nutrition-related disorders	1. By _____ the prevalence of _____ nutrition-related disorders will be reduced to _____ among target population.[a]	Prevalence of specific nutrition-related disorders
Deaths from coronary heart disease	2. By _____ (2000) reduce coronary heart disease deaths to no more than _____ (100) per 100,000 people. (Age-adjusted baseline: 135 per 100,000 in 1987) *Special population target:*	Coronary heart disease death rate

Coronary Deaths (per 100,000)

	1987 Baseline	2000 Target
a. Blacks	163	_____ (115)
b. Other	_____	_____

FOCUS	OBJECTIVE	INDICATOR
Cancer deaths	3. By _____ (2000) reverse the rise in cancer deaths to achieve a rate of no more than _____ (130) per 100,000 people. (Age-adjusted baseline: 133 per 100,000 in 1987) (*Note:* In its publications, the National Cancer Institute age-adjusts cancer death rates to the 1970 U.S. population. Using the 1970 standard, the equivalent baseline and target values for this objective would be 171 and 175 per 100,000, respectively.)	Nutritionally related cancer deaths (i.e., breast, colorectal)
Prevalence of overweight	4. By _____ (2000) reduce overweight to a prevalence of no more than _____ (20) % among people aged 20 and older and no more than 15% among adolescents aged 12 through 19. (Baseline: 26% for people aged 20 through 74 in 1976–80, 24% for men and 27% for women; 15% for adolescents aged 12 through 19 in 1976–80) *Special population targets:*	Percent overweight

Overweight Prevalence	1976–80 Baseline[b]	2000 Target
a. Low-income women aged 20 and older	37%	____ (25%)
b. Black women aged 20 and older	44%	____ (30%)
c. Hispanic women aged 20 and older		____ (25%)
◆ Mexican-American women	39%[c]	
◆ Cuban women	34%[c]	
◆ Puerto Rican women	37%[c]	
d. American Indians/ Alaska Natives	29–75%[d]	____ (30%)
e. People with disabilities	36%[e]	____ (25%)
f. Women with high blood pressure	50%	____ (41%)

Continued

TABLE
H-1   *Model Standards* **Goal for Nutrition—Continued**

FOCUS	OBJECTIVE	INDICATOR
	g. Men with high blood pressure 39% _____ (35%)	
	h. Other — —	
	(*Note:* For people aged 20 and older, overweight is defined as body mass index (BMI) equal to or greater than 27.8 for men and 27.3 for women. For adolescents, overweight is defined as BMI equal to or greater than 23 for males aged 12 through 14, 24.3 for males aged 15 through 17, 25.8 for males aged 18 through 19, 23.4 for females aged 12 through 14, 24.8 for females aged 15 through 17, and 25.7 for females aged 18 through 19. The values for adolescents are the age- and gender-specific 85th percentile values of the 1976–80 National Health and Nutrition Examination Survey (NHANES II), corrected for sample variation. BMI is calculated by dividing weight in kilograms by the square of height in meters. The cut-points used to define overweight approximate the 120% of desirable body weight definition used in the 1990 objectives.)	
Low birth weight	5. Reduce low birth weight to an incidence of no more than _____ % of live births. (*Model standards note:* The community may wish to develop special population targets, for example, by age, race, sex, income, handicapping conditions, etc., for community relevant subpopulations.)	Incidence of low and very low birth weights
Weight gain during pregnancy	6. Increase to at least _____ % the proportion of mothers who achieve the minimum recommended weight gain during their pregnancies. (*Model standards note:* All pregnancy weight gain should be adjusted for weight status prior to pregnancy. Recommended weight gain is defined as recommended in the 1990 report by the National Academy of Science, *Nutrition during Pregnancy.*)	Precent achieving appropriate weight gain
Growth retardation among low-income children	7. By _____ (2000) reduce growth retardation among low-income children aged 5 and younger to less than _____ (10)% (Baseline: Up to 16% among low-income children in 1988, depending on age and race/ethnicity)	Prevalence of growth retardation
		Continued

TABLE
H-1   *Model Standards* **Goal for Nutrition—*Continued***

FOCUS	OBJECTIVE	INDICATOR

Special population targets:
Prevalence of

	Short Stature	**1988 Baseline**	**2000 Target**
a.	Low-income black children <age 1	15%	____ (10%)
b.	Low-income Hispanic children <age 1	13%	____ (10%)
c.	Low-income Hispanic children aged 1	16%	____ (10%)
d.	Low-income Asian/ Pacific Islander children aged 1	14%	____ (10%)
e.	Low-income Asian/ Pacific Islander children aged 2–4	16%	____ (10%)
f.	Other	—	—

(*Note*: Growth retardation is defined as height for age below the fifth percentile of children in the National Center for Health Statistics' reference population.)

[a]Insert specific nutrition-related disorder, e.g., obesity, anemia, retarded growth, elevated serum cholesterol, coronary artery disease, colon cancer, hypertension, and osteoporosis.
[b]Baseline for people aged 20–74.
[c]1982–84 baseline for Hispanics aged 20–74.
[d]1984–88 estimates for different tribes.
[e]1985 baseline for people aged 20–74 who report any limitation in activity due to chronic conditions.

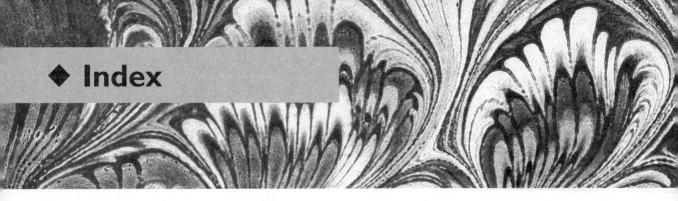

◆ Index